Diagnosis, Treatment, and Management of COPD and Asthma

Diagnosis, Treatment, and Management of COPD and Asthma

Editor

Koichi Nishimura

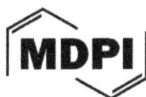

Basel • Beijing • Wuhan • Barcelona • Belgrade • Novi Sad • Cluj • Manchester

Editor
Koichi Nishimura
Visiting Researcher
National Center for Geriatrics
and Gerontology
Obu, Japan

Editorial Office
MDPI
St. Alban-Anlage 66
4052 Basel, Switzerland

This is a reprint of articles from the Special Issue published online in the open access journal *Diagnostics* (ISSN 2075-4418) (available at: https://www.mdpi.com/journal/diagnostics/special_issues/COPD_Asthma_Diagnosis%EF%BB%BF).

For citation purposes, cite each article independently as indicated on the article page online and as indicated below:

Lastname, A.A.; Lastname, B.B. Article Title. *Journal Name* **Year**, *Volume Number*, Page Range.

ISBN 978-3-0365-8965-7 (Hbk)
ISBN 978-3-0365-8964-0 (PDF)
doi.org/10.3390/books978-3-0365-8964-0

© 2023 by the authors. Articles in this book are Open Access and distributed under the Creative Commons Attribution (CC BY) license. The book as a whole is distributed by MDPI under the terms and conditions of the Creative Commons Attribution-NonCommercial-NoDerivs (CC BY-NC-ND) license.

Contents

About the Editor vii

Preface ix

Koichi Nishimura
Special Issue "Diagnosis, Treatment, and Management of COPD and Asthma"
Reprinted from: *Diagnostics* **2023**, *13*, 2634, doi:10.3390/diagnostics13162634 1

Peter M. A. Calverley and Paul Phillip Walker
ACO (Asthma–COPD Overlap) Is Independent from COPD: The Case Against
Reprinted from: *Diagnostics* **2021**, *11*, 1189, doi:10.3390/diagnostics11071189 3

Naoya Fujino and Hisatoshi Sugiura
ACO (Asthma–COPD Overlap) Is Independent from COPD, a Case in Favor: A Systematic Review
Reprinted from: *Diagnostics* **2021**, *11*, 859, doi:10.3390/diagnostics11050859 23

Akira Yamasaki, Ryota Okazaki and Tomoya Harada
Neutrophils and Asthma
Reprinted from: *Diagnostics* **2022**, *12*, 1175, doi:10.3390/diagnostics12051175 41

Naozumi Hashimoto, Keiko Wakahara and Koji Sakamoto
The Importance of Appropriate Diagnosis in the Practical Management of Chronic Obstructive Pulmonary Disease
Reprinted from: *Diagnostics* **2021**, *11*, 618, doi:10.3390/diagnostics11040618 71

Keisuke Miki
Motor Pathophysiology Related to Dyspnea in COPD Evaluated by Cardiopulmonary Exercise Testing
Reprinted from: *Diagnostics* **2021**, *11*, 364, doi:10.3390/diagnostics11020364 81

Howraman Meteran, Pradeesh Sivapalan and Jens-Ulrik Stæhr Jensen
Treatment Response Biomarkers in Asthma and COPD
Reprinted from: *Diagnostics* **2021**, *11*, 1668, doi:10.3390/diagnostics11091668 93

Athanasios Konstantinidis, Christos Kyriakopoulos, Georgios Ntritsos, Nikolaos Giannakeas, Konstantinos I. Gourgoulianis, Konstantinos Kostikas and Athena Gogali
The Role of Digital Tools in the Timely Diagnosis and Prevention of Acute Exacerbations of COPD: A Comprehensive Review of the Literature
Reprinted from: *Diagnostics* **2022**, *12*, 269, doi:10.3390/diagnostics12020269 109

Shih-Lung Cheng and Ching-Hsiung Lin
COPD Guidelines in the Asia-Pacific Regions: Similarities and Differences
Reprinted from: *Diagnostics* **2021**, *11*, 1153, doi:10.3390/diagnostics11071153 133

Koichi Nishimura, Masaaki Kusunose, Ryo Sanda, Mio Mori, Ayumi Shibayama and Kazuhito Nakayasu
Is Blood Eosinophil Count a Biomarker for Chronic Obstructive Pulmonary Disease in a Real-World Clinical Setting? Predictive Property and Longitudinal Stability in Japanese Patients
Reprinted from: *Diagnostics* **2021**, *11*, 404, doi:10.3390/diagnostics11030404 145

Koichi Nishimura, Kazuhito Nakayasu, Mio Mori, Ryo Sanda, Ayumi Shibayama and Masaaki Kusunose
Are Fatigue and Pain Overlooked in Subjects with Stable Chronic Obstructive Pulmonary Disease?
Reprinted from: *Diagnostics* **2021**, *11*, 2029, doi:10.3390/diagnostics11112029 157

Milena-Adina Man, Lavinia Davidescu, Nicoleta-Stefania Motoc, Ruxandra-Mioara Rajnoveanu, Cosmina-Ioana Bondor, Carmen-Monica Pop and Claudia Toma
Diagnostic Value of the Neutrophil-to-Lymphocyte Ratio (NLR) and Platelet-to-Lymphocyte Ratio (PLR) in Various Respiratory Diseases: A Retrospective Analysis
Reprinted from: *Diagnostics* **2022**, *12*, 81, doi:10.3390/diagnostics12010081 169

Ching-Hsiung Lin, Shih-Lung Cheng, Hao-Chien Wang, Wu-Huei Hsu, Kang-Yun Lee, Diahn-Warng Perng, et al.
Novel App-Based Portable Spirometer for the Early Detection of COPD
Reprinted from: *Diagnostics* **2021**, *11*, 785, doi:10.3390/diagnostics11050785 181

Ana L. Fernandes, Inês Neves, Graciete Luís, Zita Camilo, Bruno Cabrita, Sara Dias, et al.
Is the 1-Minute Sit-to-Stand Test a Good Tool to Evaluate Exertional Oxygen Desaturation in Chronic Obstructive Pulmonary Disease?
Reprinted from: *Diagnostics* **2021**, *11*, 159, doi:10.3390/diagnostics11020159 197

Cristiano Carlomagno, Alice Gualerzi, Silvia Picciolini, Francesca Rodà, Paolo Innocente Banfi, Agata Lax and Marzia Bedoni
Characterization of the COPD Salivary Fingerprint through Surface Enhanced Raman Spectroscopy: A Pilot Study
Reprinted from: *Diagnostics* **2021**, *11*, 508, doi:10.3390/diagnostics11030508 209

Iva Hlapčić, Daniela Belamarić, Martina Bosnar, Domagoj Kifer, Andrea Vukić Dugac and Lada Rumora
Combination of Systemic Inflammatory Biomarkers in Assessment of Chronic Obstructive Pulmonary Disease: Diagnostic Performance and Identification of Networks and Clusters
Reprinted from: *Diagnostics* **2020**, *10*, 1029, doi:10.3390/diagnostics10121029 225

Lyudmila V. Bel'skaya, Elena A. Sarf, Denis V. Solomatin and Victor K. Kosenok
Salivary Metabolic Profile of Patients with Lung Cancer, Chronic Obstructive Pulmonary Disease of Varying Severity and Their Comorbidity: A Preliminary Study
Reprinted from: *Diagnostics* **2020**, *10*, 1095, doi:10.3390/diagnostics10121095 241

Alejandro Ortega-Martínez, Gloria Pérez-Rubio, Alejandra Ramírez-Venegas, María Elena Ramírez-Díaz, Filiberto Cruz-Vicente, María de Lourdes Martínez-Gómez, et al.
Participation of *HHIP* Gene Variants in COPD Susceptibility, Lung Function, and Serum and Sputum Protein Levels in Women Exposed to Biomass-Burning Smoke
Reprinted from: *Diagnostics* **2020**, *10*, 734, doi:10.3390/diagnostics10100734 259

About the Editor

Koichi Nishimura

Dr. Nishimura has more than 30 years of experience in the practice of COPD and asthma in Japan since the early 1990s. Under the supervision of Professor Paul Jones, Dr. Nishimura spent six months researching at St. George's University in London in 2012. Dr. Nishimura retired from the National Center for Geriatrics and Gerontology (NCGG) of Japan in March 2023 and currently serves as a visiting researcher at NCGG while contributing to community health care in his own clinic.

Preface

Chronic obstructive pulmonary disease (COPD) is a disorder characterized by airflow limitation and is one of the major causes of mortality and morbidity across the globe. Although several guidelines have been published over the past three decades, they were generated in response to the fact that COPD is a major cause of mortality and morbidity and remains an important social problem. In the 20th century, forced expiratory volume in one second (FEV_1) was the single most important measure in patients with COPD from discriminative, evaluative, and predictive standpoints. We found that dyspnea is a better mortality predictor than FEV_1 in 2002 and exercise capacity in 2003. Subsequently, it has become apparent that physical activity is more predictive of mortality. Furthermore, we have recently developed the tendency to use the reduction of the future risk of exacerbation as the endpoint of relatively large-scale clinical trials rather than the improvement of FEV_1. Many researchers have continued to seek better outcome markers and have also discussed what should be used as primary or secondary endpoints in clinical trials in subjects with COPD. We have undoubtedly made great progress but still have a lot of work to do for the best interests of patients.

Koichi Nishimura
Editor

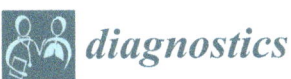

Editorial

Special Issue "Diagnosis, Treatment, and Management of COPD and Asthma"

Koichi Nishimura [1,2]

1 Visiting Researcher, National Center for Geriatrics and Gerontology, 7-430, Morioka-cho, Obu 474-8511, Japan; koichinishimura1@gmail.com
2 Clinic Nishimura, 4-3 Kohigashi, Kuri-cho, Ayabe 623-0222, Japan

It has been my great pleasure to publish 17 papers in the Special Issue "Diagnosis, Treatment, and Management of COPD and Asthma". I would like to sincerely thank all the contributing authors for submitting their manuscripts. I am proud to have served as Guest Editor for this Special Issue.

On 15 July 2020, I was suddenly offered the job of Guest Editor. I have had more than 30 years of experience in the practice of COPD and asthma since the early 1990s, but since I work in a corner of Asia, I was unsure if I would be able to serve as the Guest Editor of a publication from across the globe. Japan tends to treat respiratory medicine as a unique discipline with a reclusive tendency, and all my life I have been plagued by the closed nature of the field in Japan [1]. My opinion that globalization should be promoted has often been ignored. I have begun this work in the hope that accepting the position of Guest Editor will lead to further exploration of this path.

In Japan, the concept of ACO (Asthma–COPD Overlap) is widespread. For example, when discussing the treatment of stable COPD, it is assumed that inhaled corticosteroids (ICS) should be administered to treat ACO and not for COPD. In other words, in Western countries COPD and asthma are often discussed as two diseases and as one disease group, while in Japan there is a tendency to classify this disease group as three separate diseases: COPD, ACO and asthma. This is one reason why a pro–con discussion on ACO was organized here. Historically, there have been only two pro–con debates regarding whether ICS should be given in COPD, published in the *American Journal of Respiratory and Critical Care Medicine* in 2000 [2,3] and the *European Respiratory Journal* in 2009 [4,5]. Although not identical, the third debate was published based on more than a decade of knowledge on similar issues. We believe that it is possible to produce a paper of great interest to readers. I express my deepest gratitude to the two groups of authors, Peter Calverley and Paul Walker from Liverpool, UK [6] and Naoya Fujino and Hisatoshi Sugiura from Sendai, Japan [7], who gave us the opportunity to publish pro–con reviews in this Special Issue.

Between August 2020 and September 2021, a total of 17 papers were published, comprising 10 original articles and 7 reviews: 12 addressing COPD only, 1 addressing asthma alone, and 4 that addressed both diseases. It has been a pleasure to help facilitate this issue, and I hope that readers will find the articles interesting and informative. I am delighted to have had the opportunity to devote some of my time to writing and to have submitted two original papers [8,9]. As a Guest Editor, I issued a multifaceted call for manuscripts to attract submissions. Some manuscripts were also submitted in response to the call but were not accepted after undergoing peer review, and thus were not published. We thank all those who contributed to this Special Issue. I am very grateful to the Managing Editor, Mr. Dennis Zhu, for giving me the opportunity to serve as a Guest Editor and for his continued support and assistance.

Conflicts of Interest: The author declares no conflict of interest.

Citation: Nishimura, K. Special Issue "Diagnosis, Treatment, and Management of COPD and Asthma". *Diagnostics* 2023, 13, 2634. https://doi.org/10.3390/diagnostics13162634

Received: 27 July 2023
Accepted: 28 July 2023
Published: 9 August 2023

Copyright: © 2023 by the author. Licensee MDPI, Basel, Switzerland. This article is an open access article distributed under the terms and conditions of the Creative Commons Attribution (CC BY) license (https://creativecommons.org/licenses/by/4.0/).

References

1. Nishimura, K. Lung health in Japan. *Chronic Respir. Dis.* **2006**, *3*, 104–105. [CrossRef] [PubMed]
2. Barnes, P.J. Inhaled corticosteroids are not beneficial in chronic obstructive pulmonary disease. *Am. J. Respir. Crit. Care Med.* **2000**, *161*, 342–344; discussion 344. [CrossRef] [PubMed]
3. Calverley, P.M. Inhaled corticosteroids are beneficial in chronic obstructive pulmonary disease. *Am. J. Respir. Crit. Care Med.* **2000**, *161*, 341–342; discussion 344. [CrossRef] [PubMed]
4. Postma, D.S.; Calverley, P. Inhaled corticosteroids in COPD: A case in favour. *Eur. Respir. J.* **2009**, *34*, 10–12. [CrossRef]
5. Suissa, S.; Barnes, P.J. Inhaled corticosteroids in COPD: The case against. *Eur. Respir. J.* **2009**, *34*, 13–16. [CrossRef]
6. Calverley, P.M.A.; Walker, P.P. ACO (Asthma-COPD Overlap) Is Independent from COPD: The Case in Favour. *Diagnostics* **2021**, *11*, 1189. [CrossRef] [PubMed]
7. Fujino, N.; Sugiura, H. ACO (Asthma-COPD Overlap) Is Independent from COPD, a Case in Favor: A Systematic Review. *Diagnostics* **2021**, *11*, 859. [CrossRef] [PubMed]
8. Nishimura, K.; Kusunose, M.; Sanda, R.; Mori, M.; Shibayama, A.; Nakayasu, K. Is Blood Eosinophil Count a Biomarker for Chronic Obstructive Pulmonary Disease in a Real-World Clinical Setting? Predictive Property and Longitudinal Stability in Japanese Patients. *Diagnostics* **2021**, *11*, 404. [CrossRef] [PubMed]
9. Nishimura, K.; Nakayasu, K.; Mori, M.; Sanda, R.; Shibayama, A.; Kusunose, M. Are Fatigue and Pain Overlooked in Subjects with Stable Chronic Obstructive Pulmonary Disease? *Diagnostics* **2021**, *11*, 2029. [CrossRef] [PubMed]

Disclaimer/Publisher's Note: The statements, opinions and data contained in all publications are solely those of the individual author(s) and contributor(s) and not of MDPI and/or the editor(s). MDPI and/or the editor(s) disclaim responsibility for any injury to people or property resulting from any ideas, methods, instructions or products referred to in the content.

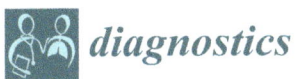

Review

ACO (Asthma–COPD Overlap) Is Independent from COPD: The Case Against

Peter M. A. Calverley [1] and Paul Phillip Walker [2,3,*]

[1] Department of Clinical Science, University of Liverpool, Liverpool L9 7AL, UK; pmacal@liverpool.ac.uk
[2] Liverpool University Hospitals Foundation NHS, University of Liverpool, Liverpool L9 7AL, UK
[3] Department of Respiratory Medicine, Aintree Hospital, Lower Lane, Liverpool L9 7AL, UK
* Correspondence: ppwalker@liverpool.ac.uk

Abstract: Over the last decade interest has been shown in people with symptomatic lung disease who have features both of COPD and asthma. In this review we examine how COPD and asthma are defined and examine clinical characteristics of people defined by researchers as having asthma-COPD overlap (ACO). We look at pathological and physiological features along with symptoms and consider the impact of each diagnosis upon therapeutic management. We highlight challenges in the diagnosis and management of airway disease and the various phenotypes that could be part of ACO, in so doing suggesting ways for the clinician to manage patients with features of both asthma and COPD.

Keywords: COPD; asthma; asthma–COPD overlap; respiratory pathophysiology; bronchodilator reversibility

Citation: Calverley, P.M.A.; Walker, P.P. ACO (Asthma–COPD Overlap) Is Independent from COPD: The Case Against. *Diagnostics* 2021, 11, 1189. https://doi.org/10.3390/diagnostics11071189

Academic Editor: Koichi Nishimura

Received: 14 May 2021
Accepted: 21 June 2021
Published: 30 June 2021

Publisher's Note: MDPI stays neutral with regard to jurisdictional claims in published maps and institutional affiliations.

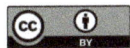

Copyright: © 2021 by the authors. Licensee MDPI, Basel, Switzerland. This article is an open access article distributed under the terms and conditions of the Creative Commons Attribution (CC BY) license (https://creativecommons.org/licenses/by/4.0/).

1. Introduction

Chronic obstructive pulmonary disease (COPD) is now recognised to be a major cause of ill health, increased health care expenditure and premature mortality internationally [1]. The current definition of COPD advocated by the Global initiative for Obstructive Lung Disease (GOLD) highlights the importance of persistent airflow obstruction as a defining characteristic of this condition [2]. Clinically this presents a simple decision. Airflow obstruction is either present or it is not when the patient performs a technically satisfactory spirogram. However, the underlying biology of this apparently simple proposition is more complex.

Longitudinal studies measuring lung function prospectively and cross sectionally over time [3–5] have shown that both the FEV_1 and FVC decrease with age and this is accelerated when people smoke tobacco or are exposed to other noxious inhaled insults [4–6]. Moreover, it is now clear that early life events impact significantly on lung growth and subsequent decline, resulting in a range of trajectories which the patient may follow up to the point where a diagnosis of COPD is confirmed by spirometry [7]. Traditionally, airflow obstruction is defined by the ratio of the FEV_1 to FVC with a value of 0.7 or less signifying that obstructed airflow is present. This simple measurement identifies the presence of emphysema on CT scanning [8] and people at risk of accelerated lung function loss, at least in the earlier stages of COPD [9]. However, this ratio decreases with age and apparently healthy elderly people can be classified as having COPD based on this measurement [10]. This has led physiologists to propose that the lower limit of normal should be used to identify people where the ratio is below that expected by age [11]. This classifies people rather differently with more young people and fewer elderly ones being considered to have airflow obstruction. In practice, this changes relatively little at least in terms of the results of clinical trials [12] and there are now data suggesting that the fixed ratio of FEV_1/FVC of 0.7 is the best predictor of subsequent ill health [13].

If it has proven difficult to define airflow obstruction, it has been even harder to decide what the term 'persistent' means. This term could imply that obstruction did not resolve when measured over time, but whether this could include significant improvements in lung function that were still below the normal predicted value, as is seen in some patients with chronic asthma, was not clear. These differences in interpretation were soon recognised as having therapeutic significance. In the 1990s an important paper from the Netherlands suggested that inhaled corticosteroids (ICS) could produce significant improvements in symptoms and lung function in COPD patients [14]. Subsequently these data were challenged, especially by physicians in the UK, who argued that the improvements seen were due to the inclusion of patients who would normally be diagnosed as having bronchial asthma. This led to an intense debate about how to best define bronchodilator reversibility in order to separate COPD from asthma. In Europe, a very tight definition of irreversible disease was proposed which precluded almost any lung function change after exposure to an inhaled bronchodilator [15]. This created a 'Catch 22' situation where any patient where lung function improved with treatment could not have COPD because treatment had improved their lung function! Such a tight definition is not used today but illustrates evolution over time.

As a result, rather than consider in more detail what bronchodilator reversibility might signify in a patient with structural lung damage due to cigarette (or any other relevant) exposure, the tendency has been to assign patients to mutually exclusive silos—either COPD or asthma. Clinicians have always realised that this is an oversimplification and that some typical COPD patients would show larger than expected benefit from treatment of various types. What has been less clear is whether this behaviour represents a variation within an established diagnosis or is a discrete condition which consistently behaves differently from 'true' asthma or COPD.

Over the last decade there has been renewed interest in the idea of an asthma–COPD overlap (ACO) state in part driven by the desire of the pharmaceutical industry to identify a subset of COPD patients who might respond better to the existing anti-inflammatory treatments and to explain why some asthmatic patients did not improve to the degree anticipated when given them. The most cogent rational academic exploration of this idea came from Gibson et al. in 2009 [16]. Subsequently there have been many publications reporting data in patients believed to be exhibiting ACO and suggestions have been made about how best to operationalise this concept [17–19]. In this review we will consider what has been proposed and outline our reasons for believing that ACO is not a helpful way to understand the variation seen in the way that disease develops in patients with asthma or COPD.

2. Defining ACO

A key issue limiting the usefulness of the ACO concept is the lack of a consistent definition. This not only hinders academic study but also confuses the clinician. This problem is not restricted to ACO but has bedeviled the field of 'airways disease' for the last 60 years. Indeed, the portmanteau term 'airways disease' to describe asthma, COPD and related conditions is itself unsatisfactory as it fails to account for airflow obstruction due to emphysema. Clearly if we have issues defining asthma and COPD, it is going to be hard to identify overlaps between them.

As has been noted before, defining both asthma and COPD is like love—everyone knows what it is when it happens, but it is hard to explain to other people. By the 1980s advances in pulmonary pathology and physiology meant that definitions based only on symptoms such as chronic bronchitis were superseded by approaches using structural and/or lung function criteria. The CIBA symposium in 1959, perhaps the most famous of the meetings which attempted to re-define these conditions, proposed definitions based on variability in lung function for asthma, the presence of enlarged airspaces due to tissue loss for emphysema and symptoms of chronic cough [20]. Helpful as these definitions were in providing a focus for further study, they contained a fundamental weakness, namely that each relied on a different domain—physiology, pathology or symptomatology—to characterise the disease, building in the study of overlap states from the outset.

In the 1970s and 1980s, attention was paid to whether chronic bronchitis or physiology, in the form of the FEV_1, identified discrete natural histories of disease and whether this differed from that seen with patients diagnosed in life with emphysema. The famous longitudinal study of British postal workers led by Charles Fletcher provided the unexpected answer that it was lung function that identified individuals whose lung disease progressed with smoking, rather than the symptoms of bronchitis [21]. Thereafter symptoms were seen to be secondary to lung pathology identified by abnormal lung function rather than identifying a discrete condition. While this is likely to be true, the importance of symptoms like mucous hypersecretion as a marker for respiratory infection and exacerbation [22] and lung disease in the earliest phases of COPD [23] has been neglected until relatively recently.

The overlap between emphysema and bronchitis (clinically defined) seemed to have an international dimension with workers in the USA reporting most of their patients with chronic airflow obstruction as having emphysema (based on CXR appearances) while in Britain similar patients were defined as being bronchitic [24]. Eventually these semantic problems were resolved, but there was still a belief that patients with emphysema without bronchitis maintained normal arterial blood gas tensions while those reporting bronchitis were more likely be hypoxaemic [25]. Again, subsequent pathology studies showed that emphysema could be associated with hypoxaemia [26]. With hindsight it is likely that some of the 'blue and bloated' patients had undetected bronchiectasis and/or left ventricular dysfunction, but this illustrates the way in which ideas about airflow obstructive disorders has been refracted through the tools available for their study rather than any intellectual limitation of those leading the investigations.

The contrast between asthma and bronchitis was not immune from the debate between 'lumpers and splitters'. Unlike the British who felt that chronic bronchitis was a discrete disorder of prognostic significance, the Dutch group in Groningen led by Dick Orie advocated the concept of chronic non-specific lung disease which recognised the heterogeneous nature of conditions others would describe as bronchitis, emphysema or asthma, and grouped them together [27]. In this approach we have the origin of the concept we now consider as ACO and, as noted already, it received considerable push back when the results of their clinical trial of inhaled corticosteroids was first published [14]. However, the conceptual framework developed in the Netherlands was taken up by Gordon Snider in Boston and led to his visual representation of COPD in a non-proportional Venn diagram which was adopted by the American Thoracic Society in its original Standards of Care for COPD document [28]. Thus, a potential for ACO was recognized, but its nature was not clarified.

Longitudinal studies in the Netherlands and New Zealand in young people who have the clinical and physiological characteristics of asthma have shown how over time they can develop fixed airflow obstruction which is often diagnosed as being COPD [29,30]. Whether these people have the same pattern of structural damage seen in typical smoking induced COPD is unclear as is their response to therapy. By contrast, much less information is available about whether people with typical COPD go on to develop disease features more typical of chronic asthma.

Although interest in this topic subsequently declined, the 2009 article by Gibson et al. reignited old uncertainties about whether a discrete phenotype of patients with features of both asthma and COPD existed [16]. These authors approached this from an asthmatic perspective and placed significant emphasis on the role of the bronchodilator response in identifying these patients, as well as emphasising the increased sputum neutrophilia seen in their ACO subjects compared with asthmatics and healthy older adults. Coming at a time of concerns about the risk of pneumonia developing in COPD patients treated with ICS, this approach offered a way of identifying a subgroup for which the benefit of ICS treatment was easier to justify.

In response to these concerns, the Global Initiative in Asthma (GINA) and Global Initiative in Obstructive Lung Disease (GOLD) produced a joint consensus document highlighting practical approaches to the management of ACO [31]. Subsequently the report of workshops convened by the ATS and ERS were published [19,32]. The GOLD/GINA approach was not to offer a specific set of criteria on which a diagnosis of ACO was based but to suggest that ACO could be considered when features usually considered typical of asthma or COPD were present in the same patient [31]. This group offered a series of choices to the clinician about clinical and laboratory features they felt were important, and more detail can be found on the respective websites. There was no attempt to weight the features for their relative importance, a task sensibly left to the individual clinician to decide, from what is basically advice on what to consider in managing patients presenting with atypical clinical findings. However, this level of individual decision makes it hard to draw conclusions about the nature and management of this condition and assumes that treatment approaches valid for the individual diseases are as effective in someone exhibiting these 'overlap' findings.

By contrast, the ATS workshop considered a wider range of issues and raised a series of research questions which needed to be addressed before the nature of ACO could be considered finalised [32]. The European consensus group reviewed the entry criteria used in a range of clinical trials of asthma and COPD and developed a series of major and minor diagnostic criteria summarised in Table 1. This group provided the clearest operational definition of ACO but, to date, this has not been widely accepted, with other groups adapting it to local perceptions of what the key features of ACO might be. The resulting plethora of reported definitions is summarised in the helpful review of Cazzola and Rogliani [33]. It is no surprise in this setting that the type of patients included in what are mainly observational studies appear to be rather different in their nature, illustrated by Barczyk et al. [34].

Table 1. A Consensus Definition of ACO proposed from an ERS Sponsored Round-table Discussion [19]. Diagnosis requires the presence of all 3 major criteria plus 1 minor criteria. LLN = lower limit of normal, BDR = bronchodilator reversibility.

Major Criteria	Minor Criteria
• Persistent airflow limitation (post-bronchodilator FEV1/FVC <0.70 or LLN) in individuals 40 years of age or older; LLN is preferred • At least 10 pack-years of tobacco smoking or equivalent indoor or outdoor air pollution exposure (e.g., biomass) • Documented history of asthma before 40 years of age or BDR of >400 mL in FEV1	• Documented history of atopy or allergic rhinitis • BDR of FEV1 $\geq$200 mL and 12% from baseline values on 2 or more visits • Peripheral blood eosinophil count of $\geq$300 cells/μL

These problems in definition raise several concerns about the utility of the term ACO as an aid to both academic and clinical understanding of people with objectively defined airflow obstruction. In the following sections we will examine what evidence we have for a discrete overlap of pulmonary pathology between asthma and COPD, whether patients meeting the definition of ACO behave differently from others not diagnosed in this way and whether objective physiological tests which are often the main driver of an ACO diagnosis can be relied on to distinguish these patients from others with chronic airflow obstruction.

3. A Pathology of ACO?

There is a dearth of evidence for a discrete pathology occurring in ACO patients. This reflects the lack of a clear definition discussed above and the fragmented nature of the data about structural and immunological features of those who do meet whatever definition is considered appropriate. The issue is not just whether the pathologies typical of asthma or COPD co-exist in the same person, but in how many people such features are present without them exhibiting the defining conditions of the overlap state.

In most cases it is accepted that a prior clinical diagnosis of asthma indicates the continuing presence of that condition. However, this is not necessarily the case. Often the diagnosis is not confirmed by any objective measurement and, in the case of the overlap between asthma and obesity, an asthma diagnosis is often made in patients without any evidence of enhanced airway responsiveness or spontaneous fluctuation in lung function [35]. The clearest evidence for a common set of pathological characteristics in asthmatics has come from biopsy studies largely conducted in milder disease and autopsy data in the relatively few people who die from the disease. In most cases there are features of Th-2 inflammatory changes, increased numbers of eosinophils in the tissue and airway lumen and, as the disease worsens more neutrophils accumulate. A striking finding is the increase in bulk of the airway smooth muscle which helps explain several of the physiological features of the disease [36–38].

For many years there was a consensus based on chest X-ray studies that emphysema only rarely occurs in asthmatic patients but was a frequent finding in those presenting with COPD. It is now clear that in most COPD patients the loss of the small airways precedes the development of emphysema which becomes a more prominent feature as lung function loss worsens [39,40]. The advent of quantitative CT scanning has allowed the relationship between structure and function to be explored in life. One of the best studies is that of Hartley et al. who studied 171 asthmatics, 81 COPD patients and 49 healthy subjects [41]. Patients met standardised diagnostic criteria and were not classified as being ACO or non-ACO in nature. These workers found that airway wall thickness increased as FEV_1 decreased in asthmatics, but the degree of air trapping, a measure of pulmonary hyperinflation, was the main driver of a low FEV_1 in COPD patients. The degree of emphysema contributed to the decreased FEV_1 in COPD patients but was infrequent in patients with asthma. Thus, different pathological changes contribute to the impaired physiology, but airways disease plays a role either directly or indirectly in both asthma and COPD.

These pathological issues have been more directly addressed by a Japanese group who report 3D CT imaging in COPD patients with and without a diagnosis of ACO based on the presence of a bronchodilator response and matched for their smoking history [42]. In this study an FEV_1 change of more than 12% baseline and 200mL after an unspecified bronchodilator or 4 weeks of anti-inflammatory treatment together with variable symptoms were used to define ACO. Patients exhibiting a positive response had thicker proximal airways and less evidence of emphysema than those who did not. However, the mean FEV_1 in this study was relatively high at 70% predicted, so extrapolation to more severe COPD should be done with caution.

Direct study of the nature of airway inflammation in ACO subjects should help resolve matters. One of the few studies to report data on this topic came from a group in Basel who systematically collected biopsies from 129 COPD patients without features of asthma, 19 smoking asthmatics and 18 COPD patients with ACO, all of whom were undergoing diagnostic bronchoscopy and biopsy procedures. They defined ACO using a modified ERS consensus definition [43], but unlike other studies the ACO group did not show greater reversibility to salbutamol that the non-ACO COPD patients. The ACO patients had higher exhaled breath nitric oxide concentrations, more blood eosinophils and significantly better lung function than the COPD control group. These differences in disease severity make it difficult to interpret the greater degree of basement membrane thickening seen in the ACO patients compared with the smoking asthmatics. As the authors comment, their data is preliminary and other focused studies will be needed to address the question of what kind of pathological changes occur in what patients.

An alternative approach to establishing overlap would be to look for differences in biomarkers of tissue inflammation between ACO and non-ACO COPD patients. This would be a very helpful strategy if the biomarkers concerned were both specific and sensitive in distinguishing asthma from COPD. Many inflammatory biomarkers have been linked to asthma with fractional exhaled breath nitric oxide (FeNO), being widely used as a marker of Th-2 inflammation. Unfortunately, the inflammatory process and its attendant biomarkers change as the clinical presentation of asthma evolves, with a more neutrophilic, less eosinophilic profile being seen in severe asthma, especially among patients who are relatively resistant to systemic corticosteroid treatment [44]. Blood eosinophilia is seen as a marker of airway eosinophilia, although studies where these variables have been directly compared suggest that this relationship is relatively weak [45] and there is little agreement about what constitutes eosinophilia and how best to express the data. Unsurprisingly, a raised peripheral blood eosinophil count is not required in the diagnosis of asthma [46]. Nonetheless, the peripheral blood eosinophil count does predict the response to biological treatments in severe asthma [47] and in general population samples of COPD sufferers, those with an eosinophil count as high as 350–600 cells /μL have an increased risk of hospitalisation [48].

Attempts to use these variables to separate ACO from COPD patients who do not meet the clinical criteria for this condition have generated conflicting results. Li et al. found that in 48 patients (42% with a history of smoking and 50% taking ICS) that an FeNO >31.5 ppb identified patients with ACO who smoked with a sensitivity of 70% and a specificity of 90% [49]. However, both the reproducibility of these threshold values and their predictive power need to be replicated in other cohorts. Nonetheless, there is a growing sense that patients who have a history of asthma before the age of 40 behave differently to those whose smoking related COPD develops later in life. Data from Spain suggests that the airway responsiveness is greater, peripheral blood eosinophil count is higher and serum IgE levels are higher in COPD patients with a prior diagnosis of asthma [50]. Further work on well characterised cohorts preferably with appropriate CT imaging should help clarify these relationships. However, the largest comparative cohort study to date, NOVELTY, found no difference in blood eosinophil counts between the asthma, COPD and asthma-COPD overlap groups that they recruited [51], suggesting that blood eosinophils are not useful discriminants in routine clinical practice in identifying what physicians felt constituted ACO.

In many ways the most powerful argument for the existence of an overlap state between asthma and COPD comes from genetics. By combining data from several pathological studies in asthma and COPD, Christenson et al. found that genes associated with a Th2 phenotype in asthmatics were also expressed in patients with COPD and that blood eosinophil counts and airway responsiveness were increased when this was the case [51]. They argue that these genes might be involved in the earlier stages of the development of COPD. However, it is important to recognise that the pathological changes associated with COPD differed from those seen with asthma, with the exception of the eosinophil numbers. Clearly these findings also merit replication in patients meeting any of the current ACO definitions.

4. The Clinical Significance of ACO

It could be argued that it is not important whether or not there is a clear definition of ACO if clinicians can identify a group of patients who should be managed differently. This approach runs the risk of committing the Procrustean crime of making the facts fit the prejudice of the observer—in this case that ACO must exist.

In Table 2 [52–61] we summarise some of the many studies which have looked at the clinical characteristics of ACO (defined in a variety of ways) in clinical populations which vary by country and care setting. The reported prevalence of the condition varies as does the sample size studied, ranging from 1.5% to 27.4% of populations with asthma or COPD. As noted by Spanish workers, the very strict definition of substantial bronchodilator reversibility change excludes so many patients that the definition had to be relaxed to allow them to identify anyone with ACO [54]. This approach feels like a very uncertain way of defining a disease as the higher threshold had originally been suggested as a way of avoiding random variation in a positive BDR (see below). There is an impression that patients identified as having ACO are somewhat younger, are more symptomatic and more likely to report exacerbations than COPD patients not identified in this way. This is supported by several of the review articles which have summarised the findings in these and/or other data sets [16–18,33,62]. Two further studies are worthy of note. In a validation of the ERS symptom score, Nelsen et al. found that most of the symptoms in the battery worked as well for COPD as for ACO, i.e., clinically the patients were very similar. However, wheeze seemed to differ and was not a reproducible symptom, suggesting that reliance on this complaint, at least in COPD patients, could be misleading [63]. A different approach was used by Pascoe who reported a mathematical analysis of a health symptom questionnaire in a large population of patients with obstructive lung disease. The resulting model was accurate in distinguishing asthma and COPD but the authors suggest that patients not falling into these groups are very heterogeneous and hard to classify [64]. This heterogeneity is emphasised by the results of the NOVELTY study [52]. Here over 11,000 patients entered an observational study based on their doctor diagnosed asthma, COPD or ACO. There was substantial heterogeneity across the diagnostic groups and physician determined disease severity classes showing that, in the 'real world' diagnostic groupings are not rigidly applied.

Table 2. Selected studies reporting clinical features of people with ACO.

Study	Definition of ACO	Main Findings
Reddel et al. [52]	Physician diagnosis of asthma, COPD or both	12.4% asthma and COPD (ACO) More likely to smoke, higher blood neutrophil count, more breathless and poorer health status compared with asthma Earlier diagnosis, more upper airway disease compared with COPD Bronchodilator responsiveness and FeNO similar across groups
Morgan et al. [53]	Features of both: COPD—post-bd FEV1/FVC below LLN and Asthma—self report physician asthma diagnosis, use of asthma medication last year or wheezing last year	Prevalence of ACO 3.8% in LMIC residents People with ACO had more biomass fuel exposure, higher smoking and lower educational attainment Worse AFO than asthma or COPD groups
Toledo-Pons et al. [54]	Three groups: Diagnosed with asthma and COPD (smoking asthmatic) COPD and bronchial hyperresponsiveness (FEV1 increase >400 mL and 15%) (COPD high bronchial response) COPD and eosinophilia (eosinophils >300cells/µL) (COPD eosinophilia)	27.4% fulfilled one or more criteria for ACO 13.8% smoking asthmatic, 12.1% COPD with eosinophilia and 1.5% COPD with high bronchodilator response Smoking asthmatics were younger, more likely female and more atopic
Singh A et al. [55]	COPD—post-bronchodilator FEV1/FVC <0.7 Asthma—>200 mL and >12% improvement in FEV1 with bronchodilator ACO—both present	Prevalence of ACO 4.6% in firefighters Eosinophil count >300 cells/µL more common in ACO More likely to have accelerated decline in FEV1
Cosentino et al. [56]	ACO; either: history of asthma or hay fever, FEV1/FVC <0.7, >200 mL and >12% improvement in FEV1 with bronchodilator and less than 15% emphysema on CT, or FEV1/FVC <0.7, >400 mL and >15% improvement in FEV1 with bronchodilator and less than 15% emphysema on CT and less than 15% emphysema on CT regardless of history of asthma or hay fever	Compared to subjects with COPD and emphysema ACO subjects were younger, more likely African-American, higher BMI and more likely to still smoke

Table 2. Cont.

Study	Definition of ACO	Main Findings
Krishnan et al. [57]	ACO defined as >40 years old, current or former smoker, FEV1/FVC <0.7 and >200 mL and >12% improvement in FEV1 with bronchodilator	Prevalence of ACO of 18.2% More common in people diagnosed with both asthma and COPD Younger and higher BMI compared with COPD cohort More likely to smoke and less rhinitis than asthma cohort
Izbicki et al. [58]	COPD was defined as FEV1 <80% predicted and FEV1/FVC <0.7. ACO was defined as this plus >200 mL and >12% improvement in FEV1 with bronchodilator	No differences seen compared with the COPD cohort except lower pre-bronchodilator lung function in ACO
Barrecheguren et al. [59]	ACO defined as COPD patients reporting a previous diagnosis of asthma Classified as ACO2 if had 2 major or 1 major & 2 minor criteria: Major criteria were improvement in FEV1 >400 mL and >15% with bronchodilator, sputum eosinophilia or a previous diagnosis of asthma before the age of 40 years Minor criteria were increased total serum immunoglobulin E, previous history of atopy or FEV1 >200 mL and >12% on two or more occasions	Prevalence of ACO of 15.9% Two thirds did not fulfil ACO2 criteria ACO subjects were more likely to be female, had more exacerbations, had better lung function and higher blood eosinophilia
Llanos et al. [60]	40 years old or greater with at least 1 asthma and 1 COPD characteristic: Asthma characteristic—even given a physician diagnosis of asthma or had an 'asthma attack' in the previous year COPD characteristic—post-bd FEV1/FVC <0.7 and ever told they had emphysema or chronic bronchitis by a physician	ACO subjects had poorer lung function than those with asthma or COPD, higher eosinophil counts than those with asthma or COPD and had more 'asthma attacks' than the asthma group
Baarnes et al. [61]	At least 1 previous hospitalisation for asthma and 1 for COPD	Subjects with ACO were older, more likely to smoke, had lower educational attainment and took less regular exercise

So far, data have largely focused on the overlap of COPD and asthma, i.e., in patients who look like they have COPD, how many have some features that are atypical and would fit better with a diagnosis of asthma. There are plentiful data about what happens when a young person diagnosed with asthma continues with symptoms into adulthood. Work from the Netherlands, Aberdeen, Australia and New Zealand have shown in patients followed for up to 45 years that a significant number of asthmatics go on to develop fixed airflow obstruction which is re-defined as COPD by the clinicians managing them [29,30,65–67]. In a recent report of children followed to age 45, a diagnosis of ACO based on the presence of airflow obstruction and a history of previous asthma irrespective of smoking history was made in an estimated 3% of the population and, like COPD without an asthma diagnosis, was especially likely to do so in those with the worst lung function at the age of 7 years [65]. These data provide further support for the early origins of COPD in a significant number of patients but ACO described here represents a different entity from the COPD with asthmatic features that has fueled much of the ACO debate [68]. It is now clear that tobacco smoking decreases the effectiveness of inhaled corticosteroid treatment in both asthma [69] and COPD [70], further complicating the distinction between COPD with asthmatic features and asthma with features of COPD in longitudinal studies like that of Bui et al. [65].

5. The Physiology of ACO

Thus far, physiological measurements made in ACO patients have been largely confined to spirometry rather than collecting data about lung volumes or gas transfer. Some studies have reported the results of non-specific bronchial challenge testing with either inhaled histamine or methacholine as the inhaled agonist [71,72], but most studies restrict themselves to reporting the results of a single bronchodilator reversibility test (BDR) usually using inhaled salbutamol as the test drug. The interpretation of this apparently simple test has proven to be fraught with difficulty, especially in patients with COPD and has been reviewed in detail on several occasions [73]. As these tests are often crucial in the clinician's decision about whether the patient has ACO or COPD, it is important to consider them in some detail and to highlight why simple assumptions about how to interpret them can be misleading.

In routine laboratory practice both the measurement of airway hyperresponsiveness (AHR) and BDR rely on changes in the FEV_1, the volume that a subject can expire in one second during a forced expiration from total lung capacity. Reliable standards exist for the performance [74] which exploits the development of flow-limitation during the manoeuvre to reduce between test variation. Nonetheless there is a short term and between day physiological variation in the FEV_1, which means that tests repeated a few minutes apart can differ by chance by up to 160 mL. Rather surprisingly this between test variability is not much influenced by the initial FEV_1 of the subject, although it is somewhat lower when the pre-test FEV_1 falls below 1.5 L. By contrast the FVC is more effort dependent with a potential for more between test variation which has meant that it is less often reported during AHR and BDR tests. This is unfortunate as change in FVC gives more clinically relevant data about lung volume change in COPD and has been suggested as a better guide to AHR in asthma [75].

Although considered as being equivalent measurements of airway smooth muscle responsiveness, AHR and BDR tests are not interchangeable and often say more about the pathology of the surrounding lung than the medium sized airways where most of the inhaled stimulant is delivered. In general, AHR testing is used to diagnose asthma with a series of threshold changes identifying mild to severe degrees of airway irritability. This approach works well if the initial FEV_1 is relatively normal, but as the pre-test FEV_1 falls the same dose of agonist can produce a more dramatic fall in FEV_1 due to the altered airway geometry rather than a greater degree of airway smooth muscle contraction. In this context, absence of AHR is more informative than its presence, as has been seen when trying to interpret the diagnosis of asthma in obese subjects [34]. Relatively few groups have looked at AHR in more severe COPD. When we did, we found that this was a surprisingly frequent occurrence [76] and accompanied by increases in end-expiratory lung volume, likely reflecting worsening flow limitation with the agonist drug. Although relevant to why such patients were more symptomatic and are prone to more exacerbations of COPD, we were confident that the changes we saw were related to predictable physiological changes in patients with more severe lung damage due to typical smoking-related COPD, as these patients had no pointer to a diagnosis of asthma, either currently or in their past. Structural differences may help explain the observation in mild to moderate COPD that those with the greatest AHR show the fastest decline in FEV_1 over time [77].

The situation around interpreting bronchodilator responsiveness is, if anything, even more complex. Table 3 summarises some of the main issues that have emerged over several decades of applying this test in clinical practice. Unlike AHR testing, which examines the ease with which airway smooth muscle contraction can be induced, BDR testing looks at the effect of an inhaled drug that promotes airway smooth muscle relaxation (usually 4 puffs of salbutamol) to improve lung function over a short time, commonly 15 min. This is a satisfying test to conduct in a labile asthmatic patient where the FEV_1 can increase by 500 mL or more and often returns to values within the predicted normal range. This form of acute reversibility is diagnostic of bronchial asthma when it occurs but is not the kind of change commonly seen in patients diagnosed as having ACO.

Table 3. Problems when interpreting bronchodilator responsiveness in people with COPD [73].

Pitfall with Reversibility Testing	Reason for the Problem
The bronchodilator drug used	Additional bronchodilation with the combination of short-acting beta-agonists and short-acting anti-muscarinics compared to one bronchodilator
The timing of reversibility testing	Short-acting anti-muscarinics achieve maximum bronchodilation longer than 15 min after administration, the timing typically used for beta-agonist reversibility
The dose of bronchodilator drug	Higher doses of salbutamol (>400 mcg) will result in further small increases in FEV1 compared with lower doses
The reproducibility of result	The magnitude of reversibility, and classification of reversibility (positive or negative), varies significantly between tests
The impact of pre-test FEV1	Individuals with a lower pre-test FEV1 are less likely to shown significant reversibility
The clinical implications of reversibility	Reversibility does not predict clinical symptoms, exacerbations and subsequent decline in lung function

As with AHR testing, the physiological basis of BDR is more complex than is commonly appreciated. Airway smooth muscle (ASM) is widely present throughout the bronchial tree down to the terminal bronchioles. In health there is a normal spontaneous variation in the degree of airway smooth muscle activation (ASM tone) which can be reduced or abolished by bronchodilator drugs; hence the enthusiasm of endurance athletes to acquire a diagnosis of asthma. This spontaneous fluctuation in ASM tone is exaggerated in bronchial asthma through a combination of airway inflammation and enhanced ASM bulk [78] but is preserved in COPD. However, in these patients the baseline airway calibre is reduced and structural changes can increase the degree to which normal physiological changes in ASM translate into changes in airflow resistance which is being indirectly assessed by the FEV_1. These effects are not as dramatic as is the case in bronchial asthma but are more than enough to account for the variable bronchodilator responses that characterise many COPD patients. None of this requires there to be any 'co-existing' asthmatic pathology in the lungs of the COPD patient.

These theoretical considerations aside, there are many obstacles to the easy interpretation of a bronchodilator reversibility test. The protocol adopted will influence the result. In patients with moderate–very severe airflow obstruction the number of positive tests rises with the number of bronchodilators given to the patient [79], a fact clinically exploited in the use of long-acting inhaled dual bronchodilators [80]. There has been an extensive discussion about how to define a positive result. The simple approach of looking for a large percentage change from baseline works well if the pre-test FEV_1 is relatively preserved, but a 160 mL increase in FEV1 which is within the spontaneous variability of two FEV_1 measurements could be interpreted as 16% reversibility in a patient with a baseline FEV_1 of 1 L. This led to the current recommended volume change which must be at least 12% of the baseline value and exceed 200 mL [81]. This was derived from basic principles and experience in population studies rather than empirical data from studies of COPD patients which helps explain its problems in clinical practice. Using a very large absolute difference of 400 mL between measurements to define a positive test greatly decreases the number of positive responses, but did not abolish the between visit fluctuation in classification in those who tested positive initially as shown in Figure 1 from the ECLIPSE study [82].

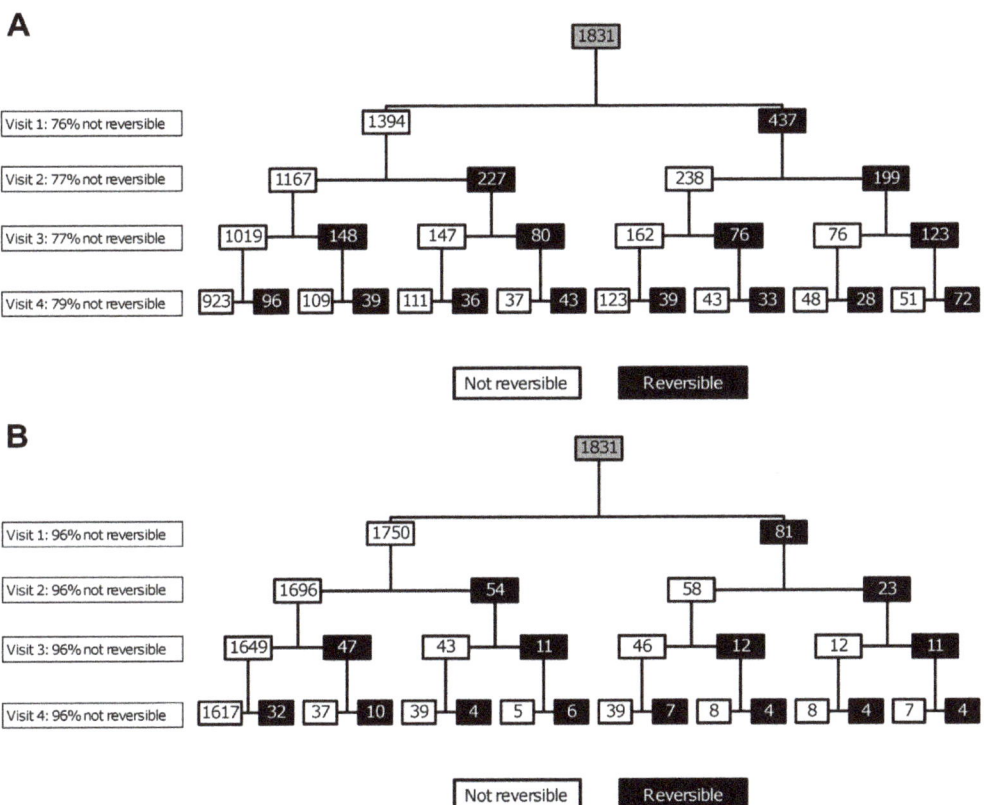

Figure 1. The reproducibility of the classification of bronchodilator reversibility in 1831 people with COPD who participated in the ECLIPSE cohort study. In (**A**) reversibility is defined by ≥12% and ≥200 mL increase from pre-bronchodilator FEV_1 and (**B**) an absolute response of >400 mL from pre-bronchodilator FEV1 [82].

To use any definition of bronchodilator reversibility to make clinical decisions requires it to be stable from day to day and this is not the case in patients without a history of asthma and diagnosed as having smoking-induced COPD. This became apparent when the reversibility testing data from the ISOLDE study conducted over 20 years ago were analysed [79] and has been confirmed in other large prospective clinical trial populations where carefully standardised reversibility testing was undertaken [82]. Figure 2 illustrates the problem. Over the 3 years of testing, significant numbers of individuals meeting the reversibility criteria at their first visit would be reclassified when tested on a subsequent visit. Overall, the percentage of people in the population testing positive at a given attendance was remarkably constant but the individuals who made up that population varied substantially. These data have to be considered when interpreting the studies described above that have classified individuals as having ACO based on a single bronchodilator test.

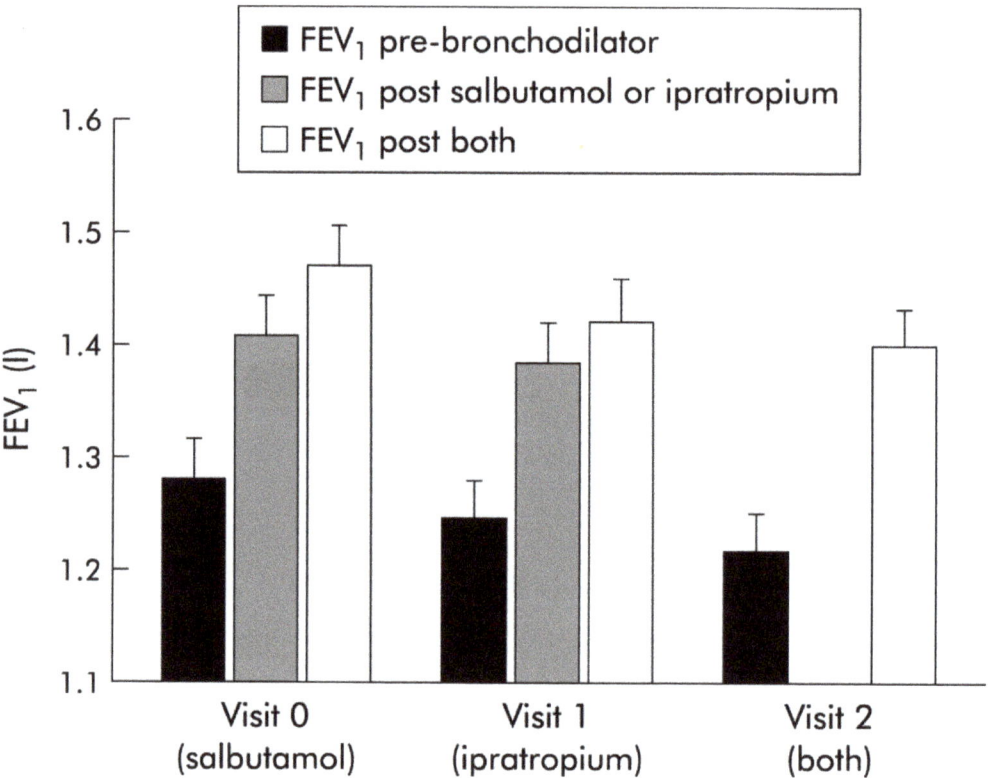

Figure 2. Response to bronchodilators in 660 people with COPD who participated in the ISOLDE study. The results presented show absolute FEV_1 pre-bronchodilator and after administration of one or more bronchodilator. At visit 0 subjects received salbutamol followed by ipratropium bromide, at visit 1 ipratropium bromide followed by salbutamol and visit 2 where both bronchodilators were administered together [79].

It would be helpful if patients with a positive BDR on one occasion behaved differently from those who did not but this does not seem to be true, at least in studies where patients did not have a history of prior asthma. The 4-year UPLIFT trial found no relationship between health status or exacerbation rate and the initial bronchodilator response [83]. This was confirmed in the ECLIPSE dataset [82]. The ECLIPSE investigators went on to look at the subset of patients who were consistently positive on testing over 3 years and compared them to those with consistently negative tests and found no difference in mortality, hospitalisation or exacerbation rates.

In summary, classification of individual patients as having an asthma–COPD overlap condition based on a single bronchodilator test is unreliable and influenced by the nature of the test conducted, the severity of pre-test lung function impairment, the way in which it is interpreted and between day fluctuations in ASM tone. How much of the apparent difference in behaviour at a group level is determined by a greater than anticipated improvement in FEV_1 after a short-term bronchodilator test remains uncertain.

6. Therapeutic Implications of ACO

One of the main reasons to identify patients as having ACO would be to vary their treatment in order to reflect the presence of a presumed dual pathology and potential treatment approaches have been reviewed before [84]. At present there is no evidence base comparing treatment efficacy in individuals meeting any of the ACO definitions with those with 'pure' COPD. Indeed, it seems unlikely that important differences would emerge in patients selected on the basis of any of the composite definitions currently proposed. Among COPD patients it is clear that even those who do not exhibit a positive response still benefit from long-acting inhaled bronchodilator treatment in terms of improved exercise capacity and reduced degrees of exertional breathlessness [85]. Hence, it would be illogical to restrict the use of these treatments to those who met the ACO criteria.

The crucial drug class where a clear distinction might be helpful is in the use of anti-inflammatory drugs. The most studied class has been ICS and here prior belief seems to trump evidence. For many working in this field it has been an item of faith that inhaled corticosteroids are ineffective in COPD and hence they need an explanation for the large body of data that show that ICS, usually combined with a long-acting inhaled bronchodilator, can improve health status, decrease exacerbation frequency, decrease the rate of decline in FEV_1 and prolong life in a large clinical trial population [86]. The suggestion that positive results reflect the presence of a 'hidden' asthmatic population overlapping with 'pure' COPD is not supported by re-analysis of the trial data [87]. However, one characteristic which is part of some definitions of ACO can properly be considered to be a treatable trait on which therapeutic choices about ICS use can be based.

As discussed above blood eosinophil counts have been proposed as a way to identify an ACO subtype of COPD. Airway eosinophilia has been studied in airways disease for almost 20 years mainly focusing on patients with asthma and reporting induced sputum data [88]. However, the relationship between induced sputum eosinophil counts and those in blood is weak in patients diagnosed with COPD [89]. The recognition that COPD patients in the highest tertile of the normal range of eosinophil counts experienced significantly fewer exacerbations when treated with ICS+LABA compared with LABA alone changed perceptions radically [90]. These data were confirmed in other data sets [91,92] as a better understanding emerged about how best to interpret the threshold where the beneficial effect of ICS on exacerbation frequency emerged. In general, this was dictated by the a priori likelihood of an exacerbation occurring and the amount of background bronchodilator treatment, with patients with a blood eosinophil count and a prior exacerbation history being likely to benefit from using ICS irrespective of the degree of concomitant therapy [93]. The extent of peripheral blood eosinophilia did not influence any positive effect of ICS on either FEV_1 or health status, but there are retrospective data suggesting that patients with higher blood eosinophil counts have a reduction in lung function loss over time when treated with ICS [94]. Rather surprisingly, the same association between blood eosinophil count and the effect of treatment on exacerbations was seen with a different agent, roflumilast [95]. Like inhaled corticosteroids [96], this drug decreases the degree of eosinophilia seen in airway biopsies [97]. Further mechanistic studies explaining these effects are needed.

The problem for the ACO concept is that the presence of a higher blood eosinophil count is not related to other proposed features of an ACO diagnosis. The distribution of blood eosinophils in COPD populations is not different from that seen in healthy patients without the disease [98], suggesting that the coexistence of a higher count and COPD occurs by chance rather than due to a specific causal mechanism. As noted already, the blood eosinophil count in the large observational NOVELTY study was not different between patients with an ACO diagnosis and those thought to have usual COPD [51], a finding that held true across the clinician-determined range of disease severity (Figure 3). The diagnostic classification did have some significance as ACO patients were more likely to receive ICS treatment in disease perceived to be mild or moderately severe than was the case if COPD alone was diagnosed. However, a similar percentage of patients with severe disease received ICS and ICS+LAMA+LABA treatment irrespective of which diagnostic label was applied.

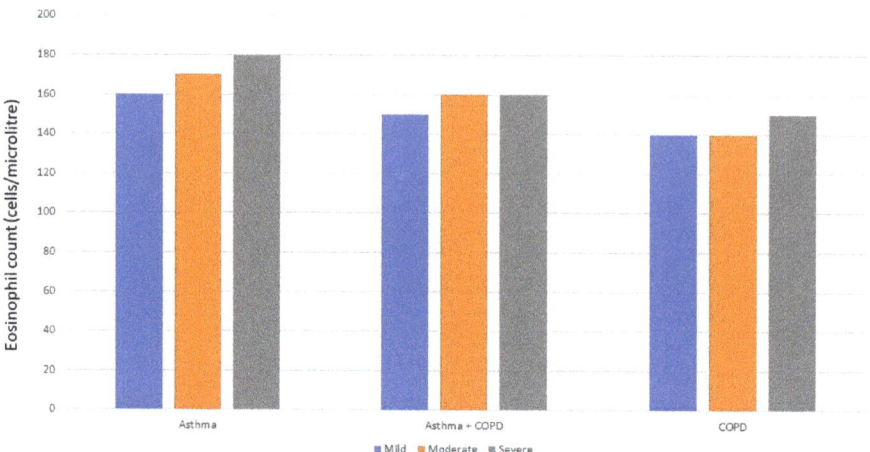

Figure 3. Mean absolute eosinophil count (cells/μL) in 11,243 patients who participated in the NOVELTY study which included 5940 with a physician diagnosis of asthma, 3907 with a physician diagnosis of COPD and 1396 with a physician diagnosis of asthma and COPD. The physician also assessed disease severity as mild, moderate or severe [51].

7. Conclusions

Doctors select medical labels for a variety of reasons—to explain to patients that their problems have a rational basis with predictable outcomes that are amenable to proven treatment, to indicate the likely clinical course and prognosis of the condition and finally, on some occasions, to conceal their diagnostic uncertainty and allow them freedom to select treatment that a more restrictive diagnosis would not necessarily allow. It is our view that most cases diagnosed as ACO fall into this last category. This is not due to any ill-intent on the part of the doctor but reflects the multidimensional way in which the diagnosis of asthma and COPD have been presented over the years with a lack of clarity about which features carry most weight in reaching a diagnostic conclusion and uncertainty about how the clinical manifestations of the illness relate to the pathological changes and disease mechanisms which cause them. It is now possible using more objective measurements made in life to categorise these processes differently but the ubiquity of both asthma and COPD, coupled with the long natural history of both conditions, make implementing this a challenging undertaking. Hence, we are likely to be left with composite diagnostic categories which will inform our clinical and academic approach to these conditions. This highlights the need for long-term cohort studies to better understand both the real-life trajectories of COPD and asthma over time, and to better identify phenotypes of patients who may experience features of COPD and asthma. The question remains in this setting—is ACO a useful diagnostic subdivision? As our review of the evidence suggests, we do not believe this is the case.

At the individual patient level, the lack of agreement about what a doctor might mean by the term ACO is a huge drawback. Extrapolating treatment algorithms for this condition based on what occurs in its better-defined progenitor conditions is not helpful. Reliance on a positive bronchodilator response means that the chance of the diagnosis being changed rises with the number of times the test is repeated, even when relatively strict definitions of a positive response are applied. Even if the response is positive, it does not preclude a useful response to the currently available inhaled therapies. Selection of patients based on relative blood eosinophilia has a better evidence base, at least for exacerbation prevention with some anti-inflammatory treatments. However, these beneficial effects are linked to the higher blood eosinophil count (which itself shows modest between day variation) rather than the other features of ACO and appear to be distributed across the general population rather than confined to a particular subset of patients with airways disease. In larger population studies, subjects identified as having ACO report more exacerbations than those with COPD alone. This may reflect the nature of their COPD pathology which increases their apparent AHR and leads to more between day fluctuation in airway calibre for reasons other than abnormal airway smooth muscle function.

Several approaches have been proposed to deal with these issues of classification. In a thoughtful article Wise and Putcha suggest four different 'phenotypes' of ACO (Table 4) which best explain associations between persistent airflow obstruction and asthma [99]. Like the other proposed definitions of ACO, there is a need for longitudinal data to prospectively determine the stability of the diagnostic groups and their subsequent outcomes. A more attractive approach is based on the approach of Agusti et al. who emphasise the treatable traits which may be present in an individual patient, where a high blood eosinophil count is seen as a biomarker of the ability of ICS to prevent exacerbations rather than a defining characteristic of a specific disease [100]. How widely this return to Orie's chronic non-specific lung disease will be accepted remains to be seen. Like others who have reviewed this issue [17–19,33] we tend to the view that it is better to ascribe a dominant likely pathology and describe the individual features that need most attention (e.g., exertional dyspnoea, frequent exacerbations, weight issues, social impacts) rather than creating a separate disease category that follows a different treatment schedule of uncertain relevance to the patient's needs.

Table 4. A suggestion for different pathways to ACO presented as 4 different 'phenotypes' of ACO described by Putcha and Wise [99].

Phenotype of ACO	Clinical and Biological Features
Smokers with airflow obstruction and eosinophilic inflammation	Exacerbations driven by eosinophilic inflammation Better lung function, less emphysema, less disease progression Better response to oral and inhaled corticosteroids Higher level of atopy
Resistant asthmatic	Asthmatics less responsive to corticosteroids Higher level of irreversible airflow obstruction Neutrophil dominated airway inflammation and exacerbations are more common
Elderly asthmatic with irreversible airflow obstruction	Long-standing asthma and irreversible airflow obstruction Neutrophil dominated airway inflammation Loss of lung elastic recoil and more hyperinflation
Childhood asthmatic who smokes and has developed COPD	Asthma as child or young adult but long-term smoking Higher number of pack years (more likely to have >20 pack years) High symptom burden and healthcare utilisation

Thus, the conclusion reached by the person who has thought most about this topic and advocated the renaissance of the term ACO in 2009, when they revisited this topic in 2015 [62], seems the most appropriate summary of the case against ACO independently of COPD:

"A precise and useful definition of asthma–COPD overlap has not been possible, and the condition itself appears to compromise several different sub-phenotypes. It is proposed that addressing disease components via a multidimensional approach to assessment and management of obstructive airway diseases will be useful to manage the heterogeneity of these conditions."

Author Contributions: P.M.A.C. and P.P.W. conceived, wrote and reviewed this manuscript without additional input or professional writing assistance. All authors have read and agreed to the published version of the manuscript.

Funding: This research received no external funding.

Institutional Review Board Statement: Not applicable.

Informed Consent Statement: Not applicable.

Data Availability Statement: Not applicable.

Conflicts of Interest: P.M.A.C. has advised many pharmaceutical companies with an interest in COPD including but not restricted to GSK, AstraZeneca, Boehringer Ingelheim, Novartis, Recipharm and Zambon. He has no connections with the tobacco industry. P.P.W. has no conflicts to declare.

References

1. GBD 2017 Disease and Injury Incidence and Prevalence Collaborators. Global, regional, and national incidence, prevalence, and years lived with disability for 354 diseases and injuries for 195 countries and territories, 1990–2017: A systematic analysis for the Global Burden of Disease Study 2017. *Lancet* **2018**, *392*, 1789–1858. [CrossRef]
2. Global Strategy for the Diagnosis, Management and Prevention of COPD; 2021 Report. Available online: https://goldcopd.org/wp-content/uploads/2020/11/GOLD-REPORT-2021-v1.1-25Nov20_WMV.pdf (accessed on 12 May 2021).
3. Fletcher, C.; Peto, R. The natural history of chronic airflow obstruction. *Br. Med. J.* **1977**, *1*, 1645–1648. [CrossRef] [PubMed]
4. Xu, X.; Dockery, D.W.; Ware, J.H.; Speizer, F.E.; Ferris, B.G. Effects of Cigarette Smoking on Rate of Loss of Pulmonary Function in Adults: A Longitudinal Assessment. *Am. Rev. Respir. Dis.* **1992**, *146*, 1345–1348. [CrossRef]
5. Anthonisen, N.R.; Connett, J.E.; Kiley, J.P.; Altose, M.D.; Bailey, W.C.; Buist, A.S.; Conway, W.A.; Enright, P.L.; Kanner, R.E.; O'Hara, P. Effects of smoking intervention and the use of an inhaled anticholinergic bronchodilator on the rate of decline of FEV1. The Lung Health Study. *JAMA* **1994**, *272*, 1497–1505. [CrossRef]
6. Burchfiel, C.M.; Marcus, E.B.; Curb, J.D.; Maclean, C.J.; Vollmer, W.M.; Johnson, L.R.; Fong, K.O.; Rodriguez, B.L.; Masaki, K.H.; Buist, A.S. Effects of smoking and smoking cessation on longitudinal decline in pulmonary function. *Am. J. Respir. Crit. Care Med.* **1995**, *151*, 1778–1785. [CrossRef]
7. Lange, P.; Celli, B.R.; Agustí, A.; Jensen, G.B.; Divo, M.; Faner, R.; Guerra, S.; Marott, J.L.; Martinez, F.D.; Martinez-Camblor, P.; et al. Lung-Function Trajectories Leading to Chronic Obstructive Pulmonary Disease. *N. Engl. J. Med.* **2015**, *373*, 111–122. [CrossRef]
8. Gelb, A.F.; Hogg, J.C.; Müller, N.L.; Schein, M.J.; Kuei, J.; Tashkin, D.P.; Epstein, J.D.; Kollin, J.; Green, R.H.; Zamel, N.; et al. Contribution of Emphysema and Small Airways in COPD. *Chest* **1996**, *109*, 353–359. [CrossRef]
9. Drummond, M.B.; Hansel, N.N.; Connett, J.E.; Scanlon, P.D.; Tashkin, N.P.; Wise, R.A. Spirometric Predictors of Lung Function Decline and Mortality in Early Chronic Obstructive Pulmonary Disease. *Am. J. Respir. Crit. Care Med.* **2012**, *185*, 1301–1306. [CrossRef] [PubMed]
10. Hardie, J.A.; Buist, A.S.; Vollmer, W.M.; Ellingsen, I.; Bakke, P.S.; Morkve, O. Risk of over-diagnosis of COPD in asymptomatic elderly never-smokers. *Eur. Respir. J.* **2002**, *20*, 1117–1122. [CrossRef] [PubMed]
11. Swanney, M.P.; Ruppel, G.; Enright, P.L.; Pedersen, O.F.; Crapo, R.O.; Miller, M.R.; Jensen, R.L.; Falaschetti, E.; Schouten, J.P.; Hankinson, J.L.; et al. Using the lower limit of normal for the FEV1/FVC ratio reduces the misclassification of airway obstruction. *Thorax* **2008**, *63*, 1046–1051. [CrossRef]
12. Calverley, P.M.A.; Mueller, A.; Fowler, A.; Metzdorf, N.; Wise, R.A. The Effect of Defining Chronic Obstructive Pulmonary Disease by the Lower Limit of Normal of FEV(1)/FVC Ratio in Tiotropium Safety and Performance in Respimat Participants. *Ann. Am. Thorac. Soc.* **2018**, *15*, 200–208. [CrossRef] [PubMed]
13. Bhatt, S.P.; Balte, P.P.; Schwartz, J.E.; Cassano, P.A.; Couper, D.; Jacobs, D.R.; Kalhan, R.; O'Connor, G.T.; Yende, S.; Sanders, J.L.; et al. Discriminative Accuracy of FEV1: FVC Thresholds for COPD-Related Hospitalization and Mortality. *JAMA* **2019**, *321*, 2438–2447. [CrossRef]
14. Kerstjens, H.A.; Brand, P.L.; Hughes, M.D.; Robinson, N.J.; Postma, D.S.; Sluiter, H.J.; Bleecker, E.R.; Dekhuijzen, P.R.; De Jong, P.M.; Mengelers, H.J.; et al. A Comparison of Bronchodilator Therapy with or without Inhaled Corticosteroid Therapy for Obstructive Airways Disease. *N. Engl. J. Med.* **1992**, *327*, 1413–1419. [CrossRef]
15. Brand, P.L.; Quanjer, P.H.; Postma, D.S.; Kerstjens, H.A.; Koeter, G.H.; Dekhuijzen, P.N.; Sluiter, H.J. Interpretation of bronchodilator response in patients with obstructive airways disease. The Dutch Chronic Non-Specific Lung Disease (CNSLD) Study Group. *Thorax* **1992**, *47*, 429–436. [CrossRef] [PubMed]
16. Gibson, P.G.; Simpson, J.L. The overlap syndrome of asthma and COPD: What are its features and how important is it? *Thorax* **2009**, *64*, 728–735. [CrossRef] [PubMed]
17. Bateman, E.D.; Reddel, H.; van Zyl-Smit, R.; Agusti, A. The asthma–COPD overlap syndrome: Towards a revised taxonomy of chronic airways diseases? *Lancet Respir. Med.* **2015**, *3*, 719–728. [CrossRef]
18. Postma, D.S.; Rabe, K.F. The Asthma-COPD Overlap Syndrome. *N. Engl. J. Med.* **2015**, *373*, 1241–1249. [CrossRef]
19. Sin, D.D.; Miravitlles, M.; Mannino, D.M.; Soriano, J.B.; Price, D.; Celli, B.R.; Leung, J.M.; Nakano, Y.; Park, H.Y.; Wark, P.; et al. What is asthma-COPD overlap syndrome? Towards a consensus definition from a round table discussion. *Eur. Respir. J.* **2016**, *48*, 664–673. [CrossRef] [PubMed]
20. Ciba Guest Symposium. Terminology, definitions, and classification of chronic pulmonary emphysema and related conditions. *Thorax* **1959**, *14*, 286–299. [CrossRef]

21. Peto, R.; Speizer, F.E.; Cochrane, A.L.; Moore, F.; Fletcher, C.M.; Tinker, C.M.; Higgins, I.T.; Gray, R.G.; Richards, S.M.; Gilliland, J.; et al. The relevance in adults of air-flow obstruction, but not of mucus hypersecretion, to mortality from chronic lung disease. Results from 20 years of prospective observation. *Am. Rev. Respir. Dis.* **1983**, *128*, 491–500. [CrossRef]
22. Vestbo, J.; Rasmussen, F.V. Respiratory symptoms and FEV1 as predictors of hospitalization and medication in the following 12 years due to respiratory disease. *Eur. Respir. J.* **1989**, *2*, 710–715.
23. Vestbo, J.; Prescott, E.; Lange, P. Association of chronic mucus hypersecretion with FEV1 decline and chronic obstructive pulmonary disease morbidity. Copenhagen City Heart Study Group. *Am. J. Respir. Crit. Care Med.* **1996**, *153*, 1530–1535. [CrossRef] [PubMed]
24. Burrows, B.; Niden, A.H.; Fletcher, C.M.; Jones, N.L. Clinical Types of Chronic Obstructive Lung Disease in London and in Chicago. A Study of One Hundred Patients. *Am. Rev. Respir. Dis.* **1964**, *90*, 14–27. [CrossRef] [PubMed]
25. Manicatide, M.A.; Teculescu, D.B.; Racoveanu, C.L. Hypoxemia in chronic bronchitis and pulmonary emphysema. *Med. Interne* **1977**, *15*, 41–48. [PubMed]
26. Jacques, J.; Cooney, T.P.; Silvers, G.W.; Petty, T.L.; Wright, J.L.; Thurlbeck, W.M. The Lungs and Causes of Death in the Nocturnal Oxygen Therapy Trial. *Chest* **1984**, *86*, 230–233. [CrossRef] [PubMed]
27. Orie, N.G.; Slutter, H.J.; Tammeling, G.J. Chronic nonspecific respiratory diseases (Dutch). *Ned. Tijdschr. Geneeskd.* **1961**, *105*, 2136–2139.
28. American Thoracic Society. Standards for the diagnosis and care of patients with chronic obstructive pulmonary disease (COPD) and asthma. *Am. Rev. Respir. Dis.* **1987**, *136*, 225–244. [CrossRef]
29. Grol, M.H.; Gerritsen, J.; Vonk, J.M.; Schouten, J.P.; Koëter, G.H.; Rijcken, B.; Postma, D.S. Risk Factors for Growth and Decline of Lung Function in Asthmatic Individuals up to Age 42 years. *Am. J. Respir. Crit. Care Med.* **1999**, *160*, 1830–1837. [CrossRef]
30. Sears, M.R.; Greene, J.M.; Willan, A.R.; Wiecek, E.M.; Taylor, D.R.; Flannery, E.M.; Cowan, J.O.; Herbison, G.P.; Silva, P.A.; Poulton, R. A Longitudinal, Population-Based, Cohort Study of Childhood Asthma Followed to Adulthood. *N. Engl. J. Med.* **2003**, *349*, 1414–1422. [CrossRef]
31. Diagnosis of Diseases of Chronic Airflow Limitation: Asthma, COPD and Asthma-COPD Overlap Syndrome (ACOS). Available online: https://goldcopd.org/wp-content/uploads/2016/04/GOLD_ACOS_2015.pdf (accessed on 13 May 2021).
32. Woodruff, P.G.; Berge, M.V.D.; Boucher, R.C.; Brightling, C.; Burchard, E.G.; Christenson, S.A.; Han, M.K.; Holtzman, M.J.; Kraft, M.; Lynch, D.A.; et al. American Thoracic Society/National Heart, Lung, and Blood Institute Asthma-Chronic Obstructive Pulmonary Disease Overlap Workshop Report. *Am. J. Respir. Crit. Care Med.* **2017**, *196*, 375–381. [CrossRef] [PubMed]
33. Cazzola, M.; Rogliani, P. Do we really need asthma-chronic obstructive pulmonary disease overlap syndrome? *J. Allergy Clin. Immunol.* **2016**, *138*, 977–983. [CrossRef]
34. Barczyk, A.; Maskey-Warzęchowska, M.; Górska, K.; Barczyk, M.; Kuziemski, K.; Śliwiński, P.; Batura-Gabryel, H.; Mróz, R.; Kania, A.; Obojski, A.; et al. Asthma-COPD Overlap-A Discordance Between Patient Populations Defined by Different Diagnostic Criteria. *J. Allergy Clin. Immunol. Pract.* **2019**, *7*, 2326–2336.e5. [CrossRef]
35. Scott, S.; Currie, J.; Albert, P.; Calverley, P.; Wilding, J. Risk of Misdiagnosis, Health-Related Quality of Life, and BMI in Patients Who Are Overweight with Doctor-Diagnosed Asthma. *Chest* **2012**, *141*, 616–624. [CrossRef] [PubMed]
36. Brightling, C.E.; Bradding, P.; Symon, F.A.; Holgate, S.T.; Wardlaw, A.J.; Pavord, I.D. Mast-Cell Infiltration of Airway Smooth Muscle in Asthma. *N. Engl. J. Med.* **2002**, *346*, 1699–1705. [CrossRef] [PubMed]
37. Perskvist, N.; Edston, E. Differential accumulation of pulmonary and cardiac mast cell-subsets and eosinophils between fatal anaphylaxis and asthma death: A post mortem comparative study. *Forensic Sci. Int.* **2007**, *169*, 43–49. [CrossRef]
38. James, A.L.; Bai, T.R.; Mauad, T.; Abramson, M.; Dolhnikoff, M.; McKay, K.O.; Maxwell, P.S.; Elliot, J.G.; Green, F.H. Airway smooth muscle thickness in asthma is related to severity but not duration of asthma. *Eur. Respir. J.* **2009**, *34*, 1040–1045. [CrossRef] [PubMed]
39. McDonough, J.; Yuan, R.; Suzuki, M.; Seyednejad, N.; Elliott, W.M.; Sanchez, P.G.; Wright, A.C.; Gefter, W.B.; Litzky, L.; Coxson, H.O.; et al. Small-Airway Obstruction and Emphysema in Chronic Obstructive Pulmonary Disease. *N. Engl. J. Med.* **2011**, *365*, 1567–1575. [CrossRef] [PubMed]
40. Koo, H.-K.; Vasilescu, D.M.; Booth, S.; Hsieh, A.; Katsamenis, O.; Fishbane, N.; Elliott, W.M.; Kirby, M.; Lackie, P.; Sinclair, I.; et al. Small airways disease in mild and moderate chronic obstructive pulmonary disease: A cross-sectional study. *Lancet Respir. Med.* **2018**, *6*, 591–602. [CrossRef]
41. Hartley, R.A.; Barker, B.L.; Newby, C.; Pakkal, M.; Baldi, S.; Kajekar, R.; Kay, R.; Laurencin, M.; Marshall, R.P.; Sousa, A.R.; et al. Relationship between lung function and quantitative computed tomographic parameters of airway remodeling, air trapping, and emphysema in patients with asthma and chronic obstructive pulmonary disease: A single-center study. *J. Allergy Clin. Immunol.* **2016**, *137*, 1413–1422.e12. [CrossRef] [PubMed]
42. Karayama, M.; Inui, N.; Yasui, H.; Kono, M.; Hozumi, H.; Suzuki, Y.; Furuhashi, K.; Hashimoto, D.; Enomoto, N.; Fujisawa, T.; et al. Physiological and morphological differences of airways between COPD and asthma-COPD overlap. *Sci. Rep.* **2019**, *9*, 7818. [CrossRef] [PubMed]
43. Papakonstantinou, E.; Savic, S.; Siebeneichler, A.; Strobel, W.; Jones, P.W.; Tamm, M.; Stolz, D. A pilot study to test the feasibility of histological characterisation of asthma-COPD overlap. *Eur. Respir. J.* **2019**, *53*, 1801941. [CrossRef]
44. Wenzel, S.E. Asthma phenotypes: The evolution from clinical to molecular approaches. *Nat. Med.* **2012**, *18*, 716–725. [CrossRef]

45. Hastie, A.T.; Martinez, F.J.; Curtis, J.L.; Doerschuk, C.M.; Hansel, N.N.; Christenson, S.; Putcha, N.; Ortega, V.E.; Li, X.; Barr, R.G.; et al. Association of sputum and blood eosinophil concentrations with clinical measures of COPD severity: An analysis of the SPIROMICS cohort. *Lancet Respir. Med.* **2017**, *5*, 956–967. [CrossRef]
46. Global Initiative for Asthma. Global Strategy for Asthma Management and Prevention. 2021. Available online: https://ginasthma.org/wp-content/uploads/2021/04/GINA-2021-Main-Report_FINAL_21_04_28-WMS.pdf (accessed on 13 May 2021).
47. Ortega, H.G.; Yancey, S.W.; Mayer, B.; Gunsoy, N.B.; Keene, O.N.; Bleecker, E.R.; Brightling, C.E.; Pavord, I.D. Severe eosinophilic asthma treated with mepolizumab stratified by baseline eosinophil thresholds: A secondary analysis of the DREAM and MENSA studies. *Lancet Respir. Med.* **2016**, *4*, 549–556. [CrossRef]
48. Vedel-Krogh, S.; Nielsen, S.F.; Lange, P.; Vestbo, J.; Nordestgaard, B.G. Blood Eosinophils and Exacerbations in Chronic Obstructive Pulmonary Disease. The Copenhagen General Population Study. *Am. J. Respir. Crit. Care Med.* **2016**, *193*, 965–974. [CrossRef] [PubMed]
49. Li, M.; Yang, T.; He, R.; Li, A.; Dang, W.; Liu, X.; Chen, M. The Value of Inflammatory Biomarkers in Differentiating Asthma–COPD Overlap from COPD. *Int. J. Chronic Obstr. Pulm. Dis.* **2020**, *15*, 3025–3037. [CrossRef] [PubMed]
50. Pérez-De-Llano, L.; On behalf of the CHACOS Study Group; Cosio, B.G. Asthma-COPD overlap is not a homogeneous disorder: Further supporting data. *Respir. Res.* **2017**, *18*, 183. [CrossRef]
51. Reddel, H.K.; Vestbo, J.; Agustí, A.; Anderson, G.P.; Bansal, A.T.; Beasley, R.; Bel, E.H.; Janson, C.; Make, B.; Pavord, I.D.; et al. Heterogeneity within and between physician-diagnosed asthma and/or COPD: NOVELTY cohort. *Eur. Respir. J.* **2021**, *25*, 2003927. [CrossRef]
52. Christenson, S.A.; Steiling, K.; van den Berge, M.; Hijazi, K.; Hiemstra, P.S.; Postma, D.S.; Lenburg, M.E.; Spira, A.; Woodruff, P.G. Asthma-COPD overlap. Clinical relevance of ge-nomic signatures of type 2 inflammation in chronic obstructive pulmonary disease. *Am. J. Respir. Crit. Care Med.* **2015**, *191*, 758–766. [CrossRef]
53. Morgan, B.W.; Grigsby, M.R.; Siddharthan, T.; Chowdhury, M.; Rubinstein, A.; Gutierrez, L.; Irazola, V.; Miranda, J.J.; Bernabe-Ortiz, A.; Alam, D.; et al. Epidemiology and risk factors of asthma-chronic obstructive pulmonary disease overlap in low- and middle-income countries. *J. Allergy Clin. Immunol.* **2019**, *143*, 1598–1606. [CrossRef]
54. Toledo-Pons, N.; van Boven, J.F.M.; Román-Rodríguez, M.; Pérez, N.; Felices, J.L.V.; Soriano, J.B.; Cosío, B.G. ACO: Time to move from the description of different phenotypes to the treatable traits. *PLoS ONE* **2019**, *14*, e0210915. [CrossRef] [PubMed]
55. Singh, A.; Liu, C.; Putman, B.; Zeig-Owens, R.; Hall, C.B.; Schwartz, T.; Webber, M.P.; Cohen, H.W.; Berger, K.I.; Nolan, A.; et al. Predictors of Asthma/COPD Overlap in FDNY Firefighters with World Trade Center Dust Exposure: A Longitudinal Study. *Chest* **2018**, *154*, 1301–1310. [CrossRef] [PubMed]
56. Cosentino, J.; Zhao, H.; Hardin, M.; Hersh, C.P.; Crapo, J.; Kim, V.; Criner, G.J. Analysis of Asthma-Chronic Obstructive Pulmonary Disease Overlap Syndrome Defined on the Basis of Bronchodilator Response and Degree of Emphysema. *Ann. Am. Thorac. Soc.* **2016**, *13*, 1483–1489. [CrossRef] [PubMed]
57. Krishnan, J.A.; Nibber, A.; Chisholm, A.; Price, D.; Bateman, E.D.; Bjermer, L.; van Boven, J.F.M.; Brusselle, G.; Costello, R.W.; Dandurand, R.J.; et al. Prevalence and Characteristics of Asthma-Chronic Obstructive Pulmonary Disease Overlap in Routine Primary Care Practices. *Ann. Am. Thorac. Soc.* **2019**, *16*, 1143–1150. [CrossRef]
58. Izbicki, G.; Teo, V.; Liang, J.; Russell, G.M.; Holland, A.E.; Zwar, N.A.; Bonevski, B.; Mahal, A.; Eustace, P.; Paul, E.; et al. Clinical Characteristics of Patients with Asthma COPD Overlap (ACO) In Australian Primary Care. *Int. J. Chronic Obstr. Pulm. Dis.* **2019**, *14*, 2745–2752. [CrossRef]
59. Miravitlles, M.; Barrecheguren, M.; Roman-Rodriguez, M. Is a previous diagnosis of asthma a reliable criterion for asthma–COPD overlap syndrome in a patient with COPD? *Int. J. Chronic Obstr. Pulm. Dis.* **2015**, *10*, 1745–1752. [CrossRef]
60. Llanos, J.-P.; Ortega, H.; Germain, G.; Duh, M.S.; Lafeuille, M.-H.; Tiggelaar, S.; Bell, C.F.; Hahn, B. Health characteristics of patients with asthma, COPD and asthma-COPD overlap in the NHANES database. *Int. J. Chronic Obstr. Pulm. Dis.* **2018**, *13*, 2859–2868. [CrossRef]
61. Baarnes, C.B.; Andersen, Z.J.; Tjønneland, A.; Ulrik, C.S. Determinants of incident asthma-COPD overlap: A prospective study of 55,110 middle-aged adults. *Clin. Epidemiol.* **2018**, *10*, 1275–1287. [CrossRef]
62. Gibson, P.G.; McDonald, V.M. Asthma-COPD overlap 2015: Now we are six. *Thorax* **2015**, *70*, 683–691. [CrossRef]
63. Nelsen, L.M.; Lee, L.A.; Wu, W.; Lin, X.; Murray, L.; Pascoe, S.J.; Leidy, N.K. Reliability, validity and responsiveness of E-RS: COPD in patients with spirometric asthma-COPD overlap. *Respir. Res.* **2019**, *20*, 107. [CrossRef] [PubMed]
64. Pascoe, S.J.; Wu, W.; Collison, K.A.; Nelsen, L.M.; Wurst, K.E.; Lee, L.A. Use of clinical characteristics to predict spirometric classification of obstructive lung disease. *Int. J. Chron. Obstruct. Pulmon. Dis.* **2018**, *13*, 889–902. [CrossRef] [PubMed]
65. Bui, D.S.; Burgess, J.A.; Lowe, A.J.; Perret, J.L.; Lodge, C.J.; Bui, M.; Morrison, S.; Thompson, B.R.; Thomas, P.S.; Giles, G.G.; et al. Childhood Lung Function Predicts Adult Chronic Obstructive Pulmonary Disease and Asthma-Chronic Obstructive Pulmonary Disease Overlap Syndrome. *Am. J. Respir. Crit. Care Med.* **2017**, *196*, 39–46. [CrossRef] [PubMed]
66. Tai, A.; Tran, H.; Roberts, M.; Clarke, N.; Wilson, J.; Robertson, C.F. The association between childhood asthma and adult chronic obstructive pulmonary disease. *Thorax* **2014**, *69*, 805–810. [CrossRef]
67. Tagiyeva, N.; Devereux, G.; Fielding, S.; Turner, S.; Douglas, G. Outcomes of Childhood Asthma and Wheezy Bronchitis. A 50-Year Cohort Study. *Am. J. Respir. Crit. Care Med.* **2016**, *193*, 23–30. [CrossRef]

68. De Marco, R.; Marcon, A.; Rossi, A.; Antó, J.M.; Cerveri, I.; Gislason, T.; Heinrich, J.; Janson, C.; Jarvis, D.; Kuenzli, N.; et al. Asthma, COPD and overlap syndrome: A longitudinal study in young European adults. *Eur. Respir. J.* **2015**, *46*, 671–679. [CrossRef] [PubMed]
69. Zheng, X.; Guan, W.; Zheng, J.; Ye, P.; Liu, S.; Zhou, J.; Xiong, Y.; Zhang, Q.; Chen, Q. Smoking influences response to inhaled corticosteroids in patients with asthma: A meta-analysis. *Curr. Med. Res. Opin.* **2012**, *28*, 1791–1798. [CrossRef]
70. Sonnex, K.; Alleemudder, H.; Knaggs, R. Impact of smoking status on the efficacy of inhaled corticosteroids in COPD: A systematic review. *BMJ Open* **2020**, *10*, e037509. [CrossRef]
71. Gao, J.; Zhou, W.; Chen, B.; Lin, W.; Wu, S.; Wu, F. Sputum cell count: Biomarkers in the differentiation of asthma, COPD and asthma-COPD overlap. *Int. J. Chronic Obstr. Pulm. Dis.* **2017**, *12*, 2703–2710. [CrossRef]
72. Brutsche, M.H.; Downs, S.H.; Schindler, C.; Gerbase, M.W.; Schwartz, J.; Frey, M.; Russi, E.W.; Ackermann-Liebrich, U.; Leuenberger, P. Bronchial hyperresponsiveness and the development of asthma and COPD in asymptomatic individuals: SAPALDIA Cohort Study. *Thorax* **2006**, *61*, 671–677. [CrossRef] [PubMed]
73. Calverley, P.M.; Albert, P.; Walker, P.P. Bronchodilator reversibility in chronic obstructive pulmonary disease: Use and limita-tions. *Lancet Respir. Med.* **2013**, *1*, 564–573. [CrossRef]
74. Miller, M.R.; Hankinson, J.; Brusasco, V.; Burgos, F.; Casaburi, R.; Coates, A.; Crapo, R.; Enright, P.; van der Grinten, C.P.M.; Gustafsson, P.; et al. Standardisation of spirometry. *Eur. Respir. J.* **2005**, *26*, 319–338. [CrossRef]
75. Gibbons, W.J.; Sharma, A.; Lougheed, D.; Macklem, P.T. Detection of excessive bronchoconstriction in asthma. *Am. J. Respir. Crit. Care Med.* **1996**, *153*, 582–589. [CrossRef]
76. Walker, P.P.; Hadcroft, J.; Costello, R.W.; Calverley, P.M. Lung function changes following methacholine inhalation in COPD. *Respir. Med.* **2009**, *103*, 535–541. [CrossRef] [PubMed]
77. Tkacova, R.; Dai, D.L.; Vonk, J.M.; Leung, J.M.; Hiemstra, P.S.; Berge, M.V.D.; Kunz, L.; Hollander, Z.; Tashkin, D.; Wise, R.; et al. Airway hyperresponsiveness in chronic obstructive pulmonary disease: A marker of asthma-chronic obstructive pulmonary disease overlap syndrome? *J. Allergy Clin. Immunol.* **2016**, *138*, 1571–1579.e10. [CrossRef]
78. Pare, P.D.; Wiggs, B.R.; James, A.; Hogg, J.C.; Bosken, C. The Comparative Mechanics and Morphology of Airways in Asthma and in Chronic Obstructive Pulmonary Disease. *Am. Rev. Respir. Dis.* **1991**, *143*, 1189–1193. [CrossRef]
79. Calverley, P.M.A.; Burge, P.S.; Spencer, S.; Anderson, J.A.; Jones, P.W. Bronchodilator reversibility testing in chronic obstructive pulmonary disease. *Thorax* **2003**, *58*, 659–664. [CrossRef]
80. Calverley, P.; Vlies, B. A rational approach to single, dual and triple therapy in COPD. *Respirology* **2016**, *21*, 581–589. [CrossRef] [PubMed]
81. Pellegrino, R.; Viegi, G.; Brusasco, V.; Crapo, R.O.; Burgos, F.; Casaburi, R.; Coates, A.; van der Grinten, C.P.M.; Gustafsson, P.; Hankinson, J.; et al. Interpretative strategies for lung function tests. *Eur. Respir. J.* **2005**, *26*, 948–968. [CrossRef] [PubMed]
82. Albert, P.; Agusti, A.; Edwards, L.; Tal-Singer, R.; Yates, J.; Bakke, P.; Celli, B.R.; Coxson, H.O.; Crim, C.; Lomas, D.A.; et al. Bronchodilator responsiveness as a phenotypic characteristic of established chronic obstructive pulmonary disease. *Thorax* **2012**, *67*, 701–708. [CrossRef]
83. Tashkin, D.P.; Celli, B.; Decramer, M.; Liu, D.; Burkhart, D.; Cassino, C.; Kesten, S. Bronchodilator responsiveness in patients with COPD. *Eur. Respir. J.* **2008**, *31*, 742–750. [CrossRef]
84. Maselli, D.J.; Hardin, M.; Christenson, S.A.; Hanania, N.A.; Hersh, C.P.; Adams, S.G.; Anzueto, A.; Peters, J.I.; Han, M.K.; Martinez, F.J. Clinical Approach to the Therapy of Asthma-COPD Overlap. *Chest* **2019**, *155*, 168–177. [CrossRef]
85. O'Donnell, D.; Voduc, N.; Fitzpatrick, M.; Webb, K. Effect of salmeterol on the ventilatory response to exercise in chronic obstructive pulmonary disease. *Eur. Respir. J.* **2004**, *24*, 86–94. [CrossRef]
86. Lipson, D.A.; Barnhart, F.; Brealey, N.; Brooks, J.; Criner, G.J.; Day, N.C.; Dransfield, M.T.; Halpin, D.M.; Han, M.K.; Jones, C.E.; et al. Once-Daily Single-Inhaler Triple versus Dual Therapy in Patients with COPD. *N. Engl. J. Med.* **2018**, *378*, 1671–1680. [CrossRef]
87. Han, M.K.; Criner, G.J.; Dransfield, M.T.; Halpin, D.M.G.; Jones, C.E.; Kilbride, S.; Lange, P.; Lettis, S.; Lipson, D.A.; Lomas, D.A.; et al. The Effect of Inhaled Corticosteroid Withdrawal and Baseline Inhaled Treatment on Exacerbations in the IMPACT Study. A Randomized, Double-Blind, Multicenter Clinical Trial. *Am. J. Respir. Crit. Care Med.* **2020**, *202*, 1237–1243. [CrossRef] [PubMed]
88. Green, R.H.; Brightling, C.E.; McKenna, S.; Hargadon, B.; Parker, D.; Bradding, P.; Wardlaw, A.J.; Pavord, I.D. Asthma exacerba-tions and sputum eosinophil counts: A randomised controlled trial. *Lancet* **2002**, *360*, 1715–1721. [CrossRef]
89. Negewo, N.A.; McDonald, V.M.; Baines, K.J.; Wark, P.A.B.; Simpson, J.L.; Jones, P.W.; Gibson, P.G. Peripheral blood eosinophils: A surrogate marker for airway eosinophilia in stable COPD. *Int. J. Chronic Obstr. Pulm. Dis.* **2016**, *11*, 1495–1504. [CrossRef] [PubMed]
90. Pascoe, S.; Locantore, N.; Dransfield, M.T.; Barnes, N.C.; Pavord, I.D. Blood eosinophil counts, exacerbations, and response to the addition of inhaled fluticasone furoate to vilanterol in patients with chronic obstructive pulmonary disease: A secondary analysis of data from two parallel randomised controlled trials. *Lancet Respir. Med.* **2015**, *3*, 435–442. [CrossRef]
91. Watz, H.; Tetzlaff, K.; Wouters, E.F.M.; Kirsten, A.; Magnussen, H.; Rodriguez-Roisin, R.; Vogelmeier, C.; Fabbri, L.M.; Chanez, P.; Dahl, R.; et al. Blood eosinophil count and exacerbations in severe chronic obstructive pulmonary disease after withdrawal of inhaled corticosteroids: A post-hoc analysis of the WISDOM trial. *Lancet Respir. Med.* **2016**, *4*, 390–398. [CrossRef]

92. Pascoe, S.; Barnes, N.; Brusselle, G.; Compton, C.; Criner, G.J.; Dransfield, M.T.; Halpin, D.M.G.; Han, M.K.; Hartley, B.; Lange, P.; et al. Blood eosinophils and treatment response with triple and dual combination therapy in chronic obstructive pulmonary disease: Analysis of the IMPACT trial. *Lancet Respir. Med.* **2019**, *7*, 745–756. [CrossRef]
93. Bafadhel, M.; Peterson, S.; de Blas, M.A.; Calverley, P.M.; Rennard, S.I.; Richter, K.; Fagerås, M. Predictors of exacerbation risk and response to budesonide in patients with chronic obstructive pulmonary disease: A post-hoc analysis of three randomised trials. *Lancet Respir. Med.* **2018**, *6*, 117–126. [CrossRef]
94. Barnes, N.C.; Sharma, R.; Lettis, S.; Calverley, P.M. Blood eosinophils as a marker of response to inhaled corticosteroids in COPD. *Eur. Respir. J.* **2016**, *47*, 1374–1382. [CrossRef]
95. Martinez, F.J.; Rabe, K.F.; Calverley, P.M.; Fabbri, L.M.; Sethi, S.; Pizzichini, E.; McIvor, A.; Anzueto, A.; Alagappan, V.K.; Siddiqui, S.; et al. Determinants of Response to Roflumilast in Severe Chronic Obstructive Pulmonary Disease. Pooled Analysis of Two Randomized Trials. *Am. J. Respir. Crit. Care Med.* **2018**, *198*, 1268–1278. [CrossRef]
96. Pignatti, P.; Visca, D.; Cherubino, F.; Zampogna, E.; Lucini, E.; Saderi, L.; Sotgiu, G.; Spanevello, A. Groningen and Leiden Universities Corticosteroids in Obstructive Lung Disease (GLUCOLD) Study Group. Predictive value of eosinophils and neutrophils on clinical effects of ICS in COPD. *Respirology* **2018**, *23*, 1023–1031.
97. Rabe, K.F.; Watz, H.; Baraldo, S.; Pedersen, F.; Biondini, D.; Bagul, N.; Hanauer, G.; Göhring, U.-M.; Purkayastha, D.; Román, J.; et al. Anti-inflammatory effects of roflumilast in chronic obstructive pulmonary disease (ROBERT): A 16-week, randomised, placebo-controlled trial. *Lancet Respir. Med.* **2018**, *6*, 827–836. [CrossRef]
98. Landis, S.; Suruki, R.; Maskell, J.; Bonar, K.; Hilton, E.; Compton, C. Demographic and Clinical Characteristics of COPD Patients at Different Blood Eosinophil Levels in the UK Clinical Practice Research Datalink. *COPD* **2018**, *15*, 177–184. [CrossRef] [PubMed]
99. Putcha, N.; Wise, R.A. Asthma-Chronic Obstructive Pulmonary Disease Overlap Syndrome: Nothing New Under the Sun. *Immunol. Allergy Clin. N. Am.* **2016**, *36*, 515–528. [CrossRef] [PubMed]
100. McDonald, V.M.; Fingleton, J.; Agusti, A.; Hiles, S.A.; Clark, V.L.; Holland, A.E.; Marks, G.B.; Bardin, P.P.; Beasley, R.; Pavord, I.D.; et al. Treatable traits: A new paradigm for 21st century management of chronic airway diseases: Treatable Traits Down Under International Workshop report. *Eur. Respir. J.* **2019**, *53*, 1802058. [CrossRef]

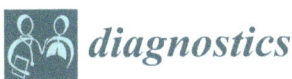

Review

ACO (Asthma–COPD Overlap) Is Independent from COPD, a Case in Favor: A Systematic Review

Naoya Fujino * and Hisatoshi Sugiura

Department of Respiratory Medicine, Tohoku University Graduate School of Medicine, Sendai 980-8574, Japan; sugiura@rm.med.tohoku.ac.jp
* Correspondence: nfujino@med.tohoku.ac.jp; Tel.: +81-22-717-8539

Abstract: Asthma and chronic obstructive pulmonary disease (COPD) are now recognized to be able to co-exist as asthma–COPD overlap (ACO). It is clinically relevant to evaluate whether patients with COPD concurrently have components of asthma in primary care. This is because: (i) ACO is a relatively common condition among asthma (over 40 years of age) or COPD irrespective of its diagnosis criteria; (ii) patients with ACO can have higher frequency of exacerbation and more rapid decline in lung function than those with asthma or COPD; and (iii) asthmatic features such as eosinophilic airway inflammation are promising indicators for prediction of inhaled corticosteroid-responsiveness in COPD. The aim of this review to evaluate diagnostic markers for ACO. We searched PubMed for articles related to ACO published until 2020. Articles associated with diagnostic biomarkers were included. We identified a total of 25 studies, some of which have revealed that a combination of biomarkers such as fractional exhaled nitric oxide and serum immunoglobulin E is useful to discern type 2 inflammation in the airways of COPD. Here, we review the current understanding of the clinical characteristics, biomarkers and molecular pathophysiology of ACO in the context of how ACO can be differentiated from COPD.

Keywords: asthma–COPD overlap; asthma; COPD; fractional exhaled nitric oxide; immunoglobulin E

Citation: Fujino, N.; Sugiura, H. ACO (Asthma–COPD Overlap) Is Independent from COPD, a Case in Favor: A Systematic Review. *Diagnostics* **2021**, *11*, 859. https://doi.org/10.3390/diagnostics11050859

Academic Editor: Koichi Nishimura

Received: 6 May 2021
Accepted: 10 May 2021
Published: 11 May 2021

Publisher's Note: MDPI stays neutral with regard to jurisdictional claims in published maps and institutional affiliations.

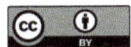

Copyright: © 2021 by the authors. Licensee MDPI, Basel, Switzerland. This article is an open access article distributed under the terms and conditions of the Creative Commons Attribution (CC BY) license (https://creativecommons.org/licenses/by/4.0/).

1. Introduction

1.1. Background of Asthma and Chronic Obstructive Pulmonary Disesase

The global burdens of asthma and chronic obstructive pulmonary disease (COPD) are increasing, each of which was estimated to affect respectively approximate 339 million and 251 million people worldwide in 2016 [1]. It has been widely accepted that asthma and COPD are strikingly different airway disorders [2,3]. Although the "Dutch hypothesis" suggested a common genetic background underlying airway obstruction with a spectrum of clinical entities from asthma to COPD, recent genetic research indicated that it was unlikely that genetic factors are shared by asthma and COPD [4].

Asthma is a heterogenous and inflammatory disease affecting large and small respiratory tracts but not the lung parenchyma, and contains clusters of demographical, clinical and pathophysiological characteristics underpinned by different pathophysiological processes [5]. This heterogeneity may be explained by the complexity of dysregulated innate and adaptive inflammatory responses to exogenous allergens and proteases leading to the spectrum of abnormal tissue remodeling, where type 2 cytokines such as interleukin (IL)-4, IL-13 and IL-5 primarily promote airway eosinophil infiltration, mucus hypersecretion, bronchial hyperresponsiveness and mast cell activation [6]. Major subpopulations of asthmatics have molecular signatures of T helper 2 (Th2)—inflammation and airway obstruction that markedly respond to inhaled corticosteroid (ICS) [7]. In line with this translational study, accumulated evidence from randomized control trials have revealed the importance of ICS usage from the early steps of asthma treatment because clinical studies have shown that ICS robustly reduced the risk of symptoms, exacerbations, hospitalization and mortality from asthma [8–10].

COPD is defined as a common, preventable and treatable disease that is characterized by persistent respiratory symptoms and airflow limitation that is due to airway and/or alveolar abnormalities usually caused by significant exposure to noxious particles or gases and influenced by host factors including abnormal lung development [11]. In addition to cigarette smoking, known as the most common COPD risk factor [12], the susceptibility could be influenced by genetic factors [13,14] and abnormal lung growth [15]. Unlike asthma, $CD4^+$ T helper 1 (Th1) cells, $CD8^+$ cytotoxic T (Tc) cells, neutrophils and macrophages predominantly affect the small airways and the lung parenchyma leading to mucus hypersecretion, alveolar wall destruction (emphysema) and small airway fibrosis in COPD [2,16]. These pro-inflammatory cell-types are functionally altered by oxidative stress and intracellular signaling pathways including activation of the proinflammatory transcription factor nuclear factor κB (NF-κB) [17], and alveolar macrophages are defective in bacterial phagocytosis, possibly via several phagocytic receptors and mitochondrial molecules related to oxidative stress [18–21]. The small airway narrowing induced by pro-inflammatory cell infiltration, luminal exudates, wall thickening, and the loss of small airways associated with emphysema increases airway obstruction [22,23]. In the wall thickening, hyperplasia of basal cells, known as airway epithelial stem cells, could be formed through several molecules such as Axl receptor tyrosine kinase [24] and Yap-Wnt7b [25]. The airflow limitation progressively leads to gas-trapping in peripheral lungs during expiration on exercise, resulting in dynamic hyperinflation which is postulated to be the main mechanism of exertional dyspnea [26,27]. Thus bronchodilators, long-acting muscarinic antagonists (LAMA) and long acting beta$_2$-agonists (LABA), are commonly used as the pharmacological therapy for COPD and are known to reduce lung hyperinflation, dyspnea and exercise endurance [28,29] leading to improvement of the quality of life and a reduction in the frequency of exacerbations [30]. Accumulated evidence indicates that LAMA significantly reduce the frequency of exacerbations and non-serious adverse events and increase the trough forced expiratory volume in one second (FEV_1) compared to LABA in patients with stable COPD [31].

1.2. Safety Issues of ICS for Airway Infection of Patients with COPD

Several lines of evidence have indicated a higher risk of pulmonary infection in COPD patients. A population-based, case-control study conducted in Spain including 859,033 inhabitants showed a strong relationship between COPD and community-acquired pneumonia, which was independent of other clinical factors (odds ratio (OR) 1.84 (95% confidence interval (CI), 1.32–2.59)) [32]. A prospective case-control study with 175,906 COPD subjects in Canada also demonstrated that current use of ICS further increased the risk of hospitalization for pneumonia (rate ratio (RR) 1.70 (95% CI, 1.63–1.77)) and pneumonia followed by death within 30 days (RR 1.53 (95% CI, 1.30–1.80)) [33]. Particularly, a subset of COPD treated with ICS who had both less than 100 cells/µL of blood eosinophils and chronic bronchial infection by potentially pathogenic microorganisms was at higher risk of pneumonia (OR 3.238 (95% CI, 1.426–7.231)) [34]. Moreover, the current use of ICS in subjects even without oral corticosteroid also increased the risk of tuberculosis (TB) in a low-prevalence country (RR 1.33 (95% CI, 1.04–1.71)) [35] as well as in an intermediate-burden setting (OR 1.20 (95% CI 1.08–1.34)) [36]. In addition, the increased risk of TB infection was significantly associated with higher doses of ICS [35,36]. These studies highlighted the importance of the risk of pulmonary infection among COPD patients who are treated with high dose ICS and provided the clinically relevant question of which subset of COPD subjects would benefit from ICS therapy.

1.3. Needs for Considering Patients with Clinical Features of Both Asthma and COPD

From the early 2000s onwards, the differential diagnosis of patients with respiratory symptoms who are more than forty years of age has been recognized to be more problematic. This is because COPD becomes more common in older adults and discriminating asthma with persistent airflow obstruction from COPD is often challenging [37,38]. In fact, in

2007, the *Canadian Thoracic Society Recommendations for Management of Chronic Obstructive Pulmonary Disease—2007 Update* described the concept of "combined COPD and asthma" to highlight the finding that early introduction of ICS could be justified if the COPD patients had prominent features of asthma [39]. In 2009, Gibson and Simpson introduced the word of "the overlap syndrome of asthma and COPD" and noted that, since these patients had been largely excluded from pivotal therapeutic trials for both asthma and COPD, its diagnosis and treatment were poorly defined and lacking firm evidence [40]. Despite a growing controversy over clinical and prognostic features of ACO, retrospective studies have provided the plausible premise showing that patients with both asthma and COPD have more respiratory symptoms [41], high frequency of exacerbations [41,42] and accelerated decline in lung function [43]. Thereafter, articles regarding asthma–COPD overlap syndrome (ACOS) have been widely reviewed [44–46]. Following these early reviews, in 2014, the Global Strategy for Asthma Management and Prevention (GINA) and the Global Initiative for Chronic Obstructive Pulmonary Disease (GOLD) jointly issued their consensus-based document on ACOS so that clinicians were able to distinguish asthma from COPD and make a diagnosis of ACOS in patients with chronic airflow limitation [47]. GINA then suggested the descriptive term asthma–COPD overlap (ACO) rather than ACOS, which had been often interpreted as implying a single disease [48].

In 2016, based on the urgent requirement of an operational definition of ACO, a global expert panel from North America, Western Europe and Asia proposed criteria for its diagnosis, which consisted of age, smoking history, the presence of persistent airflow limitation defined by spirometry, history of asthma and allergic rhinitis, bronchodilator response in FEV_1 and peripheral blood eosinophil counts [49]. Following this attempt, some guidelines, such as Spanish [50] and Japanese [51] guidelines, published diagnostic algorithms that employed objective evaluations of eosinophilic and allergic airway inflammation by quantifying the levels of fractional exhaled nitric oxide (FeNO) and serum immunoglobulin E (IgE). However, the GOLD 2020 update has stated that it no longer mentions ACO [11]. This was because asthma and COPD were different disorders, although they might share common traits and clinical features. In addition, it further documented that "if a concurrent diagnosis of asthma is suspected, pharmacotherapy should primarily follow asthma guidelines, but pharmacological and non-pharmacological approaches may be needed for their COPD". This has given rise to pro and con arguments for experts in obstructive lung diseases [52,53]. As patients with ACO have been certainly excluded from clinical studies of asthma and COPD [49], molecular mechanisms of the disease and evidence of appropriate therapies are less well understood. Considering the pro-con discussion, we still have a large, unresolved question concerning why we should have a diagnostic term of ACO and how we can distinguish between COPD and ACO. The rationale of this systematic review is to describe how ACO differs in clinical features and pathogenesis from COPD. Thus, we aimed to elaborate clinical features and diagnostic markers that enable to discriminate ACO from COPD.

2. Methods

2.1. Search Strategy and Eligibility Criteria

This systematic review adheres to the PRISMA guidelines [54]. We searched PubMed for publications until 2020 with terms of "asthma–COPD overlap" or either "diagnosis" or "biomarker". Articles were included if they indicated a total population to evaluate diagnostic biomarkers such as FeNO, IgE, humoral factors or radiographical findings to be able to differentiate ACO from COPD. We excluded articles that: (1) were not associated with diagnosis of ACO by the titles and abstracts; (2) were systematic reviews or guidelines; (3) were subset analyses in other studies; (4) did not report any biomarkers except for blood eosinophil counts and pulmonary function tests. We finally added five articles reporting FeNO-driven identification of ICS responders in patients with COPD as citation searching.

2.2. Data Collection and Risk of Bias Assessment

Two review authors (NF and HS) screened the titles and abstracts of all studies identified. Full text assessments were performed to identify studies that met inclusion criteria. The risk of bias in the eligible studies was evaluated in accordance with the recommendations in the Cochrane Handbook for Systematic Reviews of Interventions 5.1.0.

3. Results

3.1. Characteristics of Selected Studies and Risk of Bias

The literature search yielded 226 candidate studies. After excluding studies on the basis of their titles or abstracts or through examining their full texts, 20 were identified. We also included five articles reporting FeNO-driven identification of ICS responders in patients with COPD as citation searching. Thus, 25 studies were included in this review (Figure 1). These studies were summarized in Table 1. Diagnostic markers for ACO included FeNO, combination of FeNO and IgE, blood, urine or induced sputum biomarkers such as inflammatory cytokines and radiographical parameters (Table 1). There were high selection bias and performance bias in the included studies.

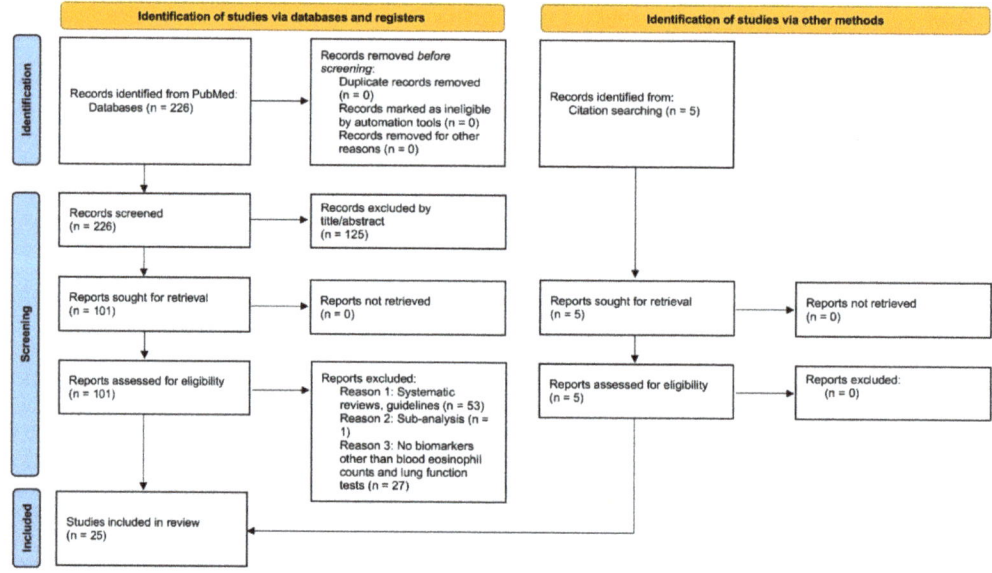

Figure 1. Study selection.

3.2. Possible Diagnostic Biomarkers for ACO: The Role of Fractional Exhaled Nitric Oxide, FeNO and IgE for the Detection of Asthmatic Features of COPD Patients

3.2.1. FeNO as a Potential Biomarker for Type 2 Inflammation for Optimal Diagnosis and to Predict the Treatment Response in Asthma.

Nitric oxide (NO) mainly originates from respiratory epithelial cells and is dominantly produced through inducible NO synthase (iNOS). Homeostatic interferon (IFN)-γ and its downstream molecule, signal transducer and activator of transcription (STAT)-1, maintains iNOS expression in the airway epithelium of healthy subjects [55]. Alving et al. firstly reported level that the FeNO of patients with mild atopic asthma was two- to three-fold higher than that of healthy control subjects [56]. A large-scale general population study supported this preliminary data by demonstrating that individuals with both increased FeNO levels and blood eosinophil counts had an increased risk of respiratory symptoms of asthma and ACO [57]. In addition, the FeNO levels were significantly increased in atopic asthma compared to non-atopic asthma [58]. The increase in the FeNO levels was underpinned by the up-regulation of iNOS mRNA and protein expression in the airway epithelium of asthmatics [59–62]. A clinical study using a selective iNOS inhibitor further confirmed that up-regulation of the FeNO levels dominantly depended on the increased iNOS expression in asthmatic patients [63]. The extent of FeNO was significantly correlated with the eosinophil counts in induced sputum [64], endobronchial biopsies [65] and bronchoalveolar fluid [66] in asthmatics, suggesting that FeNO could be used as a surrogate marker for eosinophilic airway inflammation. Although airway hyperresponsiveness (AHR) of steroid-naïve asthmatics at baseline was not associated with airway inflammation markers such as FeNO and eosinophils in induced sputum, the improvement of AHR and FEV_1 by inhaled corticosteroid therapy was significantly correlated with a reduction in the FeNO levels in those patients [67]. Researchers and clinicians in the field of asthma and allergy have given much attention to the molecular mechanisms underlying the upregulation of iNOS in asthmatic airways. Two groups reported that IL-13 induced iNOS mRNA and protein expression, which was significantly correlated with NO gas production in primary bronchial epithelial cells from healthy subjects [68] and mild-moderate asthmatics [69]. The contribution of the IL-4 and IL-13 pathway to the increase in airway NO production was further confirmed by clinical trials demonstrating that the FeNO levels were reduced in asthmatic patients treated with IL-4/IL-13 signaling blockade including nebulized soluble recombinant IL-4 receptor [70], inhaled recombinant IL-4 variant [71] and a monoclonal antibody to the alpha subunit of the IL-4 receptor alpha [72]. Collectively, these basic, translational and clinical studies have shown convincing evidence that FeNO could be a surrogate marker for type 2 inflammation of the airway.

3.2.2. How Can Feno Be Adopted to Discern ICS-Responsive, Asthmatic Phenotypes in COPD?

COPD is a highly complex and heterogenous disease, including several characteristics that could provide a rationale for the development of precision medicine [73]. Because inappropriate treatment with ICS is known to increase the risk of pneumonia for COPD patients, as discussed above, ICS should be ideally used for patients who can be expected to respond to corticosteroid therapy. Brightling et al. performed a randomized, double blind, crossover trial revealing that subjects with COPD who had higher eosinophil counts in their induced sputum exhibited increased post-bronchodilator FEV_1 after six-week-treatment with ICS [74]. Based on this research, much effort has been given to ask whether FeNO can be used to identify asthma-associated features related to a favorable ICS response among COPD patients (Table 1). These studies, despite the small numbers of patients included, produced consistent and substantial results demonstrating that the initial FeNO levels were significantly correlated with the improvement of airway obstruction evaluated by FEV_1 or ΔN_2 after additional ICS therapy [75–79]. Moreover, a recent double-blind randomized placebo-controlled trial including 214 undiagnosed subjects who had cough, wheeze or dyspnea showed that FeNO could be used in clinical practice for patients with non-specific respiratory symptoms in order to predict the ICS response [80]. Although these studies showed promise for the general use of FeNO in the clinical setting of COPD, it is still unclear whether a FeNO cut-off value could be determined to identify an ICS-responsive subset of COPD patients [81]. This question is of particular importance because the GOLD guideline limited the use of ICS to only the following types of patients: (i) Group D patients with greater than 300 cells/μL of blood eosinophils in initial pharmacological treatment or in follow-up pharmacological management post exacerbations and (ii) patients with more than 100 cells/μL of blood eosinophils when experiencing more than 2 moderate exacerbations per year or at least one severe exacerbation requiring hospitalization in the prior year [11]. Recent clinical studies compared FeNO levels between COPD and ACO and confirmed high accuracy of diagnosis to discriminate ACO from COPD [82–86].

Table 1. Characteristics of included studies.

References	Study Design	Subject Numbers	Severity of Airflow Limitation	Intervention or Measurement	Results
Studies reporting an association between baseline FeNO and improvement of airway obstruction by inhaled corticosteroid therapy					
Zietkowski, et al. [75]	Prospective	COPD 47 (current smoker 28, ex-smoker 19) Healthy control 40 (current smoker 17, non-smoker 23)	Post-bronchodilator FEV_1 47.07 ± 14.55% (smoking COPD), 48.9 ± 15.3% (ex-smoking COPD)	Budesoide 800 μg/day, 8 weeks	Initial FeNO was positively correlated with an increase in post-bronchodilator FEV_1 after ICS therapy
Kunisaki, et al. [76]	Single-arm, open-label, prospective	COPD 60 (ex-smokers)	Pre-bronchodilator FEV_1 35.6 ± 10.6%	Fluticasone propionate 500 μg + Salmeterol 50 μg, twice daily, 4 weeks	ICS responders (increase in FEV_1 > 200 mL after 4 weeks ICS) have higher baseline FeNO.
Lehtimaki, et al. [77]	Single-arm, open-label, prospective	COPD 40 (current smoker 29, ex-smoker 11)	Post-bronchodilator FEV_1 64.6 ± 2.7% (smoking COPD), 53.3 ± 4.8% (ex-smoking COPD)	Fluticasone propionate 500 μg/day, 4 weeks	Baseline FeNO was positively correlated with changes in FEV_1/FVC
Akamatsu, et al. [78]	Single-arm, open-label, prospective	COPD 14 with emphysema on high-resolution computed tomography (all ex-smokers)	Post-bronchodilator FEV_1 57.6 ± 4.4%	Fluticasone propionate 250 μg + Salmeterol 50 μg, twice daily, 12 weeks	FeNO > 35 ppb and IgE positive was correlated with airway obstruction evaluated by FEV_1 and ΔN_2.
Yamaji et al. [79]	Single-arm, open-label, prospective	COPD 44 (ex-smokers)	GOLD stage 1/2/3/4, n = 0/34/9/0	Ciclesonide 400 μg/day, 12 weeks	Baseline FeNO was positively correlated with changes in FEV_1 and correlated with improvement of COPD assessment test score.
Studies reporting FeNO for ACO diagnosis					
Alcazar-Navarrete B, et al. [82]	Cross-sectional	COPD 103 (22 ACO), never smoker 16, healthy smoker 30, asthma 43	Postbronchodilator FEV_1 95 ± 19% (never smoker), 96 ± 3% (healthy smoker), 90 ± 16% (asthma), 60 ± 21% (COPD)	FeNO	FeNO AUC 0.79 with an optimal-cut off 19 ppb (sensitivity 0.68, specificity 0.75)
Goto, et al. [83]	Cross-sectional	COPD 197 (ACO 23%)	Post-bronchodilator FEV_1 63% (95%CI, 59–67; ACO), 60% (95%CI, 60–67; COPD)	FeNO	AUC 0.63 (95% CI, 0.54–0.72)
Chen, et al. [84]	Cross-sectional	COPD 132, asthma 500, ACO 57	FEV_1 50.1 ± 19.3% (COPD), 88.5 ± 19.4% (asthma), 50.1± 18.6% (ACO)	FeNO	AUC 0.78 (cut-off 22.5 ppb, sensitivity 70%, specificity 75%)
Takayama, et al. [85]	Cross-sectional	COPD 65, ACO 56	FEV_1 69.7 ± 21.1% (COPD), 64.9 ± 17.6% (ACO)	FeNO	AUC 0.726 (FeNO cut-off level 25.0 ppb, with 60.6% sensitivity and 87.7% specificity for steroid-naïve patients)
Guo, et al. [86]	Cross-sectional	COPD 53, ACO 53	FEV_1 56.0% (IQR, 48.3–66.9; ACO), 43.0% (IQR, 34.8–57.1; COPD)	FeNO	AUC 0.815 (FeNO cut-off level 25.5 ppb, sensitivity 74%, specificity 77%
Studies reporting a combination of FeNO and IgE for ACO diagnosis					
Tamada, et al. [87]	Cross-sectional	COPD 331 (never smoker 10, ex-smoker 257, current smoker 46, unknown 18)	FEV_1 61.5 ± 20.8%	FeNO and serum IgE	7.8% of participants considered as ACO (FeNO > 35 ppb + IgE > 173 IU/L).
Kobayashi, et al. [88]	Cross-sectional	COPD 257	FEV_1 63.1 ± 32.9%	FeNO and serum IgE	AUC 0.74 (95%CI, 0.63–0.84; cut-off 23 ppb, sensitivity 73.0%, specificity 68.2%). Combination of FeNO > 23 ppb and IgE > 434 IU/mL showed 94.1% specificity and 37.8% sensitivity.

Table 1. *Cont.*

References	Study Design	Subject Numbers	Severity of Airflow Limitation	Intervention or Measurement	Results
Studies for blood biomarkers for ACO diagnosis					
Carpagnano, et al. [89]	Cross-sectional	10 ACO (Spanish guideline), 13 ACO (GINA guideline), 13 COPD, 14 asthma, 10 healthy subjects	FEV_1 72.6 ± 23.4% (ACO-Spanish), 83.6 ± 22.8% (ACO-GINA), 46.9 ± 10.7% (COPD), 88.9 ± 17.7% (asthma), 91.0 ± 6.3% (healthy)	Mitochondrial and nuclear DNA in blood cells	ACO patients showed increased mitochondrial DNA in the blood cells.
Hirai, et al. [90]	Cross-sectional	COPD 50, asthma 152	FEV_1 63.4% (95%CI, 43.1–82.7; COPD), 86.2% (95%CI, 69.3–97.1; asthma)	mRNA expression of *TBX21*, *GATA3*, *RORC* and *FOXP3* in peripheral blood mononuclear cells	AUC 0.94 (95%CI, 0.90–0.98; total serum IgE level > 310 IU/mL, blood eosinophil counts > 280 cells/μL, a higher ratio of TBX21/GATA3, FEV1/FVC ratio < 0.67 and smoking > 10 pack-years
Llano, et al. [91]	Cross-sectional	COPD 89, asthma 94, ACO 109	Post-bronchodilator FEV_1 55.1 ± 18.5% (COPD), 69.5 ± 18.9% (asthma), 58.9 ± 17.0% (ACO)	IL-6, IL-8, TNF-α, IL-13, IL-5, Periostin, IL-17, FeNO	A cutoff value of FeNO > 17 ppb showed better AUC (0.707 [0.642–0.772], p < 0.001) than the cytokines or periostin in blood
Jo, et al. [92]	Cross-sectional	COPD 60, ACO 77	Post-bronchodilator FEV_1 71.1 ± 15.8% (COPD), 77.6 ± 16.6% (ACO)	NGAL	NGAL levels (odds ratio, 1.72; 95%CI, 0.69–4.28; ACO vs. COPD)
Wang, et al. [93]	Cross-sectional	COPD 147, asthma 124, ACO 102, control 50	Post-bronchodilator FEV_1 59.0 ± 9.1% (COPD), 73.7 ± 5.5% (asthma), 70.1 ± 5.6% (ACO), 95.4 ± 7.7% (control)	YKL-40, NGAL, TSLP, periostin	YKL-40 AUC 0.71 (95%CI, 0.65–0.79), cut-off < 12.61 ng/mL, sensitivity 73.5%, specificity 67.7% for ACO vs. COPD NGAL AUC 0.75 (95%CI, 0.68–0.82), cut-off < 104.7 ng/mL, sensitivity 92.7%, specificity 58.8% for ACO vs. asthma
Shirai, et al. [94]	Cross-sectional	COPD 61, asthma 177, ACO 115	FEV_1 66.5% (IQR, 35.8–76.3; COPD), 91.0 (78.3–102.8; asthma), 65.0 (49.0–71.5; ACO)	YKL-40, periostin, IgE, FeNO	YKL-40 AUC 0.71 (95%CI, 0.64–0.77), cut-off 61.3 ng/mL, sensitivity 60.9%, specificity 73.4% for ACO vs. asthma Periostin AUC 0.61 (95%CI, 0.53–0.70), cut-off 55.1 ng/mL, sensitivity 59.1%, specificity 62.3%
Cai, et al. [95]	Cross-sectional	COPD 27, ACO 29, Healthy control 28	FEV_1 40.2 ± 6.4% (COPD), 40.6 ± 8.5% (ACO), 90.8 ± 4.6% (healthy)	Eicosanoids	15(S)- hydroxyeicosate-traenoic acid, AUC 0.96
Kubysheva, et al. [96]	Cross-sectional	COPD 58, asthma 32, ACO 57	Post-bronchodilator FEV_1 55.3 ± 21.2% (COPD), 69.5 ± 18.9% (asthma), 58.9 ± 17.0% (ACO)	IL-17, IL-18, TNF-α	No cytokines that were able to distinguish ACO from COPD
Studies for urine biomarkers for ACO					
Oh, et al. [97]	Cross-sectional	COPD 38, asthma 32, ACO 37	FEV_1 68.1% (IQR, 48.8–85.5; COPD), 92.3% (IQR, 79.1–103; asthma), 70.0% (IQR, 51.7–85.0; ACO)	L-histidine (identified from urine metabolomics)	Urinary l-histidine levels were significantly higher in patients with ACO than in those with asthma or COPD

Table 1. Cont.

References	Study Design	Subject Numbers	Severity of Airflow Limitation	Intervention or Measurement	Results
Studies for biomarkers of induced sputum differentiating ACO from COPD					
Gao, et al. [98]	Cross-sectional	Discovery cohort: 14 never smoker, 14 healthy smoker, 24 asthma, 20 COPD, 18 ACO. Replication cohort: 22 never smoker, 40 healthy smoker, 21 asthma, 35 COPD, 17 ACO	Post-bronchodilator FEV_1 105.9 ± 10.6% (never smoker), 98.5 ± 15.5% (healthy smoker), 78.8 ± 14.0% (asthma), 58.3 ± 19.1% (COPD), 51.6 ± 13.7% (ACO) in the discovery cohort.	IL-13, MPO, NGAL, YKL-40, IL-6 protein levels in induced sputum	Only sputum NGAL levels could differentiate ACOS from asthma ($p < 0.001$ and $p < 0.001$) and COPD ($p < 0.05$ and $p = 0.002$) in the discovery and replication cohorts.
Studies for radiographical analyses differentiating ACO from COPD					
Hamada, et al. [99]	Retrospective	COPD 55, asthma 39, ACO 18	FEV_1 54.1 ± 12.1% (COPD), 70.0 ± 13.8% (asthma), 55.8 ± 12.4% (ACO)	Radiographical evidence of sinonasal inflammation (Lund-Mackay staging, LMS)	In patients with ACO and COPD, total and ethmoid LMS scores were significantly lower than those in patients with asthma.
Qu, et al. [100]	Cross-sectional	COPD 123, ACO 106	Post-bronchodilator FEV_1 54.7 ± 20.8% (COPD), 64.4 ± 15.7% (ACO)	Sagittal-lung CT measurements before and after bronchodilator inhalation	Variations of all sagittal-lung CT measurements were significantly larger in patients with ACO than in patients with pure COPD (p values all < 0.001)
Karatama, et al. [101]	Cross-sectional	COPD 86, ACO 43	FEV_1 70.3 ± 20.3% (COPD), 69.4 ± 19.0% (ACO)	3 dimensional-CT	Patients with ACO had a greater wall thickness in third- to fourth-generation bronchi, smaller airway luminal area in fifth- to sixth-generation bronchi, and less emphysematous changes than did matched patients with COPD

COPD, chronic obstructive pulmonary disease; FEV_1, forced expiratory volume in one second; FeNO, fractional exhaled nitric oxide; ICS, inhaled corticosteroid; FVC, forced vital capacity; IgE, immunoglobulin E; GOLD, global initiative for COPD. CI, confidence interval; IL, interleukin; TNF, tumor necrosis factor; MPO, myeloperoxidase; NGAL, neutrophil gelatinase-associated lipocalin; YKL-40, chitinase-like protein; IQR, interquartile range; CT, computed tomography.

3.2.3. Serum IgE Elevation and Atopic Background for COPD and ACO

Atopy refers to a genetic tendency to produce IgE typically for common and environmental allergens including inhaled allergens and food allergens. The presence of IgE specific for inhaled allergens, such as dust mites, cockroach and animal dander, is known to be a risk factor for asthma [102,103]. Serum total IgE levels were significantly correlated in pairs of siblings for bronchial hyperresponsiveness to histamine, which is implicated as a coinherited trait [104]. In addition, symptoms and exacerbations of asthma were significantly associated with an elevation of serum total IgE, which was independent of specific IgE [105]. This intriguing role of total, non-specific IgE in the association with asthma may be explained by the ability of IgE to enhance mast cell survival via Fcε receptor I cross-linking [106]. Serum levels of total IgE, IL-4 and leukotriene B4 were increased in ACO compared to COPD [107]. These observational and translational studies suggest that the mast cell activation pathway is upregulated in ACO as with asthma. This hypothesis was further supported by at least two clinical studies indicating that omalizumab, a humanized monoclonal antibody for IgE, markedly improved asthma control and health-related quality of life in ACO and this observed improvement in ACO was as large as that in asthma [108,109]. Given the evidence regarding IgE biology in atopic asthma overlapping COPD, it may be sensible to evaluate asthma complications in COPD patients with atopy.

3.2.4. Combination of Type 2 Inflammation-Related Biomarkers to Define ACO

In order to maximize the benefits of ICS for COPD patients while preventing them from having pulmonary infectious diseases including pneumonia and TB caused by its inappropriate use, a combination of biomarkers may be promising for precisely defining an ICS-responsive subset. Based on this concept, our group attempted to determine whether the combination of FeNO and serum IgE had the ability to discern asthmatic, ICS-responsive features among patients with COPD. We found that the sensitivity was 1.0 and the specificity was 0.56 for the subjects who had reversibility of airway obstruction by 12-week-inhalation therapy of fluticasone propionate (FP)/Salmeterol (SAL) when FeNO > 35 parts per billion (ppb) and/or a positive result for specific IgE (atopy+) were combined [78]. Especially, all of the patients with both FeNO > 35 ppb and atopy+ responded to the additional FP/SAL therapy [78]. In addition, no patients with both less than 35 ppb of FeNO and a negative result of specific IgE responded to FP/SAL. We further reported that the prevalence of expected high ICS responders (i.e., FeNO > 35 ppb and atopy+) was 7.8 % of Japanese COPD subjects, whereas that of patients who were not likely given the benefits of ICS (i.e., FeNO $\leq$ 35 ppb and atopy−) was 54.8% [87]. Another Japanese cohort confirmed this result [88]. These clinical proof-of-concept studies may illustrate that a combination of biomarkers related to type 2 inflammation could be useful for a more precise definition of ACO. Given this concept, in 2018 the Japanese Respiratory Society (JRS) issued guidelines for new definitions and diagnostic criteria of ACO (Table 2) [51,110]. It is noteworthy that these two biomarkers (FeNO and IgE) were included in the criteria to identify the features of asthma among COPD subjects.

Table 2. Diagnostic criteria for ACO issued by the Japanese Respiratory Society [110].

Fundamental Aspects: Over 40 Years of Age, Chronic Airway Obstruction Defined By < 70% of Post-Bronchodilator FEV_1/FVC	
[Features of COPD] At least one positive features of the followings (1, 2, 3)	(Features of asthma) Two positive features of the following 1, 2, 3 items; or at least one positive features of 1, 2, 3 plus two positive features of 4
1. Smoking history > 10 pack-years or equivalent exposure to air pollution	1. Variable in diurnal, daily or seasonal symptoms, or paroxysmal respiratory symptoms (cough, sputum, dyspnea)
2. Low attenuation area indicating emphysematous changes on HRCT	2. Past history of asthma before the age of 40 years
3. Attenuated diffusion capacity (%D_{LCO} < 80% or %D_{LCO}/V_A < 80%)	3. FeNO > 35 ppb
	4-1 Comorbidity of perennial allergic rhinitis 4-2 Reversibility of airway obstruction (FEV_1 > 12% and > 200 mL) 4-3 Blood eosinophil > 5% or > 300 cells/μL 4-4 Elevated serum IgE (total IgE or specific IgE for perennial inhaled allergens)

COPD, chronic obstructive pulmonary disease; FEV_1, forced expiratory volume in one second; FeNO, fractional exhaled nitric oxide; FVC, forced vital capacity; IgE, immunoglobulin E; D_{LCO}, diffusing capacity of the lung carbon monoxide; V_A, alveolar volume.

Two recent reports used the criteria to better characterize the clinical features of ACO in the Japanese population. A retrospective study investigating 170 subjects with persistent airflow limitation indicated that the prevalence of ACO among COPD patients was 31.5% [111]. However, one of the limitations in the retrospective study was that the use of ICS was not controlled, and that the characterization of clinical phenotypes could be biased or masked by ICS. More recently, Hirai, et al. investigated the prevalence of ACO among ICS-naïve patients with COPD and compared the baseline characteristics between COPD and ACO [112]. 197 patients with COPD were included in this study and 38 (19.3%) met the ACO diagnostic criteria by the Japanese guidelines. Although they did not find statistical significance in the baseline clinical features (age, gender, pack years of smoking and pulmonary function) between ACO and COPD, symptoms and dyspnea evaluated by COPD assessment test (CAT) and modified MRC (mMRC) scale were significantly worse in ACO compared to COPD [112]. In addition, the frequency of acute exacerbations during the one year prior to the participation was three times higher in ACO than in COPD [112]. These studies with other literature [82–86] support the concept that the diagnostic criteria using biomarkers such as FeNO and IgE could be a landmark in facilitating a secure identification of ICS-responders among COPD patients. However, further worldwide research will be necessary to uncover how much the ACO diagnostic criteria could improve the clinical practice for COPD and ACO and to what extent the use of ICS could be avoided. Major problems regarding the development of diagnostic biomarkers include how biological parameters are weighed and how the cut-off values are determined. Leading-edge approach using omics and machine learning may solve this problem in an unbiased way [113–115].

3.3. Possible Biomarkers Relevant to Eosinophilic and Neutrophilic Inflammation in ACO

Christenson, et al. revealed transcriptome of airway epithelial cells in steroid-naïve subjects with mild to moderate asthma (n = 62) and control subjects without asthma (n = 43) and defined the asthma-derived gene expression signatures of Th2 inflammation [116]. The Th2-high signatures identified a clinically relevant subgroup of COPD that had a favourable response to ICS [116]. Eosinophils activated by the Th2-related priming agents, such as IL-5, IL-3, IL-33, granulocyte-macrophage colony-stimulating factor (GM-CSF) or Notch ligands acquire cell motility, increase respiratory burst and release granule proteins including eosinophil-derived neurotoxin (EDN) [117]. The serum EDN levels are known to correlate with the persistent airflow limitation with adult asthma and to be significantly decreased post eight-week treatment of omalizumab [118]. Serum EDN was significantly higher in ACO compared to asthma and COPD [119]. In addition, using a putative diagnosis biomarker for COPD, YKL-40 [120,121], combined assessment of serum EDN and YKL-40 revealed that a subset with both high serum EDN and YKL-40 levels was 45% in ACO, 14% in asthma and 30% in COPD (OR 3.85 (95% CI, 2.35–6.36); sensitivity, 45.2%; specificity 82.4%) [119]. Interestingly, this study showed other subsets of ACO based on the levels of EDN and YKL-40 (27% in high EDN and low YKL-40, 16% in low EDN and high YKL-40 and 12% in low EDN and low YKL-40), confirming that ACO was a heterogenous condition including different forms of airway diseases [47]. Since YKL-40 alone might not be reproducible for the diagnosis of ACO [93,94], combinatory evaluation might be useful.

Not only the eosinophil-related protein EDN but also a neutrophil-associated protein may be involved in the pathogenesis of ACO. Neutrophil gelatinase-associated lipocalin (NGAL) is constitutively expressed by neutrophils and has a pivotal role in antimicrobial immunity by binding bacterial siderophores and depriving bacterial iron [122]. The NGAL protein levels were elevated in induced sputum [123] and plasma [124] in patients with COPD. Moreover, the NGAL levels in bronchoalveolar lavage fluid were elevated even in subjects who had emphysematous changes with normal FEV_1 [125,126]. Considering a biochemical study demonstrating that NGAL prevented matrix metalloproteinase (MMP)-9 from being degraded and maintained the MMP-9 enzymatic activity [127], NGAL has been recognized to contribute to the development of pulmonary emphysema. However, the NGAL levels in induced sputum were significantly higher in ACO compared to COPD and asthma [128]. This might be explained by recent data indicating that NGAL is also secreted from epithelial cells of renal, intestinal and respiratory systems and is now considered to be a biomarker for acute kidney injury [122]. These data suggest that neutrophilic inflammation, emphysematous changes and epithelial injuries might contribute to the elevated levels of NGAL in induced sputum from patients with ACO [128]. However, pro-inflammatory cytokines associated with type 1 and type 2 immunity in peripheral blood might not be useful to diagnose ACO from COPD [91,96].

Recent studies using novel technologies have identified candidate molecules for biomarkers of ACO. Cai, et al. reported that several eicosanoids associated with allergic inflammation were upregulated in ACO compared to COPD and demonstrated high sensitivity and specificity to differentiate ACO from COPD [95]. Urine metabolomics approach found that L-histidine levels were significantly higher in ACO compared to COPD and asthma [97]. Computed tomographic analyses have captured characteristics of allergic airway inflammation in the upper and lower airways to predict the presence of asthma-related lesions in ACO [99–101].

4. Discussion

There are important problems yet to be addressed in clinical practice for ACO and COPD: Why should we have a diagnostic term of ACO? How can we distinguish between COPD and ACO? Since inappropriate use of ICS increases the risk of respiratory infection in COPD patients, we need to maximize the ability to identify the subset of favourable response to ICS. Our systematic review showed that FeNO was useful biomarker to identify asthmatic components in patients with COPD. In addition, a combination of biomarkers such as FeNO and IgE would be useful and provide promising diagnostic criteria for ACO, which could be validated by future studies. To define more precisely the pathophysiology of ACO, it would be essential to uncover the molecular mechanisms underlying inflammation, tissue damage/repair and oxidative/nitrosative stress that can differentiate ACO from COPD. In fact, several attempts have been done to clarify eosinophilic and neutrophilic inflammation using blood, induced sputum and urine.

Because there has been no global consensus on the diagnostic criteria of ACO, its prevalence considerably depends on how it is defined [129]. However, a recent meta-analysis of 27 studies from North America, Europe and Asia reported that the prevalence of ACO was estimated to be 2.0% (95% confidence interval (CI): 1.4–2.6%) in the general population, 26.5% (95% CI: 19.5–33.6%) among patients with asthma and 29.6% (95% CI: 19.3–33.9%) among patients with COPD [130]. In line with this meta-analysis, recent epidemiological studies confirm that ACO is a common disease in primary care [131,132]. These epidemiological data highlight the clinical importance of evaluating whether patients with airflow limitation have the features of both COPD and asthma and if patients with COPD concurrently have components of asthma in primary care. Thus, further studies are required to detect the features of asthma among patients with COPD using novel biomarkers.

One biological aspect which was not described here is genetics. Genome-wide association studies in non-Hispanic whites and African-American populations (n = 3120 in COPD; 450 in ACO) indicated that the most significant single nucleotide polymorphisms (SNPs) were in or near *GPR65* on chromosome 14 [133]. *GPP65* encodes the chief acid-sensing receptor, G protein-coupled receptor 65 (GPR65), which increased the cellular viability of eosinophils in allergic airway inflammatory settings in mice [134]. Interestingly, the GWAS study for ACO and COPD failed to identify known asthma-associated genetic loci such as *ORMDL3*, *IL1RL1* and *IL4R* [135], indicating that ACO was not just an overlapping condition of asthma and COPD but was associated with a specific genetic background independent of asthma or COPD.

Another aspect of ACO is associated with redox imbalance. Our group has recently reported a key role of oxidative and nitrosative stress in the pathogenesis of ACO. We reported that excessive nitrosative stress and lower antioxidant capability were observed in neutrophils and macrophages collected from the airways of patients with ACO [136]. This redox imbalance was associated with increases in IL-8, monocyte chemotactic protein-1 (MCP-1), tumor necrosis factor (TNF)-α in induced sputum and with a prospective clinical course of higher frequency of exacerbation and more rapid decline of FEV1 in ACO subjects compared to asthmatics [136]. These current data on the role of oxidative and nitrosative stress in ACO development may have clinical implications and provide novel insights for therapeutic strategies [137]. Future basic and translational research to define the molecular and cellular phenotypes of ACO differentiating from COPD are needed.

There are several limitations in this review. First, the number of patients included in the selected studies was relatively small. Second, diagnosis of asthma was not unified over the selected studies. Third, the selected studies were not randomized control trials. Finally, we did not examine publication bias. These suggest that the risk of selection and performance bias is high in this review. This may be due to the limited studies available regarding ACO diagnosis. Future studies are required to reduce bias and to more precisely define ACO pathogenesis.

5. Conclusions

This review demonstrates the current clinical features and diagnostic markers that enable the differentiation of ACO from COPD and discusses possible future directions that should be addressed. In conclusion, a combination of biomarkers such as FeNO and IgE is useful for ACO diagnosis to reduce airway infections in patients with COPD.

Author Contributions: Conceptualization, N.F. and H.S.; writing—original draft preparation, N.F.; writing—review and editing, N.F. and H.S. All authors have read and agreed to the published version of the manuscript.

Funding: This work was supported by MSD Life Science Foundation, Public Interest Incorporated Foundation.

Acknowledgments: We very much appreciate Brent K Bell for reading of the manuscript.

Conflicts of Interest: N.F. reports personal fees for lectures from AstraZeneca, outside the submitted work. HS reports grants from MSD and Novartis, personal fees for lectures from Astellas, KYORIN, Novartis and Sanofi, and personal fees for lectures and consulting from AstraZeneca, Boehringer Ingelheim and GlaxoSmithKline, outside the submitted work.

References

1. Vos, T.; Abajobir, A.A.; Abate, K.H.; Abbafati, C.; Abbas, K.M.; Abd-Allah, F.; Abdulkader, R.S.; Abdulle, A.M.; Abebo, T.A.; Abera, S.F.; et al. Global, regional, and national incidence, prevalence, and years lived with disability for 328 diseases and injuries for 195 countries, 1990–2016: A systematic analysis for the global burden of disease study 2016. *Lancet* **2017**, *390*, 1211–1259. [CrossRef]
2. Barnes, P.J. Immunology of asthma and chronic obstructive pulmonary disease. *Nat. Rev. Immunol.* **2008**, *8*, 183–192. [CrossRef] [PubMed]
3. Barnes, P.J. Targeting cytokines to treat asthma and chronic obstructive pulmonary disease. *Nat. Rev. Immunol.* **2018**, *18*, 454–466. [CrossRef] [PubMed]
4. Smolonska, J.; Koppelman, G.H.; Wijmenga, C.; Vonk, J.M.; Zanen, P.; Bruinenberg, M.; Curjuric, I.; Imboden, M.; Thun, G.-A.; Franke, L.; et al. Common genes underlying asthma and COPD? Genome-Wide analysis on the dutch hypothesis. *Eur. Respir. J.* **2014**, *44*, 860–872. [CrossRef] [PubMed]
5. Wenzel, S.E. Asthma phenotypes: The evolution from clinical to molecular approaches. *Nat. Med.* **2012**, *18*, 716–725. [CrossRef]
6. Lambrecht, B.N.; Hammad, H.; Fahy, J.V. The cytokines of asthma. *Immunity* **2019**, *50*, 975–991. [CrossRef]
7. Woodruff, P.G.; Modrek, B.; Choy, D.F.; Jia, G.; Abbas, A.R.; Ellwanger, A.; Arron, J.R.; Koth, L.L.; Fahy, J.V. T-Helper type 2–driven inflammation defines major subphenotypes of asthma. *Am. J. Resp. Crit. Care Med.* **2009**, *180*, 388–395. [CrossRef]
8. O'Byrne, P.M.; Barnes, P.J.; Rodriguez-Roisin, R.; Runnerstrom, E.; Sandstrom, T.; Svensson, K.; Tattersfield, A. Low dose inhaled budesonide and formoterol in mild persistent asthma. *Am. J. Resp. Crit. Care Med.* **2001**, *164*, 1392–1397. [CrossRef]
9. Pauwels, R.A.; Pedersen, S.; Busse, W.W.; Tan, W.C.; Chen, Y.-Z.; Ohlsson, S.V.; Ullman, A.; Lamm, C.J.; O'Byrne, P.M. Early intervention with budesonide in mild persistent asthma: A randomised, double-blind trial. *Lancet* **2003**, *361*, 1071–1076. [CrossRef]
10. Suissa, S.; Ernst, P.; Benayoun, S.; Baltzan, M.; Cai, B. Low-Dose inhaled corticosteroids and the prevention of death from asthma. *N. Engl. J. Med.* **2000**, *343*, 332–336. [CrossRef]
11. Global Initiative for Chronic Obstructive Lung Disease (GOLD). Global Strategy for the Diagnosis, Management and Prevention of COPD. 2020. Available online: https://goldcopd.org/wp-content/uploads/2019/12/GOLD-2020-FINAL-ver1.2-03Dec19_WMV.pdf (accessed on 1 March 2021).
12. Kohansal, R.; Martinez-Camblor, P.; Agustí, A.; Buist, A.S.; Mannino, D.M.; Soriano, J.B. The natural history of chronic airflow obstruction revisited. *Am. J. Resp. Crit. Care Med.* **2009**, *180*, 3–10. [CrossRef]
13. Hunninghake, G.M.; Cho, M.H.; Tesfaigzi, Y.; Soto-Quiros, M.E.; Avila, L.; Lasky-Su, J.; Stidley, C.; Melén, E.; Söderhäll, C.; Hallberg, J.; et al. MMP12, lung function, and COPD in high-risk populations. *N. Engl. J. Med.* **2009**, *361*, 2599–2608. [CrossRef]
14. Ding, Z.; Wang, K.; Li, J.; Tan, Q.; Tan, W.; Guo, G. Association between glutathione s-transferase gene M1 and T1 polymorphisms and chronic obstructive pulmonary disease risk: A meta-analysis. *Clin. Genet.* **2019**, *95*, 53–62. [CrossRef]
15. Lange, P.; Celli, B.; Agusti, A.; Jensen, G.B.; Divo, M.; Faner, R.; Guerra, S.; Marott, J.L.; Martinez, F.D.; Martinez-Camblor, P.; et al. Lung-Function trajectories leading to chronic obstructive pulmonary disease. *N. Engl. J. Med.* **2015**, *373*, 111–122. [CrossRef]

16. Cosio, M.G.; Saetta, M.; Agusti, A. Immunologic aspects of chronic obstructive pulmonary disease. *N. Engl. J. Med.* **2009**, *360*, 2445–2454. [CrossRef]
17. Barnes, P.J. Inflammatory mechanisms in patients with chronic obstructive pulmonary disease. *J. Allergy Clin. Immunol.* **2016**, *138*, 16–27. [CrossRef]
18. Tanno, A.; Fujino, N.; Yamada, M.; Sugiura, H.; Hirano, T.; Tanaka, R.; Sano, H.; Suzuki, S.; Okada, Y.; Ichinose, M. Decreased expression of a phagocytic receptor siglec-1 on alveolar macrophages in chronic obstructive pulmonary disease. *Respir. Res.* **2020**, *21*, 30. [CrossRef]
19. Belchamber, K.B.R.; Singh, R.; Batista, C.M.; Whyte, M.K.; Dockrell, D.H.; Kilty, I.; Robinson, M.J.; Wedzicha, J.A.; Barnes, P.J.; Donnelly, L.E.; et al. Defective bacterial phagocytosis is associated with dysfunctional mitochondria in COPD macrophages. *Eur. Respir. J.* **2019**, *54*, 1802244. [CrossRef]
20. Bewley, M.A.; Preston, J.A.; Mohasin, M.; Marriott, H.M.; Budd, R.C.; Swales, J.; Collini, P.; Greaves, D.R.; Craig, R.W.; Brightling, C.E.; et al. Impaired mitochondrial microbicidal responses in chronic obstructive pulmonary disease macrophages. *Am. J. Resp. Crit. Care Med.* **2017**, *196*, 845–855. [CrossRef]
21. Bewley, M.A.; Budd, R.C.; Ryan, E.; Cole, J.; Collini, P.; Marshall, J.; Kolsum, U.; Beech, G.; Emes, R.D.; Tcherniaeva, I.; et al. Opsonic phagocytosis in chronic obstructive pulmonary disease is enhanced by nrf2 agonists. *Am. J. Resp. Crit. Care Med.* **2018**, *198*, 739–750. [CrossRef]
22. Hogg, J.C.; Chu, F.; Utokaparch, S.; Woods, R.; Elliott, W.M.; Buzatu, L.; Cherniack, R.M.; Rogers, R.M.; Sciurba, F.C.; Coxson, H.O.; et al. The nature of small-airway obstruction in chronic obstructive pulmonary disease. *N. Engl. J. Med.* **2004**, *350*, 2645–2653. [CrossRef]
23. McDonough, J.E.; Yuan, R.; Suzuki, M.; Seyednejad, N.; Elliott, W.M.; Sanchez, P.G.; Wright, A.C.; Gefter, W.B.; Litzky, L.; Coxson, H.O.; et al. Small-Airway obstruction and emphysema in chronic obstructive pulmonary disease. *N. Engl. J. Med.* **2011**, *365*, 1567–1575. [CrossRef]
24. Fujino, N.; Brand, O.J.; Morgan, D.J.; Fujimori, T.; Grabiec, A.M.; Jagger, C.P.; Maciewicz, R.A.; Yamada, M.; Itakura, K.; Sugiura, H.; et al. Sensing of apoptotic cells through axl causes lung basal cell proliferation in inflammatory diseases. *J. Exp. Med.* **2019**, *216*, 2184–2201. [CrossRef]
25. Volckaert, T.; Yuan, T.; Chao, C.-M.; Bell, H.; Sitaula, A.; Szimmtenings, L.; Agha, E.E.; Chanda, D.; Majka, S.; Bellusci, S.; et al. Fgf10-Hippo epithelial-mesenchymal crosstalk maintains and recruits lung basal stem cells. *Dev. Cell* **2017**, *43*, 48–59.e5. [CrossRef]
26. Ofir, D.; Laveneziana, P.; Webb, K.A.; Lam, Y.-M.; O'Donnell, D.E. Mechanisms of dyspnea during cycle exercise in symptomatic patients with GOLD stage I chronic obstructive pulmonary disease. *Am. J. Resp. Crit. Care Med.* **2008**, *177*, 622–629. [CrossRef]
27. Elbehairy, A.F.; Ciavaglia, C.E.; Webb, K.A.; Guenette, J.A.; Jensen, D.; Mourad, S.M.; Neder, J.A.; O'Donnell, D.E.; Network, C.R.R. Pulmonary gas exchange abnormalities in mild chronic obstructive pulmonary disease. implications for dyspnea and exercise intolerance. *Am. J. Resp. Crit. Care Med.* **2015**, *191*, 1384–1394. [CrossRef]
28. O'Donnell, D.E.; Flüge, T.; Gerken, F.; Hamilton, A.; Webb, K.; Aguilaniu, B.; Make, B.; Magnussen, H. Effects of tiotropium on lung hyperinflation, dyspnoea and exercise tolerance in COPD. *Eur. Respir. J.* **2004**, *23*, 832–840. [CrossRef]
29. O'Donnell, D.E.; Sciurba, F.; Celli, B.; Mahler, D.A.; Webb, K.A.; Kalberg, C.J.; Knobil, K. Effect of fluticasone propionate/salmeterol on lung hyperinflation and exercise endurance in COPD. *Chest* **2006**, *130*, 647–656. [CrossRef]
30. Jones, P.W.; Donohue, J.F.; Nedelman, J.; Pascoe, S.; Pinault, G.; Lassen, C. Correlating changes in lung function with patient outcomes in chronic obstructive pulmonary disease: A pooled analysis. *Respir. Res.* **2012**, *12*, 161. [CrossRef]
31. Koarai, A.; Sugiura, H.; Yamada, M.; Ichikawa, T.; Fujino, N.; Kawayama, T.; Ichinose, M. Treatment with LABA versus LAMA for stable COPD: A systematic review and meta-analysis. *BMC Pulm. Med.* **2020**, *20*, 111. [CrossRef]
32. Almirall, J.; Bolíbar, I.; Serra-Prat, M.; Roig, J.; Hospital, I.; Carandell, E.; Agustí, M.; Ayuso, P.; Estela, A.; Torres, A.; et al. New evidence of risk factors for community-acquired pneumonia: A population-based study. *Eur. Respir. J.* **2008**, *31*, 1274–1284. [CrossRef] [PubMed]
33. Ernst, P.; Gonzalez, A.V.; Brassard, P.; Suissa, S. Inhaled corticosteroid use in chronic obstructive pulmonary disease and the risk of hospitalization for pneumonia. *Am. J. Resp. Crit. Care Med.* **2007**, *176*, 162–166. [CrossRef] [PubMed]
34. Martinez-Garcia, M.A.; Faner, R.; Osculло, G.; de La Rosa, D.; Soler-Cataluña, J.-J.; Ballester, M.; Agusti, A. Inhaled steroids, circulating eosinophils, chronic airway infection, and pneumonia risk in chronic obstructive pulmonary disease. A network analysis. *Am. J. Resp. Crit. Care Med.* **2020**, *201*, 1078–1085. [CrossRef] [PubMed]
35. Brassard, P.; Suissa, S.; Kezouh, A.; Ernst, P. Inhaled corticosteroids and risk of tuberculosis in patients with respiratory diseases. *Am. J. Resp. Crit. Care Med.* **2012**, *183*, 675–678. [CrossRef]
36. Lee, C.-H.; Kim, K.; Hyun, M.K.; Jang, E.J.; Lee, N.R.; Yim, J.-J. Use of inhaled corticosteroids and the risk of tuberculosis. *Thorax* **2013**, *68*, 1105. [CrossRef]
37. Van Schayck, C.P.; Levy, M.L.; Chen, J.C.; Isonaka, S.; Halbert, R.J. Coordinated diagnostic approach for adult obstructive lung disease in primary care. *Prim. Care Resp. J.* **2004**, *13*, 218–221. [CrossRef]
38. Guerra, S.; Sherrill, D.L.; Kurzius-Spencer, M.; Venker, C.; Halonen, M.; Quan, S.F.; Martinez, F.D. The course of persistent airflow limitation in subjects with and without asthma. *Resp. Med.* **2008**, *102*, 1473–1482. [CrossRef]

39. O'denis, D.E.; Shawn, A.; Jean, B.; Paul, H.; Marciniuk, D.D.; Meyer, B.; Gordon, F.; Andre, G.; Roger, G.; Rick, H.; et al. Canadian thoracic society recommendations for management of chronic obstructive pulmonary disease—2007 update. *Can. Respir. J.* **2007**, *14*, 5B–32B. [CrossRef]
40. Gibson, P.G.; Simpson, J.L. The overlap syndrome of asthma and COPD: What are its features and how important is it? *Thorax* **2009**, *64*, 728. [CrossRef]
41. Miravitlles, M.; Soriano, J.B.; Ancochea, J.; Muñoz, L.; Duran-Tauleria, E.; Sánchez, G.; Sobradillo, V.; García-Río, F. Characterisation of the overlap COPD–Asthma phenotype. Focus on physical activity and health status. *Resp. Med.* **2013**, *107*, 1053–1060. [CrossRef]
42. Menezes, A.M.B.; de Oca, M.M.; Pérez-Padilla, R.; Nadeau, G.; Wehrmeister, F.C.; Lopez-Varela, M.V.; Muiño, A.; Jardim, J.R.B.; Valdivia, G.; Tálamo, C.; et al. Increased risk of exacerbation and hospitalization in subjects with an overlap phenotype COPD-Asthma. *Chest* **2014**, *145*, 297–304. [CrossRef]
43. Silva, G.E.; Sherrill, D.L.; Guerra, S.; Barbee, R.A. Asthma as a risk factor for COPD in a longitudinal study. *Chest* **2004**, *126*, 59–65. [CrossRef]
44. Zeki, A.A.; Schivo, M.; Chan, A.; Albertson, T.E.; Louie, S. The Asthma-COPD overlap syndrome: A common clinical problem in the elderly. *J. Allergy* **2011**, *2011*, 861926. [CrossRef]
45. Miravitlles, M.; Soler-Cataluña, J.J.; Calle, M.; Soriano, J.B. Treatment of COPD by clinical phenotypes: Putting old evidence into clinical practice. *Eur. Respir. J.* **2012**, *41*, 1252–1256. [CrossRef]
46. Louie, S.; Zeki, A.A.; Schivo, M.; Chan, A.L.; Yoneda, K.Y.; Avdalovic, M.; Morrissey, B.M.; Albertson, T.E. The asthma–chronic obstructive pulmonary disease overlap syndrome: Pharmacotherapeutic considerations. *Expert Rev. Clin. Phar.* **2014**, *6*, 197–219. [CrossRef]
47. Global Initiative for Asthma; Global Initiative for Chronic Obstructive Lung Disease. Diagnosis of Diseases of Chronic Airflow Limitation: Asthma, COPD, and Asthma-COPD Overlap Syndrome (ACOS). Updated 2015. Available online: http://goldcopd.org/asthma-copd-asthma-copd-overlap-synd (accessed on 1 March 2021).
48. Global Initiative for Asthma. Global Strategy for Asthma Management and Prevention. Updated 2017. Available online: http://ginasthma.org/2017-gina-report-globalstrategy-for-asthma-management-andprevention/ (accessed on 1 March 2021).
49. Sin, D.D.; Miravitlles, M.; Mannino, D.M.; Soriano, J.B.; Price, D.; Celli, B.R.; Leung, J.M.; Nakano, Y.; Park, H.Y.; Wark, P.A.; et al. What Is asthma−COPD overlap syndrome? Towards a consensus definition from a round table discussion. *Eur. Respir. J.* **2016**, *48*, 664–673. [CrossRef]
50. Plaza, V.; Álvarez, F.; Calle, M.; Casanova, C.; Cosío, B.G.; López-Viña, A.; de Llano, L.P.; Quirce, S.; Román-Rodríguez, M.; Soler-Cataluña, J.J.; et al. Consensus on the Asthma–COPD Overlap (ACO) Between the Spanish COPD Guidelines (GesEPOC) and the Spanish Guidelines on the Management of Asthma (GEMA). *Arch. Bronconeumol. Engl. Ed.* **2017**, *53*, 443–449. [CrossRef]
51. Yanagisawa, S.; Ichinose, M. Definition and diagnosis of asthma–COPD overlap (ACO). *Allergol. Int.* **2018**, *67*, 172–178. [CrossRef]
52. Miravitlles, M. Asthma-COPD Overlap (ACO) PRO-CON debate. ACO: Call me by my name. *Chronic Obstr. Pulm. Dis.* **2020**, *17*, 471–473. [CrossRef]
53. Papi, A. Asthma COPD Overlap PRO-CON Debate. ACO: The mistaken term. *Chronic Obstr. Pulm Dis.* **2020**, *17*, 474–476. [CrossRef]
54. Moher, D.; Liberati, A.; Tetzlaff, J.; Altman, D.G.; Group, T.P. Preferred reporting items for systematic reviews and meta-analyses: The PRISMA statement. *PLoS Med.* **2009**, *6*, e1000097. [CrossRef] [PubMed]
55. Alving, K.; Malinovschi, A. Basic aspects of exhaled nitric oxide. *Eur. Resir. Mon.* **2010**, *49*, 1–31.
56. Alving, K.; Weitzberg, E.; Lundberg, J.M. Increased amount of nitric oxide in exhaled air of asthmatics. *Eur. Respir. J.* **1993**, *6*, 1368–1370. [PubMed]
57. Çolak, Y.; Afzal, S.; Nordestgaard, B.G.; Marott, J.L.; Lange, P. Combined value of exhaled nitric oxide and blood eosinophils in chronic airway disease: The copenhagen general population study. *Eur. Respir. J.* **2018**, *52*, 1800616. [CrossRef] [PubMed]
58. Strunk, R.C.; Szefler, S.J.; Phillips, B.R.; Zeiger, R.S.; Chinchilli, V.M.; Larsen, G.; Hodgdon, K.; Morgan, W.; Sorkness, C.A.; Lemanske, R.F.; et al. Relationship of exhaled nitric oxide to clinical and inflammatory markers of persistent asthma in children. *J. Allergy Clin. Immunol.* **2003**, *112*, 883–892. [CrossRef] [PubMed]
59. Hamid, Q.; Springall, D.R.; Polak, J.; Riveros-Moreno, V.; Chanez, P.; Bousquet, J.; Godard, P.; Holgate, S.; Howarth, P.; Redington, A. Induction of nitric oxide synthase in asthma. *Lancet* **1993**, *342*, 1510–1513. [CrossRef]
60. Ichinose, M.; Sugiura, H.; Yamagata, S.; Koarai, A.; Shirato, K. Increase in reactive nitrogen species production in chronic obstructive pulmonary disease airways. *Am. J. Resp. Crit. Care Med.* **2000**, *162*, 701–706. [CrossRef]
61. Guo, F.H.; Comhair, S.A.A.; Zheng, S.; Dweik, R.A.; Eissa, N.T.; Thomassen, M.J.; Calhoun, W.; Erzurum, S.C. molecular mechanisms of increased Nitric Oxide (NO) in asthma: Evidence for transcriptional and post-translational regulation of NO synthesis. *J. Immunol.* **2000**, *164*, 5970–5980. [CrossRef]
62. Redington, A.E.; Meng, Q.H.; Springall, D.R.; Evans, T.J.; Créminon, C.; Maclouf, J.; Holgate, S.T.; Howarth, P.H.; Polak, J.M. Increased expression of inducible nitric oxide synthase and cyclo-oxygenase-2 in the airway epithelium of asthmatic subjects and regulation by corticosteroid treatment. *Thorax* **2001**, *56*, 351–357. [CrossRef]
63. Hansel, T.T.; Kharitonov, S.A.; Donnelly, L.E.; Erin, E.M.; Currie, M.G.; Moore, W.M.; Manning, P.T.; Recker, D.P.; Barnes, P.J. A selective inhibitor of inducible nitric oxide synthase inhibits exhaled breath nitric oxide in healthy volunteers and asthmatics. *FASEB J.* **2003**, *17*, 1298–1300. [CrossRef]

64. Berlyne, G.S.; Parameswaran, K.; Kamada, D.; Efthimiadis, A.; Hargreave, F.E. A comparison of exhaled nitric oxide and induced sputum as markers of airway inflammation. *J. Allergy Clin. Immunol.* **2000**, *106*, 638–644. [CrossRef]
65. Payne, D.N.; Adcock, I.M.; Wilson, N.M.; Oates, T.; Scallan, M.; Bush, A. Relationship between exhaled nitric oxide and mucosal eosinophilic inflammation in children with difficult asthma, after treatment with oral prednisolone. *Am. J. Resp. Crit. Care Med.* **2001**, *164*, 1376–1381. [CrossRef]
66. Warke, T.J.; Fitch, P.S.; Brown, V.; Taylor, R.; Lyons, J.D.M.; Ennis, M.; Shields, M.D. Exhaled nitric oxide correlates with airway eosinophils in childhood asthma. *Thorax* **2002**, *57*, 383–387. [CrossRef]
67. Ichinose, M.; Takahashi, T.; Sugiura, H.; Endoh, N.; Miura, M.; Mashito, Y.; Shirato, K. Baseline airway hyperresponsiveness and its reversible component: Role of airway inflammation and airway calibre. *Eur. Respir. J.* **2000**, *15*, 248–253. [CrossRef]
68. Suresh, V.; Mih, J.D.; George, S.C. Measurement of IL-13–Induced INOS-Derived gas phase nitric oxide in human bronchial epithelial cells. *Am. J. Resp. Cell Mol. Biol.* **2007**, *37*, 97–104. [CrossRef]
69. Chibana, K.; Trudeau, J.B.; Mustovich, A.T.; Mustovitch, A.T.; Hu, H.; Zhao, J.; Balzar, S.; Chu, H.W.; Wenzel, S.E. IL-13 induced increases in nitrite levels are primarily driven by increases in inducible nitric oxide synthase as compared with effects on arginases in human primary bronchial epithelial cells. *Clin. Exp. Allergy* **2008**, *38*, 936–946. [CrossRef]
70. Borish, L.C.; Nelson, H.S.; Lanz, M.J.; Claussen, L.; Whitmore, J.B.; Agosti, J.M.; Garrison, L. Interleukin-4 receptor in moderate atopic asthma. *Am. J. Resp. Crit. Care Med.* **1999**, *160*, 1816–1823. [CrossRef]
71. Wenzel, S.; Wilbraham, D.; Fuller, R.; Getz, E.B.; Longphre, M. Effect of an Interleukin-4 variant on late phase asthmatic response to allergen challenge in asthmatic patients: Results of two phase 2a studies. *Lancet* **2007**, *370*, 1422–1431. [CrossRef]
72. Wenzel, S.; Ford, L.; Pearlman, D.; Spector, S.; Sher, L.; Skobieranda, F.; Wang, L.; Kirkesseli, S.; Rocklin, R.; Bock, B.; et al. Dupilumab in persistent asthma with elevated eosinophil levels. *N. Engl. J. Med.* **2013**, *368*, 2455–2466. [CrossRef]
73. Agusti, A.; Bel, E.; Thomas, M.; Vogelmeier, C.; Brusselle, G.; Holgate, S.; Humbert, M.; Jones, P.; Gibson, P.G.; Vestbo, J.; et al. Treatable traits: Toward precision medicine of chronic airway diseases. *Eur. Respir. J.* **2016**, *47*, 410–419. [CrossRef]
74. Brightling, C.E.; McKenna, S.; Hargadon, B.; Birring, S.; Green, R.; Siva, R.; Berry, M.; Parker, D.; Monteiro, W.; Pavord, I.D.; et al. Sputum eosinophilia and the short term response to inhaled mometasone in chronic obstructive pulmonary disease. *Thorax* **2005**, *60*, 193–198. [CrossRef]
75. Zietkowski, Z.; Kucharewicz, I.; Bodzenta-Lukaszyk, A. The influence of inhaled corticosteroids on exhaled nitric oxide in stable chronic obstructive pulmonary disease. *Resp. Med.* **2005**, *99*, 816–824. [CrossRef]
76. Kunisaki, K.M.; Rice, K.L.; Janoff, E.N.; Rector, T.S.; Niewoehner, D.E. Exhaled nitric oxide, systemic inflammation, and the spirometric response to inhaled fluticasone propionate in severe chronic obstructive pulmonary disease: A prospective study. *Ther Adv. Respir. Dis.* **2008**, *2*, 55–64. [CrossRef]
77. Lehtimaki, L.; Kankaanranta, H.; Saarelainen, S.; Annila, I.; Aine, T.; Nieminen, R.; Moilanen, E. Bronchial nitric oxide is related to symptom relief during fluticasone treatment in COPD. *Eur. Respir. J.* **2009**, *35*, 72–78. [CrossRef]
78. Akamatsu, K.; Matsunaga, K.; Sugiura, H.; Koarai, A.; Hirano, T.; Minakata, Y.; Ichinose, M. Improvement of airflow limitation by fluticasone propionate/salmeterol in chronic obstructive pulmonary disease: What is the specific marker? *Front. Pharmacol.* **2011**, *2*, 36. [CrossRef]
79. Yamaji, Y.; Oishi, K.; Hamada, K.; Ohteru, Y.; Chikumoto, A.; Murakawa, K.; Matsuda, K.; Suetake, R.; Murata, Y.; Ito, K.; et al. Detection of type2 biomarkers for response in COPD. *J. Breath Res.* **2020**, *14*, 026007. [CrossRef]
80. Price, D.B.; Buhl, R.; Chan, A.; Freeman, D.; Gardener, E.; Godley, C.; Gruffydd-Jones, K.; McGarvey, L.; Ohta, K.; Ryan, D.; et al. Fractional exhaled nitric oxide as a predictor of response to inhaled corticosteroids in patients with non-specific respiratory symptoms and insignificant bronchodilator reversibility: A randomised controlled trial. *Lancet Respir. Med.* **2018**, *6*, 29–39. [CrossRef]
81. Mostafavi-Pour-Manshadi, S.-M.-Y.; Naderi, N.; Barrecheguren, M.; Dehghan, A.; Bourbeau, J. Investigating fractional exhaled nitric oxide in Chronic Obstructive Pulmonary Disease (COPD) and Asthma-COPD Overlap (ACO): A scoping review. *Chronic Obstr. Pulm. Dis.* **2018**, *15*, 1–15. [CrossRef]
82. Alcázar-Navarrete, B.; Romero-Palacios, P.J.; Ruiz-Sancho, A.; Ruiz-Rodriguez, O. Diagnostic performance of the measurement of nitric oxide in exhaled air in the diagnosis of COPD phenotypes. *Nitric Oxide* **2016**, *54*, 67–72. [CrossRef]
83. Goto, T.; Camargo, C.A.; Hasegawa, K. Fractional exhaled nitric oxide levels in asthma–COPD overlap syndrome: Analysis of the national health and nutrition examination survey, 2007–2012. *Int. J. Chronic Obstr. Pulm. Dis.* **2016**, *11*, 2149–2155. [CrossRef]
84. Chen, F.; Huang, X.; Liu, Y.; Lin, G.; Xie, C. Importance of fractional exhaled nitric oxide in the differentiation of asthma–copd overlap syndrome, asthma, and COPD. *Int. J. Chronic Obstr. Pulm. Dis.* **2016**, *11*, 2385–2390. [CrossRef]
85. Takayama, Y.; Ohnishi, H.; Ogasawara, F.; Oyama, K.; Kubota, T.; Yokoyama, A. Clinical utility of fractional exhaled nitric oxide and blood eosinophils counts in the diagnosis of Asthma-COPD overlap. *Int. J. Chronic Obstr. Pulm. Dis.* **2018**, *13*, 2525–2532. [CrossRef] [PubMed]
86. Guo, Y.; Hong, C.; Liu, Y.; Chen, H.; Huang, X.; Hong, M. Diagnostic value of fractional exhaled nitric oxide for asthma-chronic obstructive pulmonary disease overlap syndrome. *Medicine* **2018**, *97*, e10857. [CrossRef] [PubMed]
87. Tamada, T.; Sugiura, H.; Takahashi, T.; Matsunaga, K.; Kimura, K.; Katsumata, U.; Takekoshi, D.; Kikuchi, T.; Ohta, K.; Ichinose, M. Biomarker-Based detection of asthma–COPD overlap syndrome in COPD populations. *Int. J. Chronic Obstr. Pulm. Dis.* **2015**, *10*, 2169–2176. [CrossRef]

88. Kobayashi, S.; Hanagama, M.; Yamanda, S.; Ishida, M.; Yanai, M. Inflammatory biomarkers in Asthma-COPD overlap syndrome. *Int. J. Chronic Obstr. Pulm. Dis.* **2016**, *11*, 2117–2123. [CrossRef]
89. Carpagnano, G.E.; Lacedonia, D.; Malerba, M.; Palmiotti, G.A.; Cotugno, G.; Carone, M.; Foschino-Barbaro, M.P. Analysis of mitochondrial DNA alteration in new phenotype ACOS. *BMC Pulm. Med.* **2016**, *16*, 31. [CrossRef]
90. Hirai, K.; Shirai, T.; Suzuki, M.; Akamatsu, T.; Suzuki, T.; Hayashi, I.; Yamamoto, A.; Akita, T.; Morita, S.; Asada, K.; et al. A clustering approach to identify and characterize the asthma and chronic obstructive pulmonary disease overlap phenotype. *Clin. Exp. Allergy* **2017**, *47*, 1374–1382. [CrossRef]
91. De Llano, L.P.; Cosío, B.G.; Iglesias, A.; de Las Cuevas, N.; Soler-Cataluña, J.J.; Izquierdo, J.L.; López-Campos, J.L.; Calero, C.; Plaza, V.; Miravitlles, M.; et al. Mixed Th2 and Non-Th2 inflammatory pattern in the Asthma–COPD overlap: A network approach. *Int. J. Chronic Obstr. Pulm. Dis.* **2018**, *13*, 591–601. [CrossRef]
92. Jo, Y.S.; Kwon, S.O.; Kim, J.; Kim, W.J. Neutrophil gelatinase-associated lipocalin as a complementary biomarker for the asthma-chronic obstructive pulmonary disease overlap. *J. Thorac. Dis.* **2018**, *10*, 5047–5056. [CrossRef]
93. Wang, J.; Lv, H.; Luo, Z.; Mou, S.; Liu, J.; Liu, C.; Deng, S.; Jiang, Y.; Lin, J.; Wu, C.; et al. Plasma YKL-40 and NGAL are useful in distinguishing ACO from asthma and COPD. *Respir. Res.* **2018**, *19*, 47. [CrossRef]
94. Shirai, T.; Hirai, K.; Gon, Y.; Maruoka, S.; Mizumura, K.; Hikichi, M.; Holweg, C.; Itoh, K.; Inoue, H.; Hashimoto, S. Combined assessment of serum periostin and YKL-40 may identify Asthma-COPD overlap. *J. Allergy Clin. Immunol. Pract.* **2019**, *7*, 134–145.e1. [CrossRef]
95. Cai, C.; Bian, X.; Xue, M.; Liu, X.; Hu, H.; Wang, J.; Zheng, S.G.; Sun, B.; Wu, J.-L. Eicosanoids metabolized through LOX Distinguish Asthma–COPD overlap from COPD by metabolomics study. *Int. J. Chronic Obstr. Pulm. Dis.* **2019**, *14*, 1769–1778. [CrossRef]
96. Kubysheva, N.; Boldina, M.; Eliseeva, T.; Soodaeva, S.; Klimanov, I.; Khaletskaya, A.; Bayrasheva, V.; Solovyev, V.; Villa-Vargas, L.A.; Ramírez-Salinas, M.A.; et al. Relationship of serum levels of IL-17, IL-18, TNF-α, and lung function parameters in patients with COPD, Asthma-COPD overlap, and bronchial asthma. *Mediat. Inflamm.* **2020**, *2020*, 1–11. [CrossRef]
97. Oh, J.Y.; Lee, Y.S.; Min, K.H.; Hur, G.Y.; Lee, S.Y.; Kang, K.H.; Rhee, C.K.; Park, S.J.; Khan, A.; Na, J.; et al. Increased urinary l-histidine in patients with Asthma–COPD overlap: A pilot study. *Int. J. Chronic Obstr. Pulm. Dis.* **2018**, *13*, 1809–1818. [CrossRef]
98. Gao, J.; Iwamoto, H.; Koskela, J.; Alenius, H.; Hattori, N.; Kohno, N.; Laitinen, T.; Mazur, W.; Pulkkinen, V. Characterization of sputum biomarkers for Asthma–COPD overlap syndrome. *Int. J. Chronic Obstr. Pulm. Dis.* **2016**, *11*, 2457–2465. [CrossRef]
99. Hamada, S.; Tatsumi, S.; Kobayashi, Y.; Matsumoto, H.; Yasuba, H. Radiographic evidence of sinonasal inflammation in asthma-chronic obstructive pulmonary disease overlap syndrome: An underrecognized association. *J. Allergy Clin. Immunol. Pract.* **2017**, *5*, 1657–1662. [CrossRef]
100. Qu, Y.; Cao, Y.; Liao, M.; Lu, Z. Sagittal-Lung CT measurements in the evaluation of Asthma-COPD overlap syndrome: A distinctive phenotype from COPD Alone. *Radiol. Med.* **2017**, *122*, 487–494. [CrossRef]
101. Karayama, M.; Inui, N.; Yasui, H.; Kono, M.; Hozumi, H.; Suzuki, Y.; Furuhashi, K.; Hashimoto, D.; Enomoto, N.; Fujisawa, T.; et al. Physiological and morphological differences of airways between COPD and Asthma–COPD overlap. *Sci. Rep.* **2019**, *9*, 7818. [CrossRef]
102. Pollart, S.M.; Chapman, M.D.; Fiocco, G.P.; Rose, G.; Platts-Mills, T.A.E. Epidemiology of acute asthma: IgE antibodies to common inhalant allergens as a risk factor for emergency room visits. *J. Allergy Clin. Immunol.* **1989**, *83*, 875–882. [CrossRef]
103. Gelber, L.E.; Seltzer, L.H.; Bouzoukis, J.K.; Pollart, S.M.; Chapman, M.D.; Platts-Mills, T.A.E. Sensitization and exposure to indoor allergens as risk factors for asthma among patients presenting to hospital. *Am. Rev. Respir. Dis.* **1993**, *147*, 573–578. [CrossRef]
104. Postma, D.S.; Bleecker, E.R.; Amelung, P.J.; Holroyd, K.J.; Xu, J.; Panhuysen, C.I.M.; Meyers, D.A.; Levitt, R.C. Genetic susceptibility to asthma—bronchial hyperresponsiveness coinherited with a major gene for atopy. *N. Engl. J. Med.* **1995**, *333*, 894–900. [CrossRef] [PubMed]
105. Sunyer, J.; Antó, J.M.; Castellsagué, J.; Soriano, J.B.; Roca, J. Total serum IgE is associated with asthma independently of specific IgE levels. *Eur. Respir. J.* **1996**, *9*, 1880–1884. [CrossRef] [PubMed]
106. Asai, K.; Kitaura, J.; Kawakami, Y.; Yamagata, N.; Tsai, M.; Carbone, D.P.; Liu, F.-T.; Galli, S.J.; Kawakami, T. regulation of mast cell survival by IgE. *Immunity* **2001**, *14*, 791–800. [CrossRef]
107. Kalinina, E.P.; Denisenko, Y.K.; Vitkina, T.I.; Lobanova, E.G.; Novgorodtseva, T.P.; Antonyuk, M.V.; Gvozdenko, T.A.; Knyshova, V.V.; Nazarenko, A.V. The mechanisms of the regulation of immune response in patients with comorbidity of chronic obstructive pulmonary disease and asthma. *Can. Respir. J.* **2016**, *2016*, 1–8. [CrossRef]
108. Maltby, S.; Gibson, P.G.; Powell, H.; McDonald, V.M. Omalizumab treatment response in a population with severe allergic asthma and overlapping COPD. *Chest* **2017**, *151*, 78–89. [CrossRef]
109. Hanania, N.A.; Chipps, B.E.; Griffin, N.M.; Yoo, B.; Iqbal, A.; Casale, T.B. Omalizumab effectiveness in asthma COPD overlap: Post hoc analysis of PROSPERO study. *J. Allergy Clin. Immunol.* **2018**, *143*, 1629–1633.e2. [CrossRef]
110. Japanese Respiratory Society. *The JRS Guidelines for the Management of ACO 2018*; Medical Review: Tokyo, Japan, 2018. (In Japanese)
111. Yamamura, K.; Hara, J.; Kobayashi, T.; Ohkura, N.; Abo, M.; Akasaki, K.; Nomura, S.; Yuasa, M.; Saeki, K.; Terada, N.; et al. The prevalence and clinical features of Asthma-COPD Overlap (ACO) definitively diagnosed according to the japanese respiratory society guidelines for the management of ACO 2018. *J. Med. Investig.* **2019**, *66*, 157–164. [CrossRef]

112. Hirai, K.; Tanaka, A.; Homma, T.; Kawahara, T.; Oda, N.; Mikuni, H.; Uchida, Y.; Uno, T.; Miyata, Y.; Inoue, H.; et al. Prevalence and clinical features of Asthma-COPD overlap in patients with COPD not using inhaled corticosteroids. *Allergol. Int.* **2020**, *70*, 134–135. [CrossRef]
113. Chatterjee, N.; Shi, J.; García-Closas, M. Developing and evaluating polygenic risk prediction models for stratified disease prevention. *Nat. Rev. Genet.* **2016**, *17*, 392–406. [CrossRef]
114. Torkamani, A.; Wineinger, N.E.; Topol, E.J. The personal and clinical utility of polygenic risk scores. *Nat. Rev. Genet.* **2018**, *19*, 581–590. [CrossRef]
115. Poss, A.M.; Maschek, J.A.; Cox, J.E.; Hauner, B.J.; Hopkins, P.N.; Hunt, S.C.; Holland, W.L.; Summers, S.A.; Playdon, M.C. Machine learning reveals serum sphingolipids as cholesterol-independent biomarkers of coronary artery disease. *J. Clin. Investig.* **2020**, *130*, 1363–1376. [CrossRef]
116. Christenson, S.A.; Steiling, K.; van den Berge, M.; Hijazi, K.; Hiemstra, P.S.; Postma, D.S.; Lenburg, M.E.; Spira, A.; Woodruff, P.G. Asthma–COPD overlap. clinical relevance of genomic signatures of type 2 inflammation in chronic obstructive pulmonary disease. *Am. J. Resp. Crit. Care Med.* **2015**, *191*, 758–766. [CrossRef]
117. Fulkerson, P.C.; Rothenberg, M.E. Targeting eosinophils in allergy, inflammation and beyond. *Nat. Rev. Drug Discov.* **2013**, *12*, 117–129. [CrossRef]
118. Gon, Y.; Ito, R.; Hattori, T.; Hiranuma, H.; Kumasawa, F.; Kozu, Y.; Endo, D.; Koyama, D.; Shintani, Y.; Eriko, T.; et al. Serum eosinophil-derived neurotoxin: Correlation with persistent airflow limitation in adults with house-dust mite allergic asthma. *Allergy Asthma Proc.* **2015**, *36*, 113–120. [CrossRef]
119. Shirai, T.; Hirai, K.; Gon, Y.; Maruoka, S.; Mizumura, K.; Hikichi, M.; Itoh, K.; Hashimoto, S. Combined assessment of serum eosinophil-derived neurotoxin and YKL-40 may identify Asthma-COPD overlap. *Allergol. Int.* **2020**, *70*, 136–139. [CrossRef]
120. James, A.J.; Reinius, L.E.; Verhoek, M.; Gomes, A.; Kupczyk, M.; Hammar, U.; Ono, J.; Ohta, S.; Izuhara, K.; Bel, E.; et al. Increased YKL-40 and chitotriosidase in asthma and chronic obstructive pulmonary disease. *Am. J. Resp. Crit. Care Med.* **2016**, *193*, 131–142. [CrossRef]
121. Gon, Y.; Maruoka, S.; Ito, R.; Mizumura, K.; Kozu, Y.; Hiranuma, H.; Hattori, T.; Takahashi, M.; Hikichi, M.; Hashimoto, S. Utility of serum YKL-40 levels for identification of patients with asthma and COPD. *Allergol. Int.* **2017**, *66*, 624–626. [CrossRef]
122. Nasioudis, D.; Witkin, S.S. Neutrophil gelatinase-associated lipocalin and innate immune responses to bacterial infections. *Med. Microbiol. Immun.* **2015**, *204*, 471–479. [CrossRef]
123. Keatings, V.M.; Barnes, P.J. Granulocyte activation markers in induced sputum: Comparison between chronic obstructive pulmonary disease, asthma, and normal subjects. *Am. J. Resp. Crit. Care Med.* **1997**, *155*, 449–453. [CrossRef]
124. Eagan, T.M.; Damås, J.K.; Ueland, T.; Voll-Aanerud, M.; Mollnes, T.E.; Hardie, J.A.; Bakke, P.S.; Aukrust, P. Neutrophil gelatinase-associated lipocalin a biomarker in COPD. *Chest* **2010**, *138*, 888–895. [CrossRef]
125. Betsuyaku, T.; Nishimura, M.; Takeyabu, K.; Tanino, M.; Venge, P.; Xu, S.; Kawakami, Y. Neutrophil granule proteins in bronchoalveolar lavage fluid from subjects with subclinical emphysema. *Am. J. Resp. Crit. Care Med.* **1999**, *159*, 1985–1991. [CrossRef]
126. Ekberg-Jansson, A.; Andersson, B.; Bake, B.; Boijsen, M.; Enanden, I.; Rosengren, A.; Skoogh, B.-E.; Tylén, U.; Venge, P.; Löfdahl, C.-G. Neutrophil-Associated activation markers in healthy smokers relates to a fall in DLCO and to emphysematous changes on high resolution CT. *Resp. Med.* **2001**, *95*, 363–373. [CrossRef]
127. Yan, L.; Borregaard, N.; Kjeldsen, L.; Moses, M.A. The high molecular weight urinary Matrix Metalloproteinase (MMP) activity is a complex of gelatinase B/MMP-9 and Neutrophil Gelatinase-Associated Lipocalin (NGAL). Modulation of MMP-9 activity by NGAL. *J. Biol. Chem.* **2001**, *276*, 37258–37265. [CrossRef]
128. Iwamoto, H.; Gao, J.; Koskela, J.; Kinnula, V.; Kobayashi, H.; Laitinen, T.; Mazur, W. Differences in plasma and sputum biomarkers between COPD and COPD-Asthma overlap. *Eur. Respir. J.* **2013**, *43*, 421–429. [CrossRef]
129. Nuñez, A.; Sarasate, M.; Loeb, E.; Esquinas, C.; Miravitlles, M.; Barrecheguren, M. Practical guide to the identification and diagnosis of Asthma-COPD Overlap (ACO). *Chronic Obstr. Pulm. Dis.* **2019**, *16*, 1–7. [CrossRef]
130. Hosseini, M.; Almasi-Hashiani, A.; Sepidarkish, M.; Maroufizadeh, S. Global prevalence of Asthma-COPD Overlap (ACO) in the general population: A systematic review and meta-analysis. *Respir. Res.* **2019**, *20*, 229. [CrossRef]
131. Krishnan, J.A.; Nibber, A.; Chisholm, A.; Price, D.; Bateman, E.D.; Bjermer, L.; van Boven, J.F.M.; Brusselle, G.; Costello, R.W.; Dandurand, R.J.; et al. Prevalence and characteristics of asthma–chronic obstructive pulmonary disease overlap in routine primary care practices. *Ann. Am. Thorac Soc.* **2019**, *16*, 1143–1150. [CrossRef]
132. Baron, A.J.; Blok, B.M.F.; van Heijst, E.; Riemersma, R.A.; der Voort, A.M.S.; Metting, E.I.; Kocks, J.W. Prevalence of asthma characteristics in COPD patients in a dutch well-established asthma/COPD service for primary care. *Int. J. Chronic Obstr. Pulm. Dis.* **2020**, *15*, 1601–1611. [CrossRef]
133. Hardin, M.; Cho, M.; McDonald, M.-L.; Beaty, T.; Ramsdell, J.; Bhatt, S.; van Beek, E.J.R.; Make, B.J.; Crapo, J.D.; Silverman, E.K.; et al. The clinical and genetic features of COPD-Asthma overlap syndrome. *Eur. Respir. J.* **2014**, *44*, 341–350. [CrossRef]
134. Kottyan, L.C.; Collier, A.R.; Cao, K.H.; Niese, K.A.; Hedgebeth, M.; Radu, C.G.; Witte, O.N.; Hershey, G.K.K.; Rothenberg, M.E.; Zimmermann, N. Eosinophil viability is increased by acidic PH in a CAMP- and GPR65-Dependent manner. *Blood* **2009**, *114*, 2774–2782. [CrossRef]
135. El-Husseini, Z.W.; Gosens, R.; Dekker, F.; Koppelman, G.H. The genetics of asthma and the promise of genomics-guided drug target discovery. *Lancet Respir. Med.* **2020**, *8*, 1045–1056. [CrossRef]

136. Kyogoku, Y.; Sugiura, H.; Ichikawa, T.; Numakura, T.; Koarai, A.; Yamada, M.; Fujino, N.; Tojo, Y.; Onodera, K.; Tanaka, R.; et al. Nitrosative stress in patients with asthma–chronic obstructive pulmonary disease overlap. *J. Allergy Clin. Immunol.* **2019**, *144*, 972–983.e14. [CrossRef] [PubMed]
137. Barnes, P.J. Nitrosative stress in patients with asthma-chronic obstructive pulmonary disease overlap. *J. Allergy Clin. Immunol.* **2019**, *144*, 928–930. [CrossRef] [PubMed]

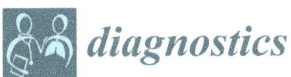

Review

Neutrophils and Asthma

Akira Yamasaki *, Ryota Okazaki and Tomoya Harada

Department of Multidisciplinary Internal Medicine, Division of Respiratory Medicine and Rheumatology, Faculty of Medicine, Tottori University, Yonago 683-8504, Japan; okazaki0222@tottori-u.ac.jp (R.O.); tomo.h.308@tottori-u.ac.jp (T.H.)
* Correspondence: yamasaki@tottori-u.ac.jp; Tel.: +81-859-38-6537

Abstract: Although eosinophilic inflammation is characteristic of asthma pathogenesis, neutrophilic inflammation is also marked, and eosinophils and neutrophils can coexist in some cases. Based on the proportion of sputum cell differentiation, asthma is classified into eosinophilic asthma, neutrophilic asthma, neutrophilic and eosinophilic asthma, and paucigranulocytic asthma. Classification by bronchoalveolar lavage is also performed. Eosinophilic asthma accounts for most severe asthma cases, but neutrophilic asthma or a mixture of the two types can also present a severe phenotype. Biomarkers for the diagnosis of neutrophilic asthma include sputum neutrophils, blood neutrophils, chitinase-3-like protein, and hydrogen sulfide in sputum and serum. Thymic stromal lymphoprotein (TSLP)/T-helper 17 pathways, bacterial colonization/microbiome, neutrophil extracellular traps, and activation of nucleotide-binding oligomerization domain-like receptor family, pyrin domain-containing 3 pathways are involved in the pathophysiology of neutrophilic asthma and coexistence of obesity, gastroesophageal reflux disease, and habitual cigarette smoking have been associated with its pathogenesis. Thus, targeting neutrophilic asthma is important. Smoking cessation, neutrophil-targeting treatments, and biologics have been tested as treatments for severe asthma, but most clinical studies have not focused on neutrophilic asthma. Phosphodiesterase inhibitors, anti-TSLP antibodies, azithromycin, and anti-cholinergic agents are promising drugs for neutrophilic asthma. However, clinical research targeting neutrophilic inflammation is required to elucidate the optimal treatment.

Keywords: asthma; biomarkers; biologics; eosinophils; inflammation; neutrophils; treatment

1. Introduction

Asthma is a common chronic airway disease that affects about 350 million people worldwide and varies in prevalence from country to country. In Japan, the prevalence is 9–10% and the number of patients with asthma was 1,177,000 in 2014 [1,2]. Diagnosis of asthma is based on a history or current symptoms, such as chest tightness, wheezing, dyspnea, and cough, together with variable expiratory airway limitation assessed by peak expiratory flow or spirometry. Chronic airway inflammation is an important feature of asthma and is characterized by the presence of eosinophils, basophils, mast cells, neutrophils, T helper 2 (Th2) cells, type 2 innate lymphoid cells (ILC2), CD8[+] T cells, B cells, and dendritic cells [3–5]. In the Japanese Guidelines for Adult Asthma, a diagnosis is based on: (I) repetitive symptoms, such as paroxysmal dyspnea, wheezing, chest tightness, and cough; (II) reversible airflow limitation; (III) airway hyper-responsiveness; (IV) airway inflammation; (V) an atopic state; and (VI) exclusion of other cardiopulmonary disease [2].

Asthma is a heterogenous airway disease, and since the 2000s, cluster analyses have identified several phenotypes [6–8]. The common phenotypes are allergic asthma; non-allergic asthma; adult-onset (late-onset) asthma; asthma with persistent airflow limitation; and asthma with obesity [9]. The Severe Asthma Research Program (SARP) identified five phenotypes in patients with severe and non-severe asthma [10]. Kuo et al. found three transcriptome-associated clusters (TACs) in patients with asthma. TAC1 is characterized by immune receptors and a sputum eosinophil increase, TAC2 is characterized by

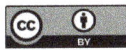

interferon-, tumor necrosis factor-, and inflammasome-associated genes and a sputum neutrophil increase, and TAC3 is characterized by genes associated with metabolic pathways, ubiquitination, and mitochondrial function, with no sputum increase [11].

Neutrophils are the most abundant cells in peripheral blood and are stored in pulmonary capillary beds [12]. These cells play important roles in the innate immune system by killing microbes, phagocytosis, granule release, and formation of neutrophil extracellular traps (NETs). The role of neutrophils in asthma has been studied, but there is much debate about the presence of neutrophilic asthma [13–16]. Since glucocorticoids enhance the survival of neutrophils, which constitutively express glucocorticoid receptor β (GRβ) [17,18], the elevation of neutrophil levels in the asthmatic airway is thought to be a consequence of corticosteroid treatment. However, neutrophils are also observed in steroid-naïve patients with asthma [19–22] and several studies have found evidence that neutrophilic inflammation is associated with severe asthma and with asthma exacerbation [23,24]. A cluster analysis has shown that sputum neutrophil counts were associated with more severe phenotypes [25]. Recently, Minchem et al. reviewed the pathology of chronic lung diseases, including asthma [26]. They described the heterogeneity of neutrophils and their interactions with several immune and structural cells, identifying anti-inflammatory, pro-resolving, and pro-repair functions via direct cell-to-cell communication as well as via soluble mediators [26]. Neutrophils also connect with other cells via exosomes and extracellular vesicles [27]. In chronic lung diseases, an overabundance of neutrophils may exacerbate inflammation and remodeling [26]. Therefore, neutrophilic inflammation is involved in the heterogeneity of asthma, and neutrophil-targeted treatment may be important for severe asthma. The pathogenesis, definition, and biomarkers of neutrophilic asthma and potential therapy for neutrophilic asthma are discussed in this review.

2. Definition of Neutrophilic Asthma

The phenotype of asthma is generally categorized by the cell profile of induced sputum. In a healthy person, this profile has $0.4 \pm 0.9\%$ eosinophils and $37.5 \pm 20.5\%$ neutrophils, with means plus 2SD and 90th percentiles of 2.2% and 1.1% for eosinophils, and 77.7% and 64.4% for neutrophils, respectively [28]. Eosinophilic asthma is defined as an increase in eosinophils to above 2% or 3% and neutrophilic asthma as an increase in neutrophils to above 60% or 76% in induced sputum [29]. Paucigranulocytic asthma is defined as neutrophils < 76% and eosinophils < 3%, and conversely, mixed granulocytic asthma is defined as neutrophils > 76% and eosinophils > 3% [30]. However, there is still no clear definition of neutrophilic asthma [13]. In children, neutrophil-predominant severe asthma is defined using a cut-off of ≥5% neutrophils in bronchial lavage fluid [31]. Alternative methods, such as nasal wash or nasal lavage, have also been used to evaluate neutrophilic asthma or non-eosinophilic asthma [32].

3. Association of Eosinophils and Neutrophils

Coexistence of neutrophils and eosinophils occurs in severe asthma [10,33,34], and recent studies have shown that patients with asthma with a mixture of neutrophilic and eosinophilic inflammation had accelerated decline of respiratory function [35–37]. In studies of the coexistence mechanism, Nagata et al. found that activation of neutrophils may induce migration of eosinophils through the basement membrane via interleukin-8 (IL-8) [38], and that leukotriene B4 (LTB4)-activated neutrophils which induced eosinophil migration and Toll-like receptor 4 (TLR4) expression on neutrophils may be involved in this mechanism [36,39]. Theophylline attenuates trans-basement membrane migration of eosinophils in vitro by suppressing superoxide anion generation [40]. Lavinskinene et al. showed that the sputum neutrophil counts after bronchial allergen challenge were related to peripheral blood neutrophil chemotaxis in patients with asthma [41].

4. Pathogenesis of Asthma

4.1. TSLP

Thymic stromal lymphopoietin (TSLP) is secreted from a variety of cells, including basophils, mast cells, and airway epithelial cells [42]. In the human airway, airway epithelial cells secrete TSLP by recognition of allergens, viruses, pollutants and cigarette smoke, bacteria, and other external stimuli by pattern recognition receptors (PRPs) [43]. TSLP triggers allergic/eosinophilic and non-allergic/eosinophilic inflammation [44,45], and is also involved in neutrophilic inflammation in asthma. TSLP and TLR3 ligands promote conversion of naïve T cells to Th17 cells [46] and subsequently induce neutrophil recruitment via IL-8 and GM-CSF from airway epithelial cells [47]. TSLP polymorphism may also be related to allergic disease and eosinophilia in patients with asthma [48].

4.2. IL-17

IL-17 is a key cytokine in neutrophilic asthma. IL-17 and IL-17A are produced by Th17 cells and ILC3 cells, and may stimulate epithelial cells and fibroblasts and induce neutrophil activation and migration via IL-6, IL-8, and tumor necrosis factor-α (TNF-α). IL-17 induces glucocorticoid receptor (GR) β on epithelial cells in patients with asthma [49]. This may be related to glucocorticoid insensitivity in neutrophilic asthma. IL-17 induces eotaxin expression in human airway smooth muscle (HASM) cells [50], which may be linked to mixed neutrophilic and eosinophilic inflammation in asthma. IL-17 is increased in bronchial biopsy in severe asthma [51] and in sputum from patients with moderate-to-severe asthma [52]. Bulles et al. showed that the *IL17* mRNA level correlated with the *IL8* mRNA level and with CD3 gamma cell and neutrophil counts, which suggested a link between IL-17 and neutrophilic inflammation [52]. IL-17 also enhances IL-1β-mediated IL-8 release from HASM cells [53], and the IL-17/Th17 axis is involved in microbiomes in the development of asthma [54].

4.3. Bacterial Colonization and Microbiome in the Airway in Neutrophilic Asthma

The intestinal and respiratory microbiomes are both thought to be associated with the pathogenesis of asthma [55]. In patients with neutrophilic asthma, 50% of patients have bacterial infection based on bronchoalveolar lavage [56], and at the time of asthma exacerbation, 87.8% of patients have bacteria in sputum, with neutrophils > 65% [13]. Recent studies have shown that bacterial microbiome profiles in the airway were associated with neutrophil inflammation in asthma [57–59] and that the Th17/IL-17 axis was involved in this process [60,61]. Microbiome-derived cluster analysis of sputum in severe asthma showed two distinct phenotypes: cluster 1 had less-severe asthma and commensal bacterial profile, and higher bacterial richness and diversity; cluster 2 had more severe asthma with a reduced commensal bacterial profile, clear deficiency of several bacterial species, and neutrophilic inflammation [57]. The intestinal microbiome has also been linked to the development of asthma, but its relationship with neutrophilic inflammation in asthma is unclear [62].

4.4. Obesity

Obesity increases the risk of asthma development [63–66], worsens asthma control and severity [8,67], increases hospitalization [68], and reduces responses to inhaled corticosteroids (ICS) alone or in conjunction with a long-acting β2 agonist (LABA) [68–70]. In cluster analyses, obesity-related asthma has been grouped into non-Th2 asthma, with later onset, female preponderance, and severe symptoms [7,8,10]. Obesity is associated with inflammatory adipokines including leptin, resistin, lipocain 2, IL-6, TNF-α, IL-1β, and IFN-γ [71–75]. These mediators induce airway inflammation. In a mouse obese asthma model, ILC3 stimulated by IL-1β, IL-6, or IL-23 produced IL-17A [76]. IL-17A alone or in combination with TNF-α has been shown to induce IL-8 production from epithelial cells [77], and cigarette smoke can also enhance IL-17A-induced IL-8 and IL-6 production [78–81]. IL-6 and IL-8 recruit and activate neutrophils in an asthmatic airway [41,81].

In obese patients with asthma, IL-17 is associated with steroid resistance by dysregulation of GRα and GRβ [82], while in human bronchial epithelial cells, IL-17A induces glucocorticoid insensitivity [83]. Insulin resistance and vitamin D deficiency related to obesity may aggravate airway remodeling and hyper-responsiveness by enhancing leptin, transforming growth factor (TGF)-β1, IL-1β, and IL-6 expression [84–87], which might then promote neutrophilic inflammation.

4.5. NETs and NETosis

Neutrophil extracellular traps (NETs) were first described by Brinkmann et al. [88]. Neutrophils stimulated by bacteria or inflammatory mediators, such as IL-8, platelet activating factor, and lipopolysaccharide (LPS), release NETs that include neutrophil elastase, cathepsin G, myeloperoxidase, defensins, lactoferrin, histones, pentraxin 3, reactive oxygen species (ROS), and DNA to captivate and kill bacteria [89]. NETosis is an active form of neutrophil death related to NETs formation [88]. Several studies have related NETs to the pathogenesis of autoimmune disease, cancer, and atherosclerosis [90,91]; dysregulation of NETs may also result in asthma pathobiology, although the mechanisms associated with NETs are not fully understood. In a mouse model, allergen exposure with endotoxin induced NETosis [92]. In severe neutrophilic asthma, Krishnamoorthy et al. determined that cytoplasts and neutrophils positively correlated with IL-17 levels in the bronchoalveolar fluid [92]. The sputum extracellular DNA (eDNA) level has been correlated with expressions of IL-8, IL-1β, and NLRP3 [93], and Lachowicz-Scroggins et al. found that high extracellular DNA (eDNA) in sputum was associated with poor asthma control, mucus hypersecretion, and oral steroid use in patients with asthma [94]. The same group also showed that the eDNA level was correlated with neutrophil inflammation, NET components, caspase-1 activity, and IL-1β. In vitro, epithelial damage caused by NETs has been prevented by DNase [94]. These studies indicate that NETs and eDNA are related to severe neutrophilic asthma.

4.6. NLRP3 Inflammasome and Asthma

Nucleotide-binding oligomerization domain-like receptor family pyrin domain-containing (NLRP) inflammasomes are a critical component of the innate immune system and they play an important role in activation of inflammation. NLRP3, an NLR family PRP, responds to pathogen-associated molecule patterns (PAMPs) or danger (damage)-associated molecular patterns (DAMPs). Activation of NLRP3 inflammasomes is mediated by two signals: the priming signal triggered by PAMPs, DAMPs, IL-1β, and TNF-α; the second (activation) signal mediated by extracellular ATP, RNA viruses, particulate matter, ionic flux, ROS, mitochondrial dysfunction, and lysosomal damage. Upon activation of NLRP3 inflammasomes, IL-1β and IL-18 are secreted [95,96]. Dysregulation of NLRP3 inflammasome activation is related to Alzheimer's disease [97], Parkinson's disease [98], diabetes mellitus, atherosclerosis [99], and pulmonary inflammatory disorders, including lung fibrosis [100], acute exacerbation of interstitial pneumonia [101], sarcoidosis [102], asbestosis, and silicosis [103]. Since human lungs are exposed to many endogenous and exogenous noxious stimuli, including viruses, bacteria, cigarette smoke, and particulate matter, the innate immune response in the airway via NLRP3 inflammasomes is important. However, excess or persistent activation of NLRP3 inflammasomes by allergens or irritants has been shown to induce persistent inflammation and tissue damage in the airway of patients with asthma [104,105]. In these patients, the sputum NLRP3 level was increased and was correlated with neutrophilic airway inflammation [106,107]. NLRP3 expression has also been shown to be increased in obese patients with asthma [108]. Kim et al. found that a high-fat diet induced airway hyper-reactivity and increased *NLRP3*, *IL17A*, and *IL1B* mRNA in an obese mouse model [76], suggesting that obesity-induced airway hypersensitivity is mediated by NLRP3 inflammasomes that are activated by fatty acids or cholesterol crystals from macrophages in adipose tissue or in the lungs [76]. In other experimental models, NLPR3 and apoptosis-associated speck-like protein containing CARD (ASC)-deficient mice exhibited reduced airway inflammation [109]. Ovalbumin (OVA) mouse models with alum [110], LPS, *Aspergillus fumigatus* [111], *Chlamydia muridarum*, or *Haemophilus influenzae* infection also have been shown to have increased NLRP3 [106]. In this latter model, neutrophil depletion suppressed IL-1β-induced airway hyper-responsiveness.

4.7. S100A8/A9, HMGB-1, RAGE, and TLR4

The S100A8/A9 complex belongs to the Ca^{2+}-binding S100 protein family and is a DAMP protein complex expressed in neutrophils, monocytes, and macrophages [112,113]. High mobility group box 1 (HMGB-1), which is also a DAMP protein, a non-histone, chromatin-associated nuclear protein is released from necrotic, inflammatory, macrophage, dendritic, natural killer, and resident cells (epithelial cells, smooth muscle cells, and fibroblasts) [114–117]. TNF-α, IL-1β, and IFN-γ induce HMBG-1 release from activated macrophages [118,119]. HMBG-1 and S100A8/S100A9 bind to two types of receptors: the receptor for advanced glycation end products (RAGE) and TLR-4. RAGE is expressed on lung [120], skeletal muscle, heart, liver, kidney [121], lung epithelial, and immune cells [122–126]. Perkins et al. showed that knockout of *RAGE* abolished type 2 cytokine-induced airway inflammation and mucus hyperplasia in a mouse model [127]. Oczypok et al. reported that RAGE induced asthma/allergic airway inflammation by promoting IL-33 expression, and that ILC2 accumulation was critical in the pathogenesis of asthma in a mouse model [128].

TLR4 is also expressed on B cells [129], T cells [130], monocytes, macrophages [131], and neutrophils [132]. S100A8/A9 and HMGB-1 might be involved in the pathobiology of remodeling in asthma by promoting inflammation and tissue repair in the airway [117]. In a mouse model, blocking HMGB-1 and TLR-4 attenuated disonoyl phthalate-induced asthma [133]. HMGB-1 is increased in OVA-induced asthma [134]. In patients with asthma, the sputum HMGB-1 level is increased and inversely correlated with the percentage predicted forced expiratory volume in 1 s (%FEV1) and FEV1/forced vital capacity (FVC) ratio. The HMGB-1 level is also associated with the severity of asthma and neutrophils in sputum [135,136]. An endogenous form of RAGE (esRAGE), which is a decoy receptor for AGE, was elevated in sputum from a patient with asthma; however, the esRAGE level was not associated with asthma severity [135], in contrast to the RAGE level [136]. Since HMGB-1 stimulates TNF-α, IL-6, and IL-8 production from monocytes [137,138], it might be a key player in inducing neutrophilic asthma. Recent studies have shown that a soluble form of RAGE prevents Th17-mediated neutrophilic asthma by blocking HMBG1/RAGE signaling in a mouse model [139]. In patients with neutrophilic asthma, decreased sRAGE was associated with asthma severity [140], and a recent study showed that sRAGE was associated with low eosinophil count and IgE in children with asthma [141]. RAGE has been linked to cigarette-smoke-induced neutrophilic inflammation and airway hyper-responsiveness in a mouse model, but TLR4, another receptor for HMGB-1 and S100A8/A, was not involved [142]. Furthermore, *AGER* (which encodes RAGE) expression, rather than TLR4 expression, was significantly correlated with the sputum neutrophil count and airway hyper-responsiveness in patients with chronic obstructive pulmonary disease (COPD) [142]. Therefore, HMGB-1 and sRAGE might be biomarkers for neutrophilic asthma.

4.8. House Dust Mites and Neutrophilic Asthma

House dust mites (HDMs) are the most important allergen for the development and worsening of allergic asthma, with 90% of cases of pediatric asthma sensitized to HDMs. Many studies of allergic and eosinophilic asthma have been conducted using a mouse model sensitized to HDMs, and several recent studies have described neutrophilic or mixed-granulocytic asthma models. Menson et al. reported a novel BALB/c female mouse model using *Mycobacterium tuberculosis* extract, complete Freund's adjuvant, and HDM, in which the bronchial alveolar lavage fluid (BALF) contained 80% neutrophils and 10% eosinophils [143]. Mack et al. described an old (9 months) C57BL/6 female mouse model sensitized to HDMs that showed elevated neutrophils in BALF as compared with young

(3 months) mice, as a model of adult-onset asthma [144]. Sadamatsu et al. found that a high-fat diet induced elevated neutrophils in BALF in an HDM-sensitized mouse model [145]. Neutrophil counts in the sputum of patients with chronic neutrophilic asthma have been shown to be correlated with the serum HDM-specific IgG levels, and these patients have HDM-derived enolase in their serum [146]. In the same study, HDM-derived enolase was shown to induce epithelial barrier disintegration and neutrophilic inflammation in a mouse model [146]. Blockade of leukotriene B4 receptor 1 (BLT1)/BLT2 by antagonists can reduce neutrophil infiltration based on findings in an HDM- and LPS-induced mouse asthma model [147]. IL-1β was found to be required to promote neutrophilic inflammation in an HDM-sensitized and viral-exacerbated model, using double-stranded RNA to mimic rhinovirus [148]. In contrast, Patel et al. found neutrophil depletion in an HDM allergic airway disease mouse, with this depletion enhancing Th2 inflammation by inducing G-colony stimulating factor-induced ILC2 activation and cytokine production [149].

4.9. Electric, Heat-Not-Burn Cigarettes, and Combustible Cigarettes

Almost one-quarter of patients with adult asthma are thought to have smoking habits. Several studies have also shown that the efficacy of ICS is reduced in patients with asthma who are exposed to smoking [150–152]. Passive smoking in a family increases the use of drugs for pediatric asthma [153]. E-cigarette or electric cigarette (vapor) exposure induces neutrophil protease, matrix metalloproteinase-2 (MMP-2), and MMP-9 in healthy subjects [154]. Schweitzer et al. showed that e-cigarette use was independently associated with asthma in adolescents [155]. A study from Korea also showed an association of e-cigarette use with asthma diagnosis and absence from school due to asthma [156]. E-cigarette liquid has been shown to induce IL-6 production from human epithelial cells and addition of nicotine further increased IL-6 production [157], while electronic nicotine delivery systems using aerosols also induced IL-6 and IL-8 secretion [158].

A 2015 internet survey showed that the use of heat-not-burn (HNB) cigarettes among patients with asthma was 0.0% in Japan [159]. The first HNB cigarette, IQOS, was released in 2014 in Japan, and the harmfulness of HNB cigarettes to asthma remains uncertain. However, HNB cigarettes contain nicotine and many other toxins [160,161], as well as particulate matter [162], and thus, may worsen asthma control by inducing neutrophilic inflammation. Further studies are needed to examine how HNB cigarettes affect asthma pathogenesis and neutrophilic inflammation [80]. In patients with mild asthma, combustible cigarette smoking increases neutrophil counts, and IL-17A, IL-6, and IL-8 levels [80]. Exposure of human epithelial cells to cigarette smoke extracts, IL-17A, and aeroallergens has been shown to induce IL-6 and IL-8 production, which may be associated with the neutrophil accumulation in asthmatic airways [80]. In a rat model, the late asthmatic response to OVA increased with cigarette smoke (CS) exposure as compared with no exposure. ICS decreased eosinophil and lymphocyte accumulation with and without CS exposure but did not decrease neutrophil accumulation with CS exposure [163]. Quitting smoking and avoiding environmental smoking can resolve neutrophil inflammation in patients with asthma who smoke. A combination of pharmacotherapy using bupropion and varenicline with counseling was most effective for smoking cessation [164]. Smoking cessation-support therapy using a smartphone application has recently been covered by insurance in Japan [165].

4.10. Air Pollution

Relationships of air pollution with asthma development or exacerbation have been reported for several years. Examples of outdoor or indoor pollution include diesel exhaust, foreign workplace matter, ozone, nitrogen dioxide, sulfur dioxide, second-hand smoke, heating sources, cooking smoke, and molds [166–168]. These pollutants induce asthma exacerbation through oxidative stress and damage, airway remodeling, inflammatory pathways, immunological responses, and enhancement of airway sensitivity [166,168]. Particulate matter induces Th2 and Th17 inflammation in allergic conditions and this induces eosinophilic and neutrophilic inflammation in asthma [169–172]. In an in vivo study, ozone exposure induced IL-8 secretion from epithelial cells [173], which was related to neutrophil accumulation in the airway after exposure to ozone in patients with asthma [174].

4.11. Gastroesophageal Reflux Disease

Gastroesophageal reflux disease (GERD) is a common comorbidity in asthma, and the severity of asthma is increased when complicated with GERD [175]. In the SARP study, a subgroup of patients with asthma defined as having a low pH in exhaled breath condensate had a high body mass index (BMI) and high neutrophilic airway inflammation, and had GERD as a complication [176]. GERD is often accompanied by mixed eosinophilic and neutrophilic inflammation (reviewed in [177]). Simpson et al. found that patients with neutrophilic asthma had a high prevalence of rhinosinusitis and symptoms of GERD as compared with patients with eosinophilic asthma [178]. The mechanism through which GERD induces or enhances airway inflammation in asthma has not been determined, but GERD is associated with obesity [179], which may lead to neutrophilic inflammation, as mentioned above. The triangle of inflammation, obesity, and GERD with sleep disordered breathing syndrome is important in children with asthma [180].

Figure 1 shows the pathology of neutrophilic asthma (Figure 1).

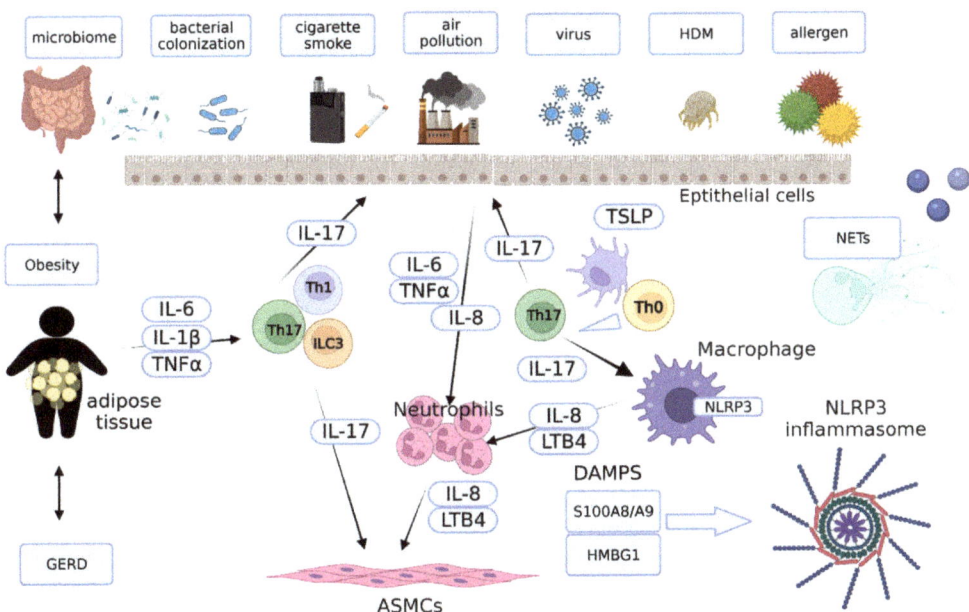

Figure 1. Pathogenesis of neutrophilic asthma. Several cells, including airway epithelial cells, macrophages, T helper (Th) cells, innate helper 3 cells (ILC3), airway smooth muscle cells (ASMCs), and neutrophils play important roles in the pathogenesis of neutrophilic asthma. Airway epithelial cells, stimulated by air pollution, cigarette smoke, bacterial colonization, virus, and allergens, secrete TSLP, IL-33, and IL-25. TSLP secreted from epithelial cells and inflammatory cells converts Th0 to Th17 cells and subsequently induced neutrophil recruitment via IL-8 and GM-CSF, induced by IL-17 from airway epithelial cells. The IL-17/Th17 axis is involved in bacterial colonization and microbiome associated neutrophilic inflammation in asthma. Obesity and GERD are related to severe, neutrophilic asthma and the IL-17/Th17 axis is involved in these conditions. Neutrophil extracellular trap (NETs) formation, damage-associated molecular patterns (DAMPs), and NLPR3 inflammasome are also involved in the pathogenesis of neutrophil asthma.

5. Biomarkers of Neutrophilic Asthma

Non-type 2 subtypes of asthma, including neutrophilic and paucigranulocytic asthma, are difficult to diagnose because of a lack of appropriate biomarkers. However, recent studies have suggested promising diagnostic biomarkers for neutrophilic asthma (Table 1).

Table 1. Possible biomarkers for neutrophilic asthma.

Biomarker	Sample	Definition	Significance	Refs.
YKL-40	Serum, sputum	Not established, but serum YKL-40 > 60.94 ng/mL showed impaired lung function and require corticosteroid	YKL-40 is released from neutrophil and epithelial cells, YKL-40 is released from neutrophils and epithelial cells Serum YKL-40 correlates with sputum neutrophil counts	[181–183]
Hydrogen sulfide (H_2S)	Serum, exhaled breath, sputum	Not established	Sputum H_2S correlates with the degree of airflow limitation Serum/sputum H_2S predicts asthma exacerbation	[184–186]
MPO	Sputum	Not established	Sputum MPO correlates with sputum YKL-40 and neutrophils	[23,187]
Neutrophil	Serum, sputum	Sputum > 60% or 76%	Associated with chronic airway obstruction, annual decline of FEV1	[188,189]
MicroRNA	Sputum, serum, and plasma	Not established	miR-199a-5p, miR142-3p, miR233-3p, and miR629-3p are increased in neutrophilic asthma miR299a-5p is negatively correlated with FEV1	[190,191]

5.1. YKL40

Chitinase-3-like protein (YKL-40) is a human glycoprotein that is released from several cell types, including neutrophils, macrophages, and epithelial cells. YKL-40 is involved in the pathogenesis of many diseases, including rheumatoid arthritis [192], multiple sclerosis [193], chronic obstructive lung disease [194,195], Alzheimer's disease [196], and asthma [181,197]. Serum YKL-40 levels are related to asthma severity, while lung YKL-40 levels are correlated with airway remodeling [181,182]. In the multicenter BIOAIR study, the serum YKL-40 level was negatively correlated with lung function (FEV1% predicted, FVC, and FEV1/FVC), but not with fraction of exhaled nitric oxide or blood and sputum eosinophil and neutrophil counts [182]. Cluster analyses have shown that high serum YKL-40 levels were associated with neutrophilic asthma and paucigranulocytic asthma [183] and that patients with high serum YKL-40 had severe airflow obstruction and near fatal or frequent exacerbation [183]. The serum YKL-40 level has been shown to be positively correlated with blood neutrophils, IL-6, and sputum IL-1β [119], while the sputum YKL-40 level has been shown to be strongly correlated with neutrophilic asthma and sputum myeloperoxidase, and was associated with sputum IL-8 and soluble IL-6 receptor levels [187]. Therefore, serum and sputum YKL-40 levels are useful biomarkers for neutrophilic asthma.

5.2. Hydrogen Sulfide

Nitric oxide is a biomarker of type 2 inflammation and carbon monoxide is a partial biomarker of asthma severity [198,199]. Hydrogen sulfide (H_2S) is the third biomarker in breath, and sputum H_2S is a novel biomarker of neutrophilic asthma. Sputum H_2S levels are correlated with neutrophils in sputum and airflow limitation [184–186], and the sputum-to-serum H_2S ratio predicts the risk of asthma exacerbation [186]. Therefore, sputum H_2S is a diagnostic marker for neutrophilic asthma and a predictor of exacerbation when combined with serum H_2S. These biomarkers are also elevated in asthma-COPD overlap [200].

5.3. Myeloperoxidase

Myeloperoxidase (MPO) is a marker of neutrophil activation. Serum MPO has been shown to be elevated in ANCA-associated vasculitis, including microscopic polyangiitis and eosinophilic granulomatous polyangiitis, while sputum MPO has been shown to correlate positively with sputum YKL-40 levels [187] and sputum neutrophils [23]. Thus, sputum MPO is a useful biomarker for neutrophilic asthma, whereas elevation of serum MPO is thought to be a marker for small vessel vasculitis.

5.4. Blood Neutrophil Count

The peripheral blood neutrophil count is not appropriate as a surrogate marker for neutrophilic asthma defined based on sputum cell differentiation [201–203]. However, neutrophilia has been shown to be associated with chronic airway obstruction [189] and an annual decline in FEV1 [188]. The sputum neutrophil count after bronchial allergen challenge has been shown to be related to peripheral blood neutrophil chemotaxis in patients with asthma [41].

5.5. MicroRNA

Several studies have shown that microRNAs (miRNAs) are biomarkers for asthma. Panganiban et al. found upregulation of miRNA-1248 in patients with asthma [204] and also showed that miRNAs in serum could be used to phenotype asthma [205]. Huang et al. revealed that miR-199a-5p in sputum and plasma was increased in neutrophilic asthma [190] and showed that levels of miRNA-199a-5p secreted from human LPS-stimulated peripheral neutrophils were inversely correlated with FEV1 [190]. A genome-wide analysis of miRNAs in sputum from patients with asthma showed that *hsa*-miR-223-3p was expressed in neutrophils and was associated with neutrophil counts in response to ozone exposure [206]. Maes et al. showed that miR-223-3p, miR-142-3p, and miR-629-3p were upregulated in severe, neutrophilic asthma [191]. Therefore, several miRNAs are biomarkers for diagnosis of neutrophilic asthma, and they are also considered to be therapeutic targets [207,208].

6. Airway Remodeling in Neutrophilic Asthma

Airway remodeling in asthma is caused by chronic airway inflammation and is a characteristic feature of chronic asthma. The pathological changes in airway remodeling involve mucous metaplasia, thickening of the reticular basement membrane, increases of goblet cells and mucus hypersecretion, shedding of epithelial cells, submucosal infiltration of inflammatory cells, extracellular matrix deposition, airway smooth muscle (ASM) cell hyperplasia, and hypertrophy. Neutrophilic asthma and airway remodeling are not fully understood, but several studies have shown that inflammatory mediators, such as LTB4, IL-6, IL-8, and TNF-α, which are related to neutrophilic inflammation, were elevated in an asthmatic airway. Several of these mediators and cytokines have also been shown to be elevated in neutrophilic asthma, of which LTB4, IL-8, TNF-α, IL-17, and IL-6 may be related to airway remodeling. Figure 2 shows neutrophilic inflammation-associated airway remodeling in asthma (Figure 2).

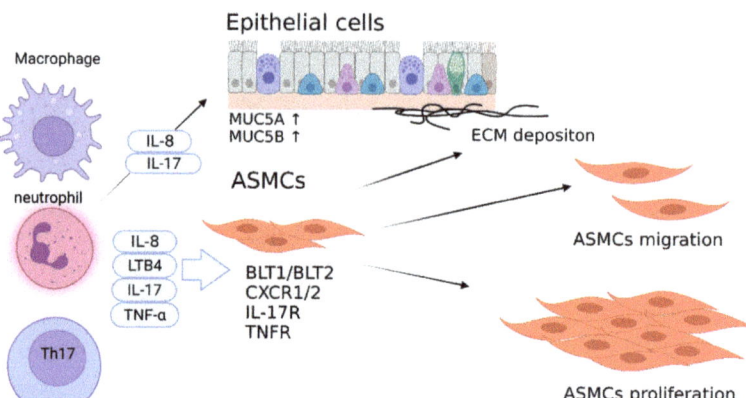

Figure 2. Airway remodeling in asthma related to neutrophilic inflammation. Airway remodeling in asthma is a characteristic feature of chronic asthma. LTB4, IL-8, LTB4, and TNF-α are elevated in an asthmatic airway and are related to airway remodeling. LTB4, IL-8, and TNF-α induce airway smooth muscle cell proliferation and migration. IL-8 and IL-17 upregulate MUC5A and MUC5B expression in epithelial cells. Abbreviations: IL, interleukin; LTB4, leukotriene B4, TNF-α; Tumor necrosis factor α, BLT1/2: leukotriene B4 receptor 1/2, IL-17R: IL-17 receptor, TNFR: TNF receptor, ASMCs: airway smooth muscle cells.

6.1. Leukotriene B4

In severe asthma, leukotriene B4 (LTB4) is increased in sputum, BALF, exhaled breath condensate, urine, and arterial blood [209]. LTB4 is a chemoattractant mediator of neutrophils [210] and has been found to recruit eosinophils in a guinea pig model [211,212]. The relationship between LTB4 and airway remodeling has not been fully studied, but BLT1 and BLT2 are expressed on HASM cells. LTB4 has been shown to induce HASM cell migration and proliferation in vitro [213]. Therefore, LTB4 might be involved in airway remodeling in asthma.

6.2. IL-8

IL-8 is increased in sputum or BALF from patients with severe asthma and is inversely correlated with %predicted FEV1 and sputum neutrophil counts [23,24,59,214–216]. A recent study showed that IL-8 in BALF was the only cytokine that distinguished controlled from uncontrolled asthma among 48 evaluated cytokines [216]. IL-8 has been shown to induce HASM cell proliferation and migration [217–219], to stimulate mucin secretion [220], and to upregulate MUC5A and MUC5B in goblet cells [221]. YKL-40 has been shown to induce IL-8 in bronchial epithelial cells and to cause HASM cell proliferation and migration [222]. Therefore, IL-8 might be related to severe neutrophilic asthma and airway remodeling in asthma.

6.3. TNF-α

TNF-α is a proinflammatory cytokine related to neutrophilic asthma. In vitro, TNF-α induced airway smooth muscle migration and proliferation [223], extracellular matrix deposition, subepithelial fibrosis, and inflammatory cytokine secretion [224,225]. In a mouse model, TNF-α was involved in glucocorticoid insensitivity in neutrophilic inflammation in asthma, which may induce chronic inflammation and lead to airway remodeling [226]. In vitro, miR874, which may be associated with the development of asthma, has been shown to inhibit TNF-α-induced IL-6, IL-8, collagen I, and collagen III production in ASM cells [224].

6.4. IL-17A

IL-17A is an independent risk factor for severe asthma and is involved in obesity-associated asthma and CS-related airway neutrophilia [82,163,227]. In a mouse model, IL-17A induced type V collagen expression, *TGFB1* mRNA expression, and SMAD3 activation in airway epithelial cells [228]. In vitro, MUC5A and MUC5B expressions have been induced by IL-17A via IL-6 and NF-κB in epithelial cells [229–231]. IL-17A has also been shown to be involved in the epithelia mesenchymal transition via expression of TGF-β1 in airway epithelial cells [232]. In a mouse model, IL-17 was involved in airway smooth muscle hyperplasia mediated by fibroblast growth factor 2 from airway epithelial cells, and neutrophil elastase played an important role in this model [233,234]. In other mouse models using OVA and LPS for exacerbation, anti-IL-17A antibody decreased extracellular matrix deposition [235] and vascular remodeling [234]. Therefore, IL-17A comodulated with TGF-β1 is involved in airway remodeling in asthma and is related to neutrophils [236].

6.5. Other Inflammatory Mediators and Cytokines

IL-1β has been shown to induce neutrophilic asthma and IL-33 expression in a mouse model of asthma with viral infection exacerbation [148], and was a key cytokine in induction of airway smooth muscle hypersensitivity [237]. IL-1β alone or with TNF superfamily members has been observed to cause airway neutrophilic inflammation and remodeling in an adult animal model [238,239]. Oncostatin M (OSM) is released from neutrophils and induces epithelial barrier dysfunction [240]. In severe asthma, there are increases in OSM in sputum and in OSM-positive neutrophils in biopsy specimens [241]. OSM is also increased in patients with asthma with fixed airway obstruction [242]. Furthermore, MMP9 and elastase may be involved in airway remodeling in asthma [243–245].

7. Treatment

Treatment with an ICS is a key approach for asthma, but corticosteroids are not effective in neutrophilic asthma [246,247]. Treatment of asthma related to neutrophilic inflammation can be categorized into non-pharmacological approaches, nonspecific treatment for neutrophil inflammation, treatment specific to neutrophils and neutrophil mediators, and biologics (Table 2).

Table 2. Summary of treatment for asthma related to neutrophilic inflammation.

	Non-Pharmacological Approach		
Approach	Patient Population	Outcomes	Ref.
Smoking cessation	Young patients with asthma (19–40 years old), steroid-free, 17% neutrophilic asthma	Improved asthma control and flung function	[248]
Weight loss	18–75-year-old, obese patients with asthma (BMI > 35 kg/m^2)	Improved asthma control, QOL, lung function, and AHR	[249]
Nonspecific treatment for neutrophilic asthma			
Therapy	Patient population	Outcomes	Ref.
Macrolide (azithromycin, clarithromycin)	Non-eosinophilic or neutrophilic severe asthma (18–75-year-old patients)	Reduced asthma exacerbation, QOL, and lung function	[250]
PDE inhibitor	Patients 18–70 years of age, moderate-to-severe asthma	Improved lung function and asthma control	[251]

Table 2. Cont.

Non-Pharmacological Approach			
Approach	Patient Population	Outcomes	Ref.
Tiotropium	Adult symptomatic patients with asthma despite treatment with medium-dose ICS	Improved lung function and asthma control, reduced risk of severe exacerbation, independent of type 2 inflammation	[252]
Tiotropium	6–17-year-old patients, symptomatic severe asthma	Improved lung function and ACQ, reduced risk of exacerbation, independent of type 2 inflammation	[253]
Specific treatment for neutrophil and mediators			
SCH527123/CXCR2	Severe asthma and sputum neutrophil >40%	Fewer mild exacerbations and a trend towards improvement in the ACQ, but not statistically significant	[254]
GSK2090915/FLAP	Persistent asthma treated with SABA only	Improved symptom score and reduced SABA use	[255]
Zileuton/5-LO	Moderate-to-severe asthma treated with low dose ICS	Improved PEF and symptoms	[256]
Biologics			
Tezepelumab/TSLP	Moderate-to-severe asthma	Reduced rate of exacerbation, improved lung function, ACQ, and AQLQ, regardless of type 2 inflammation	[257]
Golimumab/TNF-α	Uncontrolled asthma with high-dose ICS/LABA	No improvement in FEV1 and exacerbation	[258]
Etanercept/TNF-α	Moderate-to-severe persistent asthma	No improvement in FEV1 and ACQ, exacerbation, AHR, AQLQ	[259]
Brodalumab/IL-17 receptor	Inadequately controlled moderate-to-severe asthma treated with high-dose ICS ± LABA	No treatment differences were observed	[260]
Risankinumab/IL-23	Adult patients with severe asthma	No improvement in asthma exacerbation	[261]
Tocilizumab/IL-6	Mild asthma	No improvement in allergen-induced bronchoconstriction	[262]

7.1. Non-Pharmacological Approach

Smoking cessation may be the best way to reduce neutrophilic inflammation in neutrophilic asthma patients who smoke. In a clinical trial, smoking cessation in young adults with asthma improved asthma control, but with persistent eosinophil counts and little neutrophil reduction [248]. In this trial, 17% of the subjects had neutrophilic asthma. Another clinical trial showed improvements in lung function and sputum neutrophil counts [151]. Weight loss by diet, exercise, diet with exercise, or surgical intervention also improved asthma control, quality of life, lung function, and airway hyperresponsiveness [249,263–266]. Thus, smoking cessation and weight loss are good approaches for patients with severe asthma, regardless of the inflammatory phenotype.

7.2. Nonspecific Treatment for Neutrophilic Inflammation
7.2.1. Macrolides

Macrolides have various functions, in addition to their actions as antibiotics [267]. The effectiveness of clarithromycin has been shown in chronic stable asthma with *Mycoplasma pneumoniae* or *Chlamydia pneumoniae* mRNA in the airway [268]. The AMAZES study showed the effectiveness of azithromycin for persistent uncontrolled asthma [269]. In this study, 43% of the cases were eosinophilic, 11% neutrophilic, 30% paucigranulocytic, and 4% mixed, based on sputum phenotyping. A subset analysis in the AMAZES study showed that azithromycin was similarly effective for severe asthma in the cases with an eosinophilic sputum phenotype [269]. The effect of azithromycin was correlated with the abundance of *Haemophiles influenzae* colonization as assessed by quantitative polymerase chain reaction [270]. In the AMAZES study, sputum TNFR1 and TNFR2 were increased in neutrophilic asthma and azithromycin reduced sputum TNFR2 in non-eosinophilic asthma, which may be related to the therapeutic mechanism [271]. The AZISAST study showed a reduced rate of severe exacerbation by azithromycin in non-eosinophilic severe asthma [272]; in a study in severe neutrophilic asthma, 8-week administration of this drug improved quality of life and reduced airway IL-8 and neutrophils [250]. Therefore, long term macrolide treatment is a promising therapy in severe asthma, particularly for the neutrophil-dominant phenotype.

7.2.2. Phosphodiesterase Inhibitors

Roflumilast is an oral phosphodiesterase (PDE) inhibitor that has therapeutic effects on COPD [273] and asthma-COPD overlap [274]. Several studies have shown the efficacy of roflumilast alone [275,276] or in combination with a leukotriene receptor antagonist in moderate-to-severe asthma [277]. Roflumilast attenuates both eosinophilic and neutrophilic inflammation induced by allergens [251,278]. Inhaled PDE inhibitors have also been examined in patients with asthma (reviewed in [279]): CH6001 showed inhibition of the late asthmatic response induced by allergen exposure [280] and RPL554 (a PDE3 and PDE4 inhibitor) increased FEV1 in patients with asthma and reduced neutrophils and total cells in sputum from healthy individuals [281]. Studies of PDE inhibitors focusing on neutrophilic asthma are needed, but roflumilast and inhaled PDE4 inhibitors may be promising for neutrophilic asthma [282].

7.2.3. Anticholinergics

Anticholinergics have been used for treatment of COPD and asthma. Long-acting muscarinic antagonist (LAMAs) and short-acting muscarinic antagonists are both available for treatment of asthma. LAMAs decreased eosinophils in sensitized mice [283,284], and in an obstructive airway disease model in rat, tiotropium decreased neutrophil counts, IL-1β and IL-6 in bronchoalveolar lavage [285]. In an in vitro study in human epithelial cells, tiotropium reduced IL-8 production induced by IL-17A [286] or LPS [287]. In clinical studies, tiotropium has been shown to be effective as an add-on therapy to ICS [288] or ICS/LABA [289] in uncontrolled asthma, and Iwamoto et al. found that anti-cholinergics were effective in non-eosinophilic asthma [290]. Tiotropium has been shown to be effective, independent of type 2 inflammation in adults [252,291,292] and in children and adolescents [253]. However, the efficacy of ICS or tiotropium was similar to that of a placebo in patients with mild persistent asthma, including 73% with low eosinophilic asthma [293].

7.3. Specific Therapy for Neutrophils and Neutrophil Mediators
7.3.1. CXCR2 Antagonists

CXCR2 is a receptor for IL-8 that is expressed on neutrophils. A CXCR2 inhibitor, SCH527123, reduced sputum neutrophils and exacerbation in severe asthma cases in a 4-week clinical trial [254]. Another CXCR2 antagonist, AZD5069, reduced neutrophils in bronchial mucosa, sputum, and blood, but failed to reduce severe exacerbation [294,295].

7.3.2. 5-Lipoxygenase-Activating Protein Inhibitors and 5-Lipoxygenase Inhibitors

Five-lipoxygenase-activating protein (FLAP) and 5-lipoxygenase (5-LO) are required for synthesis of LTB4. GSK2190915 is a FLAP inhibitor that has been evaluated for patients with asthma in several studies [255,296,297]. In one study focused on neutrophilic asthma, a FLAP inhibitor suppressed sputum LTB4 and urine LTE4 levels, but failed to reduce neutrophil counts in sputum and had no clinical effects on FEV1, PEF, and ACQ scores [296]. Zileuton is a 5-LO inhibitor that has also been evaluated in patients with asthma [256,298] and has been shown to be effective in moderate-to-severe asthma based on improved PEF and asthma symptoms [256]. A recent retrospective study showed no associations among Th2-high or Th2-low phenotypes and a poor response rate to zileuton in association with severe asthma and obesity [298].

7.4. Biologics

Several biological agents are currently available for patients with severe asthma. There are six FDA-approved monoclonal antibodies (mAbs): omalizumab, which is anti-IgE antibody; mepolizumab and reslizumab, which are anti-IL-5 antibodies; benralizumab, which is an anti-IL-5 receptor α antibody; dupilumab, which is an anti-IL-4 receptor α antibody; and tezepelumab, which is an anti-TSLP antibody. These biologics exhibited clinical benefits for allergic/Th2-high asthma [299].

7.4.1. Targeting TSLP

Tezepelumab, a humanized mAb for TSLP, has been tested in a phase 2 clinical trial in patients with moderate-to-severe asthma [300] and in a phase 3 clinical trial in patients with severe asthma [257]. Tezepelumab reduced the rate of exacerbation and improved FEV1, ACQ, and AQLQ scores, regardless of type 2 inflammation. Therefore, tezepelumab may be effective for severe neutrophilic asthma. Biphasic antibodies for TSLP/IL-13 (zweimab and doppelmab) have recently been developed [301] and may also be evaluated for treatment of severe asthma with type 2, non-type 2, or neutrophilic inflammation.

7.4.2. Targeting TNF-α

Blocking of TNF-α by infliximab and golimumab, which are anti-TNF-α mAbs, and etanercept, which is a recombinant TNF-α receptor, has been examined as treatment for moderate and severe asthma [258,259,302–304]. In patients with severe and uncontrolled asthma under treatment with high-dose ICS and LABAs, golimumab did not improve FEV1 or the rate of exacerbation [258]. Etanercept, in several clinical trails, has been shown to improve airway hyper-responsiveness (AHR); FEV1, AQLQ, and ACQ scores; and asthma symptoms; as well as to reduce sputum macrophages and CRP levels in several clinicals trials [302–304]. However, a large, randomized clinical study of etanercept for moderate-to-severe asthma showed no efficacy for ACQ, AQLQ, FEV1, exacerbation rate, or AHR [259].

7.4.3. Targeting IL-17

Anti-IL-17 antibody has been shown to decrease airway hyper-responsiveness and airway inflammation in a mouse model of obesity, alone [305] or in combination with a Rho-kinase inhibitor [306]. Secukinumab, an mAb targeting IL-17A, was tested in a randomized clinical trial in patients with severe asthma treated with high doses of ICS alone or in combination with a LABA. In this trial, responders (defined as patients with a 5% increase in predicted FEV1) showed increased nasal epithelial neutrophilic inflammation and had decreased markers of IgE-driven systemic inflammation based on a nasal brushing pathway analysis of differentially regulated genes [307]. A randomized, double-blind, placebo-controlled study of brodalumab, a monoclonal antibody targeting IL-17 receptor A, showed no treatment effect in subjects with moderate-to-severe asthma [260]. A bispecific antibody targeting IL-13 and IL-17 showed clinical safety with no deaths or serious adverse events in a phase I study [308].

7.4.4. Targeting IL-23

As mentioned above, IL-17 is involved in neutrophilic inflammation in asthma and IL-23, an IL-12 family cytokine, is important for maintenance and recruitment of Th17 cells [309]. However, risankizumab, an IL23p19 mAb, failed to show efficacy for worsening of asthma as compared with a placebo in a phase I, randomized, double-blind, placebo-controlled study in adults with severe asthma, with no significant changes in sputum cell differentials [261].

7.4.5. Targeting IL-6

Tocilizumab, an anti-IL-6 receptor mAb, had effects on CRP, IL-6, and soluble IL-6 receptor, but did not improve allergen-induced bronchoconstriction in 11 patients with mild asthma [262].

7.5. Other Potential Therapy for Neutrophilic Asthma

Peroxisome proliferator-activated receptor-gamma agonists have been tested in a murine model of neutrophilic asthma [310]. Statins are also candidate drugs for patients with obesity and asthma [311,312]. Inhibitors of protein kinases, p38 MAPK, and phosphoinositide 3-kinase (PI3K δ and γ) have been examined for COPD or asthma [312–315]. These inhibitors might be effective in neutrophilic asthma because the PI3K pathway is involved in neutrophil migration and degranulation [316,317]. Glucagon-like peptide-1 receptor (GLP-1R) agonists inhibit aeroallergen-induced activation of ILC2 and neutrophilic airway inflammation in obese mice [318]. Fore et al. found that patients with asthma who received GLP-1R agonists had less exacerbation than those treated with sulfonylureas or insulin [319]. Some of these drugs have been tested for asthma or COPD, but not specifically for neutrophilic asthma.

8. Conclusions

Asthma is a heterogenous syndrome that includes neutrophilic asthma as one phenotype. There is still uncertainty about this phenotype, but many studies have shown the importance of neutrophils in asthma. There is no clear definition of neutrophilic asthma, but sputum and peripheral blood neutrophils, YKL-40, H_2S, MPA, and miRNAs may be useful biomarkers for this condition. Identification of new biomarkers or combinations of biomarkers will be important for future diagnosis of neutrophilic asthma. Neutrophilic inflammation is involved in airway remodeling in patients with asthma, including those with obesity and GERD. Non-pharmacological and pharmacological therapy, including targeting of neutrophils and nonspecific treatment, may be useful for neutrophilic asthma, but most treatments have yet to be tested in patients with this condition. Further studies, focused on non-type 2 cases and neutrophilic inflammation, are needed to develop treatment for severe neutrophilic asthma.

Author Contributions: Conceptualization, A.Y.; writing—original draft preparation, A.Y.; writing—review and editing, A.Y., R.O. and T.H. All authors have read and agreed to the published version of the manuscript.

Funding: This research received no external funding.

Institutional Review Board Statement: Not applicable.

Informed Consent Statement: Not applicable.

Acknowledgments: Figures are created with BioRender.com assessed on 27 April 2022 and on 4 May 2022.

Conflicts of Interest: A.Y. received speaker honorariums from Asahi Kasei Pharma, AstraZeneca, Boehringer Ingelheim, Chugai, Glaxo Smith Kline, Janssen, Kyorin, Mitsubishi Tanabe Pharma, Novartis, Ono, and Sanofi, outside of the submitted work. R.O. received speaker honorariums from Chugai, Ono, Sanofi, Jansen, and Nippon Shinyaku, outside of the submitted work. T.H. received speaker honorariums from Asahi Kasei Pharma, AstraZeneca, Glaxo Smith Kline, Janssen, Nippon Shinyaku, and Sanofi, outside of the submitted work.

References

1. Fukutomi, Y.; Nakamura, H.; Kobayashi, F.; Taniguchi, M.; Konno, S.; Nishimura, M.; Kawagishi, Y.; Watanabe, J.; Komase, Y.; Akamatsu, Y.; et al. Nationwide cross-sectional population-based study on the prevalences of asthma and asthma symptoms among Japanese adults. *Int. Arch. Allergy Immunol.* **2010**, *153*, 280–287. [CrossRef]
2. Nakamura, Y.; Tamaoki, J.; Nagase, H.; Yamaguchi, M.; Horiguchi, T.; Hozawa, S.; Ichinose, M.; Iwanaga, T.; Kondo, R.; Nagata, M.; et al. Japanese guidelines for adult asthma 2020. *Allergol. Int.* **2020**, *69*, 519–548. [CrossRef]
3. Lambrecht, B.N.; Hammad, H. The immunology of asthma. *Nat. Immunol.* **2015**, *16*, 45–56. [CrossRef]
4. Robinson, D.; Humbert, M.; Buhl, R.; Cruz, A.A.; Inoue, H.; Korom, S.; Hanania, N.A.; Nair, P. Revisiting Type 2-high and Type 2-low airway inflammation in asthma: Current knowledge and therapeutic implications. *Clin. Exp. Allergy* **2017**, *47*, 161–175. [CrossRef]
5. Hinks, T.S.C.; Hoyle, R.D.; Gelfand, E.W. CD8$^+$ Tc2 cells: Underappreciated contributors to severe asthma. *Eur. Respir. Rev.* **2019**, *28*, 190092. [CrossRef]
6. Bel, E.H. Clinical phenotypes of asthma. *Curr. Opin. Pulm. Med.* **2004**, *10*, 44–50. [CrossRef]
7. Wenzel, S.E. Asthma phenotypes: The evolution from clinical to molecular approaches. *Nat. Med.* **2012**, *18*, 716–725. [CrossRef]
8. Haldar, P.; Pavord, I.D.; Shaw, D.E.; Berry, M.A.; Thomas, M.; Brightling, C.E.; Wardlaw, A.J.; Green, R.H. Cluster analysis and clinical asthma phenotypes. *Am. J. Respir. Crit. Care Med.* **2008**, *178*, 218–224. [CrossRef]
9. Grobal Initiative for Asthma. Global Strategy for Asthma Management and Prevention 2021. Available online: www.ginasthma.org (accessed on 21 September 2021).
10. Moore, W.C.; Meyers, D.A.; Wenzel, S.E.; Teague, W.G.; Li, H.; Li, X.; D'Agostino, R., Jr.; Castro, M.; Curran-Everett, D.; Fitzpatrick, A.M.; et al. Identification of asthma phenotypes using cluster analysis in the Severe Asthma Research Program. *Am. J. Respir. Crit. Care Med.* **2010**, *181*, 315–323. [CrossRef]
11. Kuo, C.S.; Pavlidis, S.; Loza, M.; Baribaud, F.; Rowe, A.; Pandis, I.; Sousa, A.; Corfield, J.; Djukanovic, R.; Lutter, R.; et al. T-helper cell type 2 (Th2) and non-Th2 molecular phenotypes of asthma using sputum transcriptomics in U-BIOPRED. *Eur. Respir. J.* **2017**, *49*, 1602135. [CrossRef]
12. Hogg, J.C. Neutrophil kinetics and lung injury. *Physiol. Rev.* **1987**, *67*, 1249–1295. [CrossRef]
13. Nair, P.; Surette, M.G.; Virchow, J.C. Neutrophilic asthma: Misconception or misnomer? *Lancet Respir. Med.* **2021**, *9*, 441–443. [CrossRef]
14. Nair, P.; Prabhavalkar, K.S. Neutrophilic Asthma and Potentially Related Target Therapies. *Curr. Drug Targets* **2020**, *21*, 374–388. [CrossRef]
15. Nabe, T. Steroid-Resistant Asthma and Neutrophils. *Biol. Pharm. Bull.* **2020**, *43*, 31–35. [CrossRef]
16. Crisford, H.; Sapey, E.; Rogers, G.B.; Taylor, S.; Nagakumar, P.; Lokwani, R.; Simpson, J.L. Neutrophils in asthma: The good, the bad and the bacteria. *Thorax* **2021**, *76*, 835–844. [CrossRef]
17. Strickland, I.; Kisich, K.; Hauk, P.J.; Vottero, A.; Chrousos, G.P.; Klemm, D.J.; Leung, D.Y. High constitutive glucocorticoid receptor beta in human neutrophils enables them to reduce their spontaneous rate of cell death in response to corticosteroids. *J. Exp. Med.* **2001**, *193*, 585–593. [CrossRef]
18. Saffar, A.S.; Ashdown, H.; Gounni, A.S. The molecular mechanisms of glucocorticoids-mediated neutrophil survival. *Curr. Drug Targets* **2011**, *12*, 556–562. [CrossRef]
19. Shimoda, T.; Obase, Y.; Nagasaka, Y.; Nakano, H.; Kishikawa, R.; Iwanaga, T. Airway inflammation phenotype prediction in asthma patients using lung sound analysis with fractional exhaled nitric oxide. *Allergol. Int.* **2017**, *66*, 581–585. [CrossRef]
20. Berry, M.; Morgan, A.; Shaw, D.E.; Parker, D.; Green, R.; Brightling, C.; Bradding, P.; Wardlaw, A.J.; Pavord, I.D. Pathological features and inhaled corticosteroid response of eosinophilic and non-eosinophilic asthma. *Thorax* **2007**, *62*, 1043–1049. [CrossRef]
21. Toyran, M.; Bakirtas, A.; Dogruman-Al, F.; Turktas, I. Airway inflammation and bronchial hyperreactivity in steroid naive children with intermittent and mild persistent asthma. *Pediatr. Pulmonol.* **2014**, *49*, 140–147. [CrossRef]
22. Louis, R.; Sele, J.; Henket, M.; Cataldo, D.; Bettiol, J.; Seiden, L.; Bartsch, P. Sputum eosinophil count in a large population of patients with mild to moderate steroid-naive asthma: Distribution and relationship with methacholine bronchial hyperresponsiveness. *Allergy* **2002**, *57*, 907–912. [CrossRef]
23. Jatakanon, A.; Uasuf, C.; Maziak, W.; Lim, S.; Chung, K.F.; Barnes, P.J. Neutrophilic inflammation in severe persistent asthma. *Am. J. Respir. Crit. Care Med.* **1999**, *160*, 1532–1539. [CrossRef]
24. Gibson, P.G.; Simpson, J.L.; Saltos, N. Heterogeneity of airway inflammation in persistent asthma: Evidence of neutrophilic inflammation and increased sputum interleukin-8. *Chest* **2001**, *119*, 1329–1336. [CrossRef]
25. Moore, W.C.; Hastie, A.T.; Li, X.; Li, H.; Busse, W.W.; Jarjour, N.N.; Wenzel, S.E.; Peters, S.P.; Meyers, D.A.; Bleecker, E.R.; et al. Sputum neutrophil counts are associated with more severe asthma phenotypes using cluster analysis. *J. Allergy Clin. Immunol.* **2014**, *133*, 1557–1563.e5. [CrossRef]
26. Mincham, K.T.; Bruno, N.; Singanayagam, A.; Snelgrove, R.J. Our evolving view of neutrophils in defining the pathology of chronic lung disease. *Immunology* **2021**, *164*, 701–721. [CrossRef]
27. Alashkar Alhamwe, B.; Potaczek, D.P.; Miethe, S.; Alhamdan, F.; Hintz, L.; Magomedov, A.; Garn, H. Extracellular Vesicles and Asthma-More Than Just a Co-Existence. *Int. J. Mol. Sci.* **2021**, *22*, 4984. [CrossRef]
28. Belda, J.; Leigh, R.; Parameswaran, K.; O'Byrne, P.M.; Sears, M.R.; Hargreave, F.E. Induced sputum cell counts in healthy adults. *Am. J. Respir. Crit. Care Med.* **2000**, *161*, 475–478. [CrossRef]

29. Chung, K.F. Asthma phenotyping: A necessity for improved therapeutic precision and new targeted therapies. *J. Intern. Med.* **2016**, *279*, 192–204. [CrossRef]
30. Schleich, F.; Brusselle, G.; Louis, R.; Vandenplas, O.; Michils, A.; Pilette, C.; Peche, R.; Manise, M.; Joos, G. Heterogeneity of phenotypes in severe asthmatics. The Belgian Severe Asthma Registry (BSAR). *Respir. Med.* **2014**, *108*, 1723–1732. [CrossRef]
31. Grunwell, J.R.; Stephenson, S.T.; Tirouvanziam, R.; Brown, L.A.S.; Brown, M.R.; Fitzpatrick, A.M. Children with Neutrophil-Predominant Severe Asthma Have Proinflammatory Neutrophils With Enhanced Survival and Impaired Clearance. *J. Allergy Clin. Immunol. Pract.* **2019**, *7*, 516–525.e6. [CrossRef]
32. Stemmy, E.J.; Benton, A.S.; Lerner, J.; Alcala, S.; Constant, S.L.; Freishtat, R.J. Extracellular cyclophilin levels associate with parameters of asthma in phenotypic clusters. *J. Asthma* **2011**, *48*, 986–993. [CrossRef]
33. Kikuchi, S.; Nagata, M.; Kikuchi, I.; Hagiwara, K.; Kanazawa, M. Association between neutrophilic and eosinophilic inflammation in patients with severe persistent asthma. *Int. Arch. Allergy Immunol.* **2005**, *137* (Suppl. S1), 7–11. [CrossRef]
34. Jarjour, N.N.; Erzurum, S.C.; Bleecker, E.R.; Calhoun, W.J.; Castro, M.; Comhair, S.A.; Chung, K.F.; Curran-Everett, D.; Dweik, R.A.; Fain, S.B.; et al. Severe asthma: Lessons learned from the National Heart, Lung, and Blood Institute Severe Asthma Research Program. *Am. J. Respir. Crit. Care Med.* **2012**, *185*, 356–362. [CrossRef]
35. Hastie, A.T.; Mauger, D.T.; Denlinger, L.C.; Coverstone, A.; Castro, M.; Erzurum, S.; Jarjour, N.; Levy, B.D.; Meyers, D.A.; Moore, W.C.; et al. Baseline sputum eosinophil + neutrophil subgroups' clinical characteristics and longitudinal trajectories for NHLBI Severe Asthma Research Program (SARP 3) cohort. *J. Allergy Clin. Immunol.* **2020**, *146*, 222–226. [CrossRef]
36. Marc-Malovrh, M.; Camlek, L.; Skrgat, S.; Kern, I.; Flezar, M.; Dezman, M.; Korosec, P. Elevated eosinophils, IL5 and IL8 in induced sputum in asthma patients with accelerated FEV1 decline. *Respir. Med.* **2020**, *162*, 105875. [CrossRef]
37. Katz, B.; Sofonio, M.; Lyden, P.D.; Mitchell, M.D. Prostaglandin concentrations in cerebrospinal fluid of rabbits under normal and ischemic conditions. *Stroke* **1988**, *19*, 349–351. [CrossRef]
38. Kikuchi, I.; Kikuchi, S.; Kobayashi, T.; Hagiwara, K.; Sakamoto, Y.; Kanazawa, M.; Nagata, M. Eosinophil trans-basement membrane migration induced by interleukin-8 and neutrophils. *Am. J. Respir. Cell Mol. Biol.* **2006**, *34*, 760–765. [CrossRef]
39. Nishihara, F.; Nakagome, K.; Kobayashi, T.; Noguchi, T.; Araki, R.; Uchida, Y.; Soma, T.; Nagata, M. Trans-basement membrane migration of eosinophils induced by LPS-stimulated neutrophils from human peripheral blood in vitro. *ERJ Open Res.* **2015**, *1*, 00003-2015. [CrossRef]
40. Kikuchi, I.; Kikuchi, S.; Kobayashi, T.; Takaku, Y.; Hagiwara, K.; Kanazawa, M.; Nagata, M. Theophylline attenuates the neutrophil-dependent augmentation of eosinophil trans-basement membrane migration. *Int. Arch. Allergy Immunol.* **2007**, *143* (Suppl. S1), 44–49. [CrossRef]
41. Lavinskiene, S.; Bajoriuniene, I.; Malakauskas, K.; Jeroch, J.; Sakalauskas, R. Sputum neutrophil count after bronchial allergen challenge is related to peripheral blood neutrophil chemotaxis in asthma patients. *Inflamm. Res.* **2014**, *63*, 951–959. [CrossRef]
42. Gauvreau, G.M.; Sehmi, R.; Ambrose, C.S.; Griffiths, J.M. Thymic stromal lymphopoietin: Its role and potential as a therapeutic target in asthma. *Expert Opin. Ther. Targets* **2020**, *24*, 777–792. [CrossRef]
43. Menzies-Gow, A.; Wechsler, M.E.; Brightling, C.E. Unmet need in severe, uncontrolled asthma: Can anti-TSLP therapy with tezepelumab provide a valuable new treatment option? *Respir. Res.* **2020**, *21*, 268. [CrossRef]
44. Takai, T. TSLP expression: Cellular sources, triggers, and regulatory mechanisms. *Allergol. Int.* **2012**, *61*, 3–17. [CrossRef]
45. Gour, N.; Lajoie, S. Epithelial Cell Regulation of Allergic Diseases. *Curr. Allergy Asthma Rep.* **2016**, *16*, 65. [CrossRef]
46. Tanaka, J.; Watanabe, N.; Kido, M.; Saga, K.; Akamatsu, T.; Nishio, A.; Chiba, T. Human TSLP and TLR3 ligands promote differentiation of Th17 cells with a central memory phenotype under Th2-polarizing conditions. *Clin. Exp. Allergy* **2009**, *39*, 89–100. [CrossRef]
47. Gao, H.; Ying, S.; Dai, Y. Pathological Roles of Neutrophil-Mediated Inflammation in Asthma and Its Potential for Therapy as a Target. *J. Immunol. Res.* **2017**, *2017*, 3743048. [CrossRef]
48. Moorehead, A.; Hanna, R.; Heroux, D.; Neighbour, H.; Sandford, A.; Gauvreau, G.M.; Sommer, D.D.; Denburg, J.A.; Akhabir, L. A thymic stromal lymphopoietin polymorphism may provide protection from asthma by altering gene expression. *Clin. Exp. Allergy* **2020**, *50*, 471–478. [CrossRef]
49. Vazquez-Tello, A.; Semlali, A.; Chakir, J.; Martin, J.G.; Leung, D.Y.; Eidelman, D.H.; Hamid, Q. Induction of glucocorticoid receptor-beta expression in epithelial cells of asthmatic airways by T-helper type 17 cytokines. *Clin. Exp. Allergy* **2010**, *40*, 1312–1322. [CrossRef]
50. Rahman, M.S.; Yamasaki, A.; Yang, J.; Shan, L.; Halayko, A.J.; Gounni, A.S. IL-17A induces eotaxin-1/CC chemokine ligand 11 expression in human airway smooth muscle cells: Role of MAPK (Erk1/2, JNK, and p38) pathways. *J. Immunol.* **2006**, *177*, 4064–4071. [CrossRef]
51. Al-Ramli, W.; Prefontaine, D.; Chouiali, F.; Martin, J.G.; Olivenstein, R.; Lemiere, C.; Hamid, Q. T(H)17-associated cytokines (IL-17A and IL-17F) in severe asthma. *J. Allergy Clin. Immunol.* **2009**, *123*, 1185–1187. [CrossRef]
52. Bullens, D.M.; Truyen, E.; Coteur, L.; Dilissen, E.; Hellings, P.W.; Dupont, L.J.; Ceuppens, J.L. IL-17 mRNA in sputum of asthmatic patients: Linking T cell driven inflammation and granulocytic influx? *Respir. Res.* **2006**, *7*, 135. [CrossRef] [PubMed]
53. Oikawa, T.; Shimamura, M.; Ashino-Fuse, H.; Iwaguchi, T.; Ishizuka, M.; Takeuchi, T. Inhibition of angiogenesis by 15-deoxyspergualin. *J. Antibiot.* **1991**, *44*, 1033–1035. [CrossRef] [PubMed]
54. Liu, D.; Tan, Y.; Bajinka, O.; Wang, L.; Tang, Z. Th17/IL-17 Axis Regulated by Airway Microbes Get Involved in the Development of Asthma. *Curr. Allergy Asthma Rep.* **2020**, *20*, 11. [CrossRef] [PubMed]

55. Noval Rivas, M.; Crother, T.R.; Arditi, M. The microbiome in asthma. *Curr. Opin. Pediatr.* **2016**, *28*, 764–771. [CrossRef]
56. Liu, W.; Liu, S.; Verma, M.; Zafar, I.; Good, J.T.; Rollins, D.; Groshong, S.; Gorska, M.M.; Martin, R.J.; Alam, R. Mechanism of TH2/TH17-predominant and neutrophilic TH2/TH17-low subtypes of asthma. *J. Allergy Clin. Immunol.* **2017**, *139*, 1548–1558.e4. [CrossRef]
57. Abdel-Aziz, M.I.; Brinkman, P.; Vijverberg, S.J.H.; Neerincx, A.H.; Riley, J.H.; Bates, S.; Hashimoto, S.; Kermani, N.Z.; Chung, K.F.; Djukanovic, R.; et al. Sputum microbiome profiles identify severe asthma phenotypes of relative stability at 12 to 18 months. *J. Allergy Clin. Immunol.* **2021**, *147*, 123–134. [CrossRef]
58. Yang, X.; Li, H.; Ma, Q.; Zhang, Q.; Wang, C. Neutrophilic Asthma Is Associated with Increased Airway Bacterial Burden and Disordered Community Composition. *Biomed. Res. Int.* **2018**, *2018*, 9230234. [CrossRef]
59. Green, B.J.; Wiriyachaiporn, S.; Grainge, C.; Rogers, G.B.; Kehagia, V.; Lau, L.; Carroll, M.P.; Bruce, K.D.; Howarth, P.H. Potentially pathogenic airway bacteria and neutrophilic inflammation in treatment resistant severe asthma. *PLoS ONE* **2014**, *9*, e100645. [CrossRef]
60. Essilfie, A.T.; Simpson, J.L.; Horvat, J.C.; Preston, J.A.; Dunkley, M.L.; Foster, P.S.; Gibson, P.G.; Hansbro, P.M. Haemophilus influenzae infection drives IL-17-mediated neutrophilic allergic airways disease. *PLoS Pathog.* **2011**, *7*, e1002244. [CrossRef]
61. Yang, B.; Liu, R.; Yang, T.; Jiang, X.; Zhang, L.; Wang, L.; Wang, Q.; Luo, Z.; Liu, E.; Fu, Z. Neonatal Streptococcus pneumoniae infection may aggravate adulthood allergic airways disease in association with IL-17A. *PLoS ONE* **2015**, *10*, e0123010. [CrossRef]
62. Kozik, A.J.; Huang, Y.J. The microbiome in asthma: Role in pathogenesis, phenotype, and response to treatment. *Ann. Allergy Asthma Immunol.* **2019**, *122*, 270–275. [CrossRef] [PubMed]
63. Gilliland, F.D.; Berhane, K.; Islam, T.; McConnell, R.; Gauderman, W.J.; Gilliland, S.S.; Avol, E.; Peters, J.M. Obesity and the risk of newly diagnosed asthma in school-age children. *Am. J. Epidemiol.* **2003**, *158*, 406–415. [CrossRef] [PubMed]
64. Mamun, A.A.; Lawlor, D.A.; Alati, R.; O'Callaghan, M.J.; Williams, G.M.; Najman, J.M. Increasing body mass index from age 5 to 14 years predicts asthma among adolescents: Evidence from a birth cohort study. *Int. J. Obes.* **2007**, *31*, 578–583. [CrossRef] [PubMed]
65. Weinmayr, G.; Forastiere, F.; Buchele, G.; Jaensch, A.; Strachan, D.P.; Nagel, G.; Group, I.P.T.S. Overweight/obesity and respiratory and allergic disease in children: International study of asthma and allergies in childhood (ISAAC) phase two. *PLoS ONE* **2014**, *9*, e113996. [CrossRef]
66. Ho, W.C.; Lin, Y.S.; Caffrey, J.L.; Lin, M.H.; Hsu, H.T.; Myers, L.; Chen, P.C.; Lin, R.S. Higher body mass index may induce asthma among adolescents with pre-asthmatic symptoms: A prospective cohort study. *BMC Public Health* **2011**, *11*, 542. [CrossRef]
67. Schatz, M.; Hsu, J.W.; Zeiger, R.S.; Chen, W.; Dorenbaum, A.; Chipps, B.E.; Haselkorn, T. Phenotypes determined by cluster analysis in severe or difficult-to-treat asthma. *J. Allergy Clin. Immunol.* **2014**, *133*, 1549–1556. [CrossRef]
68. Holguin, F.; Bleecker, E.R.; Busse, W.W.; Calhoun, W.J.; Castro, M.; Erzurum, S.C.; Fitzpatrick, A.M.; Gaston, B.; Israel, E.; Jarjour, N.N.; et al. Obesity and asthma: An association modified by age of asthma onset. *J. Allergy Clin. Immunol.* **2011**, *127*, 1486–1493.e2. [CrossRef]
69. Peters-Golden, M.; Swern, A.; Bird, S.S.; Hustad, C.M.; Grant, E.; Edelman, J.M. Influence of body mass index on the response to asthma controller agents. *Eur. Respir. J.* **2006**, *27*, 495–503. [CrossRef]
70. Boulet, L.P.; Franssen, E. Influence of obesity on response to fluticasone with or without salmeterol in moderate asthma. *Respir. Med.* **2007**, *101*, 2240–2247. [CrossRef]
71. Hotamisligil, G.S.; Shargill, N.S.; Spiegelman, B.M. Adipose expression of tumor necrosis factor-alpha: Direct role in obesity-linked insulin resistance. *Science* **1993**, *259*, 87–91. [CrossRef]
72. Peters, U.; Dixon, A.E.; Forno, E. Obesity and asthma. *J. Allergy Clin. Immunol.* **2018**, *141*, 1169–1179. [CrossRef] [PubMed]
73. Loffreda, S.; Yang, S.Q.; Lin, H.Z.; Karp, C.L.; Brengman, M.L.; Wang, D.J.; Klein, A.S.; Bulkley, G.B.; Bao, C.; Noble, P.W.; et al. Leptin regulates proinflammatory immune responses. *FASEB J.* **1998**, *12*, 57–65. [CrossRef] [PubMed]
74. Komakula, S.; Khatri, S.; Mermis, J.; Savill, S.; Haque, S.; Rojas, M.; Brown, L.; Teague, G.W.; Holguin, F. Body mass index is associated with reduced exhaled nitric oxide and higher exhaled 8-isoprostanes in asthmatics. *Respir. Res.* **2007**, *8*, 32. [CrossRef] [PubMed]
75. Miethe, S.; Guarino, M.; Alhamdan, F.; Simon, H.U.; Renz, H.; Dufour, J.F.; Potaczek, D.P.; Garn, H. Effects of obesity on asthma: Immunometabolic links. *Pol. Arch. Intern. Med.* **2018**, *128*, 469–477. [CrossRef] [PubMed]
76. Kim, H.Y.; Lee, H.J.; Chang, Y.J.; Pichavant, M.; Shore, S.A.; Fitzgerald, K.A.; Iwakura, Y.; Israel, E.; Bolger, K.; Faul, J.; et al. Interleukin-17-producing innate lymphoid cells and the NLRP3 inflammasome facilitate obesity-associated airway hyperreactivity. *Nat. Med.* **2014**, *20*, 54–61. [CrossRef]
77. Honda, K.; Wada, H.; Nakamura, M.; Nakamoto, K.; Inui, T.; Sada, M.; Koide, T.; Takata, S.; Yokoyama, T.; Saraya, T.; et al. IL-17A synergistically stimulates TNF-alpha-induced IL-8 production in human airway epithelial cells: A potential role in amplifying airway inflammation. *Exp. Lung Res.* **2016**, *42*, 205–216. [CrossRef]
78. Prause, O.; Laan, M.; Lotvall, J.; Linden, A. Pharmacological modulation of interleukin-17-induced GCP-2-, GRO-alpha- and interleukin-8 release in human bronchial epithelial cells. *Eur. J. Pharmacol.* **2003**, *462*, 193–198. [CrossRef]
79. Lee, K.H.; Lee, C.H.; Woo, J.; Jeong, J.; Jang, A.H.; Yoo, C.G. Cigarette Smoke Extract Enhances IL-17A-Induced IL-8 Production via Up-Regulation of IL-17R in Human Bronchial Epithelial Cells. *Mol. Cells* **2018**, *41*, 282–289. [CrossRef]

80. Siew, L.Q.C.; Wu, S.Y.; Ying, S.; Corrigan, C.J. Cigarette smoking increases bronchial mucosal IL-17A expression in asthmatics, which acts in concert with environmental aeroallergens to engender neutrophilic inflammation. *Clin. Exp. Allergy* **2017**, *47*, 740–750. [CrossRef]
81. Linden, A. Role of interleukin-17 and the neutrophil in asthma. *Int. Arch. Allergy Immunol.* **2001**, *126*, 179–184. [CrossRef]
82. Al Heialy, S.; Gaudet, M.; Ramakrishnan, R.K.; Mogas, A.; Salameh, L.; Mahboub, B.; Hamid, Q. Contribution of IL-17 in Steroid Hyporesponsiveness in Obese Asthmatics Through Dysregulation of Glucocorticoid Receptors alpha and beta. *Front. Immunol.* **2020**, *11*, 1724. [CrossRef] [PubMed]
83. Zijlstra, G.J.; Ten Hacken, N.H.; Hoffmann, R.F.; van Oosterhout, A.J.; Heijink, I.H. Interleukin-17A induces glucocorticoid insensitivity in human bronchial epithelial cells. *Eur. Respir. J.* **2012**, *39*, 439–445. [CrossRef] [PubMed]
84. Park, Y.H.; Oh, E.Y.; Han, H.; Yang, M.; Park, H.J.; Park, K.H.; Lee, J.H.; Park, J.W. Insulin resistance mediates high-fat diet-induced pulmonary fibrosis and airway hyperresponsiveness through the TGF-beta1 pathway. *Exp. Mol. Med.* **2019**, *51*, 1–12. [CrossRef]
85. Cardet, J.C.; Ash, S.; Kusa, T.; Camargo, C.A., Jr.; Israel, E. Insulin resistance modifies the association between obesity and current asthma in adults. *Eur. Respir. J.* **2016**, *48*, 403–410. [CrossRef] [PubMed]
86. Sanchez Jimenez, J.; Herrero Espinet, F.J.; Mengibar Garrido, J.M.; Roca Antonio, J.; Penos Mayor, S.; Penas Boira Mdel, M.; Roca Comas, A.; Ballester Martinez, A. Asthma and insulin resistance in obese children and adolescents. *Pediatr. Allergy Immunol.* **2014**, *25*, 699–705. [CrossRef] [PubMed]
87. Han, H.; Chung, S.I.; Park, H.J.; Oh, E.Y.; Kim, S.R.; Park, K.H.; Lee, J.H.; Park, J.W. Obesity-induced Vitamin D Deficiency Contributes to Lung Fibrosis and Airway Hyperresponsiveness. *Am. J. Respir. Cell Mol. Biol.* **2021**, *64*, 357–367. [CrossRef]
88. Brinkmann, V.; Reichard, U.; Goosmann, C.; Fauler, B.; Uhlemann, Y.; Weiss, D.S.; Weinrauch, Y.; Zychlinsky, A. Neutrophil extracellular traps kill bacteria. *Science* **2004**, *303*, 1532–1535. [CrossRef] [PubMed]
89. Cheng, O.Z.; Palaniyar, N. NET balancing: A problem in inflammatory lung diseases. *Front. Immunol.* **2013**, *4*, 1. [CrossRef]
90. Liu, C.L.; Tangsombatvisit, S.; Rosenberg, J.M.; Mandelbaum, G.; Gillespie, E.C.; Gozani, O.P.; Alizadeh, A.A.; Utz, P.J. Specific post-translational histone modifications of neutrophil extracellular traps as immunogens and potential targets of lupus autoantibodies. *Arthritis Res. Ther.* **2012**, *14*, R25. [CrossRef]
91. Doring, Y.; Manthey, H.D.; Drechsler, M.; Lievens, D.; Megens, R.T.; Soehnlein, O.; Busch, M.; Manca, M.; Koenen, R.R.; Pelisek, J.; et al. Auto-antigenic protein-DNA complexes stimulate plasmacytoid dendritic cells to promote atherosclerosis. *Circulation* **2012**, *125*, 1673–1683. [CrossRef]
92. Krishnamoorthy, N.; Douda, D.N.; Bruggemann, T.R.; Ricklefs, I.; Duvall, M.G.; Abdulnour, R.E.; Martinod, K.; Tavares, L.; Wang, X.; Cernadas, M.; et al. Neutrophil cytoplasts induce TH17 differentiation and skew inflammation toward neutrophilia in severe asthma. *Sci. Immunol.* **2018**, *3*, eaao4747. [CrossRef] [PubMed]
93. Wright, T.K.; Gibson, P.G.; Simpson, J.L.; McDonald, V.M.; Wood, L.G.; Baines, K.J. Neutrophil extracellular traps are associated with inflammation in chronic airway disease. *Respirology* **2016**, *21*, 467–475. [CrossRef] [PubMed]
94. Lachowicz-Scroggins, M.E.; Dunican, E.M.; Charbit, A.R.; Raymond, W.; Looney, M.R.; Peters, M.C.; Gordon, E.D.; Woodruff, P.G.; Lefrancais, E.; Phillips, B.R.; et al. Extracellular DNA, Neutrophil Extracellular Traps, and Inflammasome Activation in Severe Asthma. *Am. J. Respir. Crit. Care Med.* **2019**, *199*, 1076–1085. [CrossRef] [PubMed]
95. Kelley, N.; Jeltema, D.; Duan, Y.; He, Y. The NLRP3 Inflammasome: An Overview of Mechanisms of Activation and Regulation. *Int. J. Mol. Sci.* **2019**, *20*, 3328. [CrossRef] [PubMed]
96. He, Y.; Hara, H.; Nunez, G. Mechanism and Regulation of NLRP3 Inflammasome Activation. *Trends Biochem. Sci.* **2016**, *41*, 1012–1021. [CrossRef]
97. Heppner, F.L.; Ransohoff, R.M.; Becher, B. Immune attack: The role of inflammation in Alzheimer disease. *Nat. Rev. Neurosci.* **2015**, *16*, 358–372. [CrossRef]
98. Wang, S.; Yuan, Y.H.; Chen, N.H.; Wang, H.B. The mechanisms of NLRP3 inflammasome/pyroptosis activation and their role in Parkinson's disease. *Int. Immunopharmacol.* **2019**, *67*, 458–464. [CrossRef]
99. Strowig, T.; Henao-Mejia, J.; Elinav, E.; Flavell, R. Inflammasomes in health and disease. *Nature* **2012**, *481*, 278–286. [CrossRef]
100. Lasithiotaki, I.; Giannarakis, I.; Tsitoura, E.; Samara, K.D.; Margaritopoulos, G.A.; Choulaki, C.; Vasarmidi, E.; Tzanakis, N.; Voloudaki, A.; Sidiropoulos, P.; et al. NLRP3 inflammasome expression in idiopathic pulmonary fibrosis and rheumatoid lung. *Eur. Respir. J.* **2016**, *47*, 910–918. [CrossRef]
101. Jager, B.; Seeliger, B.; Terwolbeck, O.; Warnecke, G.; Welte, T.; Muller, M.; Bode, C.; Prasse, A. The NLRP3-Inflammasome-Caspase-1 Pathway Is Upregulated in Idiopathic Pulmonary Fibrosis and Acute Exacerbations and Is Inducible by Apoptotic A549 Cells. *Front. Immunol.* **2021**, *12*, 642855. [CrossRef]
102. Huppertz, C.; Jager, B.; Wieczorek, G.; Engelhard, P.; Oliver, S.J.; Bauernfeind, F.G.; Littlewood-Evans, A.; Welte, T.; Hornung, V.; Prasse, A. The NLRP3 inflammasome pathway is activated in sarcoidosis and involved in granuloma formation. *Eur. Respir. J.* **2020**, *55*, 1900119. [CrossRef] [PubMed]
103. Dostert, C.; Petrilli, V.; Van Bruggen, R.; Steele, C.; Mossman, B.T.; Tschopp, J. Innate immune activation through Nalp3 inflammasome sensing of asbestos and silica. *Science* **2008**, *320*, 674–677. [CrossRef] [PubMed]
104. Pinkerton, J.W.; Kim, R.Y.; Robertson, A.A.B.; Hirota, J.A.; Wood, L.G.; Knight, D.A.; Cooper, M.A.; O'Neill, L.A.J.; Horvat, J.C.; Hansbro, P.M. Inflammasomes in the lung. *Mol. Immunol.* **2017**, *86*, 44–55. [CrossRef]
105. Lamkanfi, M. Emerging inflammasome effector mechanisms. *Nat. Rev. Immunol.* **2011**, *11*, 213–220. [CrossRef] [PubMed]

106. Kim, R.Y.; Pinkerton, J.W.; Essilfie, A.T.; Robertson, A.A.B.; Baines, K.J.; Brown, A.C.; Mayall, J.R.; Ali, M.K.; Starkey, M.R.; Hansbro, N.G.; et al. Role for NLRP3 Inflammasome-mediated, IL-1beta-Dependent Responses in Severe, Steroid-Resistant Asthma. *Am. J. Respir. Crit. Care Med.* **2017**, *196*, 283–297. [CrossRef]
107. Rossios, C.; Pavlidis, S.; Hoda, U.; Kuo, C.H.; Wiegman, C.; Russell, K.; Sun, K.; Loza, M.J.; Baribaud, F.; Durham, A.L.; et al. Sputum transcriptomics reveal upregulation of IL-1 receptor family members in patients with severe asthma. *J. Allergy Clin. Immunol.* **2018**, *141*, 560–570. [CrossRef] [PubMed]
108. Wood, L.G.; Li, Q.; Scott, H.A.; Rutting, S.; Berthon, B.S.; Gibson, P.G.; Hansbro, P.M.; Williams, E.; Horvat, J.; Simpson, J.L.; et al. Saturated fatty acids, obesity, and the nucleotide oligomerization domain-like receptor protein 3 (NLRP3) inflammasome in asthmatic patients. *J. Allergy Clin. Immunol.* **2019**, *143*, 305–315. [CrossRef]
109. Ritter, M.; Straubinger, K.; Schmidt, S.; Busch, D.H.; Hagner, S.; Garn, H.; Prazeres da Costa, C.; Layland, L.E. Functional relevance of NLRP3 inflammasome-mediated interleukin (IL)-1beta during acute allergic airway inflammation. *Clin. Exp. Immunol.* **2014**, *178*, 212–223. [CrossRef]
110. Li, H.; Willingham, S.B.; Ting, J.P.; Re, F. Cutting edge: Inflammasome activation by alum and alum's adjuvant effect are mediated by NLRP3. *J. Immunol.* **2008**, *181*, 17–21. [CrossRef]
111. Sebag, S.C.; Koval, O.M.; Paschke, J.D.; Winters, C.J.; Jaffer, O.A.; Dworski, R.; Sutterwala, F.S.; Anderson, M.E.; Grumbach, I.M. Mitochondrial CaMKII inhibition in airway epithelium protects against allergic asthma. *JCI Insight* **2017**, *2*, e88297. [CrossRef]
112. Edgeworth, J.; Gorman, M.; Bennett, R.; Freemont, P.; Hogg, N. Identification of p8,14 as a highly abundant heterodimeric calcium binding protein complex of myeloid cells. *J. Biol. Chem.* **1991**, *266*, 7706–7713. [CrossRef]
113. Bhardwaj, R.S.; Zotz, C.; Zwadlo-Klarwasser, G.; Roth, J.; Goebeler, M.; Mahnke, K.; Falk, M.; Meinardus-Hager, G.; Sorg, C. The calcium-binding proteins MRP8 and MRP14 form a membrane-associated heterodimer in a subset of monocytes/macrophages present in acute but absent in chronic inflammatory lesions. *Eur. J. Immunol.* **1992**, *22*, 1891–1897. [CrossRef] [PubMed]
114. Hamada, N.; Maeyama, T.; Kawaguchi, T.; Yoshimi, M.; Fukumoto, J.; Yamada, M.; Yamada, S.; Kuwano, K.; Nakanishi, Y. The role of high mobility group box1 in pulmonary fibrosis. *Am. J. Respir. Cell Mol. Biol.* **2008**, *39*, 440–447. [CrossRef] [PubMed]
115. Lotze, M.T.; Tracey, K.J. High-mobility group box 1 protein (HMGB1): Nuclear weapon in the immune arsenal. *Nat. Rev. Immunol.* **2005**, *5*, 331–342. [CrossRef] [PubMed]
116. Ellerman, J.E.; Brown, C.K.; de Vera, M.; Zeh, H.J.; Billiar, T.; Rubartelli, A.; Lotze, M.T. Masquerader: High mobility group box-1 and cancer. *Clin. Cancer Res.* **2007**, *13*, 2836–2848. [CrossRef]
117. Halayko, A.J.; Ghavami, S. S100A8/A9: A mediator of severe asthma pathogenesis and morbidity? *Can. J. Physiol. Pharmacol.* **2009**, *87*, 743–755. [CrossRef]
118. Ogawa, E.N.; Ishizaka, A.; Tasaka, S.; Koh, H.; Ueno, H.; Amaya, F.; Ebina, M.; Yamada, S.; Funakoshi, Y.; Soejima, J.; et al. Contribution of high-mobility group box-1 to the development of ventilator-induced lung injury. *Am. J. Respir. Crit. Care Med.* **2006**, *174*, 400–407. [CrossRef]
119. Liu, S.; Stolz, D.B.; Sappington, P.L.; Macias, C.A.; Killeen, M.E.; Tenhunen, J.J.; Delude, R.L.; Fink, M.P. HMGB1 is secreted by immunostimulated enterocytes and contributes to cytomix-induced hyperpermeability of Caco-2 monolayers. *Am. J. Physiol. Cell Physiol.* **2006**, *290*, C990–C999. [CrossRef]
120. Buckley, S.T.; Ehrhardt, C. The receptor for advanced glycation end products (RAGE) and the lung. *J. Biomed. Biotechnol.* **2010**, *2010*, 917108. [CrossRef]
121. Brett, J.; Schmidt, A.M.; Yan, S.D.; Zou, Y.S.; Weidman, E.; Pinsky, D.; Nowygrod, R.; Neeper, M.; Przysiecki, C.; Shaw, A.; et al. Survey of the distribution of a newly characterized receptor for advanced glycation end products in tissues. *Am. J. Pathol.* **1993**, *143*, 1699–1712.
122. Akirav, E.M.; Preston-Hurlburt, P.; Garyu, J.; Henegariu, O.; Clynes, R.; Schmidt, A.M.; Herold, K.C. RAGE expression in human T cells: A link between environmental factors and adaptive immune responses. *PLoS ONE* **2012**, *7*, e34698. [CrossRef] [PubMed]
123. Chen, Y.; Akirav, E.M.; Chen, W.; Henegariu, O.; Moser, B.; Desai, D.; Shen, J.M.; Webster, J.C.; Andrews, R.C.; Mjalli, A.M.; et al. RAGE ligation affects T cell activation and controls T cell differentiation. *J. Immunol.* **2008**, *181*, 4272–4278. [CrossRef]
124. Manfredi, A.A.; Capobianco, A.; Esposito, A.; De Cobelli, F.; Canu, T.; Monno, A.; Raucci, A.; Sanvito, F.; Doglioni, C.; Nawroth, P.P.; et al. Maturing dendritic cells depend on RAGE for in vivo homing to lymph nodes. *J. Immunol.* **2008**, *180*, 2270–2275. [CrossRef] [PubMed]
125. Moser, B.; Desai, D.D.; Downie, M.P.; Chen, Y.; Yan, S.F.; Herold, K.; Schmidt, A.M.; Clynes, R. Receptor for advanced glycation end products expression on T cells contributes to antigen-specific cellular expansion in vivo. *J. Immunol.* **2007**, *179*, 8051–8058. [CrossRef] [PubMed]
126. Narumi, K.; Miyakawa, R.; Ueda, R.; Hashimoto, H.; Yamamoto, Y.; Yoshida, T.; Aoki, K. Proinflammatory Proteins S100A8/S100A9 Activate NK Cells via Interaction with RAGE. *J. Immunol.* **2015**, *194*, 5539–5548. [CrossRef]
127. Perkins, T.N.; Oczypok, E.A.; Dutz, R.E.; Donnell, M.L.; Myerburg, M.M.; Oury, T.D. The receptor for advanced glycation end products is a critical mediator of type 2 cytokine signaling in the lungs. *J. Allergy Clin. Immunol.* **2019**, *144*, 796–808.e12. [CrossRef] [PubMed]
128. Oczypok, E.A.; Milutinovic, P.S.; Alcorn, J.F.; Khare, A.; Crum, L.T.; Manni, M.L.; Epperly, M.W.; Pawluk, A.M.; Ray, A.; Oury, T.D. Pulmonary receptor for advanced glycation end-products promotes asthma pathogenesis through IL-33 and accumulation of group 2 innate lymphoid cells. *J. Allergy Clin. Immunol.* **2015**, *136*, 747–756.e4. [CrossRef] [PubMed]

129. Hay, A.N.; Potter, A.; Kasmark, L.; Zhu, J.; Leeth, C.M. Rapid Communication: TLR4 expressed but with reduced functionality on equine B lymphocytes. *J. Anim. Sci.* **2019**, *97*, 2175–2180. [CrossRef]
130. Zhao, S.; Sun, M.; Meng, H.; Ji, H.; Liu, Y.; Zhang, M.; Li, H.; Li, P.; Zhang, Y.; Zhang, Q. TLR4 expression correlated with PD-L1 expression indicates a poor prognosis in patients with peripheral T-cell lymphomas. *Cancer Manag. Res.* **2019**, *11*, 4743–4756. [CrossRef]
131. Rossol, M.; Heine, H.; Meusch, U.; Quandt, D.; Klein, C.; Sweet, M.J.; Hauschildt, S. LPS-induced cytokine production in human monocytes and macrophages. *Crit. Rev. Immunol.* **2011**, *31*, 379–446. [CrossRef]
132. Alves-Filho, J.C.; Tavares-Murta, B.M.; Barja-Fidalgo, C.; Benjamim, C.F.; Basile-Filho, A.; Arraes, S.M.; Cunha, F.Q. Neutrophil function in severe sepsis. *Endocr. Metab. Immune Disord. Drug Targets* **2006**, *6*, 151–158. [CrossRef] [PubMed]
133. Hwang, Y.H.; Lee, Y.; Paik, M.J.; Yee, S.T. Inhibitions of HMGB1 and TLR4 alleviate DINP-induced asthma in mice. *Toxicol. Res.* **2019**, *8*, 621–629. [CrossRef] [PubMed]
134. Shang, L.; Wang, L.; Shi, X.; Wang, N.; Zhao, L.; Wang, J.; Liu, C. HMGB1 was negatively regulated by HSF1 and mediated the TLR4/MyD88/NF-kappaB signal pathway in asthma. *Life Sci.* **2020**, *241*, 117120. [CrossRef] [PubMed]
135. Watanabe, T.; Asai, K.; Fujimoto, H.; Tanaka, H.; Kanazawa, H.; Hirata, K. Increased levels of HMGB-1 and endogenous secretory RAGE in induced sputum from asthmatic patients. *Respir. Med.* **2011**, *105*, 519–525. [CrossRef]
136. Zhou, Y.; Jiang, Y.Q.; Wang, W.X.; Zhou, Z.X.; Wang, Y.G.; Yang, L.; Ji, Y.L. HMGB1 and RAGE levels in induced sputum correlate with asthma severity and neutrophil percentage. *Hum. Immunol.* **2012**, *73*, 1171–1174. [CrossRef]
137. Yang, H.; Hreggvidsdottir, H.S.; Palmblad, K.; Wang, H.; Ochani, M.; Li, J.; Lu, B.; Chavan, S.; Rosas-Ballina, M.; Al-Abed, Y.; et al. A critical cysteine is required for HMGB1 binding to Toll-like receptor 4 and activation of macrophage cytokine release. *Proc. Natl. Acad. Sci. USA* **2010**, *107*, 11942–11947. [CrossRef]
138. Andersson, U.; Wang, H.; Palmblad, K.; Aveberger, A.C.; Bloom, O.; Erlandsson-Harris, H.; Janson, A.; Kokkola, R.; Zhang, M.; Yang, H.; et al. High mobility group 1 protein (HMG-1) stimulates proinflammatory cytokine synthesis in human monocytes. *J. Exp. Med.* **2000**, *192*, 565–570. [CrossRef]
139. Zhang, F.; Su, X.; Huang, G.; Xin, X.F.; Cao, E.H.; Shi, Y.; Song, Y. sRAGE alleviates neutrophilic asthma by blocking HMGB1/RAGE signalling in airway dendritic cells. *Sci. Rep.* **2017**, *7*, 14268. [CrossRef]
140. Lyu, Y.; Zhao, H.; Ye, Y.; Liu, L.; Zhu, S.; Xia, Y.; Zou, F.; Cai, S. Decreased soluble RAGE in neutrophilic asthma is correlated with disease severity and RAGE G82S variants. *Mol. Med. Rep.* **2018**, *17*, 4131–4137. [CrossRef]
141. Patregnani, J.T.; Brooks, B.A.; Chorvinsky, E.; Pillai, D.K. High BAL sRAGE is Associated with Low Serum Eosinophils and IgE in Children with Asthma. *Children* **2020**, *7*, 110. [CrossRef]
142. Allam, V.; Faiz, A.; Lam, M.; Rathnayake, S.N.H.; Ditz, B.; Pouwels, S.D.; Brandsma, C.A.; Timens, W.; Hiemstra, P.S.; Tew, G.W.; et al. RAGE and TLR4 differentially regulate airway hyperresponsiveness: Implications for COPD. *Allergy* **2021**, *76*, 1123–1135. [CrossRef] [PubMed]
143. Menson, K.E.; Mank, M.M.; Reed, L.F.; Walton, C.J.; Van Der Vliet, K.E.; Ather, J.L.; Chapman, D.G.; Smith, B.J.; Rincon, M.; Poynter, M.E. Therapeutic efficacy of IL-17A neutralization with corticosteroid treatment in a model of antigen-driven mixed-granulocytic asthma. *Am. J. Physiol. Lung Cell. Mol. Physiol.* **2020**, *319*, L693–L709. [CrossRef] [PubMed]
144. Mack, S.; Shin, J.; Ahn, Y.; Castaneda, A.R.; Peake, J.; Fulgar, C.; Zhang, J.; Cho, Y.H.; Pinkerton, K.E. Age-dependent pulmonary reactivity to house dust mite allergen: A model of adult-onset asthma? *Am. J. Physiol. Lung Cell. Mol. Physiol.* **2019**, *316*, L757–L763. [CrossRef] [PubMed]
145. Sadamatsu, H.; Takahashi, K.; Tashiro, H.; Kurihara, Y.; Kato, G.; Uchida, M.; Noguchi, Y.; Kurata, K.; Omura, S.; Sunazuka, T.; et al. The Nonantibiotic Macrolide EM900 Attenuates House Dust Mite-Induced Airway Inflammation in a Mouse Model of Obesity-Associated Asthma. *Int. Arch. Allergy Immunol.* **2020**, *181*, 665–674. [CrossRef] [PubMed]
146. Lin, J.; Huang, N.; Li, J.; Liu, X.; Xiong, Q.; Hu, C.; Chen, D.; Guan, L.; Chang, K.; Li, D.; et al. Cross-reactive antibodies against dust mite-derived enolase induce neutrophilic airway inflammation. *Eur. Respir. J.* **2021**, *57*, 1902375. [CrossRef] [PubMed]
147. Kwak, D.W.; Park, D.; Kim, J.H. Leukotriene B4 receptors play critical roles in house dust mites-induced neutrophilic airway inflammation and IL-17 production. *Biochem. Biophys. Res. Commun.* **2021**, *534*, 646–652. [CrossRef]
148. Mahmutovic Persson, I.; Menzel, M.; Ramu, S.; Cerps, S.; Akbarshahi, H.; Uller, L. IL-1beta mediates lung neutrophilia and IL-33 expression in a mouse model of viral-induced asthma exacerbation. *Respir. Res.* **2018**, *19*, 16. [CrossRef]
149. Patel, D.F.; Peiro, T.; Bruno, N.; Vuononvirta, J.; Akthar, S.; Puttur, F.; Pyle, C.J.; Suveizdyte, K.; Walker, S.A.; Singanayagam, A.; et al. Neutrophils restrain allergic airway inflammation by limiting ILC2 function and monocyte-dendritic cell antigen presentation. *Sci. Immunol.* **2019**, *4*, eaax7006. [CrossRef]
150. Chalmers, G.W.; Macleod, K.J.; Little, S.A.; Thomson, L.J.; McSharry, C.P.; Thomson, N.C. Influence of cigarette smoking on inhaled corticosteroid treatment in mild asthma. *Thorax* **2002**, *57*, 226–230. [CrossRef]
151. Chaudhuri, R.; Livingston, E.; McMahon, A.D.; Lafferty, J.; Fraser, I.; Spears, M.; McSharry, C.P.; Thomson, N.C. Effects of smoking cessation on lung function and airway inflammation in smokers with asthma. *Am. J. Respir. Crit. Care Med.* **2006**, *174*, 127–133. [CrossRef]
152. Shimoda, T.; Obase, Y.; Kishikawa, R.; Iwanaga, T. Influence of cigarette smoking on airway inflammation and inhaled corticosteroid treatment in patients with asthma. *Allergy Asthma Proc.* **2016**, *37*, 50–58. [CrossRef] [PubMed]

153. Yamasaki, A.; Hanaki, K.; Tomita, K.; Watanabe, M.; Hasagawa, Y.; Okazaki, R.; Igishi, T.; Horimukai, K.; Fukutani, K.; Sugimoto, Y.; et al. Environmental tobacco smoke and its effect on the symptoms and medication in children with asthma. *Int. J. Environ. Health Res.* **2009**, *19*, 97–108. [CrossRef] [PubMed]
154. Ghosh, A.; Coakley, R.D.; Ghio, A.J.; Muhlebach, M.S.; Esther, C.R., Jr.; Alexis, N.E.; Tarran, R. Chronic E-Cigarette Use Increases Neutrophil Elastase and Matrix Metalloprotease Levels in the Lung. *Am. J. Respir. Crit. Care Med.* **2019**, *200*, 1392–1401. [CrossRef] [PubMed]
155. Schweitzer, R.J.; Wills, T.A.; Tam, E.; Pagano, I.; Choi, K. E-cigarette use and asthma in a multiethnic sample of adolescents. *Prev. Med.* **2017**, *105*, 226–231. [CrossRef] [PubMed]
156. Choi, K.; Bernat, D. E-Cigarette Use Among Florida Youth With and Without Asthma. *Am. J. Prev. Med.* **2016**, *51*, 446–453. [CrossRef] [PubMed]
157. Wu, Q.; Jiang, D.; Minor, M.; Chu, H.W. Electronic cigarette liquid increases inflammation and virus infection in primary human airway epithelial cells. *PLoS ONE* **2014**, *9*, e108342. [CrossRef]
158. Lerner, C.A.; Sundar, I.K.; Yao, H.; Gerloff, J.; Ossip, D.J.; McIntosh, S.; Robinson, R.; Rahman, I. Vapors produced by electronic cigarettes and e-juices with flavorings induce toxicity, oxidative stress, and inflammatory response in lung epithelial cells and in mouse lung. *PLoS ONE* **2015**, *10*, e0116732. [CrossRef]
159. Kioi, Y.; Tabuchi, T. Electronic, heat-not-burn, and combustible cigarette use among chronic disease patients in Japan: A cross-sectional study. *Tob. Induc. Dis.* **2018**, *16*, 41. [CrossRef]
160. Schaller, J.P.; Keller, D.; Poget, L.; Pratte, P.; Kaelin, E.; McHugh, D.; Cudazzo, G.; Smart, D.; Tricker, A.R.; Gautier, L.; et al. Evaluation of the Tobacco Heating System 2.2. Part 2: Chemical composition, genotoxicity, cytotoxicity, and physical properties of the aerosol. *Regul. Toxicol. Pharmacol.* **2016**, *81* (Suppl. S2), S27–S47. [CrossRef]
161. Smith, M.R.; Clark, B.; Ludicke, F.; Schaller, J.P.; Vanscheeuwijck, P.; Hoeng, J.; Peitsch, M.C. Evaluation of the Tobacco Heating System 2.2. Part 1: Description of the system and the scientific assessment program. *Regul. Toxicol. Pharmacol.* **2016**, *81* (Suppl. S2), S17–S26. [CrossRef]
162. Protano, C.; Manigrasso, M.; Cammalleri, V.; Biondi Zoccai, G.; Frati, G.; Avino, P.; Vitali, M. Impact of Electronic Alternatives to Tobacco Cigarettes on Indoor Air Particular Matter Levels. *Int. J. Environ. Res. Public Health* **2020**, *17*, 2947. [CrossRef] [PubMed]
163. Belvisi, M.G.; Baker, K.; Malloy, N.; Raemdonck, K.; Dekkak, B.; Pieper, M.; Nials, A.T.; Birrell, M.A. Modelling the asthma phenotype: Impact of cigarette smoke exposure. *Respir. Res.* **2018**, *19*, 89. [CrossRef] [PubMed]
164. Perret, J.L.; Bonevski, B.; McDonald, C.F.; Abramson, M.J. Smoking cessation strategies for patients with asthma: Improving patient outcomes. *J. Asthma Allergy* **2016**, *9*, 117–128. [CrossRef] [PubMed]
165. Masaki, K.; Tateno, H.; Kameyama, N.; Morino, E.; Watanabe, R.; Sekine, K.; Ono, T.; Satake, K.; Suzuki, S.; Nomura, A.; et al. Impact of a Novel Smartphone App (CureApp Smoking Cessation) on Nicotine Dependence: Prospective Single-Arm Interventional Pilot Study. *JMIR Mhealth Uhealth* **2019**, *7*, e12694. [CrossRef] [PubMed]
166. Guarnieri, M.; Balmes, J.R. Outdoor air pollution and asthma. *Lancet* **2014**, *383*, 1581–1592. [CrossRef]
167. Tiotiu, A.I.; Novakova, P.; Nedeva, D.; Chong-Neto, H.J.; Novakova, S.; Steiropoulos, P.; Kowal, K. Impact of Air Pollution on Asthma Outcomes. *Int. J. Environ. Res. Public Health* **2020**, *17*, 6212. [CrossRef] [PubMed]
168. Gowers, A.M.; Cullinan, P.; Ayres, J.G.; Anderson, H.R.; Strachan, D.P.; Holgate, S.T.; Mills, I.C.; Maynard, R.L. Does outdoor air pollution induce new cases of asthma? Biological plausibility and evidence; a review. *Respirology* **2012**, *17*, 887–898. [CrossRef]
169. Wu, J.Z.; Ge, D.D.; Zhou, L.F.; Hou, L.Y.; Zhou, Y.; Li, Q.Y. Effects of particulate matter on allergic respiratory diseases. *Chronic Dis. Transl. Med.* **2018**, *4*, 95–102. [CrossRef]
170. Wang, P.; Thevenot, P.; Saravia, J.; Ahlert, T.; Cormier, S.A. Radical-containing particles activate dendritic cells and enhance Th17 inflammation in a mouse model of asthma. *Am. J. Respir. Cell Mol. Biol.* **2011**, *45*, 977–983. [CrossRef]
171. van Voorhis, M.; Knopp, S.; Julliard, W.; Fechner, J.H.; Zhang, X.; Schauer, J.J.; Mezrich, J.D. Exposure to atmospheric particulate matter enhances Th17 polarization through the aryl hydrocarbon receptor. *PLoS ONE* **2013**, *8*, e82545. [CrossRef]
172. Brandt, E.B.; Kovacic, M.B.; Lee, G.B.; Gibson, A.M.; Acciani, T.H.; Le Cras, T.D.; Ryan, P.H.; Budelsky, A.L.; Khurana Hershey, G.K. Diesel exhaust particle induction of IL-17A contributes to severe asthma. *J. Allergy Clin. Immunol.* **2013**, *132*, 1194–1204.e2. [CrossRef] [PubMed]
173. Chang, M.M.; Wu, R.; Plopper, C.G.; Hyde, D.M. IL-8 is one of the major chemokines produced by monkey airway epithelium after ozone-induced injury. *Am. J. Physiol.* **1998**, *275*, L524–L532. [CrossRef] [PubMed]
174. Hiltermann, T.J.; Stolk, J.; Hiemstra, P.S.; Fokkens, P.H.; Rombout, P.J.; Sont, J.K.; Sterk, P.J.; Dijkman, J.H. Effect of ozone exposure on maximal airway narrowing in non-asthmatic and asthmatic subjects. *Clin. Sci.* **1995**, *89*, 619–624. [CrossRef] [PubMed]
175. Havemann, B.D.; Henderson, C.A.; El-Serag, H.B. The association between gastro-oesophageal reflux disease and asthma: A systematic review. *Gut* **2007**, *56*, 1654–1664. [CrossRef] [PubMed]
176. Liu, L.; Teague, W.G.; Erzurum, S.; Fitzpatrick, A.; Mantri, S.; Dweik, R.A.; Bleecker, E.R.; Meyers, D.; Busse, W.W.; Calhoun, W.J.; et al. Determinants of exhaled breath condensate pH in a large population with asthma. *Chest* **2011**, *139*, 328–336. [CrossRef]
177. Paoletti, G.; Melone, G.; Ferri, S.; Puggioni, F.; Baiardini, I.; Racca, F.; Canonica, G.W.; Heffler, E.; Malipiero, G. Gastroesophageal reflux and asthma: When, how, and why. *Curr. Opin. Allergy Clin. Immunol.* **2021**, *21*, 52–58. [CrossRef]
178. Simpson, J.L.; Baines, K.J.; Ryan, N.; Gibson, P.G. Neutrophilic asthma is characterised by increased rhinosinusitis with sleep disturbance and GERD. *Asian Pac. J. Allergy Immunol.* **2014**, *32*, 66–74. [CrossRef]

179. Icitovic, N.; Onyebeke, L.C.; Wallenstein, S.; Dasaro, C.R.; Harrison, D.; Jiang, J.; Kaplan, J.R.; Lucchini, R.G.; Luft, B.J.; Moline, J.M.; et al. The association between body mass index and gastroesophageal reflux disease in the World Trade Center Health Program General Responder Cohort. *Am. J. Ind. Med.* **2016**, *59*, 761–766. [CrossRef]
180. Gupta, S.; Lodha, R.; Kabra, S.K. Asthma, GERD and Obesity: Triangle of Inflammation. *Indian J. Pediatr.* **2018**, *85*, 887–892. [CrossRef]
181. Chupp, G.L.; Lee, C.G.; Jarjour, N.; Shim, Y.M.; Holm, C.T.; He, S.; Dziura, J.D.; Reed, J.; Coyle, A.J.; Kiener, P.; et al. A chitinase-like protein in the lung and circulation of patients with severe asthma. *N. Engl. J. Med.* **2007**, *357*, 2016–2027. [CrossRef]
182. James, A.J.; Reinius, L.E.; Verhoek, M.; Gomes, A.; Kupczyk, M.; Hammar, U.; Ono, J.; Ohta, S.; Izuhara, K.; Bel, E.; et al. Increased YKL-40 and Chitotriosidase in Asthma and Chronic Obstructive Pulmonary Disease. *Am. J. Respir. Crit. Care Med.* **2016**, *193*, 131–142. [CrossRef] [PubMed]
183. Liu, L.; Zhang, X.; Liu, Y.; Zhang, L.; Zheng, J.; Wang, J.; Hansbro, P.M.; Wang, L.; Wang, G.; Hsu, A.C. Chitinase-like protein YKL-40 correlates with inflammatory phenotypes, anti-asthma responsiveness and future exacerbations. *Respir. Res.* **2019**, *20*, 95. [CrossRef] [PubMed]
184. Suzuki, Y.; Saito, J.; Munakata, M.; Shibata, Y. Hydrogen sulfide as a novel biomarker of asthma and chronic obstructive pulmonary disease. *Allergol. Int.* **2021**, *70*, 181–189. [CrossRef] [PubMed]
185. Saito, J.; Zhang, Q.; Hui, C.; Macedo, P.; Gibeon, D.; Menzies-Gow, A.; Bhavsar, P.K.; Chung, K.F. Sputum hydrogen sulfide as a novel biomarker of obstructive neutrophilic asthma. *J. Allergy Clin. Immunol.* **2013**, *131*, 232–234.e3. [CrossRef]
186. Suzuki, Y.; Saito, J.; Kikuchi, M.; Uematsu, M.; Fukuhara, A.; Sato, S.; Munakata, M. Sputum-to-serum hydrogen sulphide ratio as a novel biomarker of predicting future risks of asthma exacerbation. *Clin. Exp. Allergy* **2018**, *48*, 1155–1163. [CrossRef]
187. Hinks, T.S.C.; Brown, T.; Lau, L.C.K.; Rupani, H.; Barber, C.; Elliott, S.; Ward, J.A.; Ono, J.; Ohta, S.; Izuhara, K.; et al. Multidimensional endotyping in patients with severe asthma reveals inflammatory heterogeneity in matrix metalloproteinases and chitinase 3-like protein 1. *J. Allergy Clin. Immunol.* **2016**, *138*, 61–75. [CrossRef]
188. Backman, H.; Lindberg, A.; Hedman, L.; Stridsman, C.; Jansson, S.A.; Sandstrom, T.; Lundback, B.; Ronmark, E. FEV1 decline in relation to blood eosinophils and neutrophils in a population-based asthma cohort. *World Allergy Organ. J.* **2020**, *13*, 100110. [CrossRef]
189. Backman, H.; Jansson, S.A.; Stridsman, C.; Muellerova, H.; Wurst, K.; Hedman, L.; Lindberg, A.; Ronmark, E. Chronic airway obstruction in a population-based adult asthma cohort: Prevalence, incidence and prognostic factors. *Respir. Med.* **2018**, *138*, 115–122. [CrossRef]
190. Huang, Y.; Zhang, S.; Fang, X.; Qin, L.; Fan, Y.; Ding, D.; Liu, X.; Xie, M. Plasma miR-199a-5p is increased in neutrophilic phenotype asthma patients and negatively correlated with pulmonary function. *PLoS ONE* **2018**, *13*, e0193502. [CrossRef]
191. Maes, T.; Cobos, F.A.; Schleich, F.; Sorbello, V.; Henket, M.; De Preter, K.; Bracke, K.R.; Conickx, G.; Mesnil, C.; Vandesompele, J.; et al. Asthma inflammatory phenotypes show differential microRNA expression in sputum. *J. Allergy Clin. Immunol.* **2016**, *137*, 1433–1446. [CrossRef]
192. Jafari-Nakhjavani, M.R.; Ghorbanihaghjo, A.; Bagherzadeh-Nobari, B.; Malek-Mahdavi, A.; Rashtchizadeh, N. Serum YKL-40 levels and disease characteristics in patients with rheumatoid arthritis. *Casp. J. Intern. Med.* **2019**, *10*, 92–97. [CrossRef]
193. Malmestrom, C.; Axelsson, M.; Lycke, J.; Zetterberg, H.; Blennow, K.; Olsson, B. CSF levels of YKL-40 are increased in MS and replaces with immunosuppressive treatment. *J. Neuroimmunol.* **2014**, *269*, 87–89. [CrossRef] [PubMed]
194. Przysucha, N.; Gorska, K.; Krenke, R. Chitinases and Chitinase-Like Proteins in Obstructive Lung Diseases—Current Concepts and Potential Applications. *Int. J. Chronic Obstr. Pulm. Dis.* **2020**, *15*, 885–899. [CrossRef] [PubMed]
195. Tong, X.; Wang, D.; Liu, S.; Ma, Y.; Li, Z.; Tian, P.; Fan, H. The YKL-40 protein is a potential biomarker for COPD: A meta-analysis and systematic review. *Int. J. Chronic Obstr. Pulm. Dis.* **2018**, *13*, 409–418. [CrossRef] [PubMed]
196. Olsson, B.; Lautner, R.; Andreasson, U.; Ohrfelt, A.; Portelius, E.; Bjerke, M.; Holtta, M.; Rosen, C.; Olsson, C.; Strobel, G.; et al. CSF and blood biomarkers for the diagnosis of Alzheimer's disease: A systematic review and meta-analysis. *Lancet Neurol.* **2016**, *15*, 673–684. [CrossRef]
197. Harrison, L.I.; Schuppan, D.; Rohlfing, S.R.; Hansen, A.R.; Hansen, C.S.; Funk, M.L.; Collins, S.H.; Ober, R.E. Determination of flumequine and a hydroxy metabolite in biological fluids by high-pressure liquid chromatographic, fluorometric, and microbiological methods. *Antimicrob. Agents Chemother.* **1984**, *25*, 301–305. [CrossRef] [PubMed]
198. Harnan, S.E.; Essat, M.; Gomersall, T.; Tappenden, P.; Pavord, I.; Everard, M.; Lawson, R. Exhaled nitric oxide in the diagnosis of asthma in adults: A systematic review. *Clin. Exp. Allergy* **2017**, *47*, 410–429. [CrossRef] [PubMed]
199. Zhang, J.; Yao, X.; Yu, R.; Bai, J.; Sun, Y.; Huang, M.; Adcock, I.M.; Barnes, P.J. Exhaled carbon monoxide in asthmatics: A meta-analysis. *Respir. Res.* **2010**, *11*, 50. [CrossRef]
200. Gao, J.; Iwamoto, H.; Koskela, J.; Alenius, H.; Hattori, N.; Kohno, N.; Laitinen, T.; Mazur, W.; Pulkkinen, V. Characterization of sputum biomarkers for asthma-COPD overlap syndrome. *Int. J. Chronic Obstr. Pulm. Dis.* **2016**, *11*, 2457–2465. [CrossRef]
201. Zhang, X.Y.; Simpson, J.L.; Powell, H.; Yang, I.A.; Upham, J.W.; Reynolds, P.N.; Hodge, S.; James, A.L.; Jenkins, C.; Peters, M.J.; et al. Full blood count parameters for the detection of asthma inflammatory phenotypes. *Clin. Exp. Allergy* **2014**, *44*, 1137–1145. [CrossRef]
202. Hastie, A.T.; Moore, W.C.; Li, H.; Rector, B.M.; Ortega, V.E.; Pascual, R.M.; Peters, S.P.; Meyers, D.A.; Bleecker, E.R.; National Heart, L.; et al. Biomarker surrogates do not accurately predict sputum eosinophil and neutrophil percentages in asthmatic subjects. *J. Allergy Clin. Immunol.* **2013**, *132*, 72–80. [CrossRef] [PubMed]

203. Hartjes, F.J.; Vonk, J.M.; Faiz, A.; Hiemstra, P.S.; Lapperre, T.S.; Kerstjens, H.A.M.; Postma, D.S.; van den Berge, M.; Groningen and Leiden Universities Corticosteroids in Obstructive Lung Disease (GLUCOLD) Study Group. Predictive value of eosinophils and neutrophils on clinical effects of ICS in COPD. *Respirology* **2018**, *23*, 1023–1031. [CrossRef] [PubMed]
204. Panganiban, R.P.; Pinkerton, M.H.; Maru, S.Y.; Jefferson, S.J.; Roff, A.N.; Ishmael, F.T. Differential microRNA epression in asthma and the role of miR-1248 in regulation of IL-5. *Am. J. Clin. Exp. Immunol.* **2012**, *1*, 154–165.
205. Milger, K.; Gotschke, J.; Krause, L.; Nathan, P.; Alessandrini, F.; Tufman, A.; Fischer, R.; Bartel, S.; Theis, F.J.; Behr, J.; et al. Identification of a plasma miRNA biomarker signature for allergic asthma: A translational approach. *Allergy* **2017**, *72*, 1962–1971. [CrossRef] [PubMed]
206. Gomez, J.L.; Chen, A.; Diaz, M.P.; Zirn, N.; Gupta, A.; Britto, C.; Sauler, M.; Yan, X.; Stewart, E.; Santerian, K.; et al. A Network of Sputum MicroRNAs Is Associated with Neutrophilic Airway Inflammation in Asthma. *Am. J. Respir. Crit. Care Med.* **2020**, *202*, 51–64. [CrossRef] [PubMed]
207. Canas, J.A.; Rodrigo-Munoz, J.M.; Sastre, B.; Gil-Martinez, M.; Redondo, N.; Del Pozo, V. MicroRNAs as Potential Regulators of Immune Response Networks in Asthma and Chronic Obstructive Pulmonary Disease. *Front. Immunol.* **2020**, *11*, 608666. [CrossRef]
208. Specjalski, K.; Niedoszytko, M. MicroRNAs: Future biomarkers and targets of therapy in asthma? *Curr. Opin. Pulm. Med.* **2020**, *26*, 285–292. [CrossRef]
209. Gelfand, E.W. Importance of the leukotriene B4-BLT1 and LTB4-BLT2 pathways in asthma. *Semin. Immunol.* **2017**, *33*, 44–51. [CrossRef]
210. Ford-Hutchinson, A.W.; Bray, M.A.; Doig, M.V.; Shipley, M.E.; Smith, M.J. Leukotriene B, a potent chemokinetic and aggregating substance released from polymorphonuclear leukocytes. *Nature* **1980**, *286*, 264–265. [CrossRef]
211. Teixeira, M.M.; Lindsay, M.A.; Giembycz, M.A.; Hellewell, P.G. Role of arachidonic acid in leukotriene B(4)-induced guinea-pig eosinophil homotypic aggregation. *Eur. J. Pharmacol.* **1999**, *384*, 183–190. [CrossRef]
212. Ng, C.F.; Sun, F.F.; Taylor, B.M.; Wolin, M.S.; Wong, P.Y. Functional properties of guinea pig eosinophil leukotriene B4 receptor. *J. Immunol.* **1991**, *147*, 3096–3103. [PubMed]
213. Watanabe, S.; Yamasaki, A.; Hashimoto, K.; Shigeoka, Y.; Chikumi, H.; Hasegawa, Y.; Sumikawa, T.; Takata, M.; Okazaki, R.; Watanabe, M.; et al. Expression of functional leukotriene B4 receptors on human airway smooth muscle cells. *J. Allergy Clin. Immunol.* **2009**, *124*, 59–65.e3. [CrossRef] [PubMed]
214. Lamblin, C.; Gosset, P.; Tillie-Leblond, I.; Saulnier, F.; Marquette, C.H.; Wallaert, B.; Tonnel, A.B. Bronchial neutrophilia in patients with noninfectious status asthmaticus. *Am. J. Respir. Crit. Care Med.* **1998**, *157*, 394–402. [CrossRef]
215. Wood, L.G.; Baines, K.J.; Fu, J.; Scott, H.A.; Gibson, P.G. The neutrophilic inflammatory phenotype is associated with systemic inflammation in asthma. *Chest* **2012**, *142*, 86–93. [CrossRef]
216. Hosoki, K.; Ying, S.; Corrigan, C.; Qi, H.; Kurosky, A.; Jennings, K.; Sun, Q.; Boldogh, I.; Sur, S. Analysis of a Panel of 48 Cytokines in BAL Fluids Specifically Identifies IL-8 Levels as the Only Cytokine that Distinguishes Controlled Asthma from Uncontrolled Asthma, and Correlates Inversely with FEV1. *PLoS ONE* **2015**, *10*, e0126035. [CrossRef]
217. Kuo, P.L.; Hsu, Y.L.; Huang, M.S.; Chiang, S.L.; Ko, Y.C. Bronchial epithelium-derived IL-8 and RANTES increased bronchial smooth muscle cell migration and proliferation by Kruppel-like factor 5 in areca nut-mediated airway remodeling. *Toxicol. Sci.* **2011**, *121*, 177–190. [CrossRef]
218. Govindaraju, V.; Michoud, M.C.; Al-Chalabi, M.; Ferraro, P.; Powell, W.S.; Martin, J.G. Interleukin-8: Novel roles in human airway smooth muscle cell contraction and migration. *Am. J. Physiol. Cell Physiol.* **2006**, *291*, C957–C965. [CrossRef] [PubMed]
219. Halwani, R.; Al-Abri, J.; Beland, M.; Al-Jahdali, H.; Halayko, A.J.; Lee, T.H.; Al-Muhsen, S.; Hamid, Q. CC and CXC chemokines induce airway smooth muscle proliferation and survival. *J. Immunol.* **2011**, *186*, 4156–4163. [CrossRef] [PubMed]
220. Tamaoki, J.; Nakata, J.; Tagaya, E.; Konno, K. Effects of roxithromycin and erythromycin on interleukin 8-induced neutrophil recruitment and goblet cell secretion in guinea pig tracheas. *Antimicrob. Agents Chemother.* **1996**, *40*, 1726–1728. [CrossRef]
221. Smirnova, M.G.; Birchall, J.P.; Pearson, J.P. In vitro study of IL-8 and goblet cells: Possible role of IL-8 in the aetiology of otitis media with effusion. *Acta Oto-Laryngol.* **2002**, *122*, 146–152. [CrossRef]
222. Tang, H.; Sun, Y.; Shi, Z.; Huang, H.; Fang, Z.; Chen, J.; Xiu, Q.; Li, B. YKL-40 induces IL-8 expression from bronchial epithelium via MAPK (JNK and ERK) and NF-kappaB pathways, causing bronchial smooth muscle proliferation and migration. *J. Immunol.* **2013**, *190*, 438–446. [CrossRef] [PubMed]
223. Li, X.; Zou, F.; Lu, Y.; Fan, X.; Wu, Y.; Feng, X.; Sun, X.; Liu, Y. Notch1 contributes to TNF-alpha-induced proliferation and migration of airway smooth muscle cells through regulation of the Hes1/PTEN axis. *Int. Immunopharmacol.* **2020**, *88*, 106911. [CrossRef] [PubMed]
224. Sun, M.; Huang, Y.; Li, F.; Li, H.; Zhang, B.; Jin, L. MicroRNA-874 inhibits TNF-alpha-induced remodeling in human fetal airway smooth muscle cells by targeting STAT3. *Respir. Physiol. Neurobiol.* **2018**, *251*, 34–40. [CrossRef] [PubMed]
225. Cho, J.Y.; Pham, A.; Rosenthal, P.; Miller, M.; Doherty, T.; Broide, D.H. Chronic OVA allergen challenged TNF p55/p75 receptor deficient mice have reduced airway remodeling. *Int. Immunopharmacol.* **2011**, *11*, 1038–1044. [CrossRef]
226. Dejager, L.; Dendoncker, K.; Eggermont, M.; Souffriau, J.; Van Hauwermeiren, F.; Willart, M.; Van Wonterghem, E.; Naessens, T.; Ballegeer, M.; Vandevyver, S.; et al. Neutralizing TNFalpha restores glucocorticoid sensitivity in a mouse model of neutrophilic airway inflammation. *Mucosal Immunol.* **2015**, *8*, 1212–1225. [CrossRef]

227. Agache, I.; Ciobanu, C.; Agache, C.; Anghel, M. Increased serum IL-17 is an independent risk factor for severe asthma. *Respir. Med.* **2010**, *104*, 1131–1137. [CrossRef]
228. Vittal, R.; Fan, L.; Greenspan, D.S.; Mickler, E.A.; Gopalakrishnan, B.; Gu, H.; Benson, H.L.; Zhang, C.; Burlingham, W.; Cummings, O.W.; et al. IL-17 induces type V collagen overexpression and EMT via TGF-beta-dependent pathways in obliterative bronchiolitis. *Am. J. Physiol. Lung Cell. Mol. Physiol.* **2013**, *304*, L401–L414. [CrossRef]
229. Chen, Y.; Thai, P.; Zhao, Y.H.; Ho, Y.S.; DeSouza, M.M.; Wu, R. Stimulation of airway mucin gene expression by interleukin (IL)-17 through IL-6 paracrine/autocrine loop. *J. Biol. Chem.* **2003**, *278*, 17036–17043. [CrossRef]
230. Fujisawa, T.; Chang, M.M.; Velichko, S.; Thai, P.; Hung, L.Y.; Huang, F.; Phuong, N.; Chen, Y.; Wu, R. NF-kappaB mediates IL-1beta- and IL-17A-induced MUC5B expression in airway epithelial cells. *Am. J. Respir. Cell Mol. Biol.* **2011**, *45*, 246–252. [CrossRef]
231. Fujisawa, T.; Velichko, S.; Thai, P.; Hung, L.Y.; Huang, F.; Wu, R. Regulation of airway MUC5AC expression by IL-1beta and IL-17A; the NF-kappaB paradigm. *J. Immunol.* **2009**, *183*, 6236–6243. [CrossRef]
232. Wang, T.; Liu, Y.; Zou, J.F.; Cheng, Z.S. Interleukin-17 induces human alveolar epithelial to mesenchymal cell transition via the TGF-beta1 mediated Smad2/3 and ERK1/2 activation. *PLoS ONE* **2017**, *12*, e0183972. [CrossRef]
233. Ogawa, H.; Azuma, M.; Tsunematsu, T.; Morimoto, Y.; Kondo, M.; Tezuka, T.; Nishioka, Y.; Tsuneyama, K. Neutrophils induce smooth muscle hyperplasia via neutrophil elastase-induced FGF-2 in a mouse model of asthma with mixed inflammation. *Clin. Exp. Allergy* **2018**, *48*, 1715–1725. [CrossRef] [PubMed]
234. Camargo, L.D.N.; Dos Santos, T.M.; de Andrade, F.C.P.; Fukuzaki, S.; Dos Santos Lopes, F.; de Arruda Martins, M.; Prado, C.M.; Leick, E.A.; Righetti, R.F.; Tiberio, I. Bronchial Vascular Remodeling Is Attenuated by Anti-IL-17 in Asthmatic Responses Exacerbated by LPS. *Front. Pharmacol.* **2020**, *11*, 1269. [CrossRef]
235. Camargo, L.D.N.; Righetti, R.F.; Aristoteles, L.; Dos Santos, T.M.; de Souza, F.C.R.; Fukuzaki, S.; Cruz, M.M.; Alonso-Vale, M.I.C.; Saraiva-Romanholo, B.M.; Prado, C.M.; et al. Effects of Anti-IL-17 on Inflammation, Remodeling, and Oxidative Stress in an Experimental Model of Asthma Exacerbated by LPS. *Front. Immunol.* **2017**, *8*, 1835. [CrossRef]
236. Ramakrishnan, R.K.; Al Heialy, S.; Hamid, Q. Role of IL-17 in asthma pathogenesis and its implications for the clinic. *Expert Rev. Respir. Med.* **2019**, *13*, 1057–1068. [CrossRef] [PubMed]
237. Liao, Z.; Xiao, H.T.; Zhang, Y.; Tong, R.S.; Zhang, L.J.; Bian, Y.; He, X. IL-1beta: A key modulator in asthmatic airway smooth muscle hyper-reactivity. *Expert Rev. Respir. Med.* **2015**, *9*, 429–436. [CrossRef] [PubMed]
238. Lappalainen, U.; Whitsett, J.A.; Wert, S.E.; Tichelaar, J.W.; Bry, K. Interleukin-1beta causes pulmonary inflammation, emphysema, and airway remodeling in the adult murine lung. *Am. J. Respir. Cell Mol. Biol.* **2005**, *32*, 311–318. [CrossRef]
239. Mehta, A.K.; Doherty, T.; Broide, D.; Croft, M. Tumor necrosis factor family member LIGHT acts with IL-1beta and TGF-beta to promote airway remodeling during rhinovirus infection. *Allergy* **2018**, *73*, 1415–1424. [CrossRef]
240. Pothoven, K.L.; Norton, J.E.; Hulse, K.E.; Suh, L.A.; Carter, R.G.; Rocci, E.; Harris, K.E.; Shintani-Smith, S.; Conley, D.B.; Chandra, R.K.; et al. Oncostatin M promotes mucosal epithelial barrier dysfunction, and its expression is increased in patients with eosinophilic mucosal disease. *J. Allergy Clin. Immunol.* **2015**, *136*, 737–746.e4. [CrossRef]
241. Pothoven, K.L.; Norton, J.E.; Suh, L.A.; Carter, R.G.; Harris, K.E.; Biyasheva, A.; Welch, K.; Shintani-Smith, S.; Conley, D.B.; Liu, M.C.; et al. Neutrophils are a major source of the epithelial barrier disrupting cytokine oncostatin M in patients with mucosal airways disease. *J. Allergy Clin. Immunol.* **2017**, *139*, 1966–1978.e9. [CrossRef]
242. Simpson, J.L.; Baines, K.J.; Boyle, M.J.; Scott, R.J.; Gibson, P.G. Oncostatin M (OSM) is increased in asthma with incompletely reversible airflow obstruction. *Exp. Lung Res.* **2009**, *35*, 781–794. [CrossRef] [PubMed]
243. Ventura, I.; Vega, A.; Chacon, P.; Chamorro, C.; Aroca, R.; Gomez, E.; Bellido, V.; Puente, Y.; Blanca, M.; Monteseirin, J. Neutrophils from allergic asthmatic patients produce and release metalloproteinase-9 upon direct exposure to allergens. *Allergy* **2014**, *69*, 898–905. [CrossRef] [PubMed]
244. Cundall, M.; Sun, Y.; Miranda, C.; Trudeau, J.B.; Barnes, S.; Wenzel, S.E. Neutrophil-derived matrix metalloproteinase-9 is increased in severe asthma and poorly inhibited by glucocorticoids. *J. Allergy Clin. Immunol.* **2003**, *112*, 1064–1071. [CrossRef] [PubMed]
245. Nadel, J.A. Role of enzymes from inflammatory cells on airway submucosal gland secretion. *Respiration* **1991**, *58* (Suppl. S1), 3–5. [CrossRef]
246. McGrath, K.W.; Icitovic, N.; Boushey, H.A.; Lazarus, S.C.; Sutherland, E.R.; Chinchilli, V.M.; Fahy, J.V.; Asthma Clinical Research Network of the National Heart, Lung, and Blood Institute. A large subgroup of mild-to-moderate asthma is persistently noneosinophilic. *Am. J. Respir. Crit. Care Med.* **2012**, *185*, 612–619. [CrossRef]
247. Barnes, P.J. Therapeutic approaches to asthma-chronic obstructive pulmonary disease overlap syndromes. *J. Allergy Clin. Immunol.* **2015**, *136*, 531–545. [CrossRef]
248. Westergaard, C.G.; Porsbjerg, C.; Backer, V. The effect of smoking cessation on airway inflammation in young asthma patients. *Clin. Exp. Allergy* **2014**, *44*, 353–361. [CrossRef]
249. Pakhale, S.; Baron, J.; Dent, R.; Vandemheen, K.; Aaron, S.D. Effects of weight loss on airway responsiveness in obese adults with asthma: Does weight loss lead to reversibility of asthma? *Chest* **2015**, *147*, 1582–1590. [CrossRef]
250. Simpson, J.L.; Powell, H.; Boyle, M.J.; Scott, R.J.; Gibson, P.G. Clarithromycin targets neutrophilic airway inflammation in refractory asthma. *Am. J. Respir. Crit. Care Med.* **2008**, *177*, 148–155. [CrossRef]

251. Bardin, P.; Kanniess, F.; Gauvreau, G.; Bredenbroker, D.; Rabe, K.F. Roflumilast for asthma: Efficacy findings in mechanism of action studies. *Pulm. Pharmacol. Ther.* **2015**, *35*, S4–S10. [CrossRef]
252. Casale, T.B.; Aalbers, R.; Bleecker, E.R.; Meltzer, E.O.; Zaremba-Pechmann, L.; de la Hoz, A.; Kerstjens, H.A.M. Tiotropium Respimat(R) add-on therapy to inhaled corticosteroids in patients with symptomatic asthma improves clinical outcomes regardless of baseline characteristics. *Respir. Med.* **2019**, *158*, 97–109. [CrossRef] [PubMed]
253. Szefler, S.J.; Vogelberg, C.; Bernstein, J.A.; Goldstein, S.; Mansfield, L.; Zaremba-Pechmann, L.; Engel, M.; Hamelmann, E. Tiotropium Is Efficacious in 6- to 17-Year-Olds with Asthma, Independent of T2 Phenotype. *J. Allergy Clin. Immunol. Pract.* **2019**, *7*, 2286–2295.e4. [CrossRef] [PubMed]
254. Nair, P.; Gaga, M.; Zervas, E.; Alagha, K.; Hargreave, F.E.; O'Byrne, P.M.; Stryszak, P.; Gann, L.; Sadeh, J.; Chanez, P.; et al. Safety and efficacy of a CXCR2 antagonist in patients with severe asthma and sputum neutrophils: A randomized, placebo-controlled clinical trial. *Clin. Exp. Allergy* **2012**, *42*, 1097–1103. [CrossRef] [PubMed]
255. Follows, R.M.; Snowise, N.G.; Ho, S.Y.; Ambery, C.L.; Smart, K.; McQuade, B.A. Efficacy, safety and tolerability of GSK2190915, a 5-lipoxygenase activating protein inhibitor, in adults and adolescents with persistent asthma: A randomised dose-ranging study. *Respir. Res.* **2013**, *14*, 54. [CrossRef] [PubMed]
256. O'Connor, B.J.; Lofdahl, C.G.; Balter, M.; Szczeklik, A.; Boulet, L.P.; Cairns, C.B. Zileuton added to low-dose inhaled beclomethasone for the treatment of moderate to severe persistent asthma. *Respir. Med.* **2007**, *101*, 1088–1096. [CrossRef] [PubMed]
257. Menzies-Gow, A.; Corren, J.; Bourdin, A.; Chupp, G.; Israel, E.; Wechsler, M.E.; Brightling, C.E.; Griffiths, J.M.; Hellqvist, A.; Bowen, K.; et al. Tezepelumab in Adults and Adolescents with Severe, Uncontrolled Asthma. *N. Engl. J. Med.* **2021**, *384*, 1800–1809. [CrossRef]
258. Wenzel, S.E.; Barnes, P.J.; Bleecker, E.R.; Bousquet, J.; Busse, W.; Dahlen, S.E.; Holgate, S.T.; Meyers, D.A.; Rabe, K.F.; Antczak, A.; et al. A randomized, double-blind, placebo-controlled study of tumor necrosis factor-alpha blockade in severe persistent asthma. *Am. J. Respir. Crit. Care Med.* **2009**, *179*, 549–558. [CrossRef]
259. Holgate, S.T.; Noonan, M.; Chanez, P.; Busse, W.; Dupont, L.; Pavord, I.; Hakulinen, A.; Paolozzi, L.; Wajdula, J.; Zang, C.; et al. Efficacy and safety of etanercept in moderate-to-severe asthma: A randomised, controlled trial. *Eur. Respir. J.* **2011**, *37*, 1352–1359. [CrossRef]
260. Busse, W.W.; Holgate, S.; Kerwin, E.; Chon, Y.; Feng, J.; Lin, J.; Lin, S.L. Randomized, double-blind, placebo-controlled study of brodalumab, a human anti-IL-17 receptor monoclonal antibody, in moderate to severe asthma. *Am. J. Respir. Crit. Care Med.* **2013**, *188*, 1294–1302. [CrossRef]
261. Brightling, C.E.; Nair, P.; Louis, R.; Singh, D. Risankizumab in severe asthma: A Phase IIa, placebo-controlled study. *Eur. Respir. J.* **2020**, *56*, 3699.
262. Revez, J.A.; Bain, L.M.; Watson, R.M.; Towers, M.; Collins, T.; Killian, K.J.; O'Byrne, P.M.; Gauvreau, G.M.; Upham, J.W.; Ferreira, M.A. Effects of interleukin-6 receptor blockade on allergen-induced airway responses in mild asthmatics. *Clin. Transl. Immunol.* **2019**, *8*, e1044. [CrossRef] [PubMed]
263. Scott, H.A.; Gibson, P.G.; Garg, M.L.; Pretto, J.J.; Morgan, P.J.; Callister, R.; Wood, L.G. Dietary restriction and exercise improve airway inflammation and clinical outcomes in overweight and obese asthma: A randomized trial. *Clin. Exp. Allergy* **2013**, *43*, 36–49. [CrossRef] [PubMed]
264. Boulet, L.P.; Turcotte, H.; Martin, J.; Poirier, P. Effect of bariatric surgery on airway response and lung function in obese subjects with asthma. *Respir. Med.* **2012**, *106*, 651–660. [CrossRef] [PubMed]
265. Freitas, P.D.; Ferreira, P.G.; Silva, A.G.; Stelmach, R.; Carvalho-Pinto, R.M.; Fernandes, F.L.; Mancini, M.C.; Sato, M.N.; Martins, M.A.; Carvalho, C.R. The Role of Exercise in a Weight-Loss Program on Clinical Control in Obese Adults with Asthma. A Randomized Controlled Trial. *Am. J. Respir. Crit. Care Med.* **2017**, *195*, 32–42. [CrossRef]
266. da Silva, P.L.; de Mello, M.T.; Cheik, N.C.; Sanches, P.L.; Correia, F.A.; de Piano, A.; Corgosinho, F.C.; Campos, R.M.; do Nascimento, C.M.; Oyama, L.M.; et al. Interdisciplinary therapy improves biomarkers profile and lung function in asthmatic obese adolescents. *Pediatr. Pulmonol.* **2012**, *47*, 8–17. [CrossRef]
267. Crosbie, P.A.; Woodhead, M.A. Long-term macrolide therapy in chronic inflammatory airway diseases. *Eur. Respir. J.* **2009**, *33*, 171–181. [CrossRef]
268. Kraft, M.; Cassell, G.H.; Pak, J.; Martin, R.J. Mycoplasma pneumoniae and Chlamydia pneumoniae in asthma: Effect of clarithromycin. *Chest* **2002**, *121*, 1782–1788. [CrossRef]
269. Gibson, P.G.; Yang, I.A.; Upham, J.W.; Reynolds, P.N.; Hodge, S.; James, A.L.; Jenkins, C.; Peters, M.J.; Marks, G.B.; Baraket, M.; et al. Effect of azithromycin on asthma exacerbations and quality of life in adults with persistent uncontrolled asthma (AMAZES): A randomised, double-blind, placebo-controlled trial. *Lancet* **2017**, *390*, 659–668. [CrossRef]
270. Taylor, S.L.; Ivey, K.L.; Gibson, P.G.; Simpson, J.L.; Rogers, G.B.; Group, A.S.R. Airway abundance of Haemophilus influenzae predicts response to azithromycin in adults with persistent uncontrolled asthma. *Eur. Respir. J.* **2020**, *56*, 2000194. [CrossRef]
271. Niessen, N.M.; Gibson, P.G.; Baines, K.J.; Barker, D.; Yang, I.A.; Upham, J.W.; Reynolds, P.N.; Hodge, S.; James, A.L.; Jenkins, C.; et al. Sputum TNF markers are increased in neutrophilic and severe asthma and are reduced by azithromycin treatment. *Allergy* **2021**, *76*, 2090–2101. [CrossRef]
272. Brusselle, G.G.; Vanderstichele, C.; Jordens, P.; Deman, R.; Slabbynck, H.; Ringoet, V.; Verleden, G.; Demedts, I.K.; Verhamme, K.; Delporte, A.; et al. Azithromycin for prevention of exacerbations in severe asthma (AZISAST): A multicentre randomised double-blind placebo-controlled trial. *Thorax* **2013**, *68*, 322–329. [CrossRef] [PubMed]

273. Calverley, P.M.; Rabe, K.F.; Goehring, U.M.; Kristiansen, S.; Fabbri, L.M.; Martinez, F.J.; The M2-124 and M2-125 Study Groups. Roflumilast in symptomatic chronic obstructive pulmonary disease: Two randomised clinical trials. *Lancet* **2009**, *374*, 685–694. [CrossRef]
274. Zhang, X.; Chen, Y.; Fan, L.; Ye, J.; Fan, J.; Xu, X.; You, D.; Liu, S.; Chen, X.; Luo, P. Pharmacological mechanism of roflumilast in the treatment of asthma-COPD overlap. *Drug Des. Dev. Ther.* **2018**, *12*, 2371–2379. [CrossRef] [PubMed]
275. Timmer, W.; Leclerc, V.; Birraux, G.; Neuhauser, M.; Hatzelmann, A.; Bethke, T.; Wurst, W. The new phosphodiesterase 4 inhibitor roflumilast is efficacious in exercise-induced asthma and leads to suppression of LPS-stimulated TNF-alpha ex vivo. *J. Clin. Pharmacol.* **2002**, *42*, 297–303. [CrossRef]
276. Bousquet, J.; Aubier, M.; Sastre, J.; Izquierdo, J.L.; Adler, L.M.; Hofbauer, P.; Rost, K.D.; Harnest, U.; Kroemer, B.; Albrecht, A.; et al. Comparison of roflumilast, an oral anti-inflammatory, with beclomethasone dipropionate in the treatment of persistent asthma. *Allergy* **2006**, *61*, 72–78. [CrossRef]
277. Bateman, E.D.; Goehring, U.M.; Richard, F.; Watz, H. Roflumilast combined with montelukast versus montelukast alone as add-on treatment in patients with moderate-to-severe asthma. *J. Allergy Clin. Immunol.* **2016**, *138*, 142–149.e8. [CrossRef]
278. Gauvreau, G.M.; Boulet, L.P.; Schmid-Wirlitsch, C.; Cote, J.; Duong, M.; Killian, K.J.; Milot, J.; Deschesnes, F.; Strinich, T.; Watson, R.M.; et al. Roflumilast attenuates allergen-induced inflammation in mild asthmatic subjects. *Respir. Res.* **2011**, *12*, 140. [CrossRef]
279. Phillips, J.E. Inhaled Phosphodiesterase 4 (PDE4) Inhibitors for Inflammatory Respiratory Diseases. *Front. Pharmacol.* **2020**, *11*, 259. [CrossRef]
280. Singh, D.; Leaker, B.; Boyce, M.; Nandeuil, M.A.; Collarini, S.; Mariotti, F.; Santoro, D.; Barnes, P.J. A novel inhaled phosphodiesterase 4 inhibitor (CHF6001) reduces the allergen challenge response in asthmatic patients. *Pulm. Pharmacol. Ther.* **2016**, *40*, 1–6. [CrossRef]
281. Franciosi, L.G.; Diamant, Z.; Banner, K.H.; Zuiker, R.; Morelli, N.; Kamerling, I.M.; de Kam, M.L.; Burggraaf, J.; Cohen, A.F.; Cazzola, M.; et al. Efficacy and safety of RPL554, a dual PDE3 and PDE4 inhibitor, in healthy volunteers and in patients with asthma or chronic obstructive pulmonary disease: Findings from four clinical trials. *Lancet Respir. Med.* **2013**, *1*, 714–727. [CrossRef]
282. Luo, J.; Yang, L.; Yang, J.; Yang, D.; Liu, B.C.; Liu, D.; Liang, B.M.; Liu, C.T. Efficacy and safety of phosphodiesterase 4 inhibitors in patients with asthma: A systematic review and meta-analysis. *Respirology* **2018**, *23*, 467–477. [CrossRef] [PubMed]
283. Damera, G.; Jiang, M.; Zhao, H.; Fogle, H.W.; Jester, W.F.; Freire, J.; Panettieri, R.A., Jr. Aclidinium bromide abrogates allergen-induced hyperresponsiveness and reduces eosinophilia in murine model of airway inflammation. *Eur. J. Pharmacol.* **2010**, *649*, 349–353. [CrossRef] [PubMed]
284. Ohta, S.; Oda, N.; Yokoe, T.; Tanaka, A.; Yamamoto, Y.; Watanabe, Y.; Minoguchi, K.; Ohnishi, T.; Hirose, T.; Nagase, H.; et al. Effect of tiotropium bromide on airway inflammation and remodelling in a mouse model of asthma. *Clin. Exp. Allergy* **2010**, *40*, 1266–1275. [CrossRef] [PubMed]
285. Toumpanakis, D.; Loverdos, K.; Tzouda, V.; Vassilakopoulou, V.; Litsiou, E.; Magkou, C.; Karavana, V.; Pieper, M.; Vassilakopoulos, T. Tiotropium bromide exerts anti-inflammatory effects during resistive breathing, an experimental model of severe airway obstruction. *Int. J. Chronic Obstr. Pulm. Dis.* **2017**, *12*, 2207–2220. [CrossRef] [PubMed]
286. Anzalone, G.; Gagliardo, R.; Bucchieri, F.; Albano, G.D.; Siena, L.; Montalbano, A.M.; Bonanno, A.; Riccobono, L.; Pieper, M.P.; Gjomarkaj, M.; et al. IL-17A induces chromatin remodeling promoting IL-8 release in bronchial epithelial cells: Effect of Tiotropium. *Life Sci.* **2016**, *152*, 107–116. [CrossRef]
287. Suzaki, I.; Asano, K.; Shikama, Y.; Hamasaki, T.; Kanei, A.; Suzaki, H. Suppression of IL-8 production from airway cells by tiotropium bromide in vitro. *Int. J. Chronic Obstr. Pulm. Dis.* **2011**, *6*, 439–448. [CrossRef]
288. Peters, S.P.; Kunselman, S.J.; Icitovic, N.; Moore, W.C.; Pascual, R.; Ameredes, B.T.; Boushey, H.A.; Calhoun, W.J.; Castro, M.; Cherniack, R.M.; et al. Tiotropium bromide step-up therapy for adults with uncontrolled asthma. *N. Engl. J. Med.* **2010**, *363*, 1715–1726. [CrossRef]
289. Kerstjens, H.A.; Engel, M.; Dahl, R.; Paggiaro, P.; Beck, E.; Vandewalker, M.; Sigmund, R.; Seibold, W.; Moroni-Zentgraf, P.; Bateman, E.D. Tiotropium in asthma poorly controlled with standard combination therapy. *N. Engl. J. Med.* **2012**, *367*, 1198–1207. [CrossRef]
290. Iwamoto, H.; Yokoyama, A.; Shiota, N.; Shoda, H.; Haruta, Y.; Hattori, N.; Kohno, N. Tiotropium bromide is effective for severe asthma with noneosinophilic phenotype. *Eur. Respir. J.* **2008**, *31*, 1379–1380. [CrossRef]
291. Kerstjens, H.A.; Moroni-Zentgraf, P.; Tashkin, D.P.; Dahl, R.; Paggiaro, P.; Vandewalker, M.; Schmidt, H.; Engel, M.; Bateman, E.D. Tiotropium improves lung function, exacerbation rate, and asthma control, independent of baseline characteristics including age, degree of airway obstruction, and allergic status. *Respir. Med.* **2016**, *117*, 198–206. [CrossRef]
292. Casale, T.B.; Bateman, E.D.; Vandewalker, M.; Virchow, J.C.; Schmidt, H.; Engel, M.; Moroni-Zentgraf, P.; Kerstjens, H.A.M. Tiotropium Respimat Add-on Is Efficacious in Symptomatic Asthma, Independent of T2 Phenotype. *J. Allergy Clin. Immunol. Pract.* **2018**, *6*, 923–935.e9. [CrossRef] [PubMed]
293. Lazarus, S.C.; Krishnan, J.A.; King, T.S.; Lang, J.E.; Blake, K.V.; Covar, R.; Lugogo, N.; Wenzel, S.; Chinchilli, V.M.; Mauger, D.T.; et al. Mometasone or Tiotropium in Mild Asthma with a Low Sputum Eosinophil Level. *N. Engl. J. Med.* **2019**, *380*, 2009–2019. [CrossRef] [PubMed]

294. O'Byrne, P.M.; Metev, H.; Puu, M.; Richter, K.; Keen, C.; Uddin, M.; Larsson, B.; Cullberg, M.; Nair, P. Efficacy and safety of a CXCR2 antagonist, AZD5069, in patients with uncontrolled persistent asthma: A randomised, double-blind, placebo-controlled trial. *Lancet Respir. Med.* **2016**, *4*, 797–806. [CrossRef]
295. Watz, H.; Uddin, M.; Pedersen, F.; Kirsten, A.; Goldmann, T.; Stellmacher, F.; Groth, E.; Larsson, B.; Bottcher, G.; Malmgren, A.; et al. Effects of the CXCR2 antagonist AZD5069 on lung neutrophil recruitment in asthma. *Pulm. Pharmacol. Ther.* **2017**, *45*, 121–123. [CrossRef] [PubMed]
296. Chaudhuri, R.; Norris, V.; Kelly, K.; Zhu, C.Q.; Ambery, C.; Lafferty, J.; Cameron, E.; Thomson, N.C. Effects of a FLAP inhibitor, GSK2190915, in asthmatics with high sputum neutrophils. *Pulm. Pharmacol. Ther.* **2014**, *27*, 62–69. [CrossRef]
297. Snowise, N.G.; Clements, D.; Ho, S.Y.; Follows, R.M. Addition of a 5-lipoxygenase-activating protein inhibitor to an inhaled corticosteroid (ICS) or an ICS/long-acting beta-2-agonist combination in subjects with asthma. *Curr. Med. Res. Opin.* **2013**, *29*, 1663–1674. [CrossRef]
298. Thalanayar Muthukrishnan, P.; Nouraie, M.; Parikh, A.; Holguin, F. Zileuton use and phenotypic features in asthma. *Pulm. Pharmacol. Ther.* **2020**, *60*, 101872. [CrossRef]
299. Chiu, C.J.; Huang, M.T. Asthma in the Precision Medicine Era: Biologics and Probiotics. *Int. J. Mol. Sci.* **2021**, *22*, 4528. [CrossRef]
300. Corren, J.; Parnes, J.R.; Wang, L.; Mo, M.; Roseti, S.L.; Griffiths, J.M.; van der Merwe, R. Tezepelumab in Adults with Uncontrolled Asthma. *N. Engl. J. Med.* **2017**, *377*, 936–946. [CrossRef]
301. Venkataramani, S.; Low, S.; Weigle, B.; Dutcher, D.; Jerath, K.; Menzenski, M.; Frego, L.; Truncali, K.; Gupta, P.; Kroe-Barrett, R.; et al. Design and characterization of Zweimab and Doppelmab, high affinity dual antagonistic anti-TSLP/IL13 bispecific antibodies. *Biochem. Biophys. Res. Commun.* **2018**, *504*, 19–24. [CrossRef]
302. Howarth, P.H.; Babu, K.S.; Arshad, H.S.; Lau, L.; Buckley, M.; McConnell, W.; Beckett, P.; Al Ali, M.; Chauhan, A.; Wilson, S.J.; et al. Tumour necrosis factor (TNFalpha) as a novel therapeutic target in symptomatic corticosteroid dependent asthma. *Thorax* **2005**, *60*, 1012–1018. [CrossRef] [PubMed]
303. Berry, M.A.; Hargadon, B.; Shelley, M.; Parker, D.; Shaw, D.E.; Green, R.H.; Bradding, P.; Brightling, C.E.; Wardlaw, A.J.; Pavord, I.D. Evidence of a role of tumor necrosis factor alpha in refractory asthma. *N. Engl. J. Med.* **2006**, *354*, 697–708. [CrossRef] [PubMed]
304. Morjaria, J.B.; Chauhan, A.J.; Babu, K.S.; Polosa, R.; Davies, D.E.; Holgate, S.T. The role of a soluble TNFalpha receptor fusion protein (etanercept) in corticosteroid refractory asthma: A double blind, randomised, placebo controlled trial. *Thorax* **2008**, *63*, 584–591. [CrossRef] [PubMed]
305. Liang, L.; Hur, J.; Kang, J.Y.; Rhee, C.K.; Kim, Y.K.; Lee, S.Y. Effect of the anti-IL-17 antibody on allergic inflammation in an obesity-related asthma model. *Korean J. Intern. Med.* **2018**, *33*, 1210–1223. [CrossRef]
306. Dos Santos, T.M.; Righetti, R.F.; Camargo, L.D.N.; Saraiva-Romanholo, B.M.; Aristoteles, L.; de Souza, F.C.R.; Fukuzaki, S.; Alonso-Vale, M.I.C.; Cruz, M.M.; Prado, C.M.; et al. Effect of Anti-IL17 Antibody Treatment Alone and in Combination With Rho-Kinase Inhibitor in a Murine Model of Asthma. *Front. Physiol.* **2018**, *9*, 1183. [CrossRef]
307. Khokhlovich, E.; Grant, S.; Kazani, S.; Strieter, R.; Thornton-Wells, T.; Laramie, J.; Morgan, T.; Kennedy, S. The biological pathways underlying response to anti-IL-17A (AIN457; secukinumab) therapy differ across severe asthmatic patients. *Eur. Respir. J.* **2017**, *50*, OA2897.
308. Staton, T.L.; Peng, K.; Owen, R.; Choy, D.F.; Cabanski, C.R.; Fong, A.; Brunstein, F.; Alatsis, K.R.; Chen, H. A phase I, randomized, observer-blinded, single and multiple ascending-dose study to investigate the safety, pharmacokinetics, and immunogenicity of BITS7201A, a bispecific antibody targeting IL-13 and IL-17, in healthy volunteers. *BMC Pulm. Med.* **2019**, *19*, 5. [CrossRef]
309. Langrish, C.L.; Chen, Y.; Blumenschein, W.M.; Mattson, J.; Basham, B.; Sedgwick, J.D.; McClanahan, T.; Kastelein, R.A.; Cua, D.J. IL-23 drives a pathogenic T cell population that induces autoimmune inflammation. *J. Exp. Med.* **2005**, *201*, 233–240. [CrossRef]
310. Zhao, Y.; Huang, Y.; He, J.; Li, C.; Deng, W.; Ran, X.; Wang, D. Rosiglitazone, a peroxisome proliferator-activated receptor-gamma agonist, attenuates airway inflammation by inhibiting the proliferation of effector T cells in a murine model of neutrophilic asthma. *Immunol. Lett.* **2014**, *157*, 9–15. [CrossRef]
311. Han, W.; Li, J.; Tang, H.; Sun, L. Treatment of obese asthma in a mouse model by simvastatin is associated with improving dyslipidemia and decreasing leptin level. *Biochem. Biophys. Res. Commun.* **2017**, *484*, 396–402. [CrossRef]
312. Lee, H.Y.; Lee, E.G.; Hur, J.; Rhee, C.K.; Kim, Y.K.; Lee, S.Y.; Kang, J.Y. Pravastatin alleviates allergic airway inflammation in obesity-related asthma mouse model. *Exp. Lung Res.* **2019**, *45*, 275–287. [CrossRef] [PubMed]
313. Norman, P. Evaluation of WO2013136076: Two crystalline forms of the phosphatidylinositol 3-kinase-delta inhibitor RV-1729. *Expert Opin. Ther. Pat.* **2014**, *24*, 471–475. [CrossRef] [PubMed]
314. Leaker, B.R.; Barnes, P.J.; O'Connor, B.J.; Ali, F.Y.; Tam, P.; Neville, J.; Mackenzie, L.F.; MacRury, T. The effects of the novel SHIP1 activator AQX-1125 on allergen-induced responses in mild-to-moderate asthma. *Clin. Exp. Allergy* **2014**, *44*, 1146–1153. [CrossRef] [PubMed]
315. Cahn, A.; Hamblin, J.N.; Begg, M.; Wilson, R.; Dunsire, L.; Sriskantharajah, S.; Montembault, M.; Leemereise, C.N.; Galinanes-Garcia, L.; Watz, H.; et al. Safety, pharmacokinetics and dose-response characteristics of GSK2269557, an inhaled PI3Kdelta inhibitor under development for the treatment of COPD. *Pulm. Pharmacol. Ther.* **2017**, *46*, 69–77. [CrossRef]
316. Winkler, D.G.; Faia, K.L.; DiNitto, J.P.; Ali, J.A.; White, K.F.; Brophy, E.E.; Pink, M.M.; Proctor, J.L.; Lussier, J.; Martin, C.M.; et al. PI3K-delta and PI3K-gamma inhibition by IPI-145 abrogates immune responses and suppresses activity in autoimmune and inflammatory disease models. *Chem. Biol.* **2013**, *20*, 1364–1374. [CrossRef]

317. Kampe, M.; Lampinen, M.; Stolt, I.; Janson, C.; Stalenheim, G.; Carlson, M. PI3-kinase regulates eosinophil and neutrophil degranulation in patients with allergic rhinitis and allergic asthma irrespective of allergen challenge model. *Inflammation* **2012**, *35*, 230–239. [CrossRef]
318. Toki, S.; Newcomb, D.C.; Printz, R.L.; Cahill, K.N.; Boyd, K.L.; Niswender, K.D.; Peebles, R.S., Jr. Glucagon-like peptide-1 receptor agonist inhibits aeroallergen-induced activation of ILC2 and neutrophilic airway inflammation in obese mice. *Allergy* **2021**, *76*, 3433–3445. [CrossRef]
319. Foer, D.; Beeler, P.E.; Cui, J.; Karlson, E.W.; Bates, D.W.; Cahill, K.N. Asthma Exacerbations in Patients with Type 2 Diabetes and Asthma on Glucagon-like Peptide-1 Receptor Agonists. *Am. J. Respir. Crit. Care Med.* **2021**, *203*, 831–840. [CrossRef]

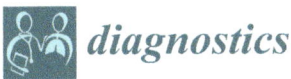

Review

The Importance of Appropriate Diagnosis in the Practical Management of Chronic Obstructive Pulmonary Disease

Naozumi Hashimoto *, Keiko Wakahara and Koji Sakamoto

Department of Respiratory Medicine, Nagoya University Graduate School of Medicine, Nagoya 466-8550, Japan; wakahara@med.nagoya-u.ac.jp (K.W.); sakakoji@med.nagoya-u.ac.jp (K.S.)
* Correspondence: hashinao@med.nagoya-u.ac.jp; Tel.: +81-52-744-2167; Fax: +81-52-744-2176

Abstract: Chronic obstructive pulmonary disease (COPD) is projected to continue to contribute to an increase in the overall worldwide burden of disease until 2030. Therefore, an accurate assessment of the risk of airway obstruction in patients with COPD has become vitally important. Although the Global Initiative for Chronic Obstructive Lung Disease (GOLD), the American Thoracic Society (ATS) and European Respiratory Society (ERS), and the Japanese Respiratory Society (JRS) provide the criteria by which to diagnose COPD, many studies suggest that it is in fact underdiagnosed. Its prevalence increases, while the impact of COPD-related systemic comorbidities is also increasingly recognized in clinical aspects of COPD. Although a recent report suggests that spirometry should not be used to screen for airflow limitation in individuals without respiratory symptoms, the early detection of COPD in patients with no, or few, symptoms is an opportunity to provide appropriate management based on COPD guidelines. Clinical advances have been made in pharmacotherapeutic approaches to COPD. This article provides a current understanding of the importance of an appropriate diagnosis in the real-world management of COPD.

Keywords: chronic obstructive pulmonary disease; spirometry; lower limit of normal

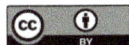

1. Introduction

Chronic obstructive pulmonary disease (COPD) is projected to continue to contribute to an increase in the worldwide burden of disease until 2030 [1]. Therefore, an accurate assessment of the risk of airway obstruction in patients with COPD has become vitally important. The Global Initiative for Chronic Obstructive Lung Disease (GOLD), the American Thoracic Society (ATS) and European Respiratory Society (ERS), and the Japanese Respiratory Society (JRS) all provide criteria with which to diagnose COPD [2–4]. Although the clinical guideline, an official statement of the American College of Physicians (ACP), American College of Chest Physicians (ACCP), ATS, and ERS, does not recommend the evaluation of airflow limitations by respiratory function testing in patients without respiratory symptoms [2], many studies suggest that COPD is under-diagnosed.

Smoking exposure also causes several systemic comorbidities in COPD patients [5]. Although severe acute respiratory syndrome coronavirus 2 (SARS-CoV-2), the virus responsible for the coronavirus disease 2019 (COVID-19) pandemic, has infected over 100.0 million people around the world and caused more than over 2.2 million deaths [6], there is mounting evidence that COPD may be a risk factor for more severe COVID-19 disease [7]. Furthermore, the coexistence of several comorbidities hinders efforts to illuminate the pathogenesis of COPD and the heterogeneity of disease progression. Mounting evidence suggests that the heterogeneity of disease progression in COPD might be due to the varying lung function trajectories [8,9].

Although, there are many critical issues for COPD-related outcomes in the real-world clinical settings, understanding whether insufficient management arising from undiagnosed COPD might affect the outcomes related to COPD has not been concisely reviewed, including COPD management (acute exacerbation, hospitalization, and mortality), development of systemic comorbidities (cardiovascular diseases and frailty), the coronavirus disease 2019 (COVID-19) pandemic, and postoperative management of resected lung cancer patients [10,11].

This article provides the current understanding of appropriate diagnosis in the real-world management of COPD.

2. Method

The aim of this study was to evaluate the clinical issues in undiagnosed COPD patients. PubMed was searched for population-based estimates published during the period 1980–2020. The search terms included "chronic obstructive pulmonary disease" and either "undiagnosis", "emphysema", "lower limit of normal", "prevalence", "exacerbation", "systemic diseases", "comorbidity", "coronavirus disease 2019", "post-operative complication", or "mortality". Articles were included if they: (1) Provided the total population for evaluating the clinical issues in undiagnosed COPD patients; and (2) gave sufficient method details to evaluate the outcomes using the criteria defined by the investigators. Studies that might not provide any conclusion on the issues were excluded. From the 436 studies, which the initial search identified, 61 articles were selected to achieve our aim for this review.

3. Results

3.1. Prevalence of COPD

World-wide cohort studies suggest that the prevalence of COPD is estimated to be about 10% to 14% [12,13]. Under the Japanese Industrial Safety and Health Act, a chest X-ray examination is included in a legal medical examination. It aids the early detection of lung cancer, as a lung cancer screening method. An evaluation of airflow limitation by spirometry examination is optional in statutory medical examinations in Japan. For the early detection of COPD, some studies evaluated airflow limitation by spirometry among subjects aged 40 years or older who had participated in community-based annual health checks in Japan [14,15]. The prevalence of COPD in adults, aged 40 and over, is estimated to be around 10% in Japan.

Although the prevalence of lung cancer is estimated to be about 3 % in COPD patients [16], the coexistence rate of COPD was more than 40% in resected lung cancer patients [17]. A therapeutic option, other than surgery, such as chemotherapy and/or radiation, might be selected for the older lung cancer patients with COPD [17–19]. To determine the substantial prevalence of COPD among Asian patients with newly diagnosed lung cancer who were sequentially registered, spirometry was performed when applying bronchoscopy for lung cancer diagnosis. The coexistence rate of COPD was 54.4% among 270 new lung cancer cases that underwent bronchoscopy, and 84.4% were diagnosed with COPD for the first time [20]. In the study population, 61.3% of men had COPD, but only 35.2% of women had COPD. In addition, 95.5% of men had a history of smoking, whereas 67.6% of women were non-smokers. The percentage of non-smokers among women with lung cancer was only 10.5% in a study by Loganathan et al. [21]. The discrepancy might be due to difference in smoking habits in each country. As the severity of airflow limitation was evaluated in these patients with COPD, the proportion of grade 1 (mild) and grade 2 (moderate) in the GOLD classification was more than 90 % of COPD cases. [20]. When the association between airflow limitation and thin-section computed tomography (TSCT)-determined emphysema was evaluated, 38.8% of subjects with airflow limitation were found to have TSCT-determined emphysema. Airflow limitation was observed in 68.1% of subjects with TSCT-determined emphysema [22]. It was also reported that the use of deep residual networks on chest CT scans for ex-smokers, and current smokers who underwent lung cancer screening, was an effective case-finding method in detecting and diagnosing COPD [23].

3.2. Clinical Significance of COPD Diagnosis

3.2.1. Management of COPD and Its Exacerbations

The Evaluation of COPD Longitudinally to identify the Predictive Surrogate Endpoints (ECLIPSE) study shows that a COPD acute exacerbation event can itself predict the next COPD acute exacerbation event in a COPD acute exacerbation risk assessment in patients with COPD GOLD grade 2 or higher [24]. Nevertheless, more than 75% of individuals with COPD, who have been symptomatic for at least five years, are not diagnosed [25]. Although more than 50% of Asian patients with newly diagnosed lung cancer had COPD, only 8.5% of the total study population had been diagnosed and managed as having COPD [20]. This finding is compatible with a retrospective analysis of a clinical cohort in the United Kingdom, which showed that of the COPD patients who had received a chest radiography in the two years before COPD diagnosis, only 33% had spirometry [26].

3.2.2. COPD and Systemic Diseases

Smoking is strongly associated with the development of chronic lung inflammation and systemic inflammation via the inflammatory mediators derived from smoking-stimulated lung tissue [5]. A recent study reported that people with accelerated FEV1 decline were at greater risk of cardiovascular disease, compared to those without accelerated decline over a more than 15-years [27]. Another study suggested that frequency of COPD exacerbation and increasing dyspnea, not a decline in FEV1, might be associated with increasing cardiac events [28]. Frailty is defined as a progressive physiological decline in multiple organ systems marked by loss of function, loss of physiological reserve, and increased vulnerability to disease [29]. Many chronic diseases are associated with frailty and functional decline in older people [30]. The prevalence of frailty might be assumed to be 6–10% in elderly patients with COPD [31,32]. More than 20% of frail elderly subjects with dyspnea might be detected using a near-home screening strategy [33]. Kennedy, et al. demonstrated that frail COPD participants reported significantly worse disease-specific symptoms and the overall quality of life [32]. Furthermore, frailty triggered by worsening of COPD might decrease the time to first hospitalization and an increased the duration of hospitalization [32]. A further understanding of how the COPD frailty phenotype can be modified or treated is warranted.

3.2.3. The Effect of COPD on the Severity and Mortality of COVID-19

For cohorts in China, America, and Italy reporting on hospitalized COVID-19 patients, the prevalence of COPD has ranged from zero to 15% [7,34]. Comparing its severity among COPD patients, the risk of development of severe COVID-19 disease might be relatively lower than the risk among asthma patients, possibly due to the use of inhaler corticosteroid (ICS) [35]. Nevertheless, a recent observational study did not support the hypothesis that regular ICS use might protect against COVID-19-related death among people with asthma or COPD [36]. A decrease in physical activity might be strongly associated with mortality in COPD patients [37]. The extensive social distancing policies and restrictions brought about by the COVID-19 pandemic often makes it difficult for individuals to visit with their physicians, resulting in fewer opportunities to receive pulmonary rehabilitation programs [34].

3.2.4. The Effect of COPD Co-Existence in Resected Lung Cancer

Most COPD patients with resected lung cancer show no or few COPD-related symptoms, due to mild airflow limitation [20]. Nevertheless, COPD patients with an FEV1/ forced vital capacity (FVC) ratio below 0.70 had a prolonged postoperative stay, and a greater need of prolonged oxygen therapy, than patients without COPD [17,38]. Although clinical guidelines recommend spirometric assessment to evaluate the optimum selection of surgical procedures, in view of the risks of mortality and post-operative complications [11,18], better risk stratification for post-operative outcomes in patients, with COPD undergoing thoracic surgery, has not been fully determined. An FEV1/FVC ratio below the lower fifth percentile of a large healthy reference group (that is, the statistically defined lower limit of normal [LLN]) is used to classify airflow obstruction [39,40]. Studies have not evaluated whether an FEV1/FVC ratio below 0.70 but above the LLN (an "inbetween" group) could identify patients at risk of adverse COPD-related clinical outcomes had not been fully evaluated (Figure 1) [41,42]. When the combined assessment of the 0.70 fixed ratio and the LLN of the FEV1/FVC ratio was used for risk stratification, the in-between group classified by a FEV1/FVC ratio below 0.70, but above the LLN included patients with mild cases of COPD patients. The LLN assessment of the FEV1/FVC ratio might provide more accurate risk stratification in COPD patients undergoing thoracic surgery [41]. In this study, the LLN of FEV1 and FVC were calculated by using the reference equations of the National Health and Nutrition Survey III (NHANESIII), due to the absences of a Japanese reference equation to calculate the LLN of FEV1/FVC [41]. A recent study suggested that the locally derived LLN criteria seem to be better at identifying high-risk individuals with COPD, compared with the LLN criteria from other regions. Whereas, COPD individuals determined by the five different LLN criteria showed similar risk of COPD exacerbations and mortality [43]. Okada, et al. stratified the risk for postoperative outcomes in COPD patients with resected lung cancer by using renewed Japanese spirometric reference variables [3,44]. The studies demonstrated that airflow obstruction, determined by a different lung function reference, had a similar risk of post-operative outcomes [41,44].

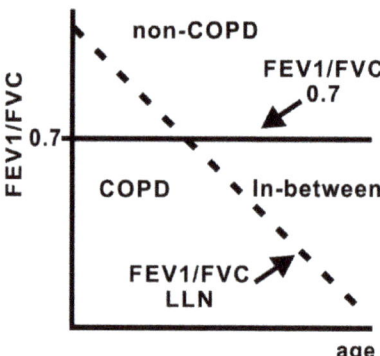

Figure 1. Diagram depicting the fixed 0.7 ratio of FEV1/ FVC and the decline of the LLN of FEV1/ FVC with aging. Modified from [42]. Solid line: The fixed 0.7 ratio. Dotted line: The LLN of FEV1/ FVC with aging.

3.2.5. The Effect of COPD Coexistence in Advanced Lung Cancer Cases

High COPD coexistence rates were shown in lung cancer cases [20], but no increase in chemotherapy-related adverse events was observed in COPD patients that underwent chemotherapy for advanced lung cancer [19,45]. Therefore, the effect of COPD on patients with lung cancer might depend on treatment options, such as surgery or chemotherapy.

3.3. Early COPD

In some cases, COPD develops from accelerated lung function decline. Other cases do not achieve the expected maximally attained lung function in early adulthood, resulting in COPD [8]. Therefore, among COPD patients, those with accelerated disease progression should be identified. Martinez, et al. suggested that a classification to distinguish between "early disease" and late "mild disease" was warranted, in order to aid individualized interventions and modify progression before irreversible damage [9]. They proposed that early COPD should be defined in individuals under 50 years of age with 10 or more pack-years of smoking history and any of these abnormalities: (1) Early airflow limitation (post-bronchodilator FEV1/FVC, LLN); (2) compatible CT abnormalities, and; (3) a rapid decline in FEV1 (> 60 mL/year); that is, accelerated relative to FVC [9,46]. Based on the definition of early COPD [9,46], a recent study demonstrated that the operational definition for early COPD may be effective in excluding individuals unlikely to develop clinical COPD later in life [47]. Furthermore, COPD that develops through a normal maximally attained FEV1 trajectory is associated with increased risks of both respiratory disease mortality and all-cause mortality, compared with COPD that develops through a low maximally attained FEV1 trajectory [48].

4. Discussion

In global setting, including Japan, the prevalence of COPD in adults aged 40 and over is estimated to be around 10%. There is a discrepancy of more than 20 times between the approximately five million individuals with COPD and 200,000 patients with COPD undergoing pharmacotherapy [49]. Spirometry was performed to determine the substantial prevalence of COPD among Asian patients with newly diagnosed lung cancer who were sequentially registered. It was found that COPD is a common comorbidity in elderly people with a smoking history [26,46,50].

Many studies point out that undiagnosed COPD patients often visit primary care for COPD-related respiratory symptoms, such as dyspnea, cough, and sputum [25]. This underlines the need for COPD management options [26,46,50]. Primary physicians might not recognize the worsening respiratory symptoms in these undiagnosed patients as involving COPD acute exacerbation. Efficacious COPD management might be provided for patients at an early stage of COPD when patients with respiratory symptoms, who visit primary care, are appropriately diagnosed with COPD by spirometry [51].

Systemic inflammation from smoking-stimulated lung tissue in COPD patients might induce the development of heart disease, osteoporosis, metabolic syndrome, skeletal muscle atrophy, frailty, and depression [5,28,30–32,52]. Nevertheless, COPD-related systemic comorbidities, including diabetes, hypertension, and ischemic cardiac disease, might not be associated with the development of post-operative outcomes in resected lung cancer patients [17,38]. Therefore, post-operative outcomes should be recognized as COPD-related outcomes, even in patients with mild cases of COPD. Although, the COPD frailty phenotype might affect COPD-related outcomes, such as respiratory and all-cause mortalities, hospitalization, acute exacerbation, poor quality of life, and depression [32]. It also remains undetermined whether the decreased physical activity in COPD patients, due to the COVID-19 pandemic, could increase the incidence of the COPD-related outcomes. If we can appropriately diagnose COPD, early detection plays a key role in improving the prognosis of patients with COPD [53]. Further investigation is warranted.

There is growing awareness of the need to identify COPD in patients at an early stage [50,53–57]. A recent systematic review suggests that pharmacotherapy is effective in altering the rate of lung function decline and that the annual decline of forced expiratory volume in one second (FEV1) modified by bronchodilators was within the decline, reported for health status and for the exacerbation rate in the clinical trials [58]. Further research efforts are warranted to verify the effectiveness of appropriate management of undiagnosed COPD patients, as mounting evidence suggest early COPD with a rapid decline in FEV1 might be a suitable target for appropriate therapy [47,48].

Two issues remain elusive for providing helpful guidance to the practicing clinicians. Firstly, when should spirometry be performed? Smoking often causes the development of lung cancer and COPD [59,60]. A chest radiography might be examined by primary physicians to screen for lung cancers among patients aged over 70 years and with smoking history [20]. The timing might provide an opportunity to use spirometry tests to detect COPD [20,25,26]. By evaluating the presence of emphysematous lesions on TSCT in individuals under 50 years of age with 10 or more pack-years of smoking history [9], diagnosing emphysema can be an indicator for assessing airflow obstruction [61,62]. Secondly, how should the data from spirometry be evaluated? The combined assessment of the 0.70 fixed ratio and the LLN of the FEV1/FVC ratio could identify patients at risk of adverse COPD-related clinical outcomes in resected lung cancer patients [41,42,44]. Although adult smokers, suspected of having COPD, were reported to be at no increased risk of respiratory morbidity or all-cause mortality until the ratio falls below the age-corrected LLN (even though it is below 0.70) [40], the combined assessment of the 0.70 fixed ratio and the LLN of the FEV1/FVC ratio might provide more accurate management in early COPD patients that develop through a low maximally attained FEV1 trajectory [48], but also COPD patients at an early disease stage [50,53–57]. Further research efforts are warranted for providing helpful guidance to the practicing clinicians.

5. Conclusions

This article provides a current understanding of the unresolved issues that arise from insufficient management of undiagnosed COPD and how they might affect the outcomes related to COPD in the real-world clinical settings. In summary, the importance of an appropriate diagnosis in the real-world management of COPD should be emphasized.

Author Contributions: Conceptualization, N.H.; review of the literature, N.H.; writing—review and editing, N.H.; supervision, K.W. and K.S. All authors have read and agreed to the published version of the manuscript.

Funding: This research received no external funding.

Acknowledgments: We are very appreciative to all staffs at the Department of Respiratory Medicine, Nagoya University School of Medicine.

Conflicts of Interest: Disclosure Statement: N.H. received speaker honorariums from AstraZeneca, Boehringer Ingelheim, Glaxo Smith Kline, and Novartis, outside the submitted work. N.H. received a research grant from Boehringer Ingelheim, outside the submitted work.

References

1. Mathers, C.D.; Loncar, D. Projections of Global Mortality and Burden of Disease from 2002 to 2030. *PLoS Med.* **2006**, *3*, e442. [CrossRef] [PubMed]
2. Qaseem, A.; Wilt, T.J.; Weinberger, S.E.; Hanania, N.A.; Criner, G.; Van Der Molen, T.; Marciniuk, D.D.; Denberg, T.; Schünemann, H.; Wedzicha, W.; et al. Diagnosis and Management of Stable Chronic Obstructive Pulmonary Disease: A Clinical Practice Guideline Update from the American College of Physicians, American College of Chest Physicians, American Thoracic Society, and European Respiratory Society. *Ann. Intern. Med.* **2011**, *155*, 179–191. [CrossRef] [PubMed]
3. Kubota, M.; Kobayashi, H.; Quanjer, P.H.; Omori, H.; Tatsumi, K.; Kanazawa, M. Reference values for spirometry, including vital capacity, in Japanese adults calculated with the LMS method and compared with previous values. *Respir. Investig.* **2014**, *52*, 242–250. [CrossRef]
4. Vogelmeier, C.F.; Criner, G.J.; Martinez, F.J.; Anzueto, A.; Barnes, P.J.; Bourbeau, J.; Celli, B.R.; Chen, R.; Decramer, M.; Fabbri, L.M.; et al. Global Strategy for the Diagnosis, Management, and Prevention of Chronic Obstructive Lung Disease 2017 Report. GOLD Executive Summary. *Am. J. Respir. Crit. Care Med.* **2017**, *195*, 557–582. [CrossRef] [PubMed]
5. Barnes, P.J.; Celli, B.R. Systemic manifestations and comorbidities of COPD. *Eur. Respir. J.* **2009**, *33*, 1165–1185. [CrossRef] [PubMed]
6. Coronavirus Worldometer. Available online: www.worldometers.info/coronavirus/ (accessed on 19 February 2021).
7. Alqahtani, J.S.; Oyelade, T.; Aldhahir, A.M.; Alghamdi, S.M.; Almehmadi, M.; Alqahtani, A.S.; Quaderi, S.; Mandal, S.; Hurst, J.R. Prevalence, Severity and Mortality associated with COPD and Smoking in patients with COVID-19: A Rapid Systematic Review and Meta-Analysis. *PLoS ONE* **2020**, *15*, e0233147. [CrossRef] [PubMed]
8. Lange, P.; Celli, B.R.; Agustí, A.; Jensen, G.B.; Divo, M.; Faner, R.; Guerra, S.; Marott, J.L.; Martinez, F.D.; Martinez-Camblor, P.; et al. Lung-Function Trajectories Leading to Chronic Obstructive Pulmonary Disease. *N. Engl. J. Med.* **2015**, *373*, 111–122. [CrossRef] [PubMed]
9. Martinez, F.J.; Han, M.K.; Allinson, J.P.; Barr, R.G.; Boucher, R.C.; Calverley, P.M.A.; Celli, B.R.; Christenson, S.A.; Crystal, R.G.; Fageras, M.; et al. At the Root: Defining and Halting Progression of Early Chronic Obstructive Pulmonary Disease. *Am. J. Respir. Crit. Care Med.* **2018**, *197*, 1540–1551. [CrossRef]
10. Turner, M.C.; Chen, Y.; Krewski, D.; Calle, E.E.; Thun, M.J. Chronic Obstructive Pulmonary Disease Is Associated with Lung Cancer Mortality in a Prospective Study of Never Smokers. *Am. J. Respir. Crit. Care Med.* **2007**, *176*, 285–290. [CrossRef] [PubMed]
11. Raviv, S.; Hawkins, K.A.; DeCamp, M.M., Jr.; Kalhan, R. Lung cancer in chronic obstructive pulmonary disease: Enhancing surgical options and outcomes. *Am. J. Respir. Crit. Care Med.* **2011**, *183*, 1138–1146. [CrossRef] [PubMed]
12. Buist, A.S.; McBurnie, M.A.; Vollmer, W.M.; Gillespie, S.; Burney, P.; Mannino, D.M.; Menezes, A.M.; Sullivan, S.D.; Lee, T.A.; Weiss, K.B.; et al. International variation in the prevalence of COPD (The BOLD Study): A population-based prevalence study. *Lancet* **2007**, *370*, 741–750. [CrossRef]

13. Fang, L.; Gao, P.; Bao, H.; Tang, X.; Wang, B.; Feng, Y.; Cong, S.; Juan, J.; Fan, J.; Lu, K.; et al. Chronic obstructive pulmonary disease in China: A nationwide prevalence study. *Lancet Respir. Med.* **2018**, *6*, 421–430. [CrossRef]
14. Osaka, D.; Shibata, Y.; Abe, S.; Inoue, S.; Tokairin, Y.; Igarashi, A.; Yamauchi, K.; Kimura, T.; Sato, M.; Kishi, H.; et al. Relationship between Habit of Cigarette Smoking and Airflow Limitation in Healthy Japanese Individuals: The Takahata Study. *Intern. Med.* **2010**, *49*, 1489–1499. [CrossRef] [PubMed]
15. Sekine, Y.; Yanagibori, R.; Suzuki, K.; Sugiyama, S.; Yamaji, H.; Ishibashi, M.; Fujisawa, T. Surveillance of chronic obstructive pulmonary disease in high-risk individuals by using regional lung cancer mass screening. *Int. J. Chronic Obstr. Pulm. Dis.* **2014**, *9*, 647–656. [CrossRef]
16. Butler, S.J.; Li, L.S.K.; Ellerton, L.; Gershon, A.S.; Goldstein, R.S.; Brooks, D. Prevalence of comorbidities and impact on pulmonary rehabilitation outcomes. *ERJ Open Res.* **2019**, *5*, 00264–02019. [CrossRef] [PubMed]
17. Matsuo, M.; Hashimoto, N.; Usami, N.; Imaizumi, K.; Wakai, K.; Kawabe, T.; Yokoi, K.; Hasegawa, Y. Inspiratory capacity as a preoperative assessment of patients undergoing thoracic surgery. *Interact. Cardiovasc. Thorac. Surg.* **2012**, *14*, 560–564. [CrossRef] [PubMed]
18. Brunelli, A.; Charloux, A.; Bolliger, C.T.; Rocco, G.; Sculier, J.-P.; Varela, G.; Licker, M.; Ferguson, M.K.; Faivre-Finn, C.; Huber, R.M.; et al. ERS/ESTS clinical guidelines on fitness for radical therapy in lung cancer patients (surgery and chemo-radiotherapy). *Eur. Respir. J.* **2009**, *34*, 17–41. [CrossRef]
19. Omote, N.; Hashimoto, N.; Morise, M.; Sakamoto, K.; Miyazaki, S.; Ando, A.; Nakahara, Y.; Hasegawa, Y. Impact of mild to moderate COPD on feasibility and prognosis in non-small cell lung cancer patients who received chemotherapy. *Int. J. Chronic Obstr. Pulm. Dis.* **2017**, *12*, 3541–3547. [CrossRef]
20. Hashimoto, N.; Matsuzaki, A.; Okada, Y.; Imai, N.; Iwano, S.; Wakai, K.; Imaizumi, K.; Yokoi, K.; Hasegawa, Y. Clinical impact of prevalence and severity of COPD on the decision-making process for therapeutic management of lung cancer patients. *BMC Pulm. Med.* **2014**, *14*, 14. [CrossRef] [PubMed]
21. Loganathan, R.S.; Stover, D.E.; Shi, W.; Venkatraman, E. Prevalence of COPD in Women Compared to Men Around the Time of Diagnosis of Primary Lung Cancer. *Chest* **2006**, *129*, 1305–1312. [CrossRef]
22. Hashimoto, N.; Ando, A.; Iwano, S.; Sakamoto, K.; Okachi, S.; Matsuzaki, A.; Okada, Y.; Wakai, K.; Yokoi, K.; Hasegawa, Y. Thin-section computed tomography-determined usual interstitial pneumonia pattern affects the decision-making process for resection in newly diagnosed lung cancer patients: A retrospective study. *BMC Pulm. Med.* **2018**, *18*, 2. [CrossRef] [PubMed]
23. Tang, L.Y.W.; Coxson, H.O.; Lam, S.; Leipsic, J.; Tam, R.C.; Sin, D.D. Towards large-scale case-finding: Training and validation of residual networks for detection of chronic obstructive pulmonary disease using low-dose CT. *Lancet Digit. Health* **2020**, *2*, e259–e267. [CrossRef]
24. Hurst, J.R.; Vestbo, J.; Anzueto, A.; Locantore, N.; Mullerova, H.; Tal-Singer, R.; Miller, B.; Lomas, D.A.; Agusti, A.; Macnee, W.; et al. Susceptibility to exacerbation in chronic obstructive pulmonary disease. *N. Engl. J. Med.* **2010**, *363*, 1128–1138. [CrossRef] [PubMed]
25. Lamprecht, B.; Soriano, J.B.; Studnicka, M.; Kaiser, B.; Vanfleteren, L.E.; Gnatiuc, L.; Burney, P.; Miravitlles, M.; García-Rio, F.; Akbari, K.; et al. Determinants of Underdiagnosis of COPD in National and International Surveys. *Chest* **2015**, *148*, 971–985. [CrossRef] [PubMed]
26. Jones, R.C.M.; Price, D.; Ryan, D.; Sims, E.J.; von Ziegenweidt, J.; Mascarenhas, L.; Burden, A.; Halpin, D.M.G.; Winter, R.; Hill, S.; et al. Opportunities to diagnose chronic obstructive pulmonary disease in routine care in the UK: A retrospective study of a clinical cohort. *Lancet Respir. Med.* **2014**, *2*, 267–276. [CrossRef]
27. Silvestre, O.M.; Nadruz, W., Jr.; Querejeta, R.G.; Claggett, B.; Solomon, S.D.; Mirabelli, M.C.; London, S.J.; Loehr, L.R.; Shah, A.M. Declining Lung Function and Cardiovascular Risk: The ARIC Study. *J. Am. Coll. Cardiol.* **2018**, *72*, 1109–1122. [CrossRef] [PubMed]
28. Whittaker, H.R.; Bloom, C.; Morgan, A.; Jarvis, D.; Kiddle, S.J.; Quint, J.K. Accelerated FEV1 decline and risk of cardiovascular disease and mortality in a primary care population of COPD patients. *Eur. Respir. J.* **2021**, *57*, 2000918. [CrossRef] [PubMed]
29. Rodriguez-Mañas, L.; Fried, L.P. Frailty in the clinical scenario. *Lancet* **2015**, *385*, e7–e9. [CrossRef]
30. Bousquet, J.; Dinh-Xuan, A.T.; Similowski, T.; Malva, J.; Ankri, J.; Barbagallo, M.; Fabbri, L.; Humbert, M.; Mercier, J.; Robalo-Cordeiro, C.; et al. Should we use gait speed in COPD, FEV1 in frailty and dyspnoea in both? *Eur. Respir. J.* **2016**, *48*, 315–319. [CrossRef] [PubMed]
31. Lahousse, L.; Ziere, G.; Verlinden, V.J.A.; Zillikens, M.C.; Uitterlinden, A.G.; Rivadeneira, F.; Tiemeier, H.; Joos, G.F.; Hofman, A.; Ikram, M.A.; et al. Risk of Frailty in Elderly With COPD: A Population-Based Study. *J. Gerontol. Ser. A Boil. Sci. Med. Sci.* **2016**, *71*, 689–695. [CrossRef]
32. Kennedy, C.C.; Novotny, P.J.; Lebrasseur, N.K.; Wise, R.A.; Sciurba, F.C.; Benzo, R.P. Frailty and Clinical Outcomes in Chronic Obstructive Pulmonary Disease. *Ann. Am. Thorac. Soc.* **2019**, *16*, 217–224. [CrossRef] [PubMed]
33. Bertens, L.C.; Reitsma, J.B.; Van Mourik, Y.; Lammers, J.-W.J.; Moons, K.G.; Hoes, A.W.; Rutten, F.H. COPD detected with screening: Impact on patient management and prognosis. *Eur. Respir. J.* **2014**, *44*, 1571–1578. [CrossRef] [PubMed]
34. Leung, J.M.; Niikura, M.; Yang, C.W.T.; Sin, D.D. COVID-19 and COPD. *Eur. Respir. J.* **2020**, *56*, 2002108. [CrossRef] [PubMed]
35. Williamson, E.J.; Walker, A.J.; Bhaskaran, K.; Bacon, S.; Bates, C.; Morton, C.E.; Curtis, H.J.; Mehrkar, A.; Evans, D.; Inglesby, P.; et al. Factors associated with COVID-19-related death using OpenSAFELY. *Nature* **2020**, *584*, 430–436. [CrossRef] [PubMed]

36. Schultze, A.; Walker, A.J.; MacKenna, B.; Morton, C.E.; Bhaskaran, K.; Brown, J.P.; Rentsch, C.T.; Williamson, E.; Drysdale, H.; Croker, R.; et al. Risk of COVID-19-related death among patients with chronic obstructive pulmonary disease or asthma prescribed inhaled corticosteroids: An observational cohort study using the OpenSAFELY platform. *Lancet Respir. Med.* **2020**, *8*, 1106–1120. [CrossRef]
37. Waschki, B.; Kirsten, A.; Holz, O.; Muller, K.C.; Meyer, T.; Watz, H.; Magnussen, H. Physical activity is the strongest predictor of all-cause mortality in patients with COPD: A prospective cohort study. *Chest* **2011**, *140*, 331–342. [CrossRef]
38. Sekine, Y.; Behnia, M.; Fujisawa, T. Impact of COPD on pulmonary complications and on long-term survival of patients undergoing surgery for NSCLC. *Lung Cancer* **2002**, *37*, 95–101. [CrossRef]
39. Hankinson, J.L.; Odencrantz, J.R.; Fedan, K.B. Spirometric reference values from a sample of the general U.S. population. *Am. J. Respir. Crit. Care Med.* **1999**, *159*, 179–187. [CrossRef] [PubMed]
40. Vaz Fragoso, C.A.; Concato, J.; McAvay, G.; Van Ness, P.H.; Rochester, C.L.; Yaggi, H.K.; Gill, T.M. The ratio of FEV1 to FVC as a basis for establishing chronic obstructive pulmonary disease. *Am. J. Respir. Crit. Care Med.* **2010**, *181*, 446–451. [CrossRef]
41. Osuka, S.; Hashimoto, N.; Sakamoto, K.; Wakai, K.; Yokoi, K.; Hasegawa, Y. Risk stratification by the lower limit of normal of FEV1/FVC for postoperative outcomes in patients with COPD undergoing thoracic surgery. *Respir. Investig.* **2015**, *53*, 117–123. [CrossRef]
42. Matsuzaki, A.; Hashimoto, N.; Okachi, S.; Taniguchi, T.; Kawaguchi, K.; Fukui, T.; Wakai, K.; Yokoi, K.; Hasegawa, Y. Clinical impact of the lower limit of normal of FEV1/FVC on survival in lung cancer patients undergoing thoracic surgery. *Respir. Investig.* **2016**, *54*, 184–192. [CrossRef]
43. Çolak, Y.; Nordestgaard, B.G.; Vestbo, J.; Lange, P.; Afzal, S. Comparison of five major airflow limitation criteria to identify high-risk individuals with COPD: A contemporary population-based cohort. *Thorax* **2020**, *75*, 944–954. [CrossRef]
44. Okada, Y.; Hashimoto, N.; Iwano, S.; Kawaguchi, K.; Fukui, T.; Sakamoto, K.; Wakai, K.; Yokoi, K.; Hasegawa, Y. ⟨Editors' Choice⟩ Renewed Japanese spirometric reference variables and risk stratification for postoperative outcomes in COPD patients with resected lung cancer. *Nagoya J. Med. Sci.* **2019**, *81*, 427–438.
45. Izquierdo, J.L.; Resano, P.; El Hachem, A.; Graziani, D.; Almonacid, C.; Sánchez, I.M. Impact of COPD in patients with lung cancer and advanced disease treated with chemotherapy and/or tyrosine kinase inhibitors. *Int. J. Chronic Obstr. Pulm. Dis.* **2014**, *9*, 1053–1058. [CrossRef] [PubMed]
46. Ritchie, A.I.; Martinez, F.J. The Challenges of Defining Early COPD in the General Population. *Am. J. Respir. Crit. Care Med.* **2020**. [CrossRef] [PubMed]
47. Çolak, Y.; Afzal, S.; Nordestgaard, B.G.; Vestbo, J.; Lange, P. Prevalence, Characteristics, and Prognosis of Early Chronic Obstructive Pulmonary Disease. The Copenhagen General Population Study. *Am. J. Respir. Crit. Care Med.* **2020**, *201*, 671–680. [CrossRef] [PubMed]
48. Marott, J.L.; Ingebrigtsen, T.S.; Çolak, Y.; Vestbo, J.; Lange, P. Lung Function Trajectories Leading to Chronic Obstructive Pulmonary Disease as Predictors of Exacerbations and Mortality. *Am. J. Respir. Crit. Care Med.* **2020**, *202*, 210–218. [CrossRef] [PubMed]
49. Fukuchi, Y.; Nishimura, M.; Ichinose, M.; Adachi, M.; Nagai, A.; Kuriyama, T.; Takahashi, K.; Nishimura, K.; Ishioka, S.; Aizawa, H.; et al. COPD in Japan: The Nippon COPD Epidemiology study. *Respirology* **2004**, *9*, 458–465. [CrossRef] [PubMed]
50. Labonté, L.E.; Tan, W.C.; Li, P.Z.; Mancino, P.; Aaron, S.D.; Benedetti, A.; Chapman, K.R.; Cowie, R.; Fitzgerald, J.M.; Hernandez, P.; et al. Undiagnosed Chronic Obstructive Pulmonary Disease Contributes to the Burden of Health Care Use. Data from the CanCOLD Study. *Am. J. Respir. Crit. Care Med.* **2016**, *194*, 285–298. [CrossRef] [PubMed]
51. Press, V.G.; Cifu, A.S.; White, S.R. Screening for Chronic Obstructive Pulmonary Disease. *JAMA* **2017**, *318*, 1702–1703. [CrossRef] [PubMed]
52. Rabe, K.F.; Hurst, J.R.; Suissa, S. Cardiovascular disease and COPD: Dangerous liaisons? *Eur. Respir. Rev.* **2018**, *27*, 180057. [CrossRef] [PubMed]
53. Laucho-Contreras, M.E.; Cohen-Todd, M. Early diagnosis of COPD: Myth or a true perspective. *Eur. Respir. Rev.* **2020**, *29*, 200131. [CrossRef]
54. Zhou, Y.; Zhong, N.-S.; Li, X.; Chen, S.; Zheng, J.; Zhao, D.; Yao, W.; Zhi, R.; Wei, L.; He, B.; et al. Tiotropium in Early-Stage Chronic Obstructive Pulmonary Disease. *N. Engl. J. Med.* **2017**, *377*, 923–935. [CrossRef] [PubMed]
55. Di Marco, F.; Balbo, P.; de Blasio, F.; Cardaci, V.; Crimi, N.; Girbino, G.; Pelaia, G.; Pirina, P.; Roversi, P.; Santus, P.; et al. Early management of COPD: Where are we now and where do we go from here? A Delphi consensus project. *Int. J. Chronic Obstruct. Pulm. Dis.* **2019**, *14*, 353–360. [CrossRef]
56. Agusti, A.; Alcazar, B.; Cosio, B.; Echave, J.M.; Faner, R.; Izquierdo, J.L.; Marin, J.M.; Soler-Cataluña, J.J.; Celli, B. Time for a change: Anticipating the diagnosis and treatment of COPD. *Eur. Respir. J.* **2020**, *56*, 2002104. [CrossRef] [PubMed]
57. Yawn, B.P.; Martinez, F.J. POINT: Can Screening for COPD Improve Outcomes? Yes. *Chest* **2020**, *157*, 7–9. [CrossRef]
58. Celli, B.R.; Anderson, J.A.; Cowans, N.J.; Crim, C.; Hartley, B.F.; Martinez, F.J.; Morris, A.N.; Quasny, H.; Yates, J.; Vestbo, J.; et al. Pharmacotherapy and Lung Function Decline in Patients with Chronic Obstructive Pulmonary Disease. A Systematic Review. *Am. J. Respir. Crit. Care Med.* **2021**, *203*, 689–698. [CrossRef]
59. Young, R.P.; Hopkins, R.J.; Christmas, T.; Black, P.N.; Metcalf, P.; Gamble, G.D. COPD prevalence is increased in lung cancer, independent of age, sex and smoking history. *Eur. Respir. J.* **2009**, *34*, 380–386. [CrossRef] [PubMed]
60. Houghton, A.M. Mechanistic links between COPD and lung cancer. *Nat. Rev. Cancer* **2013**, *13*, 233–245. [CrossRef]

61. Mets, O.M.; Buckens, C.F.M.; Zanen, P.; Isgum, I.; Van Ginneken, B.; Prokop, M.; Gietema, H.A.; Lammers, J.-W.J.; Vliegenthart, R.; Oudkerk, M.; et al. Identification of Chronic Obstructive Pulmonary Disease in Lung Cancer Screening Computed Tomographic Scans. *JAMA* **2011**, *306*, 1775–1781. [CrossRef] [PubMed]
62. Labaki, W.W.; Xia, M.; Murray, S.; Hatt, C.R.; Al-Abcha, A.; Ferrera, M.C.; Meldrum, C.A.; Keith, L.A.; Galbán, C.J.; Arenberg, D.A.; et al. Quantitative Emphysema on Low-Dose CT Imaging of the Chest and Risk of Lung Cancer and Airflow Obstruction. *Chest* **2020**. [CrossRef] [PubMed]

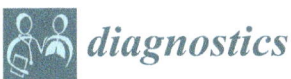

Review

Motor Pathophysiology Related to Dyspnea in COPD Evaluated by Cardiopulmonary Exercise Testing

Keisuke Miki

Department of Respiratory Medicine, National Hospital Organization Osaka Toneyama Medical Center, 5-1-1 Toneyama, Toyonaka, Osaka 560-8552, Japan; miki.keisuke.pu@mail.hosp.go.jp

Abstract: In chronic obstructive pulmonary disease (COPD), exertional dyspnea, which increases with the disease's progression, reduces exercise tolerance and limits physical activity, leading to a worsening prognosis. It is necessary to understand the diverse mechanisms of dyspnea and take appropriate measures to reduce exertional dyspnea, as COPD is a systemic disease with various comorbidities. A treatment focusing on the motor pathophysiology related to dyspnea may lead to improvements such as reducing dynamic lung hyperinflation, respiratory and metabolic acidosis, and eventually exertional dyspnea. However, without cardiopulmonary exercise testing (CPET), it may be difficult to understand the pathophysiological conditions during exercise. CPET facilitates understanding of the gas exchange and transport associated with respiration-circulation and even crosstalk with muscles, which is sometimes challenging, and provides information on COPD treatment strategies. For respiratory medicine department staff, CPET can play a significant role when treating patients with diseases that cause exertional dyspnea. This article outlines the advantages of using CPET to evaluate exertional dyspnea in patients with COPD.

Keywords: acidosis; breathing; cardiopulmonary exercise testing; dynamic hyperinflation; muscle; ventilation

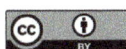

1. Introduction

Globally, chronic obstructive pulmonary disease (COPD) was the third leading cause of death in 2018 [1], and countermeasures against COPD are required. The most frequent and important complaint of patients with COPD is exertional dyspnea, the pathophysiology of which is known to includes several etiological factors [2–5]. There can be no improvement in exercise tolerance and physical activity for patients without mitigating dyspnea, which is difficult to bear. Customized treatment suitable for the condition must be provided to alleviate exertional dyspnea after exploring the causes of COPD, given that COPD is a systemic disease with comorbidities [6,7] and that exertional dyspnea can have diverse etiologies.

This article discusses the motor pathophysiology of COPD, which is directly related to the treatment of exertional dyspnea, based on previous insights into how dyspnea in COPD can be evaluated using cardiopulmonary exercise testing (CPET) [8]. Briefly, two types of protocols are used in CPET: a maximum (symptom-limited) incremental exercise test, and a constant work rate exercise test. Numerous exertional parameters are included, all of which are calculated using the ventilation amount, and the concentration of oxygen and carbon dioxide during inspiration or expiration [8–10]. CPET facilitates diagnosis and determination of the patient's exertional pathophysiological condition and can help in the choice of treatment, evaluation of the response to treatment, and determination of the prognosis [8,11]. Although the interpretation of data obtained from CPET sometimes requires a comprehensive understanding of this test method, CPET can quickly provide deep insights into pathophysiological responses to exercise, reflecting crosstalk between the functions of the cardiopulmonary system and peripheral muscles [10]. This article also examines how CPET can facilitate the implementation of treatment strategies to further alleviate exertional dyspnea, with a particular focus on respiratory patterns.

2. Exercise Tolerance and Exercise-Limiting Factors

The forced expiratory volume in one second (FEV_1) is an important indicator that correlates well with minute ventilation (V'_E), but has a weak relationship with exercise tolerance [12]. This distinction reflects the fact that the ventilatory efficiency is related to wasted ventilation [13–15] and to the fact that the difference between inspired and expired oxygen concentrations (measured as the difference between average inspired oxygen concentration and average expired oxygen concentration) [9,10], not just the ventilation amount, is related to exercise tolerance. In this context, it is worth noting that oxygen uptake (V'_{O2}) is determined using an equation that includes the product of V'_E and the difference between inspired and expired oxygen concentrations, and that the average expired oxygen concentration is dependent on the collective cardiac, pulmonary and muscular metabolism [9,10]. Although many factors define the daily activity level of patients with COPD, this activity level is often influenced by dyspnea. Predicting the level of daily activity based on resting pulmonary function alone is difficult because other exercise limiting factors, such as cardiovascular disorders and lower limb fatigue, are not evaluated. Evaluation of exercise tolerance by CPET indicates the level of daily activity more directly and is also useful in predicting the patient's prognosis [16–20]. Adequate measures are needed, mainly for patients who can engage only in activities of approximately 3 metabolic equivalents (METs) (maximal oxygen uptake of 10.5 mL/min/Kg) [18,21,22]. The pathophysiology of exertional dyspnea can be understood in due course, including the exercise-limiting factors concerned with dyspnea treatment.

Accurate evaluation during the CPET of leg fatigue, in addition to dyspnea during CPET, is important for determining the treatment plan. The evaluation must be performed while the patient is not talking, thereby ensuring that there is no interference with exhaled gas evaluation. The 10-point modified Borg Scale, with 0 corresponding to no dyspnea and 10 corresponding to maximal dyspnea or leg fatigue, is often used [23]. When dyspnea and leg fatigue are evaluated during CPET, dyspnea alone, leg fatigue alone, or the combination of both dyspnea and leg fatigue is commonly reported at the end of exercise. On this scale of dyspnea, scores of 2 or 3 correspond to the anaerobic metabolism threshold and are associated with an elevated threshold of sympathetic nerve activity not only in COPD but also in interstitial pneumonia [3,24]. Therefore, it is useful to instruct people to engage, as part of their self-range, in activities for which dyspnea is 2–3 points on the modified Borg scale, thereby avoiding excessive exercise in daily life. If the causes of dyspnea are examined closely, the exercise-limiting factors among these causes can be classified broadly into three categories, namely: dyspnea due to ventilatory impairment, lower limb fatigue, and cardiovascular impairment (Figure 1).

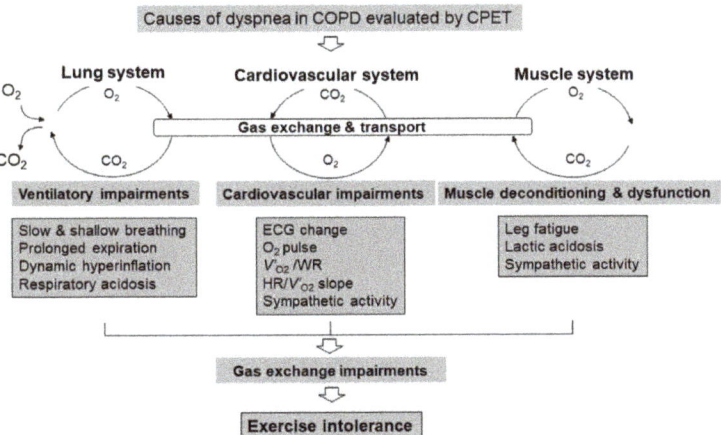

Figure 1. Schematic pathophysiologic pathway exertional dyspnea in chronic obstructive pulmonary disease. CO_2: carbon dioxide; CPET: cardiopulmonary exercise testing; ECG: electrocardiogram; HR: heart rate; O_2: oxygen; O_2 pulse: V'_{O2}/heart rate; V'_{O2}: oxygen uptake; WR: work rate. This is an original figure (no permission is required).

2.1. Exertional Dyspnea Due to Cardiovascular Disorders

In previous studies of patients with COPD who exhibit exertional dyspnea [12,25], 10–17% of patients with exertional dyspnea were subjects whose dyspnea was due to cardiovascular disorders; many of these patients were observed to have abnormalities as assessed by electrocardiogram (ECG). Reports from the United States and Europe indicate that the percentage of ischemic heart disease and heart failure is higher among patients with COPD complications [26]. According to reports from Japanese cardiovascular facilities, the percentage of patients with COPD who also exhibited cardiovascular diseases represented 27% of individuals with COPD complications [27]. Determining that the heart is the limiting factor for exercise may be difficult if the ECG does not indicate an abnormality. In such cases, limitation due to the heart is indicated if (during CPET) the slope of V'_{O2} versus work rate (measured in watts) is reduced (Figure 1). Alternatively, a plateau phenomenon of the oxygen pulse (V'_{O2}/heart rate (HR)), which is almost equivalent to the stroke volume, may be occurring (Figure 1). In either instance, a steep slope of HR versus V'_{O2} can be used as a reference to assess whether cardiovascular disorders are limiting factors for exercise (Figure 1) [28]. If the oxygen pulse plateaus during exercise, but there are no abnormalities in the ECG during exercise, then the pathological condition may be clarified using an echocardiogram to test for the existence of a valve disease, possibly including that of the mitral valve [29]. In addition, evaluating impairments of the pulmonary microvasculature may be informative, given that such impairments already can be seen in mild-stage COPD; indeed, reduced pulmonary blood flow during exercise has been reported in such patients [30,31]. Furthermore, the evaluation of sympathetic activity during exercise may provide important information on the pathophysiologic conditions underlying not only cardiovascular disease but also COPD during exercise (Figure 1). Elevated sympathetic activity already will be apparent in the resting condition in patients with advanced COPD, and the change of sympathetic activity has been shown to correlate with exertional dyspnea in patients with stable COPD [3,20,22]. Therefore, respiratory medicine department staff need to remember that cardiovascular diseases may be a cause of exertional dyspnea.

2.2. Measures and Treatment of Lower Limb Fatigue

Work by the author and colleagues has revealed that, in 20% of the patients with exertional dyspnea as the chief complaint, lower limb fatigue, not dyspnea, was actually the exercise-limiting factor (Figure 1); in such patients, resting pulmonary function was relatively preserved [12]. With the progression of respiratory or cardiovascular diseases, ventilatory disorders, circulatory disorders, or muscle sympathetic overactivity develop in addition to the lower limb fatigue, leading to the progression of dyspnea as the pathological condition worsens. Furthermore, aside from the case where dyspnea is the only exercise-limiting factor, if dyspnea and lower limb fatigue are of approximately the same intensity, then ventilation must compensate for exercise-induced acidosis (due to lactic acid production by the muscles). In such cases, exercise therapy focusing on the lower limbs may improve exertional dyspnea by suppressing excessive lactic acid production and consequently lowering the need for ventilation [32,33]. In any case, exercise therapy for the lower limbs should be performed from an early stage. The staff of respiratory medicine or cardiovascular departments often tend to neglect exercise therapy for the lower limbs in favor of their department's respective specialty. Increasing physical activity at an earlier stage of COPD is associated with a better prognosis, and it is important to teach exercise habits that make use of hobbies from an earlier stage, thereby promoting behavioral changes [34]. Unfortunately, however, as COPD advances, the related functional impairments lead to muscle weakness and body weight loss [35,36]. Indeed, loss of muscle mass and muscle strength are greater in patients in the advanced stages of COPD [37], the progress of which particularly affects the lower limbs [36,38]. In patients that are underweight or have sarcopenia, exertional dyspnea can become very severe, because such patients must compensate for muscle impairments as well as for ventilatory impairments [39–41]. To treat such patients, it may be important to choose suitable therapies based on cardiopulmonary-peripheral muscle crosstalk. Ghrelin, first discovered in 1999 as a novel growth-hormone-releasing peptide isolated from the stomach [42], has a variety of effects, such as causing a positive energy balance and weight gain by decreasing fat utilization [43], stimulating food intake [44], and inhibiting sympathetic nerve activity [45]. The author and colleagues reported that, in cachectic patients with COPD, ghrelin administration with exercise training provided improvements in exertional dyspnea [39,46], respiratory strength [39], and exertional intolerance [47] in randomized, double-blind, placebo-controlled trials.

In the future, as the population ages, the number of patients who are immobilized due to lower limb fatigue is expected to increase, and the need for exercise therapy of the lower limbs based on the cardiopulmonary-peripheral muscle crosstalk will increase further. CPET will be useful for identifying patients who are candidates for exercise therapy of the lower limbs.

2.3. Exertional Dyspnea Due to Ventilatory Impairment

In a study by the author and colleagues [12], exertional dyspnea due to ventilatory impairment accounted for 70% of patients with exertional dyspnea as the chief complaint (Figure 1). Here, the author considers the mechanism of exertional dyspnea due to ventilatory impairment and the relevant remedies that focus on respiratory patterns. Although tachypnea [48] is often considered to be a cause of dyspnea and a target of treatment, tachypnea is observed during maximal exercise in patients with COPD who exhibit a preserved exercise tolerance, and even in healthy individuals [49], and is considered to be a standard physiological mechanism used by the body to increase the amount of ventilation. On the other hand, it should be noted that, among patients with COPD who exhibit exercise intolerance, a surprisingly large number of subjects have a slow-shallow pattern with prolonged expiration (Figure 2a–c), where expiratory tidal volume ($V_T$ex) is reduced without an increase in the respiratory frequency. Typically, such patients do not demonstrate a rapid-shallow pattern, where a rise in the $V_T$ex is limited and is compensated by tachypnea [12]. The worsening of these mechanical ventilatory abnormalities during exercise is explained by i) high elastic load, ii) decreased dynamic lung compliance, and iii) increased resistive load of respiratory muscles, all of which lead to dynamic lung hyperinflation in COPD [50–54]. Studies of dynamic blood gas show that, in healthy individuals and patients with COPD who retain ventilation capacity, metabolic acidosis (resulting from elevated levels of lactic acid) progresses during exercise; ventilation compensation for such acidosis is detected as a decrease in bicarbonate ions, and exercise is terminated when metabolic acidosis is no longer compensated [12]. On the other hand, in patients with poor ventilation compensation capacity and decreased exercise tolerance, exercise is terminated when the patient develops respiratory acidosis (Figure 2d), which does not lead to an elevation in lactic acid levels but rather to an elevation in the partial pressure of arterial carbon dioxide and bicarbonate ions [12]. These observations explain why patients with dynamic lung hyperinflation [55,56] may become breathless. Dyspnea is an exercise-limiting factor in a high percentage of these patients [12], and an increase in ventilation capacity, ideally by increasing $V_T$ex, or using a treatment to improve ventilatory efficiency, is expected to yield successful results. Interestingly, in patients with COPD who possess various resting pulmonary functions, ventilation limitations, and exercise tolerances, exercise was terminated when exercise-induced acidosis (pH) and dyspnea during maximal exercise (Figure 2e) were comparable [12]. This observation suggests that, though dyspnea is caused by complex factors, including the central nervous network and peripheral muscles [5], one of the common mechanisms in exertional dyspnea involves a compensatory mechanism that maintains acid-base homeostasis in the blood [3,12,57]. In the body, CO_2 transport is affected by the exertional pH change that accompanies CO_2 production due to ventilatory impairments or lactate production during exercise. Furthermore, in a study examining exercise-limiting factors in patients with idiopathic pulmonary fibrosis and COPD [3,58], exercise-induced acidosis was a limiting factor for exercise regardless of the concentration of oxygen administered. In addition, exertional hypoxemia was not a normal feature in heathy subjects who also felt exertional dyspnea at the end of exercise [24,59]. In other words, exertional dyspnea is associated with exercise-induced acidosis rather than with hypoxia, and ventilation may be an important compensatory mechanism for maintaining acid-base homeostasis, the mechanism of which may lead to optimal exercise performance. Therefore, adequate ventilation, especially exhalation, is fundamental to the treatment of COPD. As mentioned above, the slow-shallow pattern during exertion in patients with exercise intolerance is often accompanied by prolonged expiration (Figure 2c). Laveneziana et al. [60] reported that expiratory muscle activity in COPD was relatively increased during exercise but did not mitigate dynamic lung hyperinflation. More recently, it has been reported that expiratory muscle strength often increases in patients with COPD, perhaps to compensate for inadequate ventilation [61]; a negative correlation has been observed between maximal expiratory muscle strength at rest and maximal oxygen uptake, especially in patients with COPD who have prolonged expiration [61,62]. In other words, although the slow-shallow pattern prolongs expiration (Figure 2a–c), this ventilation pattern requires high expiratory muscle strength but does not raise oxygen uptake, making breathing difficult for the patient. Inadequate exhalation leading to prolonged expiration results in a large amount of air remaining in the lung after expiration ($V_T$in-$V_T$ex), expressed as the difference between the inspiratory tidal volume ($V_T$in) and $V_T$ex [61,62]. Excess expiratory muscle recruitment might be a compensatory mechanism to improve exercise intolerance. Further studies are necessary to clarify the implications for the COPD of excess expiratory muscle recruitment.

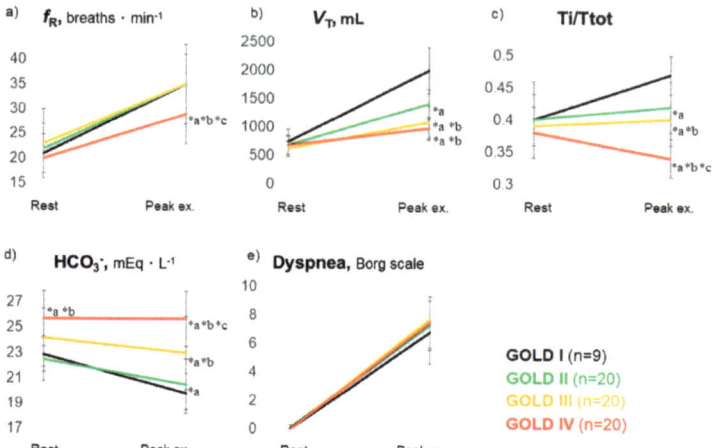

Figure 2. Typical responses to incremental exercise by patients with chronic obstructive pulmonary disease. Data are presented as mean ± SD. ex.: exercise; f_R: respiratory frequency; HCO_3^-: bicarbonate ion; Ti/Ttot: inspiratory duty cycle; Vex: tidal volume. The 10-point modified Borg Scale, with 0 corresponding to no dyspnea and 10 corresponding to maximal dyspnea was used to evaluate the exertional dyspnea. Among the four Global Initiative for Chronic Obstructive Lung Disease (GOLD) stages, despite the different breathing patterns ((**a**): f_R, (**b**): Vex, and (**c**): Ti/Ttot) during exercise, patients with COPD did not regulate the exertional acidosis ((**d**): HCO_3^-) to stop exercise, reaching a similar exertional dyspnea level (**e**). Using the Kruskal-Wallis test to compare the groups consisting of the four GOLD stages, there was a significant difference in f_R ($p = 0.0021$), V_T ($p < 0.0001$), Ti/Ttot ($p < 0.0001$), and HCO_3^- ($p < 0.0001$) at peak exercise, and HCO_3^- ($p < 0.0001$) at rest. Using the Steel-Dwass test to carry out between-group comparisons, *a, $p < 0.05$ versus GOLD I; *b, $p < 0.05$ versus GOLD II; *c, $p < 0.05$ versus GOLD III. This is an original figure (no permission is required).

2.3.1. Improving Ventilatory Impairments to Reduce Exertional Dyspnea

Reducing the air remaining in the lung after the expiration of each exhaled breath is expected to improve dynamic hyperinflation, respiratory acidosis, and eventually dyspnea. COPD is recognized as a disease that primarily involves pulmonary parenchyma and obstructs the peripheral respiratory tract, which affects the exertional dyspnea [63]. Interestingly, however, collapse of the respiratory tract during forced expiration was reported in the 1960s among patients with COPD [64]. In addition, since its first description in the 1980s, exercise-induced laryngeal obstruction has been considered problematic because this condition may affect young adults and can mimic exercise-induced asthma [65–68]. Although there is no standardized methodology for confirming exertional laryngeal obstruction and dyspnea severity, continuous laryngoscopy during CPET has been reported to improve diagnostic sensitivity [69]. Furthermore, Baz et al. [70] recently reported that the central respiratory tract outside the mediastinum, namely, the vocal cords, is obstructed during exercise. As the obstruction intensifies, the degree of prolonged expiration also increases. The expiratory airflow limitation in patients with COPD involves obstruction of the peripheral respiratory tract and of the central respiratory tract, including the vocal cords, which affects exertional dyspnea and breathing patterns. In a preliminary study, the author and colleagues observed that expiratory pressure load training in patients with severe and very severe COPD increased the expiratory tidal volume, reduced the air remaining in the lung after expiration, and improved prolonged expiration. In other words, the slow-shallow pattern with prolonged expiration improved, which in turn resulted in improvements in subjective symptoms and exercise tolerance [62]. In contrast, inspiratory pressure load training, which is also referred to as inspiratory muscle training, has been recommended as a pulmonary rehabilitation (PR) program [71]. However, at least in patients with advanced COPD, no large studies have reported the adjunctive effects of inspiratory pressure load training added to PR [72–74]. In addition, Yamamoto et al. reported that, especially in underweight patients with advanced COPD, inspiratory pressure load training might lead to tachypnea and wasted ventilation, which would in turn decrease exercise performance; however, this point was made as part of a case report [75]. Further studies are needed to evaluate the effect of expiratory or inspiratory pressure load training on exertional dyspnea in patients with COPD. In the future, the author hopes to develop therapies for the slow-shallow pattern with prolonged expiration, which is the cause of exertional dyspnea in patients with advanced COPD.

2.3.2. Reducing Ventilatory Demand to Reduce Exertional Dyspnea

In contrast to providing adequate ventilation, reducing ventilatory demand or increasing oxygen utilization may be of help in improving exertional dyspnea in COPD. Especially in patients who exhibit exercise intolerance due to the reduced capability to increase ventilation during exercise, a strategy related to oxygen utilization may be useful in reducing exertional dyspnea. Acupuncture, an Eastern medical practice, has been reported to improve exercise intolerance, dyspnea, and quality of life in patients with COPD [76,77]. In addition, the physiological benefits of acupuncture have been reported to include the relaxation of muscle tension, along with improvements of muscle/anti-muscle fatigue, muscle blood flow, and sympathetic control [78,79]. However, to date, little is known about the mechanism whereby acupuncture improves exertional dyspnea. Using CPET, Maekura et al. [80] investigated the effect and mechanism of acupuncture on exercise intolerance and exertional dyspnea in patients with COPD. Their findings demonstrated that the effects of acupuncture on exertional dyspnea were associated primarily with improved oxygen utilization and reduced ventilation during exercise.

A similar mechanism explains how PR improves exercise performance and exertional dyspnea [81–84]. Using CPET, the author and colleagues [83] investigated how PR reduces exertional dyspnea; the results demonstrated that the reduced exertional dyspnea obtained from PR was associated with reduced ventilatory demand due to the economized oxygen requirements. In addition, although the mechanisms underlying meditative movement (tai chi, yoga, and qigong) on COPD are unclear, a systematic review and meta-analysis reported that the application of meditative movement as non-conventional therapies might improve exercise capacity, dyspnea, and health-related quality of life in COPD patients [85].

3. Conclusions

Diverse exertional dyspnea is related to the crosstalk between the heart, lungs, and muscles; further exploration of the exertional dyspnea patterns, which are related to cardiovascular disorders, ventilatory impairment, and/or lower limb fatigue, will not only facilitate elucidation of the dynamic pathophysiology of COPD but will also contribute directly to the treatment of patients with this disease. Reducing the air remaining in the lungs after the expiration of each exhaled breath is expected to improve dynamic hyperinflation, respiratory acidosis, and eventually dyspnea. Furthermore, reducing ventilatory demand or increasing oxygen utilization may also facilitate improvements in exertional dyspnea in COPD. Considering that CPET can provide key information on specific dysfunctions in COPD patients that can be used to help them maintain daily living activities and allow them to feel that they can "walk with a little more ease", staff providing respiratory care should make the most of CPET as a more approachable test.

Funding: This research received no external funding.

Institutional Review Board Statement: Not applicable.

Acknowledgments: The author would like to thank R. Maekura, M. Miki, K. Tsujino, H. Hashimoto, Y. Yamamoto, H. Kagawa, T. Matsuki, T. Kawasaki, T. Kuge, H. Kida, J. Ikeda, S. Sakaguchi, and S. Ito for help with the CPET measurements.

Conflicts of Interest: The author declares no conflict of interest.

References

1. World Health Organization. The Top 10 Causes of Death. Available online: https://www.who.int/news-room/fact-sheets/detail/the-top-10-causes-of-death (accessed on 29 December 2020).
2. Laveneziana, P.; Webb, K.A.; Ora, J.; Wadell, K.; O'Donnell, D.E. Evolution of dyspnea during exercise in chronic obstructive pulmonary disease: Impact of critical volume constraints. *Am. J. Respir. Crit. Care Med.* **2011**, *184*, 1367–1373. [CrossRef] [PubMed]
3. Miki, K.; Maekura, R.; Hiraga, T.; Kitada, S.; Miki, M.; Yoshimura, K.; Tateishi, Y. Effects of oxygen on exertional dyspnoea and exercise performance in patients with chronic obstructive pulmonary disease. *Respirology* **2012**, *17*, 149–154. [CrossRef]
4. O'Donnell, D.E.; Lam, M.; Webb, K.A. Measurement of symptoms, lung hyperinflation, and endurance during exercise in chronic obstructive pulmonary disease. *Am. J. Respir. Crit. Care Med.* **1998**, *158*, 1557–1565. [CrossRef] [PubMed]
5. O'Donnell, D.E.; Milne, K.M.; James, M.D.; de Torres, J.P.; Neder, J.A. Dyspnea in COPD: New Mechanistic Insights and Management Implications. *Adv. Ther.* **2020**, *37*, 41–60. [CrossRef]
6. Gan, W.Q.; Man, S.F.; Senthilselvan, A.; Sin, D.D. Association between chronic obstructive pulmonary disease and systemic inflammation: A systematic review and a meta-analysis. *Thorax* **2004**, *59*, 574–580. [CrossRef]
7. Vanfleteren, L.E.; Spruit, M.A.; Groenen, M.; Gaffron, S.; van Empel, V.P.; Bruijnzeel, P.L.; Rutten, E.P.; Roodt, J.O.; Wouters, E.F.; Franssen, F.M. Clusters of comorbidities based on validated objective measurements and systemic inflammation in patients with chronic obstructive pulmonary disease. *Am. J. Respir. Crit. Care Med.* **2013**, *187*, 728–735. [CrossRef] [PubMed]
8. Radtke, T.; Crook, S.; Kaltsakas, G.; Louvaris, Z.; Berton, D.; Urquhart, D.S.; Kampouras, A.; Rabinovich, R.A.; Verges, S.; Kontopidis, D.; et al. ERS statement on standardisation of cardiopulmonary exercise testing in chronic lung diseases. *Eur. Respir. Rev.* **2019**, *28*, 180101. [CrossRef]
9. Laviolette, L.; Laveneziana, P. Exercise Testing in the prognostic evaluation of patients with lung and heart diseases. In *Clinical Exercise Testing (ERS Monograph)*; Palange, P., Laveneziana, P., Neder, J.A., Ward, S.A., Eds.; European Respiratory Society: Sheffield, UK, 2018; pp. 222–234.
10. Wasserman, K.; Hansen, J.; Sue, D.; Stringer, W.; Sietsema, K.; Sun, X.-G. *Principles of Exercise Testing and Interpretation: Including Pathophysiology and Clinical Applications*, 5th ed.; Lippincott Williams and Wilkins: Philadelphia, PA, USA, 2012.
11. Puente-Maestu, L.; Palange, P.; Casaburi, R.; Laveneziana, P.; Maltais, F.; Neder, J.A.; O'Donnell, D.E.; Onorati, P.; Porszasz, J.; Rabinovich, R.; et al. Use of exercise testing in the evaluation of interventional efficacy: An official ERS statement. *Eur. Respir. J.* **2016**, *47*, 429–460. [CrossRef]
12. Kagawa, H.; Miki, K.; Kitada, S.; Miki, M.; Yoshimura, K.; Oshitani, Y.; Nishida, K.; Sawa, N.; Tsujino, K.; Maekura, R. Dyspnea and the Varying Pathophysiologic Manifestations of Chronic Obstructive Pulmonary Disease Evaluated by Cardiopulmonary Exercise Testing With Arterial Blood Analysis. *Front. Physiol.* **2018**, *9*, 1293. [CrossRef]
13. Neder, J.A.; Berton, D.C.; Arbex, F.F.; Alencar, M.C.; Rocha, A.; Sperandio, P.A.; Palange, P.; O'Donnell, D.E. Physiological and clinical relevance of exercise ventilatory efficiency in COPD. *Eur. Respir. J.* **2017**, *49*, 1602036. [CrossRef]
14. Phillips, D.B.; Collins, S.; Stickland, M.K. Measurement and Interpretation of Exercise Ventilatory Efficiency. *Front. Physiol.* **2020**, *11*, 659. [CrossRef]
15. Weatherald, J.; Sattler, C.; Garcia, G.; Laveneziana, P. Ventilatory response to exercise in cardiopulmonary disease: The role of chemosensitivity and dead space. *Eur. Respir. J.* **2018**, *51*, 1700860. [CrossRef]
16. Hiraga, T.; Maekura, R.; Okuda, Y.; Okamoto, T.; Hirotani, A.; Kitada, S.; Yoshimura, K.; Yokota, S.; Ito, M.; Ogura, T. Prognostic predictors for survival in patients with COPD using cardiopulmonary exercise testing. *Clin. Physiol. Funct. Imaging* **2003**, *23*, 324–331. [CrossRef]
17. Oga, T.; Nishimura, K.; Tsukino, M.; Hajiro, T.; Ikeda, A.; Mishima, M. Relationship between different indices of exercise capacity and clinical measures in patients with chronic obstructive pulmonary disease. *Heart Lung* **2002**, *31*, 374–381. [CrossRef]
18. Oga, T.; Nishimura, K.; Tsukino, M.; Sato, S.; Hajiro, T. Analysis of the factors related to mortality in chronic obstructive pulmonary disease: Role of exercise capacity and health status. *Am. J. Respir Crit Care Med.* **2003**, *167*, 544–549. [CrossRef]
19. Ozgür, E.S.; Nayci, S.A.; Özge, C.; Taşdelen, B. An integrated index combined by dynamic hyperinflation and exercise capacity in the prediction of morbidity and mortality in COPD. *Respir. Care* **2012**, *57*, 1452–1459. [CrossRef]
20. Yoshimura, K.; Maekura, R.; Hiraga, T.; Miki, K.; Kitada, S.; Miki, M.; Tateishi, Y.; Mori, M. Identification of three exercise-induced mortality risk factors in patients with COPD. *COPD* **2014**, *11*, 615–626. [CrossRef] [PubMed]
21. Guazzi, M.; Adams, V.; Conraads, V.; Halle, M.; Mezzani, A.; Vanhees, L.; Arena, R.; Fletcher, G.F.; Forman, D.E.; Kitzman, D.W.; et al. EACPR/AHA Scientific Statement. Clinical recommendations for cardiopulmonary exercise testing data assessment in specific patient populations. *Circulation* **2012**, *126*, 2261–2274. [CrossRef]
22. Maekura, R.; Hiraga, T.; Miki, K.; Kitada, S.; Yoshimura, K.; Miki, M.; Tateishi, Y. Differences in physiological response to exercise in patients with different COPD severity. *Respir. Care* **2014**, *59*, 252–262. [CrossRef] [PubMed]
23. Wilson, R.C.; Jones, P.W. A comparison of the visual analogue scale and modified Borg scale for the measurement of dyspnoea during exercise. *Clin. Sci.* **1989**, *76*, 277–282. [CrossRef]
24. Miki, K.; Maekura, R.; Hiraga, T.; Hashimoto, H.; Kitada, S.; Miki, M.; Yoshimura, K.; Tateishi, Y.; Fushitani, K.; Motone, M. Acidosis and raised norepinephrine levels are associated with exercise dyspnoea in idiopathic pulmonary fibrosis. *Respirology* **2009**, *14*, 1020–1026. [CrossRef]

25. Hirotani, A.; Maekura, R.; Okuda, Y.; Yoshimura, K.; Moriguchi, K.; Kitada, S.; Hiraga, T.; Ito, M.; Ogura, T.; Ogihara, T. Exercise-induced electrocardiographic changes in patients with chronic respiratory diseases: Differential diagnosis by 99mTc-tetrofosmin SPECT. *J. Nucl. Med.* **2003**, *44*, 325–330.
26. Rutten, F.H.; Cramer, M.J.; Grobbee, D.E.; Sachs, A.P.; Kirkels, J.H.; Lammers, J.W.; Hoes, A.W. Unrecognized heart failure in elderly patients with stable chronic obstructive pulmonary disease. *Eur. Heart J.* **2005**, *26*, 1887–1894. [CrossRef]
27. Onishi, K.; Yoshimoto, D.; Hagan, G.W.; Jones, P.W. Prevalence of airflow limitation in outpatients with cardiovascular diseases in Japan. *Int. J. Chron. Obs. Pulmon. Dis.* **2014**, *9*, 563–568. [CrossRef]
28. Agostoni, P.; Casaburi, R. *Patterns of cariopulmonary response to exercise in cardiac diseses In Clinical Exercise Testing (ERS Monograph)*; Palange, P., Laveneziana, P., Neder, J.A., Ward, S.A., Eds.; European Respiratory Society: Sheffield, UK, 2018; pp. 160–174.
29. Nery, L.E.; Wasserman, K.; French, W.; Oren, A.; Davis, J.A. Contrasting cardiovascular and respiratory responses to exercise in mitral valve and chronic obstructive pulmonary diseases. *Chest* **1983**, *83*, 446–453. [CrossRef]
30. Barr, R.G.; Bluemke, D.A.; Ahmed, F.S.; Carr, J.J.; Enright, P.L.; Hoffman, E.A.; Jiang, R.; Kawut, S.M.; Kronmal, R.A.; Lima, J.A.; et al. Percent emphysema, airflow obstruction, and impaired left ventricular filling. *N. Engl. J. Med.* **2010**, *362*, 217–227. [CrossRef] [PubMed]
31. Grau, M.; Barr, R.G.; Lima, J.A.; Hoffman, E.A.; Bluemke, D.A.; Carr, J.J.; Chahal, H.; Enright, P.L.; Jain, A.; Prince, M.R.; et al. Percent emphysema and right ventricular structure and function: The Multi-Ethnic Study of Atherosclerosis-Lung and Multi-Ethnic Study of Atherosclerosis-Right Ventricle Studies. *Chest* **2013**, *144*, 136–144. [CrossRef]
32. Coppoolse, R.; Schols, A.M.; Baarends, E.M.; Mostert, R.; Akkermans, M.A.; Janssen, P.P.; Wouters, E.F. Interval versus continuous training in patients with severe COPD: A randomized clinical trial. *Eur. Respir. J.* **1999**, *14*, 258–263. [CrossRef] [PubMed]
33. Ward, T.J.C.; Lindley, M.R.; Ferguson, R.A.; Constantin, D.; Singh, S.J.; Bolton, C.E.; Evans, R.A.; Greenhaff, P.L.; Steiner, M.C. Submaximal Eccentric Cycling in People With COPD: Acute Whole-Body Cardiopulmonary and Muscle Metabolic Responses. *Chest* **2020**, *159*, 564–574. [CrossRef] [PubMed]
34. Watz, H.; Pitta, F.; Rochester, C.L.; Garcia-Aymerich, J.; ZuWallack, R.; Troosters, T.; Vaes, A.W.; Puhan, M.A.; Jehn, M.; Polkey, M.I.; et al. An official European Respiratory Society statement on physical activity in COPD. *Eur. Respir. J.* **2014**, *44*, 1521–1537. [CrossRef]
35. Agusti, A.; Soriano, J.B. COPD as a systemic disease. *COPD* **2008**, *5*, 133–138. [CrossRef]
36. Rabe, K.F.; Watz, H. Chronic obstructive pulmonary disease. *Lancet* **2017**, *389*, 1931–1940. [CrossRef]
37. Celli, B.R.; Locantore, N.; Tal-Singer, R.; Riley, J.; Miller, B.; Vestbo, J.; Yates, J.C.; Silverman, E.K.; Owen, C.A.; Divo, M.; et al. Emphysema and extrapulmonary tissue loss in COPD: A multi-organ loss of tissue phenotype. *Eur. Respir. J.* **2018**, *51*, 1702146. [CrossRef]
38. Maltais, F.; Decramer, M.; Casaburi, R.; Barreiro, E.; Burelle, Y.; Debigaré, R.; Dekhuijzen, P.N.; Franssen, F.; Gayan-Ramirez, G.; Gea, J.; et al. An official American Thoracic Society/European Respiratory Society statement: Update on limb muscle dysfunction in chronic obstructive pulmonary disease. *Am. J. Respir. Crit. Care Med.* **2014**, *189*, e15–e62. [CrossRef] [PubMed]
39. Miki, K.; Maekura, R.; Nagaya, N.; Nakazato, M.; Kimura, H.; Murakami, S.; Ohnishi, S.; Hiraga, T.; Miki, M.; Kitada, S.; et al. Ghrelin treatment of cachectic patients with chronic obstructive pulmonary disease: A multicenter, randomized, double-blind, placebo-controlled trial. *PLoS ONE* **2012**, *7*, e35708. [CrossRef]
40. Rosenberg, I.H. Sarcopenia: Origins and clinical relevance. *J. Nutr.* **1997**, *127*, 990s–991s. [CrossRef] [PubMed]
41. Studenski, S.A.; Peters, K.W.; Alley, D.E.; Cawthon, P.M.; McLean, R.R.; Harris, T.B.; Ferrucci, L.; Guralnik, J.M.; Fragala, M.S.; Kenny, A.M.; et al. The FNIH sarcopenia project: Rationale, study description, conference recommendations, and final estimates. *J. Gerontol. A Biol. Sci. Med. Sci.* **2014**, *69*, 547–558. [CrossRef] [PubMed]
42. Kojima, M.; Hosoda, H.; Date, Y.; Nakazato, M.; Matsuo, H.; Kangawa, K. Ghrelin is a growth-hormone-releasing acylated peptide from stomach. *Nature* **1999**, *402*, 656–660. [CrossRef]
43. Tschöp, M.; Smiley, D.L.; Heiman, M.L. Ghrelin induces adiposity in rodents. *Nature* **2000**, *407*, 908–913. [CrossRef]
44. Nakazato, M.; Murakami, N.; Date, Y.; Kojima, M.; Matsuo, H.; Kangawa, K.; Matsukura, S. A role for ghrelin in the central regulation of feeding. *Nature* **2001**, *409*, 194–198. [CrossRef]
45. Matsumura, K.; Tsuchihashi, T.; Fujii, K.; Abe, I.; Iida, M. Central ghrelin modulates sympathetic activity in conscious rabbits. *Hypertension* **2002**, *40*, 694–699. [CrossRef]
46. Miki, K.; Maekura, R.; Nagaya, N.; Miki, M.; Kitada, S.; Yoshimura, K.; Mori, M.; Kangawa, K. Effects of ghrelin treatment on exertional dyspnea in COPD: An exploratory analysis. *J. Physiol. Sci.* **2015**, *65*, 277–284. [CrossRef] [PubMed]
47. Miki, K.; Maekura, R.; Nagaya, N.; Kitada, S.; Miki, M.; Yoshimura, K.; Tateishi, Y.; Motone, M.; Hiraga, T.; Mori, M.; et al. Effects of ghrelin treatment on exercise capacity in underweight COPD patients: A substudy of a multicenter, randomized, double-blind, placebo-controlled trial of ghrelin treatment. *BMC Pulm. Med.* **2013**, *13*, 37. [CrossRef]
48. Macklem, P.T. Therapeutic implications of the pathophysiology of COPD. *Eur. Respir. J.* **2010**, *35*, 676–680. [CrossRef]
49. Neder, J.A.; Arbex, F.F.; Alencar, M.C.; O'Donnell, C.D.; Cory, J.; Webb, K.A.; O'Donnell, D.E. Exercise ventilatory inefficiency in mild to end-stage COPD. *Eur. Respir. J.* **2015**, *45*, 377–387. [CrossRef]
50. Dodd, D.S.; Brancatisano, T.; Engel, L.A. Chest wall mechanics during exercise in patients with severe chronic air-flow obstruction. *Am. Rev. Respir. Dis.* **1984**, *129*, 33–38. [CrossRef] [PubMed]
51. Faisal, A.; Alghamdi, B.J.; Ciavaglia, C.E.; Elbehairy, A.F.; Webb, K.A.; Ora, J.; Neder, J.A.; O'Donnell, D.E. Common Mechanisms of Dyspnea in Chronic Interstitial and Obstructive Lung Disorders. *Am. J. Respir. Crit. Care Med.* **2016**, *193*, 299–309. [CrossRef]

52. Jolley, C.J.; Luo, Y.M.; Steier, J.; Rafferty, G.F.; Polkey, M.I.; Moxham, J. Neural respiratory drive and breathlessness in COPD. *Eur. Respir. J.* **2015**, *45*, 355–364. [CrossRef]
53. O'Donnell, D.E.; Guenette, J.A.; Maltais, F.; Webb, K.A. Decline of resting inspiratory capacity in COPD: The impact on breathing pattern, dyspnea, and ventilatory capacity during exercise. *Chest* **2012**, *141*, 753–762. [CrossRef] [PubMed]
54. Potter, W.A.; Olafsson, S.; Hyatt, R.E. Ventilatory mechanics and expiratory flow limitation during exercise in patients with obstructive lung disease. *J. Clin. Investig.* **1971**, *50*, 910–919. [CrossRef]
55. O'Donnell, D.E.; Revill, S.M.; Webb, K.A. Dynamic hyperinflation and exercise intolerance in chronic obstructive pulmonary disease. *Am. J. Respir. Crit. Care Med.* **2001**, *164*, 770–777. [CrossRef]
56. O'Donnell, D.E.; Webb, K.A. Exertional breathlessness in patients with chronic airflow limitation. *Am. Rev. Respir. Dis.* **1993**, *148*, 1351–1357. [CrossRef]
57. Wasserman, K.; Cox, T.A.; Sietsema, K.E. Ventilatory regulation of arterial H(+) (pH) during exercise. *Respir. Physiol. Neurobiol.* **2014**, *190*, 142–148. [CrossRef]
58. Miki, K.; Maekura, R.; Miki, M.; Kitada, S.; Yoshimura, K.; Tateishi, Y.; Mori, M. Exertional acidotic responses in idiopathic pulmonary fibrosis: The mechanisms of exertional dyspnea. *Respir. Physiol. Neurobiol.* **2013**, *185*, 653–658. [CrossRef]
59. Dempsey, J.A.; Wagner, P.D. Exercise-induced arterial hypoxemia. *J. Appl. Physiol.* **1999**, *87*, 1997–2006. [CrossRef]
60. Laveneziana, P.; Webb, K.A.; Wadell, K.; Neder, J.A.; O'Donnell, D.E. Does expiratory muscle activity influence dynamic hyperinflation and exertional dyspnea in COPD? *Respir. Physiol. Neurobiol.* **2014**, *199*, 24–33. [CrossRef] [PubMed]
61. Miki, K.; Tsujino, K.; Edahiro, R.; Kitada, S.; Miki, M.; Yoshimura, K.; Kagawa, H.; Oshitani, Y.; Ohara, Y.; Hosono, Y.; et al. Exercise tolerance and balance of inspiratory-to-expiratory muscle strength in relation to breathing timing in patients with chronic obstructive pulmonary disease. *J. Breath Res.* **2018**, *12*, 036008. [CrossRef]
62. Miki, K.; Tsujino, K.; Miki, M.; Yoshimura, K.; Kagawa, H.; Oshitani, Y.; Fukushima, K.; Matsuki, T.; Yamamoto, Y.; Kida, H. Managing COPD with expiratory or inspiratory pressure load training based on a prolonged expiration pattern. *ERJ Open Res.* **2020**, *6*. [CrossRef] [PubMed]
63. McDonough, J.E.; Yuan, R.; Suzuki, M.; Seyednejad, N.; Elliott, W.M.; Sanchez, P.G.; Wright, A.C.; Gefter, W.B.; Litzky, L.; Coxson, H.O.; et al. Small-airway obstruction and emphysema in chronic obstructive pulmonary disease. *N. Engl. J. Med.* **2011**, *365*, 1567–1575. [CrossRef]
64. Rainer, W.G.; Hutchinson, D.; Newby, J.P.; Hamstra, R.; Durrance, J. Major Airway Collapsibility in the Pathogenesis of Obstructive Emphysema. *J. Thorac. Cardiovasc. Surg.* **1963**, *46*, 559–567. [CrossRef]
65. Johansson, H.; Norlander, K.; Berglund, L.; Janson, C.; Malinovschi, A.; Nordvall, L.; Nordang, L.; Emtner, M. Prevalence of exercise-induced bronchoconstriction and exercise-induced laryngeal obstruction in a general adolescent population. *Thorax* **2015**, *70*, 57–63. [CrossRef]
66. Lakin, R.C.; Metzger, W.J.; Haughey, B.H. Upper airway obstruction presenting as exercise-induced asthma. *Chest* **1984**, *86*, 499–501. [CrossRef]
67. Landwehr, L.P.; Wood, R.P.; Blager, F.B.; Milgrom, H. Vocal cord dysfunction mimicking exercise-induced bronchospasm in adolescents. *Pediatrics* **1996**, *98*, 971–974.
68. McFadden, E.R., Jr.; Zawadski, D.K. Vocal cord dysfunction masquerading as exercise-induced asthma. a physiologic cause for "choking" during athletic activities. *Am. J. Respir. Crit. Care Med.* **1996**, *153*, 942–947. [CrossRef]
69. Olin, J.T.; Clary, M.S.; Fan, E.M.; Johnston, K.L.; State, C.M.; Strand, M.; Christopher, K.L. Continuous laryngoscopy quantitates laryngeal behaviour in exercise and recovery. *Eur. Respir. J.* **2016**, *48*, 1192–1200. [CrossRef]
70. Baz, M.; Haji, G.S.; Menzies-Gow, A.; Tanner, R.J.; Hopkinson, N.S.; Polkey, M.I.; Hull, J.H. Dynamic laryngeal narrowing during exercise: A mechanism for generating intrinsic PEEP in COPD? *Thorax* **2015**, *70*, 251–257. [CrossRef]
71. Gosselink, R.; De Vos, J.; van den Heuvel, S.P.; Segers, J.; Decramer, M.; Kwakkel, G. Impact of inspiratory muscle training in patients with COPD: What is the evidence? *Eur. Respir. J.* **2011**, *37*, 416–425. [CrossRef]
72. Ambrosino, N. Inspiratory muscle training in stable COPD patients: Enough is enough? *Eur. Respir. J.* **2018**, *51*, 1702285. [CrossRef]
73. Charususin, N.; Gosselink, R.; Decramer, M.; Demeyer, H.; McConnell, A.; Saey, D.; Maltais, F.; Derom, E.; Vermeersch, S.; Heijdra, Y.F.; et al. Randomised controlled trial of adjunctive inspiratory muscle training for patients with COPD. *Thorax* **2018**, *73*, 942–950. [CrossRef]
74. Schultz, K.; Jelusic, D.; Wittmann, M.; Krämer, B.; Huber, V.; Fuchs, S.; Lehbert, N.; Wingart, S.; Stojanovic, D.; Göhl, O.; et al. Inspiratory muscle training does not improve clinical outcomes in 3-week COPD rehabilitation: Results from a randomised controlled trial. *Eur. Respir. J.* **2018**, *51*, 1702000. [CrossRef]
75. Yamamoto, Y.; Miki, K.; Matsuki, T.; Fukushima, K.; Oshitani, Y.; Kagawa, H.; Tsujino, K.; Yoshimura, K.; Miki, M.; Kida, H. Intolerance to and limitations of inspiratory muscle training in patients with advanced chronic obstructive pulmonary disease: A report of two cases. *Respir. Med. Case Rep.* **2020**, *31*, 101210. [CrossRef]
76. Jobst, K.; Chen, J.H.; McPherson, K.; Arrowsmith, J.; Brown, V.; Efthimiou, J.; Fletcher, H.J.; Maciocia, G.; Mole, P.; Shifrin, K.; et al. Controlled trial of acupuncture for disabling breathlessness. *Lancet* **1986**, *2*, 1416–1419. [CrossRef]
77. Suzuki, M.; Muro, S.; Ando, Y.; Omori, T.; Shiota, T.; Endo, K.; Sato, S.; Aihara, K.; Matsumoto, M.; Suzuki, S.; et al. A randomized, placebo-controlled trial of acupuncture in patients with chronic obstructive pulmonary disease (COPD): The COPD-acupuncture trial (CAT). *Arch. Intern. Med.* **2012**, *172*, 878–886. [CrossRef]

78. Cagnie, B.; Barbe, T.; De Ridder, E.; Van Oosterwijck, J.; Cools, A.; Danneels, L. The influence of dry needling of the trapezius muscle on muscle blood flow and oxygenation. *J. Manip. Physiol. Ther.* **2012**, *35*, 685–691. [CrossRef]
79. Shinbara, H.; Okubo, M.; Sumiya, E.; Fukuda, F.; Yano, T.; Kitade, T. Effects of manual acupuncture with sparrow pecking on muscle blood flow of normal and denervated hindlimb in rats. *Acupunct. Med.* **2008**, *26*, 149–159. [CrossRef] [PubMed]
80. Maekura, T.; Miki, K.; Miki, M.; Kitada, S.; Maekura, R. Clinical Effects Of Acupuncture On The Pathophysiological Mechanism Of Chronic Obstructive Pulmonary Disease During Exercise. *Int. J. Chron. Obs. Pulmon. Dis.* **2019**, *14*, 2787–2798. [CrossRef] [PubMed]
81. Casaburi, R.; Porszasz, J.; Burns, M.R.; Carithers, E.R.; Chang, R.S.; Cooper, C.B. Physiologic benefits of exercise training in rehabilitation of patients with severe chronic obstructive pulmonary disease. *Am. J. Respir. Crit. Care Med.* **1997**, *155*, 1541–1551. [CrossRef] [PubMed]
82. Laveneziana, P.; Palange, P. Physical activity, nutritional status and systemic inflammation in COPD. *Eur. Respir. J.* **2012**, *40*, 522–529. [CrossRef]
83. Miki, K.; Maekura, R.; Kitada, S.; Miki, M.; Yoshimura, K.; Yamamoto, H.; Kawabe, T.; Kagawa, H.; Oshitani, Y.; Satomi, A.; et al. Pulmonary rehabilitation for COPD improves exercise time rather than exercise tolerance: Effects and mechanisms. *Int. J. Chron. Obs. Pulmon. Dis.* **2017**, *12*, 1061–1070. [CrossRef]
84. Rochester, C.L.; Vogiatzis, I.; Holland, A.E.; Lareau, S.C.; Marciniuk, D.D.; Puhan, M.A.; Spruit, M.A.; Masefield, S.; Casaburi, R.; Clini, E.M.; et al. An Official American Thoracic Society/European Respiratory Society Policy Statement: Enhancing Implementation, Use, and Delivery of Pulmonary Rehabilitation. *Am. J. Respir. Crit. Care Med.* **2015**, *192*, 1373–1386. [CrossRef]
85. Wu, L.L.; Lin, Z.K.; Weng, H.D.; Qi, Q.F.; Lu, J.; Liu, K.X. Effectiveness of meditative movement on COPD: A systematic review and meta-analysis. *Int. J. Chron. Obs. Pulmon. Dis.* **2018**, *13*, 1239–1250. [CrossRef] [PubMed]

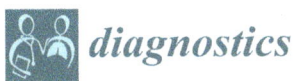

Review

Treatment Response Biomarkers in Asthma and COPD

Howraman Meteran [1,2,*], Pradeesh Sivapalan [1,3] and Jens-Ulrik Stæhr Jensen [1,4]

1. Department of Internal Medicine, Respiratory Medicine Section, Copenhagen University Hospital—Herlev and Gentofte, 2900 Hellerup, Denmark; pradeesh.sivapalan.02@regionh.dk (P.S.); jens.ulrik.jensen@regionh.dk (J.-U.S.J.)
2. Department of Microbiology and Immunology, University of Copenhagen, 1353 Copenhagen, Denmark
3. Department of Internal Medicine, Zealand University Hospital, 4000 Roskilde, Denmark
4. Department of Clinical Medicine, Faculty of Health Sciences, University of Copenhagen, 1353 Copenhagen, Denmark
* Correspondence: hmeteran@gmail.com; Tel.: +45-60-67-72-96

Abstract: Chronic obstructive pulmonary disease (COPD) and asthma are two of the most common chronic diseases worldwide. Both diseases are heterogenous and complex, and despite their similarities, they differ in terms of pathophysiological and immunological mechanisms. Mounting evidence supports the presence of several phenotypes with various responses to treatment. A systematic and thorough assessment concerning the diagnosis of both asthma and COPD is crucial to the clinical management of the disease. The identification of different biomarkers can facilitate targeted treatment and monitoring. Thanks to the presence of numerous immunological studies, our understanding of asthma phenotypes and mechanisms of disease has increased markedly in the last decade, and several treatments with monoclonal antibodies are available. There are compelling data that link eosinophilia with an increased risk of COPD exacerbations but a greater treatment response and lower all-cause mortality. Eosinophilia can be considered as a treatable trait, and the initiation of inhaled corticosteroid in COPD patients with eosinophilia is supported in many studies. In spite of advances in our understanding of both asthma and COPD in terms pathophysiology, disease mechanisms, biomarkers, and response to treatment, many uncertainties in the management of obstructive airways exist.

Keywords: COPD; asthma; biomarker treatment; response

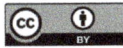

1. Introduction

Chronic obstructive pulmonary disease (COPD) and asthma affect more than 600 million individuals globally. Although COPD and asthma are heterogenous and complex diseases that share similarities concerning symptoms, inflammation, and airflow limitation, they also differ with regard to certain key features. Asthma is characterized by variable airflow limitation, airway hyperresponsiveness, and airway inflammation [1]. It has several phenotypes with distinct aetiologies that can be classified based on triggers, clinical presentation, and inflammatory type [2]. Asthma was previously thought to be characterized by eosinophilic inflammation, but it is now recognized that characteristics of asthma can be present without eosinophilic inflammation [2,3]. COPD is characterized by chronic inflammation of the lungs with the presence of neutrophils, macrophages, and T-lymphocytes. The T-lymphocytes consist mostly of TH1, TH17, and cytotoxic T cells [4]. Based on the idea that COPD is characterized by neutrophilic inflammation, the presence of eosinophilic airway inflammation has been used to discriminate between asthma and COPD. However, this notion is flawed because around 40% of COPD patients exhibit eosinophilic inflammation even when adjusting for asthma [5]. These patients exhibit characteristics similar to those of asthma patients, and the term asthma–COPD overlap (ACO) has been used to describe this subset of patients who simultaneously exhibit characteristics of both diseases [6].

This overlap between asthma and COPD presents many challenges, as different aetiologies with different treatment needs can present with similar symptoms. Thus, distinguishing between allergic inflammation, bacterial infection, and other disease phenotypes is crucial to providing optimal treatment as well as reducing the burden and side effects of ineffective treatment.

The identification of the various phenotypes makes it possible to take an individualized approach to clinical decision making when treating patients with asthma and COPD. The need for predictive biomarkers has become increasingly vital to identifying patients who are most likely to achieve clinical benefit and minimum side effects [7]. Thus, the aim of this study is to review the identified treatment response biomarkers in asthma and COPD.

2. Biomarkers in Asthma

Asthma has long been classified as either atopic ("extrinsic") or non-atopic ("intrinsic") asthma but is now considered an umbrella diagnosis for various diseases with different endotypes (underlying immunological mechanisms) and phenotypes (e.g., atopy, obesity and age). Cluster analyses of data from large cohorts have led to two major asthma endotypes, T2-high and non-T2-high asthma [8,9].

2.1. T2-High Asthma

Reduced barrier function in the respiratory epithelium seems to play an important role in T2-high asthma, as microbes and allergens activate epithelial-derived alarmins, such as thymic stromal lymphopoietin (TSLP), interleukin (IL)-25, and IL-33 [10]. Activation of these upstream cytokines results in several type 2 immune responses. TLSP activates T- and B-cell responses, while IL-25 and IL-33 activate innate lymphoid cells (ILCs), which play a crucial role in the production of IL-5 and IL-13 [11]. The principal cytokines produced by Th2-cells are IL-4, IL-5, and IL-13 [12]. These cytokines are involved in numerous immunological processes, such as the production of downstream cytokines (IL13 and IL-4), activation of mast cells (IL-13), B-cell activation to undergo immunoglobulin E (IgE) isotype switching (IL-4), and maturation and survival of eosinophils (IL-5) [13] and subsequently promote pathophysiological changes, such as increased mucus secretion, airway hyperresponsiveness, inflammation, and tissue remodelling [3,14]. Thus, both Th2-cells and ILCs are involved in type 2 inflammation, which is manifested as high IgE and eosinophils in asthma.

Corticosteroids are the cornerstone of asthma treatment and result in clinically significant improvements in lung function, symptom control, and reduction of asthma exacerbations [15]. However, approximately 10% of asthma patients remain uncontrolled in terms of symptoms and exacerbations despite treatment with high-dose, inhaled corticosteroids in combination with long-acting β-2-agonists and long-acting muscarinic-antagonists. For this group of patients, treatment with monoclonal antibodies targeting some of the cytokines can significantly improve various clinical outcomes in patients with severe asthma [16]. Omalizumab (humanized, monoclonal antibody that binds to circulating IgE molecules) was the first approved treatment for patients with allergic asthma, followed by treatments targeting the IL-5 pathway: mepolizumab (monoclonal antibody that binds to IL-5), reslizumab (also a monoclonal antibody that binds specifically to IL-5), and benralizumab (monoclonal antibody that binds directly to the IL-5-receptorα on eosinophils) [17]. Dupilumab is the most recently approved biological treatment for severe asthma. Dupilumab blocks the α-subunit of the IL-4-receptor, which is used by both IL-4 and IL-13 and thus inhibits signal transduction from these key mediators of type 2 inflammation [18].

2.1.1. Eosinophilia

The prevalence of eosinophilic inflammation among the asthmatic population is 50% but might be underestimated [19]. Eosinophils are the most important cells associated with type 2 inflammation, and when activated, they release a number of inflammatory mediators from intracellular granules [20], resulting in airway remodelling and bronchoconstriction [21]. Eosinophil inflammation in asthma is associated with poor prognosis [22] and, moreover, predicts response to treatment with corticosteroids [23]. Thus, several biomarkers have been identified and utilized to quantify eosinophilic airway inflammation and will be discussed in the following sections.

Sputum and Blood Eosinophils

Eosinophilic airway inflammation in induced sputum (cut-off > 3%) is considered to be a more accurate biomarker of T2-inflammation than absolute eosinophil count in peripheral blood [24]. An inconsistent association between airway and peripheral eosinophils has been observed in several studies and might be due to heterogenous study populations [25,26]. The correlation between sputum and blood eosinophils was investigated in a clinical study including both asthma and COPD patients and showed that the correlation was better in the asthmatic population [27]. Another study using data from the SPIROMICS (Subpopulation and Intermediate Outcome Measures In COPD Study) cohort found that stratification by sputum eosinophils but not blood eosinophils was associated with an increased risk of COPD exacerbations [28]. However, the presence of blood eosinophils in both asthma and COPD is associated with accelerated lung function decline and increased risk of exacerbations [29–31] and serves as a useful biomarker to identity patients with severe eosinophilic asthma [32] and response to inhaled corticosteroids in COPD [33].

Moreover, as induced sputum for daily clinical practice is laborious and can be bothersome for the patient, the use of blood eosinophils as a marker of T2-inflammation is more widely used.

Various cut-off values between 150–400 cells/µL have been used in the definition of blood eosinophilia and are able to predict response to treatment with anti-IL-5 in asthmatic individuals [34–36]. However, mounting evidence suggests that eosinophil count should be deemed a continuous variable and that higher levels predict a greater response [33].

Furthermore, a post-hoc study examining the stability of blood eosinophils in asthmatic individuals found that a single measurement might be insufficient in the diagnosis and management of asthma and that the instability was more pronounced for eosinophil counts between 150–299 cells/µL [37].

A study comprising stable COPD patients showed that using a threshold of ≥300 cells/µL in peripheral blood enabled the identification of sputum eosinophilia in 71% of the patients [38].

Eosinophils and Response to Treatment

Based on the last two decades of research, it is now established that eosinophilia can be used as a predictive biomarker for both the initiation and discontinuation of treatment with inhaled corticosteroids [39–42]. A retrospective study of asthmatics from a secondary care centre showed that inhaled corticosteroids (ICS) reduced both sputum and blood eosinophils, and clinical improvements were observed in terms of quality of life, forced expiratory volume in first second (FEV1), airway hyperresponsiveness, and exacerbation rate in those asthma patients with eosinophilic inflammation [42]. In addition, reducing ICS among patients with non-eosinophilic inflammation resulted in improved asthma control. In a 16-week trial with mild-to-moderate asthmatic individuals, sputum eosinophil counts two weeks after discontinuation of ICS and the change in eosinophil counts from before and after cessation of ICS predicted subsequent loss of asthma control [39]. A Cochrane review concluded that the frequency of asthma exacerbations can be reduced by tailoring the asthma treatment based on sputum eosinophils [41].

Randomized clinical trials have shown that a higher baseline eosinophil count predicts a greater reduction of severe asthma exacerbations in patients treated with inhaled corticosteroids [43]. A systematic review and meta-analysis including 61 studies found that oral corticosteroids improved lung function and reduced asthma symptoms and markers of type 2 inflammation and that patients with increased sputum and blood eosinophils at baseline were more responsive to treatment with oral corticosteroids [44]. In a clinical study of OCS-dependent asthmatic individuals, several type-2-related biomarkers returned to baseline levels after month after treatment (0.5 mg/kg prednisolone for 7 days) [45].

The level of blood eosinophils is also the key biomarker in selecting patients for treatment with monoclonal antibodies targeting the IL-5 pathway. In both the DREAM (Mepolizumab For Severe Eosinophilic Asthma) and MENSA (Mepolizumab Treatment for Patients With Severe Eosinophilic Asthma) studies, an eosinophil count of $\geq$150 cells/µL at baseline predicted a better response to treatment with mepolizumab in severe asthma patients [35]. The pooled analyses of the CALIMA (randomized, double-blind, placebo-controlled phase 3 trial with benralizumab) and SIROCCO (randomized, multicentre, placebo-controlled phase 3 trial with benralizumab) studies showed that in severe asthma patients, blood eosinophils $\geq$300 cells/µL and exacerbations in the previous year were predictors of a greater treatment response compared with those patients with eosinophils <300 cells/µL [46].

The early efficacy studies on reslizumab included patients with persistent asthma and blood eosinophils $\geq$400 cells/µL and observed significant improvements in the annual frequency of asthma exacerbations [47] and FEV1 [48].

2.1.2. Fraction of Exhaled Nitrogen Oxide (FeNO)

Nitric oxide is produced in the bronchial airway by inducible nitric oxide synthase (iNOS) and is mediated by type 2 inflammatory cytokines, such as IL-4 and IL-13 [49]. The measurement of FeNO is widely used as a marker of eosinophilic inflammation in the airways [50], and when combined with blood eosinophils, it might be useful for differentiating between COPD and asthma–COPD overlap [51].

A study including steroid-naive asthma patients and healthy individuals found that the level of FeNO was highest among patients with allergic asthma, followed by non-allergic asthma and healthy individuals [52]. FeNO is associated with reversibility of airway obstruction, blood eosinophils [52], and bronchial hyperresponsiveness [53]. Various cut-off values have been suggested, but it has become evident that values below 25 ppb are not associated with eosinophil inflammation, whereas values above 50 are strongly associated with eosinophilic inflammation (Table 1) [54].

A number of factors, such as sex, smoking, atopy, BMI, and chronic rhinosinusitis with nasal polyps, even in the absence of asthma, can affect the level of FeNO and should be taken into account in clinical evaluation [55,56].

A three-year follow-up study including severe asthma patients found an association between patients with sustained high levels of FeNO ($\geq$50 ppb) and an increased risk of asthma exacerbations (shorter exacerbation-free survival time and number of exacerbations) compared with those with sustained low levels of FeNO (<25 ppb) [57]. Another study that used data from the same cohort found that among a number of type-2-related biomarkers, only FeNO was associated with an increased risk of exacerbations [58]. Interestingly, the association was independent of past exacerbation status.

An early randomized, placebo-controlled trial showed that treatment with inhaled corticosteroids significantly decreased the level of FeNO compared with placebo after only two weeks of treatment [59]. The decreased level was sustained during the treatment period (four weeks) and increased significantly after a (two-week) washout period. Another randomized, open-label clinical trial examined FeNO in relation to spirometry and sequential changes in relation to inhaled corticosteroids [60] and found that FeNO but not spirometry was able to differentiate between patients treated with or without ICS. Moreover, the reduction in FeNO correlated significantly with patients' adherence to ICS.

In a more recent double-blind, randomized, placebo-controlled multicentre study, the baseline level of FeNO predicted the response to treatment with extrafine ICS in terms of significant changes in Asthma Control Questionnaire 7 (ACQ-7): for every 10-ppb increase in baseline FeNO, the change in ACQ-7 was greater in the treatment group than in the placebo group (difference between groups 0.071 (0.002–0.139), p = 0.04) [61].

Table 1. Summary table of biomarkers in asthma and COPD.

Biomarker	Method of Measurement	Indicates	Predicts
Eosinophilia	Sputum and blood sampling	- Type 2 inflammation - Eosinophilic inflammation: - Various cut-off values have been suggested, but the vast majority suggest ≥3% in sputum or ≥300 cells cells/µL in blood. However, the general conception is that eosinophilia should be considered as a continuous rather than a binary biomarker	- Risk of exacerbations - Response to inhaled corticosteroids - Response to biologics (anti-IgE, anti-IL-5, and anti-IL-4R)
Neutrophilia	Sputum and blood sampling	- Neutrophilic inflammation - Non-type 2 inflammation - Associated with obesity and air pollution	- Smaller response to inhaled corticosteroids compared with eosinophilic inflammation
FeNO	- Non-invasive device to measure the concentration of fractional nitric oxide in exhaled breath	- Type 2 inflammation - Eosinophilic inflammation: - FeNO levels <25 ppb: normal (eosinophilia is unlikely) 25–50 ppb: intermediate (eosinophilia is possible) >50 ppb: high (eosinophilia is very likely)	- Exacerbation history - Response to inhaled corticosteroids - Response to anti-IgE and anti-IL-4R
IgE	Blood sample or skin prick test	- Atopy	- Response to inhaled corticosteroids (levels ≥350 K/µL) - Response to anti-IgE
Periostin	Blood sample	- Type 2 inflammation and airway remodelling - Fixed airflow limitation	- Response to anti-IL-13 (in asthmatic individuals with high levels of periostin)
Procalcitonin	Blood sample	Bacterial infection	- Shorter duration of antibiotic treatment, fewer antibiotics - Side effects and lower mortality when used as a tool to guide the prescription of antibiotics

A number of randomized, clinical trials (RCTs) have assessed FeNO as a tool for guiding asthma treatment [62,63]. In an Australian RCT including 220 pregnant, non-smoking asthmatic women, the exacerbation rate was lower in the FeNO-group than in the control group in which the treatment was adjusted according to clinical symptoms, incidence rate ratio 0.47 (0.33–0.76), $p = 0.001$ [62]. A 36-week RCT including 80 asthmatic Danish adults assessed the utility of a FeNO-guided versus symptom-based treatment algorithm [63]. The decrease in airway hyperresponsiveness (AHR) from week 8 to 24 was significantly different in the FeNO-group compared with the control group, suggesting that the use of FeNO resulted in an earlier lowering of AHR. However, no differences were observed in week 36.

The data to support a universal use of FeNO to tailor the asthma treatment are lacking, but FeNO might be useful for guiding treatment for asthma patients with frequent exacerbations. In the most recent Cochrane review on this subject, Petsky et al. found significant differences in asthma exacerbations between the FeNO-group versus non-FeNO-group, rate ratio 0.59 (0.45–0.77), but no differences were observed for symptoms, lung function, or inhaled corticosteroids [64].

2.1.3. Immunoglobin E (IgE)

It has been known for decades that the level of immunoglobin E (IgE) is elevated in allergic asthma patients compared with non-allergic asthma patients [65] and is significantly related to atopic status [66]. Longitudinal studies have shown an association between high levels of IgE and impaired lung function in both asthmatic individuals [67] and non-asthmatic and non-COPD individuals [68]. In a small study including nonsteroid-dependent asthmatic individuals, treatment with corticosteroids during an exacerbation resulted in an initial elevation of total IgE and a subsequent decrease [69], whereas serum IgG was decreased. In a more recent, 44-week randomized controlled trial, asthmatic individuals with baseline serum IgE $\geq$ 350 K/µL obtained greater benefit from inhaled corticosteroids compared with those with baseline serum IgE < 350 K/µL (Table 1) [70].

Treatment with anti-IgE (omalizumab) in patients with allergic asthma has been shown to significantly improve asthma control and lung function as well as reduce ICS use and exacerbations (Table 1) [71,72]. A high baseline level of IgE is a strong predictor of response to treatment with anti-IgE in both allergic asthma [73] and chronic spontaneous urticaria [74]. However, a small, retrospective case-control study showed that treatment response to omalizumab was similar in asthma patients with baseline IgE levels between 30 and 700 UI/mL and IgE levels >700 IU/mL [75].

Although immunological changes in terms of an initial increase in total IgE and decrease in free serum IgE had already been observed in the first clinical studies with omalizumab [76,77], the underlying mechanisms have yet to be fully elucidated [78,79]. However, it has been suggested that total IgE, after the initial accumulation, can serve as a biomarker to monitor IgE production and guide treatment on an individual level [80].

Similar changes in total IgE levels are observed upon treatment with allergen immunotherapy, but these changes are not related to the subsequent reduced response to an allergen [72], whereas an increase in immunoglobin G (especially IgG1 and IgG4) seems to play an important role in clinical outcomes, as these subclasses of antibodies compete with IgE in binding the specific allergen [81].

2.1.4. Periostin

Periostin is a matricellular protein present in the extracellular matrix [82]. Periostin is considered to be a type-2-related biomarker [83] that is influenced by IL-4 and IL-13. Moreover, periostin differs from other type 2 inflammatory markers in that it is involved in airway remodelling and thus can be considered a chronic rather than an acute biomarker. Serum periostin has been shown to be a biomarker of persistent eosinophilic inflammation and fixed airflow limitation in asthmatic individuals treated with inhaled corticosteroids [84].

A randomized controlled trial comparing the effect of ICS on serum periostin level and the association with inflammation found that ICS significantly lowered serum periostin [85] and that the decrease in periostin was associated with improved lung function, decreased sputum eosinophils, and airway remodelling. The association between periostin and lung function has been confirmed in other clinical studies [86].

Anti-IL-13 has not yet been approved for the treatment of severe asthma. A phase 2, double-blind, placebo-controlled trial including 219 asthmatic adults found that lebrikizumab significantly increased FEV1 compared with placebo and that the improvement in lung function occurred only in patients with high baseline serum periostin [87]. These findings are in line with subgroup analyses from other large RCTs with anti-IL-13. In a 52-week RCT with tralokinumab, patients with pre-treatment levels of periostin had improvements in asthma exacerbation rate, lung function, and ACQ-6 [88].

2.2. Non-T2-High Asthma

Although many asthmatic patients have signs of type 2 inflammation, a large group of patients does not. Roughly half of asthma patients show no signs eosinophilic inflammation [15], and this inflammatory state seems to be stable for at least five years [89]. Non-eosinophilic asthma is recognized as a diverse phenotype. It is described as neutrophilic asthma if neutrophils are elevated in sputum and as pauci-granulocytic asthma if neither neutrophils nor eosinophils are elevated [15]. Non-eosinophilic asthma is also associated with a poor response to inhaled and oral corticosteroid treatment [89,90]. Furthermore, it was shown that the ICS dose could be reduced in two-thirds of non-eosinophilic patients (defined as sputum eosinophils <3% and blood eosinophils <400/μL) [91].

Neutrophilic inflammation is a phenotype where the TH2-driven response is replaced by a TH17-driven inflammatory response. This phenotype is only recently being acknowledged and was previously thought to be a misdiagnosis of COPD or induced by corticosteroid treatment because it promotes neutrophilic inflammation [92]. No clear definition of neutrophilic asthma exists, and studies in healthy individuals have shown that the normal range of neutrophils in induced sputum is between 30–50% [93]. Multiple measurements and a cut-off value above 5×10^9/L are suggested [94]. Furthermore, as airway neutrophilia is related to age in adults, the use of age-specific reference values is recommended [95]. Neutrophilia is present in 20–30% of the asthmatic population, although the prevalence varies across regions [96]. This phenotype is more often associated with smoking [97], obesity [98], and various forms of pollution, air pollution, ozone, and other pollutants [99,100]. Neutrophilic inflammation may also be caused by acute airway infections [101], particularly in children [102]. Elevated neutrophil counts have also been associated with a decrease in microbial diversity [103].

A range of treatment strategies has been suggested for this subset of patients, with varying efficacy [91]. Smoking cessation has been shown to benefit asthma patients independent of inflammatory phenotype, but it could be hypothesized that this benefit would be even more significant for patients with neutrophilic inflammation [104]. Obesity has also been associated with neutrophilic asthma, and weight loss has been shown to reduce asthmatic symptoms without changes in inflammatory markers, indicating an inflammation-independent mechanism for asthma [98,105]. TH2-blocking drugs, such as anti-IL-5 or anti-IgE, are not viable for non-eosinophilic asthma. A range of other specific biologics-targeting cytokines, such as TNFα, IL-1, IL-6, and IL-17, have been tried, but none have yet seen widespread use, and more research is needed to identify safe and effective drugs [106]. Systemic inflammation has been associated with neutrophilic asthma, and a microarray analysis has revealed more than 400 genes that are involved in IL-1, TNF-α/nuclear factor-κB, and Kit receptor pathway [107]. These findings may enable a novel treatment strategy for neutrophilic asthma. The AMAZES study (Effect of Azithromycin on Asthma Exacerbations and Quality of Life) showed that oral azithromycin significantly decreased exacerbations and improved quality of life in patients with uncontrolled asthma despite medium-to-high-dose inhaled corticosteroids + long acting β-2 agonist (LABA) [108]. A recent analysis in an AMAZES sub-population showed that baseline sputum TNF-receptors 1 and 2 were significantly increased in neutrophilic versus non-neutrophilic asthma and were related to increased age, lower lung function, and worse asthma control [109]. Azithromycin significantly reduced sputum TNF-receptor 2 and TNF compared with placebo, particularly in non-eosinophilic asthma.

3. Biomarkers in COPD

3.1. Eosinophil Counts to Guide Use of Systemic Corticosteroids

As seen in asthma, increased levels of blood eosinophils have been associated with worse clinical outcomes in a range of parameters, such as length of hospital admission, risk of readmission, and risk of future exacerbation [110–113]. Furthermore, blood eosinophil counts predict response to corticosteroids [31,114]. Systemic corticosteroids, such as prednisolone, are used in the treatment of acute exacerbations. These drugs can alleviate symptoms in many cases, but they do not reduce mortality [115]. Corticosteroids are, however, associated with significant side effects [116]. For this reason, there has recently been a great deal of interest in using blood eosinophil counts to predict which patients will benefit from systemic corticosteroid treatment. One study categorized exacerbation as being either eosinophilic or non-eosinophilic and showed non-inferiority when replacing systemic corticosteroids with placebo in the non-eosinophilic group. This algorithm reduced total corticosteroid use by 49% in the eosinophil-guided group [117]. The CORTICO-COP trial (Eosinophil-guided Corticosteroid Therapy In Patients Admitted To Hospital With COPD Exacerbation) used daily blood eosinophil counts to guide corticosteroid use and compared these patients to a control group receiving a five-day prednisolone treatment. This algorithm led to a reduction of median treatment duration from five to two days with no change in the number of days alive and out of hospital within 14 days or the 30-day mortality [118]. The authors also reported a decreased risk of worsening of pre-existing diabetes in the eosinophil-guided group compared to the control group.

3.2. Eosinophil Counts to Guide Use of Inhaled Corticosteroids

While systemic corticosteroids are typically used to treat patients admitted with acute exacerbations, ICS are often used to treat COPD patients to alleviate symptoms and reduce risk of exacerbation [119]. While ICS are generally thought to be safer than systemic corticosteroids, they have been associated with an increased risk of infection and pneumonia [120]. ICS have also been indicated to cause many of the known systemic side effects of oral corticosteroids, such as cataracts [121,122] and bone demineralization. No randomized clinical trials have currently shown that blood eosinophil counts can be used to guide prescription of ICS. However, several post-hoc studies of large clinical trials have shown that blood eosinophil count might be used as a predictor of response to treatment with ICS [123,124] These results have made it into GOLD guidelines 2019, which recommend ICS only for patients with blood eosinophil counts $\geq$100 /μL [125]. A post-hoc analysis of three randomized controlled trials found a greater response to ICS/LABA compared with both placebo and long acting muscarine antagonist (LAMA) in COPD patients with baseline blood eosinophils $\geq$2% [126]. In another study, Siddiqui and colleagues conducted post-hoc predictive modelling using data from the FORWARD trial and externally validated data to examine the association between baseline eosinophils and the effect of ICS in exacerbations [127]. The authors found that ICS/LABA across all eosinophil levels reduced COPD exacerbations compared with LABA, and the difference in exacerbation rate was more pronounced with increasing level of baseline blood eosinophils. Two studies have investigated the safety of withdrawing ICS, and post-hoc analyses have been done on the effects of blood eosinophil counts. The SUNSET study found negative effects on lung function when withdrawing ICS from long-term ICS/LAMA/LABA treatment, but they found that the negative effects of withdrawal were much less apparent in patients with blood eosinophil counts of $\leq$300/μL [128]. The WISDOM trial showed no difference in the risk of COPD exacerbation when withdrawing ICS [129]. However, a post-hoc analysis of the WISDOM trial showed a higher exacerbation rate after ICS withdrawal in patients with blood eosinophil counts $\geq$300/μL [130]. There is currently one ongoing multi-centre trial, the COPERNICOS trial (NCT04481555), which aims to assess whether blood eosinophil counts can be used to guide ICS usage in patients with severe or very severe COPD, the results of which are expected by 2025 [131]. The intervention group will have their ICS adjusted every three months based on whether blood eosinophils count is $\leq$300/μL with the aim of reducing corticosteroid exposure while being non-inferior to the current treatment regime (COPERNICUS).

3.3. IL-5-Targeted Therapy and Blood Eosinophils

Since a subset of COPD patients present with eosinophilic airway inflammation, it can be hypothesized that these patients may benefit from the same therapies used in the treatment of asthma. In the METREX and METREO randomized trials, the efficacy and safety of mepolizumab were investigated in a population of COPD patients [132]. In METREX, patients were randomized to placebo or 100 mg mepolizumab every four weeks. In METREO, patients were randomized to either placebo, 100 mg or 400 mg every five weeks. Neither trial was able to show a significant difference in exacerbation rates or secondary outcomes in the whole population, but a post-hoc analysis on patients from both trials with blood eosinophils ≥300 /μL showed a statistically significant reduction of exacerbation rate by 23% in patients receiving 100 mg mepolizumab versus placebo. Future studies investigating the effect of mepolizumab in the subgroup of COPD patients are warranted.

A phase 2a randomized trial investigated whether benralizumab could reduce acute exacerbation in COPD with ≥ 3% eosinophils in sputum [133]. No statistically significant effect was seen on exacerbation rates, but the sample size of the study was low, and a numerical reduction was seen in patients with blood eosinophils ≥200/μL. The GALATHEA (Benralizumab Efficacy in Moderate to Very Severe COPD With Exacerbation History) and TERRANOVA (Benralizumab for the Prevention of COPD Exacerbations) randomized phase 3 trials further investigated the effect of benralizumab and were unable to show a reduction in exacerbation frequency in patients with moderate to very severe COPD with blood eosinophil counts ≥220/μL. To date, no trials with reslizumab in COPD patients have been conducted.

Thus, there are no current indications that IL-5-targeted therapies are a viable strategy for treating COPD.

4. Procalcitonin as a Tool to Guide Antibiotic Treatment for Respiratory Tract Infections

Procalcitonin (PCT) is a fast-acting biomarker of bacterial infection [134]. Thus, it has been suggested that PCT could be used in the early detection of bacterial infections and to guide antibiotic therapy [135]. Antibiotic resistance is a growing concern and threatens both human health and food security. While the causes of resistance are many, overuse of antibiotics in humans and livestock is a central component in accelerating the development of resistance [136]. It is therefore crucial to administer antibiotics only when the expected clinical benefits overweigh the risk of side effects and resistance. Bacteria can be isolated from sputum in 40–60% of acute exacerbations of COPD, while acute exacerbations of asthma are more commonly triggered by other factors, such as allergens, gastro-oesophageal reflux, and viral infections, though bacterial infection occasionally occurs as well [137].

Although bacterial infections are uncommon in asthma exacerbations, antibiotics are heavily prescribed. From 2006 to 2012, 51% of patients admitted with asthma to 383 US hospitals were prescribed antibiotics [138]. Two clinical trials have looked at PCT-guided therapy, specifically in the context of asthma exacerbations.

PCT has been used to guide antibiotic usage in both mild [139] and severe [140] asthma exacerbations without being inferior on clinical outcomes. Both studies used a protocol where antibiotics were strongly discouraged when PCT was below 0.1 μg/L, discouraged when between 0.1 μg/L and 0.25 μg/L, and encouraged above 0.25 μg/L. Antibiotics were prescribed to 80–90% of the control group but to only around half of the intervention group, leading to a significant reduction in antibiotics. Although bacterial infections in COPD are estimated to account for roughly half of acute exacerbations, antibiotics are commonly prescribed, along with systemic corticosteroids, to most patients presenting with moderate to severe acute exacerbations [31]. This suggests that antibiotics are overprescribed. Corticosteroids, on the other hand, are known to increase the risk of pneumonia [120], so it could be hypothesized that systemic corticosteroids are ineffective or even harmful in patients with acute exacerbations caused by bacterial airway infections. Research on this topic is limited, but one study found that corticosteroids did not improve outcomes in patients with diagnosed pneumonia [141]. This finding accords with the previously discussed fact that corticosteroid response is worse in patients presenting with neutrophilic inflammation, which is the typical inflammatory pattern of bacterial infections [142].

A patient-level meta-analysis on 26 trials including a total of 6708 patients investigated whether PCT was useful as a tool to guide antibiotic usage in all airway infections. This analysis showed that PCT-guided therapy was effective in reducing antibiotic prescription rates, antibiotic side effects, and even mortality (Table 1) [143].

A systematic review from 2017 of 32 RCTs examining procalcitonin to guide antibiotic usage in airway infections in general found that procalcitonin-guided algorithms led to lower mortality, shorter duration of antibiotic treatment, and fewer antibiotic side effects [144].

5. Conclusions

Asthma and COPD compose a great burden for public health worldwide, and the need for early identification of cases and intervention is still of great importance. Obstructive airway diseases are a group of complex and heterogeneous diseases. Our knowledge has evolved markedly due to research over the past 15 to 20 years, and several distinct phenotypes and endotypes are now described in the literature. The advantages of conducting a systematic assessment of asthma and COPD become evident when specific and reliable biomarkers enable the possibility of precision medicine. While type 2-high asthma is the most well-described endotype, our understanding of non-type-2 is now increasing, and if specific biomarkers for non-type 2 asthma can be identified, it is reasonable to expect better treatment options for this group of patients. The role of eosinophilia in COPD is now established as a valuable biomarker to predict both prognosis and treatment response and serves as a tool for tailoring the use of corticosteroids for maintenance therapy and during an exacerbation. To date, evidence for the clinical benefits of monoclonal antibodies in COPD-patients has not been overwhelming. However, future studies using biomarkers to identify patients who are most likely to respond are warranted.

Author Contributions: Conceptualization, H.M., P.S. and J.-U.S.J.; writing—original draft preparation, H.M. and P.S.; writing—review and editing, H.M., P.S. and J.-U.S.J.; final approval: H.M., P.S. and J.-U.S.J. All authors have read and agreed to the published version of the manuscript.

Funding: This study was funded by the Danish Regions Medical Fund (grant no. 5894/16) and the Danish Council for Independent Research (grant no. 6110-00268B). The research salary of PS was sponsored by Herlev and Gentofte Hospital, University of Copenhagen.

Institutional Review Board Statement: Not applicable.

Informed Consent Statement: Not applicable.

Conflicts of Interest: H.M. reports fees from GSK, Teva, Novartis, and ALK-Abéllo Nordic A/S outside the submitted work. P.S. reports fees from Boehringer Ingelheim, GSK, and AstraZeneca outside the submitted work. J.-U.S.J. reports no conflicts of interest. All authors have completed wthe ICMJE uniform disclosure form describing any conflicts of interest. The funders had no role in the design of the study; in the collection, analyses, or interpretation of data; in the writing of the manuscript, or in the decision to publish the results.

References

1. Bousquet, J.; Chanez, P.; Lacoste, J.Y.; Barnéon, G.; Ghavanian, N.; Enander, I.; Venge, P.; Ahlstedt, S.; Simony-Lafontaine, J.; Godard, P.; et al. Eosinophilic Inflammation in Asthma. *N. Engl. J. Med.* **1990**, *323*, 1033–1039. [CrossRef] [PubMed]
2. Barnes, P.J. Immunology of asthma and chronic obstructive pulmonary disease. *Nat. Rev. Immunol.* **2008**, *8*, 183–192. [CrossRef]
3. Bradding, P.; Walls, A.; Holgate, S.T. The role of the mast cell in the pathophysiology of asthma. *J. Allergy Clin. Immunol.* **2006**, *117*, 1277–1284. [CrossRef] [PubMed]
4. Kumar, B.V.; Connors, T.; Farber, D.L. Human T Cell Development, Localization, and Function throughout Life. *Immunity* **2018**, *48*, 202–213. [CrossRef] [PubMed]
5. Saha, S.; Brightling, C.E. Eosinophilic airway inflammation in COPD. *Int. J. Chronic Obstr. Pulm. Dis.* **2006**, *1*, 39–47. [CrossRef]
6. George, L.; Brightling, C. Eosinophilic airway inflammation: Role in asthma and chronic obstructive pulmonary disease. *Ther. Adv. Chronic Dis.* **2016**, *7*, 34–51. [CrossRef]
7. Chung, K.F. Personalised medicine in asthma: Time for action: Number 1 in the Series "Personalised medicine in respiratory diseases" Edited by Renaud Louis and Nicolas Roche. *Eur. Respir. Rev.* **2017**, *26*, 145. [CrossRef] [PubMed]
8. Moore, W.C.; Meyers, D.A.; Wenzel, S.E.; Teague, W.G.; Li, H.; Li, X.; D'Agostino, R., Jr.; Castro, M.; Curran-Everett, D.; Fitzpatrick, A.M.; et al. Identification of Asthma Phenotypes Using Cluster Analysis in the Severe Asthma Research Program. *Am. J. Respir. Crit. Care Med.* **2010**, *181*, 315–323. [CrossRef]

9. Shaw, D.E.; Sousa, A.R.; Fowler, S.; Fleming, L.; Roberts, G.; Corfield, J.; Pandis, I.; Bansal, A.T.; Bel, E.H.; Auffray, C.; et al. Clinical and inflammatory characteristics of the European U-BIOPRED adult severe asthma cohort. *Eur. Respir. J.* **2015**, *46*, 1308–1321. [CrossRef]
10. Calvén, J.; Ax, E.; Rådinger, M. The Airway Epithelium—A Central Player in Asthma Pathogenesis. *Int. J. Mol. Sci.* **2020**, *21*, 8907. [CrossRef]
11. Chen, R.; Smith, S.; Salter, B.; El-Gammal, A.; Oliveria, J.P.; Obminski, C.; Watson, R.; O'Byrne, P.M.; Gauvreau, G.M.; Sehmi, R. Allergen-induced Increases in Sputum Levels of Group 2 Innate Lymphoid Cells in Subjects with Asthma. *Am. J. Respir. Crit. Care Med.* **2017**, *196*, 700–712. [CrossRef]
12. Murphy, K.M.; Reiner, S.L. The lineage decisions of helper T cells. *Nat. Rev. Immunol.* **2002**, *2*, 933–944. [CrossRef]
13. Singh, V.; Agrewala, J.N. Regulatory role of pro-Th1 and pro-Th2 cytokines in modulating the activity of Th1 and Th2 cells when B cell and macrophages are used as antigen presenting cells. *BMC Immunol.* **2006**, *7*, 17. [CrossRef] [PubMed]
14. Barrett, N.A.; Austen, K.F. Innate Cells and T Helper 2 Cell Immunity in Airway Inflammation. *Immunity* **2009**, *31*, 425–437. [CrossRef] [PubMed]
15. Global Initiative for Asthma. Global Strategy for Asthma Management and Prevention. 2020. Available online: https://ginasthma.org/wp-content/uploads/2021/05/GINA-Main-Report-2021-V2-WMS.pdf (accessed on 20 January 2021).
16. Meteran, H.; Meteran, H.; Porsbjerg, C.; Backer, V. Novel monoclonal treatments in severe asthma. *J. Asthma* **2017**, *54*, 991–1011. [CrossRef] [PubMed]
17. Menzella, F.; Ruggiero, P.; Ghidoni, G.; Fontana, M.; Bagnasco, D.; Livrieri, F.; Scelfo, C.; Facciolongo, N. Anti-IL5 Therapies for Severe Eosinophilic Asthma: Literature Review and Practical Insights. *J. Asthma Allergy* **2020**, *13*, 301–313. [CrossRef] [PubMed]
18. Corren, J.; Castro, M.; O'Riordan, T.; Hanania, N.A.; Pavord, I.D.; Quirce, S.; Chipps, B.E.; Wenzel, S.; Thangavelu, K.; Rice, M.S.; et al. Dupilumab Efficacy in Patients with Uncontrolled, Moderate-to-Severe Allergic Asthma. *J. Allergy Clin. Immunol. Pr.* **2020**, *8*, 516–526. [CrossRef] [PubMed]
19. Kulkarni, N.S.; Hollins, F.; Sutcliffe, A.; Saunders, R.; Shah, S.; Siddiqui, S.; Gupta, S.; Haldar, P.; Green, R.; Pavord, I.; et al. Eosinophil protein in airway macrophages: A novel biomarker of eosinophilic inflammation in patients with asthma. *J. Allergy Clin. Immunol.* **2010**, *126*, 61–69.e3. [CrossRef] [PubMed]
20. Persson, C. Lysis of primed eosinophils in severe asthma. *J. Allergy Clin. Immunol.* **2013**, *132*, 1459–1460. [CrossRef]
21. Chung, K.F. Airway smooth muscle cells: Contributing to and regulating airway mucosal inflammation? *Eur. Respir. J.* **2000**, *15*, 961–968. [CrossRef]
22. Schleich, F.N.; Chevremont, A.; Paulus, V.; Henket, M.; Manise, M.; Seidel, L.; Louis, R. Importance of concomitant local and systemic eosinophilia in uncontrolled asthma. *Eur. Respir. J.* **2014**, *44*, 97–108. [CrossRef]
23. Rhyou, H.I.; Nam, Y.H. Predictive factors of response to inhaled corticosteroids in newly diagnosed asthma: A real-world observational study. *Ann. Allergy Asthma Immunol.* **2020**, *125*, 177–181. [CrossRef]
24. Pizzichini, M.; Efthimiadis, A.; Dolovich, J.; Hargreave, F.E. Measuring airway inflammation in asthma: Eosinophils and eosinophilic cationic protein in induced sputum compared with peripheral blood. *J. Allergy Clin. Immunol.* **1997**, *99*, 539–544. [CrossRef]
25. Hastie, A.T.; Moore, W.C.; Li, H.; Rector, B.M.; Ortega, V.E.; Pascual, R.M.; Peters, S.P.; Meyers, D.A.; Bleecker, E.R. Biomarker surrogates do not accurately predict sputum eosinophil and neutrophil percentages in asthmatic subjects. *J. Allergy Clin. Immunol.* **2013**, *132*, 72–80.e12. [CrossRef]
26. Wagener, A.H.; De Nijs, S.B.; Lutter, R.; Sousa, A.R.; Weersink, E.J.M.; Bel, E.H.; Sterk, P.J. External validation of blood eosinophils, FENO and serum periostin as surrogates for sputum eosinophils in asthma. *Thorax* **2015**, *70*, 115–120. [CrossRef]
27. Pignatti, P.; Visca, D.; Cherubino, F.; Zampogna, E.; Lucini, E.; Saderi, L.; Sotgiu, G.; Spanevello, A. Do blood eosinophils strictly reflect airway inflammation in COPD? Comparison with asthmatic patients. *Respir. Res.* **2019**, *20*, 145. [CrossRef]
28. Hastie, A.T.; Martinez, F.J.; Curtis, J.L.; Doerschuk, C.M.; Hansel, N.N.; Christenson, S.; Putcha, N.; Ortega, V.E.; Li, X.; Barr, R.G.; et al. Association of sputum and blood eosinophil concentrations with clinical measures of COPD severity: An analysis of the SPIROMICS cohort. *Lancet Respir. Med.* **2017**, *5*, 956–967. [CrossRef]
29. Tan, W.C.; Bourbeau, J.; Nadeau, G.; Wang, W.; Barnes, N.; Landis, S.H.; Kirby, M.; Hogg, J.C.; Sin, D.D.; CanCOLD Collaborative Research Group; et al. High eosinophil counts predict decline in FEV_1: Results from the CanCOLD study. *Eur. Respir. J.* **2021**, *57*, 2000838. [CrossRef] [PubMed]
30. Price, D.B.; Rigazio, A.; Campbell, J.D.; Bleecker, E.R.; Corrigan, C.; Thomas, M.; Wenzel, S.; Wilson, A.M.; Small, M.B.; Gopalan, G.; et al. Blood eosinophil count and prospective annual asthma disease burden: A UK cohort study. *Lancet Respir. Med.* **2015**, *3*, 849–858. [CrossRef]
31. Bafadhel, M.; Greening, N.; Harvey-Dunstan, T.C.; Williams, J.E.; Morgan, M.D.; Brightling, C.; Hussain, S.F.; Pavord, I.; Singh, S.J.; Steiner, M. Blood Eosinophils and Outcomes in Severe Hospitalized Exacerbations of COPD. *Chest* **2016**, *150*, 320–328. [CrossRef]
32. Katz, L.E.; Gleich, G.J.; Hartley, B.F.; Yancey, S.W.; Ortega, H.G. Blood Eosinophil Count Is a Useful Biomarker to Identify Patients with Severe Eosinophilic Asthma. *Ann. Am. Thorac. Soc.* **2014**, *11*, 531–536. [CrossRef] [PubMed]
33. Bafadhel, M.; Peterson, S.; De Blas, M.A.; Calverley, P.M.; Rennard, S.I.; Richter, K.; Fagerås, M. Predictors of exacerbation risk and response to budesonide in patients with chronic obstructive pulmonary disease: A post-hoc analysis of three randomised trials. *Lancet Respir. Med.* **2018**, *6*, 117–126. [CrossRef]

34. FitzGerald, J.M.; Bleecker, E.R.; Nair, P.; Korn, S.; Ohta, K.; Lommatzsch, M.; Ferguson, G.T.; Busse, W.W.; Barker, P.; Sproule, S.; et al. Benralizumab, an anti-interleukin-5 receptor α monoclonal antibody, as add-on treatment for patients with severe, uncontrolled, eosinophilic asthma (CALIMA): A randomised, double-blind, placebo-controlled phase 3 trial. *Lancet* **2016**, *388*, 2128–2141. [CrossRef]
35. Ortega, H.G.; Yancey, S.W.; Mayer, B.; Gunsoy, N.B.; Keene, O.; Bleecker, E.R.; Brightling, C.; Pavord, I. Severe eosinophilic asthma treated with mepolizumab stratified by baseline eosinophil thresholds: A secondary analysis of the DREAM and MENSA studies. *Lancet Respir. Med.* **2016**, *4*, 549–556. [CrossRef]
36. Corren, J.; Weinstein, S.; Janka, L.; Zangrilli, J.; Garin, M. Phase 3 Study of Reslizumab in Patients With Poorly Controlled Asthma: Effects Across a Broad Range of Eosinophil Counts. *Chest* **2016**, *150*, 799–810. [CrossRef] [PubMed]
37. Chipps, B.E.; Jarjour, N.; Calhoun, W.J.; Iqbal, A.; Haselkorn, T.; Yang, M.; Brumm, J.; Corren, J.; Holweg, C.T.; Bafadhel, M. A Comprehensive Analysis of the Stability of Blood Eosinophil Levels. *Ann. Am. Thorac. Soc.* **2021**. Online ahead of print. [CrossRef]
38. Negewo, N.A.; McDonald, V.M.; Baines, K.J.; Wark, P.A.; Simpson, J.L.; Jones, P.W.; Gibson, P.G. Peripheral blood eosinophils: A surrogate marker for airway eosinophilia in stable COPD. *Int. J. Chronic Obstr. Pulm. Dis.* **2016**, *11*, 1495–1504. [CrossRef]
39. Deykin, A.; Lazarus, S.C.; Fahy, J.V.; Wechsler, M.E.; Boushey, H.A.; Chinchilli, V.M.; Craig, T.J.; Dimango, E.; Kraft, M.; Leone, F.; et al. Sputum eosinophil counts predict asthma control after discontinuation of inhaled corticosteroids. *J. Allergy Clin. Immunol.* **2005**, *115*, 720–727. [CrossRef]
40. Li, A.M.; Tsang, T.W.T.; Lam, H.S.; Sung, R.Y.T.; Chang, A.B. Predictors for failed dose reduction of inhaled corticosteroids in childhood asthma. *Respirology* **2008**, *13*, 400–407. [CrossRef]
41. Petsky, H.L.; Li, A.; Chang, A.B. Tailored interventions based on sputum eosinophils versus clinical symptoms for asthma in children and adults. *Cochrane Database Syst. Rev.* **2017**, *8*, CD005603. [CrossRef]
42. Demarche, S.F.; Schleich, F.N.; Henket, M.A.; Paulus, V.A.; Van Hees, T.; Louis, R.E. Effectiveness of inhaled corticosteroids in real life on clinical outcomes, sputum cells and systemic inflammation in asthmatics: A retrospective cohort study in a secondary care centre. *BMJ Open* **2017**, *7*, e018186. [CrossRef] [PubMed]
43. Brusselle, G.; Nicolini, G.; Santoro, L.; Guastalla, D.; Papi, A. BDP/formoterol MART asthma exacerbation benefit increases with blood eosinophil level. *Eur. Respir. J.* **2021**, *58*, 2004098. [CrossRef]
44. Busby, J.; Khoo, E.; Pfeffer, P.; Mansur, A.H.; Heaney, L.G. The effects of oral corticosteroids on lung function, type-2 biomarkers and patient-reported outcomes in stable asthma: A systematic review and meta-analysis. *Respir. Med.* **2020**, *173*, 106156. [CrossRef]
45. Busby, J.; Holweg, C.T.J.; Chai, A.; Bradding, P.; Cai, F.; Chaudhuri, R.; Mansur, A.H.; Lordan, J.L.; Matthews, J.G.; Menzies-Gow, A.; et al. Change in type-2 biomarkers and related cytokines with prednisolone in uncontrolled severe oral corticosteroid dependent asthmatics: An interventional open-label study. *Thorax* **2019**, *74*, 806–809. [CrossRef]
46. FitzGerald, J.M.; Bleecker, E.R.; Menzies-Gow, A.; Zangrilli, J.G.; Hirsch, I.; Metcalfe, P.; Newbold, P.; Goldman, M. Predictors of enhanced response with benralizumab for patients with severe asthma: Pooled analysis of the SIROCCO and CALIMA studies. *Lancet Respir. Med.* **2018**, *6*, 51–64. [CrossRef]
47. Castro, M.; Zangrilli, J.; Wechsler, M.E.; Bateman, E.D.; Brusselle, G.; Bardin, P.; Murphy, K.; Maspero, J.F.; O'Brien, C.; Korn, S. Reslizumab for inadequately controlled asthma with elevated blood eosinophil counts: Results from two multicentre, parallel, double-blind, randomised, placebo-controlled, phase 3 trials. *Lancet Respir. Med.* **2015**, *3*, 355–366. [CrossRef]
48. Bjermer, L.; Lemiere, C.; Maspero, J.; Weiss, S.; Zangrilli, J.; Germinaro, M. Reslizumab for Inadequately Controlled Asthma with Elevated Blood Eosinophil Levels: A Randomized Phase 3 Study. *Chest* **2016**, *150*, 789–798. [CrossRef]
49. Lane, C.; Knight, D.; Burgess, S.; Franklin, P.; Horak, F.; Legg, J.; Moeller, A.; Stick, S. Epithelial inducible nitric oxide synthase activity is the major determinant of nitric oxide concentration in exhaled breath. *Thorax* **2004**, *59*, 757–760. [CrossRef] [PubMed]
50. Mattes, J.; Storm van's Gravesande, K.; Reining, U.; Alving, K.; Ihorst, G.; Henschen, M.; Kuehr, J. NO in exhaled air is correlated with markers of eosinophilic airway inflammation in corticosteroid-dependent childhood asthma. *Eur. Respir. J.* **1999**, *13*, 1391–1395. [PubMed]
51. Takayama, Y.; Ohnishi, H.; Ogasawara, F.; Oyama, K.; Kubota, T.; Yokoyama, A. Clinical utility of fractional exhaled nitric oxide and blood eosinophils counts in the diagnosis of asthma-COPD overlap. *Int. J. Chronic Obstr. Pulm. Dis.* **2018**, *13*, 2525–2532. [CrossRef]
52. Zietkowski, Z.; Bodzenta-Lukaszyk, A.; Tomasiak, M.M.; Skiepko, R.; Szmitkowski, M. Comparison of exhaled nitric oxide measurement with conventional tests in steroid-naive asthma patients. *J. Investig. Allergol. Clin. Immunol.* **2006**, *16*, 239–246.
53. Sverrild, A.; Porsbjerg, C.; Thomsen, S.F.; Backer, V. Airway hyperresponsiveness to mannitol and methacholine and exhaled nitric oxide: A random-sample population study. *J. Allergy Clin. Immunol.* **2010**, *126*, 952–958. [CrossRef] [PubMed]
54. Dweik, R.A.; Boggs, P.B.; Erzurum, S.C.; Irvin, C.G.; Leigh, M.W.; Lundberg, J.O.; Olin, A.-C.; Plummer, A.L.; Taylor, D.R. An Official ATS Clinical Practice Guideline: Interpretation of Exhaled Nitric Oxide Levels (FeNO) for Clinical Applications. *Am. J. Respir. Crit. Care Med.* **2011**, *184*, 602–615. [CrossRef] [PubMed]
55. Taylor, D.R.; Mandhane, P.; Greene, J.M.; Hancox, R.J.; Filsell, S.; McLachlan, C.R.; Williamson, A.J.; Cowan, J.O.; Smith, A.D.; Sears, M.R. Factors affecting exhaled nitric oxide measurements: The effect of sex. *Respir. Res.* **2007**, *8*, 82. [CrossRef] [PubMed]
56. Frendø, M.; Hakansson, K.; Schwer, S.; Ravn, A.; Meteran, H.; Porsbjerg, C.; Backer, V.; von Buchwald, C. Exhaled and nasal nitric oxide in chronic rhinosinusitis patients with nasal polyps in primary care. *Rhinol. J.* **2018**, *56*, 59–64. [CrossRef]

57. Abe, Y.; Suzuki, M.; Kimura, H.; Shimizu, K.; Makita, H.; Nishimura, M.; Konno, S. Annual Fractional Exhaled Nitric Oxide Measurements and Exacerbations in Severe Asthma. *J. Asthma Allergy* **2020**, *13*, 731–741. [CrossRef]
58. Kimura, H.; Konno, S.; Makita, H.; Taniguchi, N.; Shimizu, K.; Suzuki, M.; Goudarzi, H.; Nakamaru, Y.; Ono, J.; Ohta, S.; et al. Prospective predictors of exacerbation status in severe asthma over a 3-year follow-up. *Clin. Exp. Allergy* **2018**, *48*, 1137–1146. [CrossRef]
59. van Rensen, E.L.; Straathof, K.C.; Veselic-Charvat, M.A.; Zwinderman, A.H.; Bel, E.H.; Sterk, P.J. Effect of inhaled steroids on airway hyperresponsiveness, sputum eosinophils, and exhaled nitric oxide levels in patients with asthma. *Thorax* **1999**, *54*, 403–408. [CrossRef]
60. Beck-Ripp, J.; Griese, M.; Arenz, S.; Köring, C.; Pasqualoni, B.; Bufler, P. Changes of exhaled nitric oxide during steroid treatment of childhood asthma. *Eur. Respir. J.* **2002**, *19*, 1015–1019. [CrossRef]
61. Price, D.B.; Buhl, R.; Chan, A.; Freeman, D.; Gardener, E.; Godley, C.; Gruffydd-Jones, K.; McGarvey, L.; Ohta, K.; Ryan, D.; et al. Fractional exhaled nitric oxide as a predictor of response to inhaled corticosteroids in patients with non-specific respiratory symptoms and insignificant bronchodilator reversibility: A randomised controlled trial. *Lancet Respir. Med.* **2018**, *6*, 29–39. [CrossRef]
62. Powell, H.; Murphy, V.E.; Taylor, D.R.; Hensley, M.J.; McCaffery, K.; Giles, W.; Clifton, V.L.; Gibson, P.G. Management of asthma in pregnancy guided by measurement of fraction of exhaled nitric oxide: A double-blind, randomised controlled trial. *Lancet* **2011**, *378*, 983–990. [CrossRef]
63. Bernholm, K.F.; Homøe, A.S.; Meteran, H.; Jensen, C.B.; Porsbjerg, C.; Backer, V. FeNO-based asthma management results in faster improvement of airway hyperresponsiveness. *ERJ Open Res.* **2018**, *4*, 00147-02017. [CrossRef]
64. Petsky, H.L.; Kew, K.M.; Turner, C.; Kynaston, J.A.; Chang, A.B. Exhaled nitric oxide levels to guide treatment for adults with asthma. *Cochrane Database Syst. Rev.* **2015**, *9*, CD011440. [CrossRef]
65. Johansson, S. Raised levels of a new immunoglobulin class (ignd) in asthma. *Lancet* **1967**, *290*, 951–953. [CrossRef]
66. Sharma, S.; Kathuria, P.C.; Gupta, C.K.; Nordling, K.; Ghosh, B.; Singh, A.B. Total serum immunoglobulin E levels in a case–control study in asthmatic/allergic patients, their family members, and healthy subjects from India. *Clin. Exp. Allergy* **2006**, *36*, 1019–1027. [CrossRef]
67. Sherrill, D.L.; Lebowitz, M.D.; Halonen, M.; Barbee, R.A.; Burrows, B. Longitudinal evaluation of the association between pulmonary function and total serum IgE. *Am. J. Respir. Crit. Care Med.* **1995**, *152*, 98–102. [CrossRef]
68. Hizawa, N.; Masuko, H.; Sakamoto, T.; Kaneko, Y.; Iijima, H.; Naito, T.; Noguchi, E.; Hirota, T.; Tamari, M. Lower FEV1 in non-COPD, nonasthmatic subjects: Association with smoking, annual decline in FEV1, total IgE levels, and TSLP genotypes. *Int. J. Chronic Obstr. Pulm. Dis.* **2011**, *6*, 181–189. [CrossRef] [PubMed]
69. Posey, W.; Nelson, H.; Branch, B.; Pearlman, D. The effects of acute corticosteroid therapy for asthma on serum immunoglobulin levels. *J. Allergy Clin. Immunol.* **1978**, *62*, 340–348. [CrossRef]
70. Gerald, J.K.; Gerald, L.B.; Vasquez, M.M.; Morgan, W.J.; Boehmer, S.J.; Lemanske, R.F.; Mauger, D.T.; Strunk, R.C.; Szefler, S.J.; Zeiger, R.S.; et al. Markers of Differential Response to Inhaled Corticosteroid Treatment Among Children with Mild Persistent Asthma. *J. Allergy Clin. Immunol. Pr.* **2015**, *3*, 540–546.e3. [CrossRef]
71. Busse, W.; Corren, J.; Lanier, B.Q.; McAlary, M.; Fowler-Taylor, A.; Cioppa, G.D.; van As, A.; Gupta, N. Omalizumab, anti-IgE recombinant humanized monoclonal antibody, for the treatment of severe allergic asthma. *J. Allergy Clin. Immunol.* **2001**, *108*, 184–190. [CrossRef]
72. Meteran, H.; Backer, V. SQ house dust mite sublingual immunotherapy for the treatment of adults with house dust mite-induced allergic rhinitis. *Expert Rev. Clin. Immunol.* **2019**, *15*, 1127–1133. [CrossRef]
73. Peters, J.; Singh, H.; Kaur, Y.; Diaz, J.D. Response to Omalizumab Therapy Based on Level of IgE: A Two Year Observational Study (REALITY Study). *J. Allergy Clin. Immunol.* **2016**, *137*, AB16. [CrossRef]
74. Ertas, R.; Ozyurt, K.; Atasoy, M.; Hawro, T.; Maurer, M. The clinical response to omalizumab in chronic spontaneous urticaria patients is linked to and predicted by IgE levels and their change. *Allergy* **2017**, *73*, 705–712. [CrossRef]
75. Maselli, D.; Diaz, J.; Peters, J. Omalizumab in asthmatics with IgE levels > 700 IU/mL. *Eur. Respir. J.* **2011**, *38*, 266.
76. Boulet, L.P.; Chapman, K.R.; Cote, J.; Kalra, S.; Bhagat, R.; Swystun, V.A.; Laviolette, M.; Cleland, L.D.; Deschesnes, F.; Su, J.Q.; et al. Inhibitory effects of an anti-IgE antibody E25 on allergen-induced early asthmatic response. *Am. J. Respir. Crit. Care Med.* **1997**, *155*, 1835–1840. [CrossRef] [PubMed]
77. Milgrom, H.; Fick, R.B., Jr.; Su, J.Q.; Reimann, J.D.; Bush, R.K.; Watrous, M.L.; Metzger, W.J. Treatment of allergic asthma with monoclonal anti-IgE antibody. rhuMAb-E25 Study Group. *N. Engl. J. Med.* **1999**, *341*, 1966–1973. [CrossRef] [PubMed]
78. Bousquet, J.; Rabe, K.; Humbert, M.; Chung, K.F.; Berger, W.; Fox, H.; Ayre, G.; Chen, H.; Thomas, K.; Blogg, M.; et al. Predicting and evaluating response to omalizumab in patients with severe allergic asthma. *Respir. Med.* **2007**, *101*, 1483–1492. [CrossRef]
79. Chu, S.Y.; Horton, H.M.; Pong, E.; Leung, I.W.; Chen, H.; Nguyen, D.-H.; Bautista, C.; Muchhal, U.S.; Bernett, M.J.; Moore, G.L.; et al. Reduction of total IgE by targeted coengagement of IgE B-cell receptor and FcγRIIb with Fc-engineered antibody. *J. Allergy Clin. Immunol.* **2012**, *129*, 1102–1115. [CrossRef] [PubMed]
80. Lowe, P.; Renard, D. Omalizumab decreases IgE production in patients with allergic (IgE-mediated) asthma; PKPD analysis of a biomarker, total IgE. *Br. J. Clin. Pharmacol.* **2011**, *72*, 306–320. [CrossRef] [PubMed]

81. Reisinger, J.; Horak, F.; Pauli, G.; van Hage, M.; Cromwell, O.; König, F.; Valenta, R.; Niederberger, V. Allergen-specific nasal IgG antibodies induced by vaccination with genetically modified allergens are associated with reduced nasal allergen sensitivity. *J. Allergy Clin. Immunol.* **2005**, *116*, 347–354. [CrossRef]
82. Bornstein, P.; Sage, E. Matricellular proteins: Extracellular modulators of cell function. *Curr. Opin. Cell Biol.* **2002**, *14*, 608–616. [CrossRef]
83. Izuhara, K.; Nunomura, S.; Nanri, Y.; Ono, J.; Takai, M.; Kawaguchi, A. Periostin: An emerging biomarker for allergic diseases. *Allergy* **2019**, *74*, 2116–2128. [CrossRef]
84. Takahashi, K.; Meguro, K.; Kawashima, H.; Kashiwakuma, D.; Kagami, S.-I.; Ohta, S.; Ono, J.; Izuhara, K.; Iwamoto, I. Serum periostin levels serve as a biomarker for both eosinophilic airway inflammation and fixed airflow limitation in well-controlled asthmatics. *J. Asthma* **2018**, *56*, 236–243. [CrossRef]
85. Hoshino, M.; Ohtawa, J.; Akitsu, K. Effect of treatment with inhaled corticosteroid on serum periostin levels in asthma. *Respirology* **2015**, *21*, 297–303. [CrossRef]
86. Mansur, A.H.; Srivastava, S.; Sahal, A. Disconnect of type 2 biomarkers in severe asthma; dominated by FeNO as a predictor of exacerbations and periostin as predictor of reduced lung function. *Respir. Med.* **2018**, *143*, 31–38. [CrossRef] [PubMed]
87. Corren, J.; Lemanske, R.F.; Hanania, N.A.; Korenblat, P.E.; Parsey, M.V.; Arron, J.; Harris, J.M.; Scheerens, H.; Wu, L.C.; Su, Z.; et al. Lebrikizumab Treatment in Adults with Asthma. *N. Engl. J. Med.* **2011**, *365*, 1088–1098. [CrossRef]
88. Brightling, C.; Chanez, P.; Leigh, R.; O'Byrne, P.; Korn, S.; She, D.; May, R.; Streicher, K.; Ranade, K.; Piper, E. Efficacy and safety of tralokinumab in patients with severe uncontrolled asthma: A randomised, double-blind, placebo-controlled, phase 2b trial. *Lancet Respir. Med.* **2015**, *3*, 692–701. [CrossRef]
89. McGrath, K.W.; Icitovic, N.; Boushey, H.A.; Lazarus, S.C.; Sutherland, E.R.; Chinchilli, V.M.; Fahy, J.V. A Large Subgroup of Mild-to-Moderate Asthma Is Persistently Noneosinophilic. *Am. J. Respir. Crit. Care Med.* **2012**, *185*, 612–619. [CrossRef]
90. Berry, M.; Morgan, A.; Shaw, D.; Parker, D.; Green, R.; Brightling, C.; Bradding, P.; Wardlaw, A.; Pavord, I. Pathological features and inhaled corticosteroid response of eosinophilic and non-eosinophilic asthma. *Thorax* **2007**, *62*, 1043–1049. [CrossRef]
91. Sze, E.; Bhalla, A.; Nair, P. Mechanisms and therapeutic strategies for non-T2 asthma. *Allergy* **2020**, *75*, 311–325. [CrossRef]
92. Gibson, P.G.; Foster, P.S. Neutrophilic asthma: Welcome back! *Eur. Respir. J.* **2019**, *54*, 1901846. [CrossRef]
93. Belda, J.; Leigh, R.; Parameswaran, K.; O'Byrne, P.M.; Sears, M.R.; Hargreave, F.E. Induced Sputum Cell Counts in Healthy Adults. *Am. J. Respir. Crit. Care Med.* **2000**, *161*, 475–478. [CrossRef] [PubMed]
94. Nair, P.; Aziz-Ur-Rehman, A.; Radford, K. Therapeutic implications of 'neutrophilic asthma'. *Curr. Opin. Pulm. Med.* **2015**, *21*, 33–38. [CrossRef] [PubMed]
95. Brooks, C.R.; Gibson, P.; Douwes, J.; Van Dalen, C.J.; Simpson, J.L. Relationship between airway neutrophilia and ageing in asthmatics and non-asthmatics. *Respirology* **2013**, *18*, 857–865. [CrossRef] [PubMed]
96. Crisford, H.; Sapey, E.; Rogers, G.B.; Taylor, S.; Nagakumar, P.; Lokwani, R.; Simpson, J.L. Neutrophils in asthma: The good, the bad and the bacteria. *Thorax* **2021**, *76*, 835–844. [CrossRef]
97. Chalmers, G.W.; MacLeod, K.J.; Thomson, L.; Little, S.A.; McSharry, C.; Thomson, N. Smoking and Airway Inflammation in Patients With Mild Asthma. *Chest* **2001**, *120*, 1917–1922. [CrossRef] [PubMed]
98. Telenga, E.; Tideman, S.W.; Kerstjens, H.; Hacken, N.H.T.T.; Timens, W.; Postma, D.S.; Berge, M.V.D. Obesity in asthma: More neutrophilic inflammation as a possible explanation for a reduced treatment response. *Allergy* **2012**, *67*, 1060–1068. [CrossRef]
99. Nightingale, J.; Rogers, D.F.; Barnes, P.J. Effect of inhaled ozone on exhaled nitric oxide, pulmonary function, and induced sputum in normal and asthmatic subjects. *Thorax* **1999**, *54*, 1061–1069. [CrossRef]
100. Guarnieri, M.; Balmes, J.R. Outdoor air pollution and asthma. *Lancet* **2014**, *383*, 1581–1592. [CrossRef]
101. Wang, F.; He, X.Y.; Baines, K.; Gunawardhana, L.P.; Simpson, J.L.; Li, F.; Gibson, P.G. Different inflammatory phenotypes in adults and children with acute asthma. *Eur. Respir. J.* **2011**, *38*, 567–574. [CrossRef]
102. Robinson, P.; Pattaroni, C.; Cook, J.; Gregory, L.; Alonso, A.M.; Fleming, L.; Lloyd, C.; Bush, A.; Marsland, B.; Saglani, S. Lower Airway Microbiota Associates with Inflammatory Phenotype in Severe Preschool Wheeze. *J. Allergy Clin. Immunol.* **2019**, *143*, 1607–1610.e3. [CrossRef]
103. Taylor, S.; Leong, L.E.X.; Choo, J.M.; Wesselingh, S.; Yang, I.; Upham, J.; Reynolds, P.N.; Hodge, S.; James, A.L.; Jenkins, C.; et al. Inflammatory phenotypes in patients with severe asthma are associated with distinct airway microbiology. *J. Allergy Clin. Immunol.* **2018**, *141*, 94–103.e15. [CrossRef] [PubMed]
104. Chaudhuri, R.; Livingston, E.; McMahon, A.D.; Lafferty, J.; Fraser, I.; Spears, M.; McSharry, C.P.; Thomson, N. Effects of Smoking Cessation on Lung Function and Airway Inflammation in Smokers with Asthma. *Am. J. Respir. Crit. Care Med.* **2006**, *174*, 127–133. [CrossRef] [PubMed]
105. Dias-Júnior, S.A.; Reis, M.; de Carvalho-Pinto, R.M.; Stelmach, R.; Halpern, A.; Cukier, A. Effects of weight loss on asthma control in obese patients with severe asthma. *Eur. Respir. J.* **2014**, *43*, 1368–1377. [CrossRef]
106. Esteban-Gorgojo, I.; Antolín-Amérigo, D.; Domínguez-Ortega, J.; Quirce, S. Non-eosinophilic asthma: Current perspectives. *J. Asthma Allergy* **2018**, *11*, 267–281. [CrossRef] [PubMed]
107. Fu, J.-J.; Baines, K.J.; Wood, L.; Gibson, P. Systemic Inflammation Is Associated with Differential Gene Expression and Airway Neutrophilia in Asthma. *OMICS* **2013**, *17*, 187–199. [CrossRef] [PubMed]

108. Gibson, P.G.; Yang, I.; Upham, J.; Reynolds, P.N.; Hodge, S.; James, A.L.; Jenkins, C.; Peters, M.; Marks, G.B.; Baraket, M.; et al. Effect of azithromycin on asthma exacerbations and quality of life in adults with persistent uncontrolled asthma (AMAZES): A randomised, double-blind, placebo-controlled trial. *Lancet* **2017**, *390*, 659–668. [CrossRef]
109. Niessen, N.M.; Gibson, P.G.; Baines, K.J.; Barker, D.; Yang, I.A.; Upham, J.W.; Reynolds, P.N.; Hodge, S.; James, A.L.; Jenkins, C.; et al. Sputum TNF markers are increased in neutrophilic and severe asthma and are reduced by azithromycin treatment. *Allergy* **2021**, *76*, 2090–2101. [CrossRef] [PubMed]
110. Vedel-Krogh, S.; Nielsen, S.F.; Lange, P.; Vestbo, J.; Nordestgaard, B.G. Blood Eosinophils and Exacerbations in Chronic Obstructive Pulmonary Disease. The Copenhagen General Population Study. *Am. J. Respir. Crit. Care Med.* **2016**, *193*, 965–974. [CrossRef]
111. Couillard, S.; Larivée, P.; Courteau, J.; Vanasse, A. Eosinophils in COPD Exacerbations Are Associated With Increased Readmissions. *Chest* **2017**, *151*, 366–373. [CrossRef]
112. Zeiger, R.S.; Tran, T.N.; Butler, R.K.; Schatz, M.; Li, Q.; Khatry, D.; Martin, U.; Kawatkar, A.A.; Chen, W. Relationship of Blood Eosinophil Count to Exacerbations in Chronic Obstructive Pulmonary Disease. *J. Allergy Clin. Immunol. Pr.* **2018**, *6*, 944–954.e5. [CrossRef] [PubMed]
113. Yun, J.; Lamb, A.; Chase, R.; Singh, D.; Parker, M.M.; Saferali, A.; Vestbo, J.; Tal-Singer, R.; Castaldi, P.J.; Silverman, E.K.; et al. Blood eosinophil count thresholds and exacerbations in patients with chronic obstructive pulmonary disease. *J. Allergy Clin. Immunol.* **2018**, *141*, 2037–2047.e10. [CrossRef]
114. Duman, D.; Aksoy, E.; Agca, M.C.; Kocak, N.D.; Ozmen, I.; Akturk, U.A.; Gungor, S.; Tepetam, F.M.; Eroglu, S.A.; Oztas, S.; et al. The utility of inflammatory markers to predict readmissions and mortality in COPD cases with or without eosinophilia. *Int. J. Chron. Obs. Pulmon. Dis.* **2015**, *10*, 2469–2478. [CrossRef] [PubMed]
115. Walters, J.A.; Tan, D.J.; White, C.J.; Gibson, P.G.; Wood-Baker, R.; Walters, E.H. Systemic corticosteroids for acute exacerbations of chronic obstructive pulmonary disease. *Cochrane Database Syst. Rev.* **2014**, *9*, CD001288. [CrossRef]
116. Waljee, A.K.; Rogers, M.; Lin, P.; Singal, A.G.; Stein, J.; Marks, R.M.; Ayanian, J.Z.; Nallamothu, B.K. Short term use of oral corticosteroids and related harms among adults in the United States: Population based cohort study. *BMJ* **2017**, *357*, j1415. [CrossRef] [PubMed]
117. Bafadhel, M.; McKenna, S.; Terry, S.; Mistry, V.; Pancholi, M.; Venge, P.; Lomas, D.A.; Barer, M.R.; Johnston, S.L.; Pavord, I.D.; et al. Blood eosinophils to direct corticosteroid treatment of exacerbations of chronic obstructive pulmonary disease: A randomized placebo-controlled trial. *Am. J. Respir. Crit. Care Med.* **2012**, *186*, 48–55. [CrossRef]
118. Sivapalan, P.; Lapperre, T.S.; Janner, J.; Laub, R.R.; Moberg, M.; Bech, C.S.; Eklöf, J.; Holm, F.S.; Armbruster, K.; Sivapalan, P.; et al. Eosinophil-guided corticosteroid therapy in patients admitted to hospital with COPD exacerbation.(CORTICO-COP): A multicentre, randomised, controlled, open-label, non-inferiority trial. *Lancet Respir. Med.* **2019**, *7*, 699–709. [CrossRef]
119. Vogelmeier, C.F.; Criner, G.J.; Martinez, F.J.; Anzueto, A.; Barnes, P.J.; Bourbeau, J.; Celli, B.R.; Chen, R.; Decramer, M.; Fabbri, L.M.; et al. Global Strategy for the Diagnosis, Management, and Prevention of Chronic Obstructive Lung Disease 2017 Report. GOLD Executive Summary. *Am. J. Respir. Crit. Care Med.* **2017**, *195*, 557–582. [CrossRef]
120. Kew, K.M.; Seniukovich, A. Inhaled steroids and risk of pneumonia for chronic obstructive pulmonary disease. *Cochrane Database Syst. Rev.* **2014**, *2014*, CD010115. [CrossRef]
121. Ernst, P.; Baltzan, M.; Deschênes, J.; Suissa, S. Low-dose inhaled and nasal corticosteroid use and the risk of cataracts. *Eur. Respir. J.* **2006**, *27*, 1168–1174. [CrossRef]
122. Smeeth, L.; Boulis, M.; Hubbard, R.; Fletcher, A.E. A population based case-control study of cataract and inhaled corticosteroids. *Br. J. Ophthalmol.* **2003**, *87*, 1247–1251. [CrossRef] [PubMed]
123. Lipson, D.; Barnhart, F.; Brealey, N.; Brooks, J.; Criner, G.J.; Day, N.C.; Dransfield, M.T.; Halpin, D.M.; Han, M.K.; Jones, C.E.; et al. Once-Daily Single-Inhaler Triple versus Dual Therapy in Patients with COPD. *N. Engl. J. Med.* **2018**, *378*, 1671–1680. [CrossRef] [PubMed]
124. Calverley, P.M.A.; Tetzlaff, K.; Vogelmeier, C.; Fabbri, L.M.; Magnussen, H.; Wouters, E.F.M.; Mezzanotte, W.; Disse, B.; Finnigan, H.; Asijee, G.; et al. Eosinophilia, Frequent Exacerbations, and Steroid Response in Chronic Obstructive Pulmonary Disease. *Am. J. Respir. Crit. Care Med.* **2017**, *196*, 1219–1221. [CrossRef]
125. Singh, D.; Agusti, A.; Anzueto, A.; Barnes, P.J.; Bourbeau, J.; Celli, B.R.; Criner, G.J.; Frith, P.; Halpin, D.M.G.; Han, M.; et al. Global Strategy for the Diagnosis, Management, and Prevention of Chronic Obstructive Lung Disease: The GOLD science committee report 2019. *Eur. Respir. J.* **2019**, *53*, 1900164. [CrossRef] [PubMed]
126. Pavord, I.; Lettis, S.; Locantore, N.; Pascoe, S.; Jones, P.W.; Wedzicha, J.A.; Barnes, N.C. Blood eosinophils and inhaled corticosteroid/long-acting β-2 agonist efficacy in COPD. *Thorax* **2016**, *71*, 118–125. [CrossRef] [PubMed]
127. Siddiqui, S.H.; Pavord, I.D.; Barnes, N.C.; Guasconi, A.; Lettis, S.; Pascoe, S.; Petruzzelli, S. Blood eosinophils: A biomarker of COPD exacerbation reduction with inhaled corticosteroids. *Int. J. Chronic Obstr. Pulm. Dis.* **2018**, *13*, 3669–3676. [CrossRef]
128. Chapman, K.R.; Hurst, J.R.; Frent, S.-M.; Larbig, M.; Fogel, R.; Guerin, T.; Banerji, D.; Patalano, F.; Goyal, P.; Pfister, P.; et al. Long-Term Triple Therapy De-escalation to Indacaterol/Glycopyrronium in Patients with Chronic Obstructive Pulmonary Disease (SUNSET): A Randomized, Double-Blind, Triple-Dummy Clinical Trial. *Am. J. Respir. Crit. Care Med.* **2018**, *198*, 329–339. [CrossRef] [PubMed]
129. Magnussen, H.; Disse, B.; Rodriguez-Roisin, R.; Kirsten, A.; Watz, H.; Tetzlaff, K.; Towse, L.; Finnigan, H.; Dahl, R.; Decramer, M.; et al. Withdrawal of Inhaled Glucocorticoids and Exacerbations of COPD. *N. Engl. J. Med.* **2014**, *371*, 1285–1294. [CrossRef]

130. Watz, H.; Tetzlaff, K.; Wouters, E.F.M.; Kirsten, A.; Magnussen, H.; Rodriguez-Roisin, R.; Vogelmeier, C.; Fabbri, L.; Chanez, P.; Dahl, R.; et al. Blood eosinophil count and exacerbations in severe chronic obstructive pulmonary disease after withdrawal of inhaled corticosteroids: A post-hoc analysis of the WISDOM trial. *Lancet Respir. Med.* **2016**, *4*, 390–398. [CrossRef]
131. Eosinophil-guided Reduction of Inhaled Corticosteroids (COPERNICOS). Available online: https://.ClinicalTrials.gov/show/NCT04481555 (accessed on 20 January 2021).
132. Pavord, I.D.; Chanez, P.; Criner, G.J.; Kerstjens, H.; Korn, S.; Lugogo, N.; Martinot, J.-B.; Sagara, H.; Albers, F.C.; Bradford, E.S.; et al. Mepolizumab for Eosinophilic Chronic Obstructive Pulmonary Disease. *N. Engl. J. Med.* **2017**, *377*, 1613–1629. [CrossRef] [PubMed]
133. Brightling, C.E.; Bleecker, E.R.; Panettieri, R.A.; Bafadhel, M.; She, D.; Ward, C.K.; Xu, X.; Birrell, C.; van der Merwe, R. Benralizumab for chronic obstructive pulmonary disease and sputum eosinophilia: A randomised, double-blind, placebo-controlled, phase 2a study. *Lancet Respir. Med.* **2014**, *2*, 891–901. [CrossRef]
134. Assicot, M.; Bohuon, C.; Gendrel, D.; Raymond, J.; Carsin, H.; Guilbaud, J. High serum procalcitonin concentrations in patients with sepsis and infection. *Lancet* **1993**, *341*, 515–518. [CrossRef]
135. Ventetuolo, C.; Levy, M.M. Biomarkers: Diagnosis and Risk Assessment in Sepsis. *Clin. Chest Med.* **2008**, *29*, 591–603. [CrossRef] [PubMed]
136. Aslam, B.; Wang, W.; Arshad, M.I.; Khurshid, M.; Muzammil, S.; Rasool, M.H.; Nisar, M.A.; Alvi, R.F.; Aslam, M.A.; Qamar, M.U.; et al. Antibiotic resistance: A rundown of a global crisis. *Infect. Drug Resist.* **2018**, *11*, 1645–1658. [CrossRef] [PubMed]
137. Cukic, V.; Lovre, V.; Dragisic, D.; Ustamujic, A. Asthma and Chronic Obstructive Pulmonary Disease (Copd) and #8211; Differences and Similarities. *Mater. Socio Medica* **2012**, *24*, 100–105. [CrossRef]
138. Baggs, J.; Fridkin, S.K.; Pollack, L.A.; Srinivasan, A.; Jernigan, J.A. Estimating National Trends in Inpatient Antibiotic Use Among US Hospitals From 2006 to 2012. *JAMA Intern. Med.* **2016**, *176*, 1639–1648. [CrossRef] [PubMed]
139. Tang, J.; Long, W.; Yan, L.; Zhang, Y.; Xie, J.; Lu, G.; Yang, C. Procalcitonin guided antibiotic therapy of acute exacerbations of asthma: A randomized controlled trial. *BMC Infect. Dis.* **2013**, *13*, 596. [CrossRef]
140. Long, W.; Li, L.-J.; Huang, G.-Z.; Zhang, X.-M.; Zhang, Y.-C.; Tang, J.-G.; Zhang, Y.; Lu, G. Procalcitonin guidance for reduction of antibiotic use in patients hospitalized with severe acute exacerbations of asthma: A randomized controlled study with 12-month follow-up. *Crit. Care* **2014**, *18*, 471. [CrossRef]
141. Scholl, T.; Kiser, T.H.; Vondracek, S.F. Evaluation of Systemic Corticosteroids in Patients With an Acute Exacerbation of COPD and a Diagnosis of Pneumonia. *Chronic Obstr. Pulm. Dis. J. COPD Found.* **2018**, *5*, 57–65. [CrossRef]
142. Barnes, P.J. Inflammatory mechanisms in patients with chronic obstructive pulmonary disease. *J. Allergy Clin. Immunol.* **2016**, *138*, 16–27. [CrossRef] [PubMed]
143. Schuetz, P.; Wirz, Y.; Sager, R.; Christ-Crain, M.; Stolz, D.; Tamm, M.; Bouadma, L.; Luyt, C.E.; Wolff, M.; Chastre, J.; et al. Effect of procalcitonin-guided antibiotic treatment on mortality in acute respiratory infections: A patient level meta-analysis. *Lancet Infect. Dis.* **2018**, *18*, 95–107. [CrossRef]
144. Schuetz, P.; Wirz, Y.; Sager, R.; Christ-Crain, M.; Stolz, D.; Tamm, M.; Bouadma, L.; Luyt, C.E.; Wolff, M.; Chastre, J.; et al. Procalcitonin to initiate or discontinue antibiotics in acute respiratory tract infections. *Cochrane Database Syst. Rev.* **2017**, *10*, CD007498. [CrossRef] [PubMed]

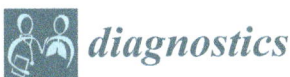

Review

The Role of Digital Tools in the Timely Diagnosis and Prevention of Acute Exacerbations of COPD: A Comprehensive Review of the Literature

Athanasios Konstantinidis [1], Christos Kyriakopoulos [1,*], Georgios Ntritsos [2,3], Nikolaos Giannakeas [3], Konstantinos I. Gourgoulianis [4], Konstantinos Kostikas [1] and Athena Gogali [1]

1. Respiratory Medicine Department, Faculty of Medicine, University of Ioannina, 45500 Ioannina, Greece; akonstan@uoi.gr (A.K.); ktkostikas@gmail.com (K.K.); athenagogali@yahoo.com (A.G.)
2. Department of Hygiene and Epidemiology, Faculty of Medicine, University of Ioannina, 45500 Ioannina, Greece; gntritsos@uoi.gr
3. Department of Informatics and Telecommunications, School of Informatics and Telecommunications, University of Ioannina, 47100 Arta, Greece; giannakeas@uoi.gr
4. Department of Respiratory Medicine, Faculty of Medicine, University of Thessaly, 41110 Larissa, Greece; kgourg@med.uth.gr
* Correspondence: ckyriako123@gmail.com; Tel.: +30-6974332047

Abstract: Chronic obstructive pulmonary disease (COPD) is a chronic inflammatory disease of the airways and lung parenchyma with multiple systemic manifestations. Exacerbations of COPD are important events during the course of the disease, as they are associated with increased mortality, severe impairment of health-related quality of life, accelerated decline in lung function, significant reduction in physical activity, and substantial economic burden. Telemedicine is the use of communication technologies to transmit medical data over short or long distances and to deliver healthcare services. The need to limit in-person appointments during the COVID-19 pandemic has caused a rapid increase in telemedicine services. In the present review of the literature covering published randomized controlled trials reporting results regarding the use of digital tools in acute exacerbations of COPD, we attempt to clarify the effectiveness of telemedicine for identifying, preventing, and reducing COPD exacerbations and improving other clinically relevant outcomes, while describing in detail the specific telemedicine interventions used.

Keywords: telemedicine; telehealth; telemonitoring; COPD; acute exacerbation COPD; diagnosis; prevention

Citation: Konstantinidis, A.; Kyriakopoulos, C.; Ntritsos, G.; Giannakeas, N.; Gourgoulianis, K.I.; Kostikas, K.; Gogali, A. The Role of Digital Tools in the Timely Diagnosis and Prevention of Acute Exacerbations of COPD: A Comprehensive Review of the Literature. *Diagnostics* **2022**, *12*, 269. https://doi.org/10.3390/diagnostics12020269

Academic Editor: Koichi Nishimura

Received: 19 December 2021
Accepted: 19 January 2022
Published: 21 January 2022

Publisher's Note: MDPI stays neutral with regard to jurisdictional claims in published maps and institutional affiliations.

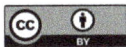

Copyright: © 2022 by the authors. Licensee MDPI, Basel, Switzerland. This article is an open access article distributed under the terms and conditions of the Creative Commons Attribution (CC BY) license (https://creativecommons.org/licenses/by/4.0/).

1. Introduction

Chronic obstructive pulmonary disease (COPD) is a chronic debilitating disease of the airways and lung parenchyma with a prevalence of approximately 380 million cases worldwide [1]. It is currently the third leading cause of death, responsible for approximately 6% of the world's total deaths (approximately 3.3 million annually) [2]. An exacerbation of COPD (AECOPD) is defined as an acute worsening of respiratory symptoms requiring additional therapy, usually caused by a viral or bacterial lung infection [3]. AECOPDs are important events during the course of the disease because they are associated with increased mortality, severe impairment of health-related quality of life, accelerated decline in lung function, significant reduction in physical activity, and substantial economic burden [4–6].

Telemedicine is defined as the use of communication technologies to transmit medical data over long and short distances and to deliver healthcare services [7]. The term telemedicine (from the Greek term "tele" and the Latin "medicus") was devised in the 1970s by the American Thomas Bird and actually means "treating from a distance" [8]. The origins of telemedicine date back to 1905, when Willem Einthoven successfully transmitted both the first electrocardiogram and the heart sounds of a volunteer between his lab and the Academic Hospital in Leiden, the Netherlands by a telephone line [9]. Progress in telemedicine has been expedited due to recent technological advances that offer user-friendly and reliable applications, as depicted in Figure 1. In addition, the need to limit in-person appointments during the COVID-19 pandemic has caused a rapid increase in telemedicine services.

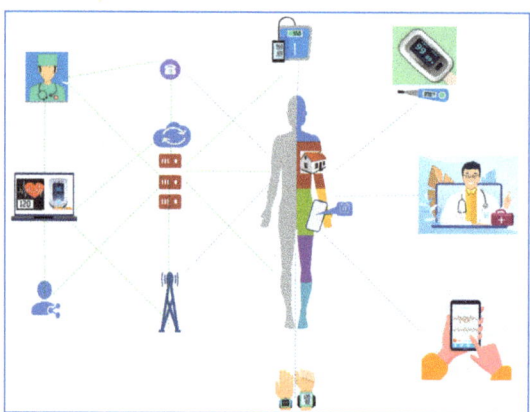

Figure 1. The telemedicine ecosystem.

Telemedicine applications in COPD were introduced more than 20 years ago but have rapidly expanded over the last decade [10]. These applications include tracking COPD patients for earlier detection of disease exacerbations and early intervention to prevent deterioration and the need for hospitalization [11]. Given that exacerbations of COPD are associated with high mortality and morbidity as well as substantial healthcare expenditures, well-designed telemedicine applications might become a valuable tool for reducing AECOPDs.

A number of systematic reviews and meta-analyses have evaluated the role of telemedicine in various clinical outcomes in patients with COPD [7,12–17]. A recent systematic review and meta-analysis of 22 randomized controlled trials (RCTs) involving 2906 participants in telemonitoring (TM) interventions for severe COPD exacerbations suggested that the addition of TM to usual care decreased avoidable emergency department (ED) visits but was unlikely to prevent hospitalizations due to COPD exacerbations [18]. However, the authors underline the fact that there was 'high' bias in the 'blinding of participants and personnel' in the included studies because it might have been difficult for the participants and personnel to remain unaware of the interventions due to the nature of TM interventions. In addition, they comment that there was significant clinical heterogeneity between trials in terms of the study duration, study population, patient recruitment setting, type of technology used, and TM interventions [18]. Similar diversity in outcomes has been found among meta-analyses involving various telemedicine interventions in patients with COPD, attributed to the complexity of telemedicine applications, lack of validated data collection instruments, and lack of high-quality reporting [11].

The evidence as to whether digital tools are actually effective in early detection and prevention of AECOPDs seems inconclusive and contradictory. In our comprehensive review of the literature, we attempt to clarify the effectiveness of telemedicine for the identification, prevention or reduction in AECOPDs. Specifically, we aim to classify the studies into those reporting significant improvement in outcomes and those reporting non-significant ones, and to describe in detail the specific telemedicine interventions used in each study.

2. Methods

We conducted a search of EMBASE, PubMed, and Scopus databases using the following search algorithm ("chronic obstructive pulmonary disease" OR "chronic obstructive airway disease" OR "chronic obstructive lung disease" OR "chronic obstructive bronchitis" OR "COPD") AND ("telemonitoring" OR "telehealth" OR "telemedicine" OR "telecommunication" OR "remote consultation") AND ("random" OR "trial" OR "randomised controlled trial" OR "randomized controlled trial" OR "clinical trial" OR "RCT"). Papers published between 2006 and October 2021 in the English language were considered. C. K. and A. G. assessed the identified randomized controlled trials (RCTs) studies for suitability. Among the 325 identified studies, 35 RCTs containing a TM and control group reported results regarding digital tools in AECOPDs and were considered appropriate for inclusion in the review.

3. Studies with Positive Results
3.1. Telemedicine Involving Close Healthcare Monitoring

An RCT conducted in Taiwan by Ho et al. [19] including 106 COPD patients showed a beneficial effect of TM in preventing AECOPDs and related admissions, using an electronic diary for the intervention group, which was easy to fill, consisting of 8 questions about symptoms, vital signs, and weight. Based on an algorithm, data were scored and transmitted to the medical team, while warnings related to the scores achieved generated notifications if appropriate. TM took place for 2 months, with atotal follow-up of 6 months, while the control group received the usual care. The time to first readmission for AECOPD was increased in the TM group as compared with the usual care group ($p = 0.026$). The probability of COPD-related readmission was significantly lower in the TM group (hazard ratio 0.42, 95% CI: 0.19–0.92), and there was a trend for fewer episodes of COPD-related readmissions (0.19 vs. 0.49; $p = 0.11$) or ED visits (0.23 vs. 0.55; $p = 0.16$) in this group. The first COPD-related ED visit was also delayed (hazard ratio = 0.50). Finally, TM intervention was associated with significant reductions in the numbers of all-cause readmissions and ED visits for all causes compared to the usual care group. Investigators attributed the effectiveness of TM to the items monitored and corresponding algorithm [19].

Kessler et al. [20] included 319 COPD patients with a mean forced expiratory volume in one second (FEV1) of 37.1% predicted and at least one severe exacerbation in the previous year. Patients in the telehealth (TH) group were under home monitoring and an e-health telephone and web platform was applied that transmitted FEV1, heart rate (HR), pulse arterial oxygen saturation (SPO_2) plus daily oxygen use, and respiratory ratio (RR) data for patients on long-term oxygen therapy (LTOT). Upon deterioration, patients were contacted by the investigators. No significant difference was observed regarding hospitalization days, hospital admissions, AECOPDs, six minute walking test (6MWT), Saint George's respiratory questionnaire (SGRQ), or hospital anxiety and depression scale (HADS) scores. Nevertheless in the TH group, acute care hospitalizations and mortality rate were significantly lower (1.9% vs. 14.2%, $p < 0.001$), with greater improvements in body mass index, airflow obstruction, dyspnea, and exercise capacity (BODE) index score and a higher proportion of patients who quit smoking. One possible explanation for the mortality rate reduction is that the TH management program may have promoted earlier intervention, thereby preventing fatal complications of AECOPDs [20].

Koff et al. [21] recruited 40 GOLD COPD stage III or IV patients, administering in the TM group a pulse oximeter, a FEV1 monitor, a pedometer, and a technology platform for delivery of education and transmission of the results for 3 months. When a clinical problem emerged, the coordinator would help facilitate its resolution by providing the appropriate instructions. Patients receiving integrated care demonstrated a lower number of hospitalizations and ED visits, improvement of SGRQ, and reduced healthcare costs. However, the generalizability of the results is limited by the small number of participants and the short duration of the study [21].

Pedone et al. [22], in an RCT including elderly patients with COPD in stages II and III, used a simple, fully automated system that required no effort on the patient's side and was able to monitor vital signs several times a day and transmit them to a skilled physician that could contact and advise the patient when appropriate. In total, 50 patients received the intervention and 49 received usual care, who were followed for 9 months. Although statistical significance was not reached due to the lower incidence of events than expected, a beneficial effect of home telemonitoring was shown, with a 33% reduction in exacerbations (incidence rate ratio 0.67, 95% CI: 0.32–1.36) and related admissions (incidence rate ratio 0.66, 95% CI: 0.21–1.86). The only parameter monitored able to identify timely AECOPD was oxygen saturation. Surprisingly, the average length of stay was shorter for the control group, possibly because TM helped patients dealing with less severe exacerbations at home [22].

Similarly, Segrelles-Calvo et al. [23] recruited 60 COPD GOLD stage III–IV patients on LTOT in order to assess the efficacy and effectiveness of a home TH program for COPD patients with severe or very severe airflow obstruction. TM parameters included oxygen saturation, HR, and blood pressure (BP) daily and peak expiratory flow (PEF) results three times a week. In the TH group, reductions in the number of ED visits, hospital admissions, length of hospitalization, and mortality were observed. The positive results of this study could be attributed to the combination of TH resources with conventional care and prompt interventions after an early detection of an AECOPD, together with the coordination of primary care, pneumologists, and nursing staff. Moreover, the accessibility of the TM device and the overall satisfaction rate, which was high, led to no withdrawals [23].

Shanny et al. [24] assessed the effects of TM in 42 COPD patients with severe or very severe airflow obstruction. The TH intervention included measurements of pulse saturation, temperature, HR, BP, and weight, daily symptoms, electrocardiogram, and spirometry, with telephone support and home visits. Reductions in the total length of stay for all admissions, time to first hospitalization, relative risk of ED visit or hospital admission, and hospitalization costs were observed, while there was also a trend towards reductions in the numbers of ED visits and hospital admissions [24].

In an RCT with a different design, Sink et al. [25] recruited 168 COPD patients with mild to very severe airflow obstruction. Patients allocated to the treatment group received a daily message regarding their breathing status. If a patient responded "worse", then the EpxCOPD system immediately triggered an alert to the assigned medical resident provider, while if they were experiencing a medical emergency, they were advised to present to the emergency department to seek care. The time to hospitalization was significantly different between the two groups, favoring the TM group (hazard ratio 2.36, 95% CI: 1.02–5.45; $p = 0.043$), while the same applied for the number of hospital admissions. The positive results were associated with the early intervention and proper consultation by the health staff, leading to the prompt detection and treatment of AECOPDs and finally to the reduction in hospital admissions [25].

Vitacca et al. [26] studied 101 COPD patients with the need for home mechanical ventilation (HMV) or LTOT and at least one hospitalization for AECOPD in the previous year, with a mean FEV1 of 39% pred. Patients allocated to the TH group received a pulse oximetry device that transmitted pulse saturation data via a telephone modem to a receiving station, where a nurse was available to provide a real-time teleconsultation, for 12 months. The on-duty respiratory physician was informed for unscheduled calls and provided a consultation. The study demonstrated that patients in the intervention group had fewer hospital admissions per month compared with controls (mean (SD) 0.17 (0.23) vs. 0.30 (0.30); $p = 0.019$), experienced fewer hospitalizations ($p = 0.018$), and had a higher probability of avoiding hospitalization ($p = 0.012$). Moreover, patients in the TM group had a significantly higher probability of remaining free from AECOPDs ($p = 0.0001$), from further urgent general practitioner (GP) calls ($p = 0.013$), and from further ED visits ($p = 0.003$). However, the mortality rates did not differ between the two groups ($p = 0.148$) [26].

Clemente et al. [27] performed a randomized clinical trial to examine the role of telemedicine in monitoring early-discharged and home-hospitalized COPD patients after an exacerbation. The intervention group underwent TM during home hospitalization using a multiparametric recording unit. Data on vital constants (electrocardiogram (ECG), SPO2, HR, BP, temperature, and RR) were transmitted twice per day to the physician in charge with a subsequent phone call by him concerning their clinical situation, and only

2 home visits by healthcare staff were performed (intermediate and at discharge). The control group received daily visits by nursing staff and a final visit from the physician. Both groups were then followed for six months without TM. The main outcome was time until first exacerbation; no difference was observed, with a median of 48 days in the control group and 47 days in the intervention group ($p = 0.52$). Additionally, during the follow-up period, no significant difference was observed in the numbers of AECOPDs that both groups experienced. Notably, the durations of home hospitalization were similar in the two groups (median 7 days), as were the numbers of readmissions observed. Thus, in this study, home hospitalization using telemedicine after early discharge proved non-inferior to conventional home follow-up [27].

A different aspect of how telemedicine can improve the health of COPD patients is given by the study of de Toledo et al. [28], who used a technological platform called the Chronic Care Management Center, which consists of a telephone center and a telemedicine server that gives access to the electronic chronic patient records to all the members of the care team from any location (patient's home, hospital, primary care center). The study lasted for a year and a total of 157 COPD patients were recruited during hospital admission due to an exacerbation. The intervention group had telephone access to the system's center, while the multidisciplinary team caring for these patients had access to the platform. Follow-up of the control group did not involve phone calls or telemedicine support for the health providers. Care coordination and telephone support to patients led to a significant reduction in readmissions (number of patients that did not need a readmission: 51% intervention vs. 33% control; $p = 0.04$), possibly due to early detection of AECOPD symptoms. No difference in ED visit number or mortality was demonstrated [28].

3.2. Telemedicine Involving Primarily Self-Management Techniques

Casas et al. [29] showed that integrated care intervention could prevent COPD-related hospitalizations. Here, 155 COPD patients from two different centers, Barcelona and Leuven, who had an exacerbation, were recruited immediately after discharge, and 65 of them were offered integrated care, which consisted of an individual well-defined care plan shared between the primary care and hospital team, as well as accessibility to a specialized nurse through a web-based call center. Patients in the intervention arm were educated before discharge on several issues, including self-management techniques, receiving an early joint visit from the specialized nurse and the primary care team or regular visits from their GP, who had been contacted by the primary investigator. They also received weekly reinforcement calls from the specialized nurse in the first month, while a chronic platform (a call center coupled to a web-based application providing access to the patients' records) was accessible by them and primary care providers. Patients in the control arm were visited by their own physician, usually every six months, without additional support. During 12-month follow-up, a significantly lower readmission rate was observed in the intervention group (hazard ratio 0.55, 95% CI: 0.35–0.88; $p = 0.01$), the percentage of patients without admissions was greater, while the difference in the rate of admissions per patient between the follow-up and the previous year was also lower. No survival differences were found. This positive result was possibly due to a combination of the effectiveness of patient education programs along with the personalized health plan and higher accessibility to healthcare professionals [29].

In a different approach, Jehn et al. [30] monitored 32 patients specifically during the summer period (9 months in total), showing that climate change (heat stress) has a negative impact on the clinical status, lung function, and exercise capacity of COPD stage II–IV patients. Interesting remarks were made regarding exacerbations when the TM group was compared to the control group. More specifically, the TM intervention included a daily COPD assessment test (CAT), spirometry, and a weekly 6MWT measured by accelerometry performed at home. Data were transmitted and reviewed daily, although the study had an observational character. The intervention group exhibited significantly fewer AECOPDs during summer (3 for TM vs. 14 for control group; $p = 0.006$) and over the rest of the year. Over the whole 9-month follow-up period, the intervention group had a significantly lower number of exacerbation-related hospital admissions (7 vs. 22; $p = 0.012$), spent significantly less time in hospital due to COPD (34 vs. 97 days), and performed significantly fewer visits to the pulmonologist (24 vs. 42; $p = 0.042$). As there had been no medical intervention, positive results were attributed to better disease awareness and improved physical condition, possibly due to weekly performance of the 6MWT [30].

Paré et al. [31] included 120 COPD patients with a FEV1 under 45% pred. and at least one hospitalization in the previous year. A digital device was provided to the intervention group and the patients had to complete a daily data entry table documenting symptoms and adherence to prescribed medication for 6 months. Patients were afterwards under surveillance for the next 6 months, after the initial 6-month period. During the initial 6-month period, the TM group exhibited less ED visits (36% vs. 13% reduction, without statistical significance) and hospital admissions, shorter length of hospitalization, less home visits by nurses, and lower healthcare costs [31].

3.3. Telemedicine Involving Telerehabilitation

Dinesen et al. [32] constructed an RCT that showed that telerehabilitation using a TM device could significantly reduce hospital admissions in patients with COPD. In total, 111 stage III and IV patients were randomized and 60 of them were instructed to use digital equipment in order to measure, monitor, and transmit vital signs, training inputs of the rehabilitation program, and spirometry values. All healthcare professionals (GP, nurses, and hospital doctors), patients, and relatives had access to the data, while once a month a video meeting was held between healthcare teams to coordinate the individual rehabilitation programs of the patients. The control group performed home exercises by themselves, without any contact. The TM program had a duration of 4 months and patients were followed-up for 10 months in total, resulting in a reduction in admission rate to 0.48 over 10 months compared to 1.17 for the control group ($p = 0.041$). A trend towards a longer time to first admission was also observed in the telerehabilitation group. A positive preventative impact of the study was attributed to the improved self-management of the illness and interactions among healthcare professionals and the patients with the help of technology [32].

Tabak et al. [33] performed a pilot RCT including 29 COPD patients with three or more AECOPDs or one hospitalization for respiratory disease in the preceding 2 years. Patients in the TH group received a web-based exercise program, an activity coach, a self-management module, and a teleconsultation module on the web portal for 9 months. The TH group showed a lower number of hospital admissions, shorter hospitalization stay, and improvement in the quality of life satisfaction with received care. These findings are limited in their generalizability by the fact that it was a pilot study, the small number of participants, and the significantly worse dyspnea levels in the control group [33].

Vasilopoulou et al. [34] recruited 147 GOLD COPD stage II or IV patients with at least one AECOPD in the year prior to the study. Following the completion of an initial 2-month pulmonary rehabilitation program, this RCT compared 12 months of home-based maintenance telerehabilitation ($n = 47$) with 12 months of hospital-based outpatient maintenance rehabilitation ($n = 50$) and also 12 months of usual care treatment ($n = 50$), without initial pulmonary rehabilitation. Patients in the TM group received an oximeter, a spirometer, a pedometer, and a video demonstration of the home exercises. The TH intervention led to lower rates of AECOPDs, hospital admissions, and ED visits; improvement of health-related quality of life (HRQL); higher functional capacity; and higher daily physical activity compared to the usual care group. Notably, the results were comparable with the hospital-based rehabilitation program for all parameters, while the reduction in ED visits was even greater in the telerehabilitation arm [34]. Table 1 summarizes the characteristics of the RCTs for TM, which showed positive results.

Table 1. Telemedicine studies showing positive results.

Author (Year)	Country	Primary Objective	Secondary Objectives	COPD Severity	TM Duration	n Telemonitoring Group	n Control Group	Patient Effort Required	Telemonitoring Intervention	Telemonitoring Data	Exacerbation Outcomes	Other Study Outcomes
Casas (2006) [29]	Spain, Belgium	Rehospitalization rate, mortality	-	Discharge after AECOPD	12 m	65	90	Mild	Web-based call center	-	Readmission rate-	Mortality=
De Toledo (2006) [28]	Spain	Readmissions, ED visits, mortality	Acceptability to professionals, characterization of the patterns of use of the system, costs	Discharge after AECOPD	12 m	67	90	Mild	Chronic care telemedicine system, phone calls by patients	Electronic chronic patient record accessible to the care team	Readmissions-; ED visits=; mortality=	Acceptability+
Koff (2009) [21]	USA	HRQL	AECOPDs, healthcare costs	COPD GOLD stage III-IV	3 m	20	20	High	Telemonitoring plus self-management plus phone contact	PFTs, SPO2, 6MWT, shortness of breath, cough	Hospital admissions-; ER visits-	SGRQ; costs-
Vitacca (2009) [26]	Italy	Reduction in hospital admissions	Reduction in AECOPDs, ED visits, urgent GP calls, cost-effectiveness	Need for HMV and/or need of LTOT and at least one hospitalization for AECOPD in the previous year, FEV1 % pred. 39%	12 m	57	44	Mild	Telemonitoring plus telenursing and doctor on demand	SPO2	Hospital admissions-; AECOPDs-; urgent GP calls-; mortality=	Cost-effectiveness=
Dinesen (2012) [32]	Denmark	Readmissions, costs	-	COPD GOLD stage III-IV	4 m/10 m follow-up	60	51	High	Remote TM	PFTs, HR, SPO2, BP, weight	Hospital readmissions-; time to first exacerbation + (trend)	Costs-
Jehn (2013) [30]	Germany	FEV1, 6MWT, CAT score, AECOPD	-	COPD GOLD stage II-IV, at least one AECOPD during the previous year	9 m	32	30	High	Remote TM	PFTs, CAT, 6MWT	AECOPD-; hospital stay-; specialist consultations-	PFTs=; CAT; 6MWT+

Table 1. Cont.

Author (Year)	Country	Primary Objective	Secondary Objectives	COPD Severity	TM Duration	n Telemonitoring Group	n Control Group	Patient Effort Required	Telemonitoring Intervention	Telemonitoring Data	Exacerbation Outcomes	Other Study Outcomes
Paré (2013) [31]	Canada	ED visits, hospital admissions, length of hospitalization, home visits by nurses and respiratory therapists, and economic viability of the program	-	FEV1 < 45%, at least one hospitalization in the previous year	6 m/6 m follow-up	60	60	Mild	Remote TM patient health status and adherence to therapy plus self-management plus telenursing and doctor on demand	Symptoms and medication consumed	ED visits-; hospital admissions-; length of hospitalization-	Cost-effectiveness=; home visits by nurses=; home visits by respiratory physicians=
Pedone (2013) [22]	Italy	AECOPD, related admissions	-	Patients > 65, COPD GOLD stage II and III	9 m	50	49	Mild	Remote TM	HR, SPO2, TEMP, overall physical activity	AECOPD, hospital admissions— (not statistically significant); length of hospitalization+	-
Segrelles Calvo (2014) [23]	Spain	ED visits, hospital admissions, length of hospitalization, mortality	-	COPD GOLD stage III-IV and LTOT	7 m	30	30	High	Telemonitoring plus teleconsultation plus home visits	PEF, SPO2, HR, BP	ED visits-; hospital admissions-; length of hospitalization-; mortality-	Satisfaction+
Tabak (2014) [33]	Netherlands	Hospital admissions, length of hospitalization, and ED visits	Functional capacity, HRQL, daily physical activity	≥3 AECOPDs or 1 hospitalization for respiratory problems in the 2 years preceding study entry	9 m	15	14	High	Exercising plus self-management plus teleconsultation	-	Hospital admissions-; length of hospitalization-	HRQL+; 6MWT=; satisfaction+
Ho (2016) [19]	Taiwan	Time to first readmission for AECOPD	Time to first ER visit for AECOPD, number of all-cause hospital readmissions, number of all-cause ER visits	Discharge after AECOPD	2 m/6 m follow-up	53	53	Mild	Remote TM, e-diary	SPO2, HR, BP, symptoms, TEMP, weight	Time to first readmission for AECOPD+; time to first ER visit for AECOPD+	Number of all-cause hospital re-admissions-; the number of all-cause ER visits-

Table 1. *Cont.*

Author (Year)	Country	Primary Objective	Secondary Objectives	COPD Severity	TM Duration	n Telemonitoring Group	n Control Group	Patient Effort Required	Telemonitoring Intervention	Telemonitoring Data	Exacerbation Outcomes	Other Study Outcomes
Shany (2017) [24]	Australia	ED visits, hospital admissions, length of hospitalization	HRQL, anxiety, depression, costs	COPD GOLD stage III-IV	12 m	21	21	High	Telemonitoring plus e-questionnaire plus telephone support and home visits	PFTs, SPO2, HR, TEMP, BP, ECG, weight, symptoms	ED visits=; hospital admissions=; length of hospitalization-; TTFH+	HRQL=; HADS=; costs-
Vasilopoulou (2017) [34]	Greece	Rate of moderate to severe AECOPDs, hospital admissions, ED visits	Functional capacity, HRQL, daily physical activity	GOLD COPD stage II-IV, and a history of acute exacerbations of COPD 1 year prior to entering the study	2 m/12 m	47	50/50	High	TM plus self-management plus phone contact	SPO2, HR, PFTs, 6MWD, questionnaire	AECOPDs-; hospital admissions-; ED visits-	HRQL+; 6MWT; SGRQ-; CAT-; mMRC-
Kessler (2018) [20]	France, Germany, Italy, Spain	Length of hospitalization	Number of AECOPDs, acute care hospitalizations, mortality, 6MWT, BODE, HADS, SGQR	COPD GOLD stage III-IV and at least one severe exacerbation in the previous year	12 m	157	162	High	TM plus self-management plus phone contact	PFTs, HR, SPO2, questionnaire plus for patients on LTOT daily oxygen use and RR	Length of hospitalization=; AECOPDs=; acute care hospitalizations=; mortality=; hospital admissions=	BODE=; 6MWT=; SGRQ=; HADS=; quit smoking+
Sink (2020) [25]	USA	TTFH	Hospital admissions	COPD GOLD stage I-IV	8 m	83	85	Low	E-questionnaire plus teleconsultation	Symptoms	TTFH+; hospital admissions-	
Clemente (2021) [27]	Spain	Time to first exacerbation	Number of exacerbations, use of healthcare resources, satisfaction, HRQL anxiety–depression, therapeutic adherence	Early discharge after AECOPD	7 d/6 m follow-up	58	58	Mild	Remote TM	ECG (leads I, II and III), SPO2, HR, BP, TEMP, and RR	Time to first exacerbation=; number of exacerbations=; costs = (non-inferiority proven)	Use of healthcare resources=; satisfaction+; quality of life+; anxiety-depression=; therapeutic adherence-

BODE: body mass index, airflow obstruction, dyspnea, and exercise capacity; CAT: COPD Assessment Tool; CSQ8: Client Satisfaction Questionnaire-8; COPD: chronic obstructive pulmonary disease; ECG: electrocardiogram; ED: emergency department; FEV1: forced expiratory volume in one second; FOT: forced oscillation technique; HRQL: health-related quality of life; HR: heart rate; HMV: home mechanical ventilation; HADS: hospital anxiety and depression scale; LTOT: long-term oxygen therapy; PEF: peak expiratory flow; PHQ-9: Patient Health Questionnaire; PFTs: pulmonary function tests; RR: respiration rate; SGRQ: Saint George's Respiratory Questionnaire; SPO2: pulse arterial oxygen saturation; SES: COPD Self-Efficacy Scale; TEMP: temperature; TH: telehealth; TM: telemonitoring; TTFH: time to first hospitalization; 6MWT: six minute walking test.

4. Studies with Negative Results

4.1. Telemedicine Involving Primarily Close Healthcare Monitoring

Antoniades et al. [35], in a pilot study including 44 patients with moderate to severe COPD, aimed to explore the feasibility of remote monitoring and a possible reduction in healthcare use when this intervention is added to the standard of care (SOC). Multiple parameters were monitored daily over a 12-month period (spirometry, weight, temperature, BP, SPO2, ECG, sputum color and volume, symptoms, and medication usage) with close revision by a nurse and frequent reminders. Adherence of up to 80% was observed, although the addition of TM did not achieve a significant reduction in admission rate (SOC 1.5 ± 1.8 vs. TM 1.3 ± 1.7, $p = 0.76$) or length of hospitalization (SOC 15.6 ± 19.4 vs. TM 11.4 ± 19.6, $p = 0.66$). Possible explanations are that the SOC was not usual but was a very high-quality multidisciplinary referral institution approach to COPD management, as well as the small size of the study. Nevertheless, patients who received TM exhibited a significant trend toward fewer admissions during the study period compared with the previous year (1 (0–2) admission/year during study period compared to 2 (1–4) admissions/year during the year before, $p = 0.052$), implying that matching in terms of history of prior admissions instead of disease severity and smoking habit may have altered conclusions [35].

Boer et al. [36] recruited 87 patients with two or more AECOPDs, comparing exacerbation self-management strategies using either a paper exacerbation action plan (control group) or an innovative mobile health tool (mHealth group), consisting of a mobile phone, a pulse oximeter, a spirometer, a thermometer, and a question–answer system, which provided automated advice based on a decision tree manufactured by experts and with the help of a Bayesian prediction model (intervention group). In terms of exacerbation-related outcomes, no differences were found between the two groups in the number of exacerbation-free weeks, in the number of symptom-based exacerbations, the exacerbations treated with antibiotics or prednisone, the unscheduled healthcare contacts, or the hospital admissions. Furthermore, no difference in timely action that would prevent an exacerbation was identified between the two groups. Apart from the small size of the study, this result could be explained by the small room of improvement left, as both groups were provided an introductive education session based on the recognition and treatment of exacerbations [36].

Chau et al. [37] conducted a small 8-week study including 40 older COPD patients with moderate or severe disease and history of at least one hospital admission for exacerbation in the past year. Twenty-two patients in the intervention group received a telecare device kit that monitored SPO2, HR, and RR indices transmitted to a health provider via an online platform that could act promptly. A high level of user satisfaction was reported but no significant differences in the numbers of ED visits and hospital readmissions between the groups were observed. Nevertheless, the very small duration and size of the study did not permit extraction of safe conclusions [37].

Cordova et al. [38] focused their research on daily symptom reporting using telemedicine in a 24-month randomized control trial with 79 participants that had been hospitalized for an AECOPD within the past year or were using supplemental O_2. While the 40 patients in the control group were provided with peak flow meters and electronic diaries for symptom reporting and had been advised to seek medical assistance if they worsened, the 39 patients in the intervention group received a telecommunication device for symptom reporting and scoring via a computerized algorithm that included a score "alert". The alert was generated when the symptom score reflected a significant alteration of the baseline symptoms, initiating appropriate medical intervention that was available 24 h/day. The symptom assessment included PEF; dyspnea; and sputum quantity, color, and consistency. Coughing, wheezing, sore throat, nasal congestion, and temperature were considered minor symptoms. Although there were no differences in hospitalization rates, hospitalization durations, times to first hospitalization, or mortality rates between groups, acute exacerbation symptoms were significantly different, with the intervention group reporting significantly fewer moderate and severe symptom days ($p < 0.0001$). The failure to show either a mortality benefit or reduction in hospitalization days was attributed by the authors to the slow recruitment rate and to a lower hospitalization rate observed across both groups due to the optimized care [38].

De San Miguel and colleagues [39] attempted to show that self-monitoring combined with remote monitoring via a TH instrument that measured COPD patients' vital signs could make a difference in health service utilization. In this RCT, which had a duration of 6 months and included 80 patients, BP, weight, temperature, HR, and oxygen saturation levels were measured and transmitted automatically to the Internet, along with patients' daily answers related to their health, which became available to the TH nurse daily. Information triggered an intervention when appropriate, while the parameters were also made available to each participant's physician. The intervention group had fewer hospitalizations and ED presentations (almost half), as well as a reduced length of in-hospital stay (77 fewer days in total), with a significant impact on health costs. However, the study did not reach statistical significance, possibly due to the fact that it was performed in the summer period, when the hospital admission rate was lower than expected [39].

Jakobsen et al. [40] compared home-based TH hospitalization in patients with severe COPD that were admitted with an acute exacerbation and had an expected hospitalization of more than 2 days to standard in-hospital treatment. Patients needing non-invasive or invasive mechanical ventilation or intravenous antibiotics, had pH < 7.35, or with serious comorbidities were excluded. This was a non-inferiority study and treatment failure was defined as readmission due to COPD within 30 days after discharge. The intervention group (29 patients) were provided with a touch screen with a webcam, pulse oximeter, spirometer, thermometer, and medicines, and participated in daily scheduled virtual ward rounds, while acute contacts were possible through a "call hospital" button. The control group (28 patients) was hospitalized as usual. The study did not meet the primary endpoint, which was a treatment failure rate less than 20% higher than that of the control group. A possible explanation for this is the small sample size. No participants died within 30 days of the discharge and 3 patients returned to the hospital due to technical failure, hyponatremia, and nebulizer failure [40].

Another Spanish study by Jodar-Sanchez et al. [41], including 45 GOLD stage III–IV patients with at least one severe exacerbation in the previous year, showed no benefit from TM in terms of preventing serious exacerbations. The investigators included patients with advanced COPD treated with long-term oxygen therapy. The intervention group measured daily vital signs and spirometry twice a week, while transmitted measurements were followed and evaluated and clinical responses were generated by alerts. Although a small, non-significant reduction was observed in the number of ED visits, hospital admissions were not fewer and most of the patients admitted had previously visited the ED. It was noted that 33% of the serious exacerbations leading to hospitalization occurred during weekends and holidays when the TH program was interrupted, a fact that should be taken into consideration in future studies [41].

McDowell et al. [42] recruited 110 GOLD stage II–III patients with at least two ED admissions, hospital admissions, or emergency GP contacts in the 12 months before the study. The TM device recorded BP, HR, and SPO2 for six months and patients answered questions relating to symptoms (difficulty in breathing, cough, sputum, tiredness). If an alert occurred, a nurse contacted the patient and provided advice; if further escalation was necessary, the nurse contacted the respiratory physician, who decided whether a home visit or an ED admission was required. There were no significant differences between the two groups in exacerbations, hospital admissions, ED visits, total GP calls, EQ-5D quality of life scores, or HADS depression scores, and the intervention was not cost-effective. However, the SGRQ score improved significantly in the TM group compared to usual care, exceeding the minimum clinically important difference of at least four units (mean difference 5.75, 95% CI: 2.32–9.18; $p = 0.001$), and the same applied for the HADS anxiety score ($p = 0.01$).

The negative results regarding AECOPDs, hospital admissions, ED visits, and total GP calls could be attributed to the short duration of the TM (6 months) [42].

Pinnock et al. [43] included 256 COPD patients with admission to the hospital with an AECOPD in the previous year. Patients in the TM group completed a daily questionnaire regarding symptoms and use of treatment, and SPO2 was monitored. For the symptom scores, the patients were asked to assess whether their dyspnea, cough, wheeze sputum purulence, and volume had increased and if they had a fever or had developed an upper respiratory tract infection. No significant difference was observed in the time to first hospitalization, time to first hospitalization with an AECOPD or all cause death, number and duration of hospital admissions with an AECOPD, number and duration of admissions for any cause, number of exacerbations self-reported by participants, HRQL, anxiety, or depression. However, patients in the TM group exhibited a significantly lower number of deaths and higher use of healthcare resources [43].

Rose et al. [44] evaluated the effectiveness of a multi-component intervention including individualized care action plans and telephone consults (12-weekly then 9-monthly) for reducing emergency department visits. In total, 470 COPD patients with one or more ED visits or hospital admissions for AECOPD in the previous 12 months and two or more prognostically important COPD-associated comorbidities were randomized. The TH intervention had no impact on either the number of ED visits or the number of hospital admissions. However, TH significantly reduced mortality, a finding that could not be fully explained by the authors [44].

Rinbaek et al. [45] recruited 281 COPD GOLD stage III–IV patients with one hospital admission due to AECOPD within the previous 36 months or treated with LTOT for at least 3 months. Patients allocated to the TM group were provided a tablet computer with a web camera, a microphone, and measurement equipment (spirometer, pulse oximeter, and mMRC scale), while patients reported changes in dyspnea and sputum color, volume, and purulence. There was no significant difference between the two groups in number of hospitalizations, AECOPDs, ED visits, length of hospitalization, all-cause hospital admissions, time to first hospital admission, or all-cause mortality. Patients in the TM group demonstrated a significantly lower number of visits to the outpatient clinic and a significantly higher number of AECOPDs requiring treatment with systemic steroids and antibiotics but not admission to hospital. The negative results of the study could be attributed to the short duration of the TM (6 months) [45].

In a similar RCT, Soriano et al. [46] recruited 229 COPD GOLD stage III–IV patients with LTOT and two or more moderate or severe AECOPDs in the previous year, with or without hospitalization. Patients in the TM group received a pulse oximeter, a blood pressure gauge, a spirometer, a respiratory rate, and an oxygen therapy compliance monitor connected to the oxygen feed from their main oxygen source. No significant difference in number of AECOPDs, ED visits, hospital admissions, mortality, health related costs, or quality of life was observed. However, there was a trend towards shorter lengths of hospitalization and days in intensive care unit. The negative results of the study could be attributed to the fact that patients in the TM group had more hospital admissions in the previous year, the reduced primary care integration (since it was a multicenter study), and the high sensitivity of the clinical alert threshold applied to the TH group, which may have increased ED visits and hospital admissions due to false alerts [46].

Vianello et al. [47] recruited 315 COPD GOLD stage III–IV patients with a mean FEV1 of 41.9% pred. at the time of discharge from hospital after an AECOPD episode or while attending the outpatient respiratory medicine clinic. A finger pulse oximeter and a gateway device for data transmission over a telephone line to a central data management unit were applied to the patients for a 12-months period. When the transmitted values were considered out-of-range, the clinical staff were alerted and the patient was contacted. The readmission rate for AECOPD was significantly lower in the TM group compared to the standard care group (incidence rate ratio 0.43, 95% CI: 0.19–0.98; p = 0.01), and the same applied for the number of appointments with a pulmonary specialist (incidence rate ratio 0.82,

95% CI: 0.67–1; $p = 0.049$). However, the number and duration of hospitalizations due to AECOPD or any other cause, the number of ED visits, and the number of deaths did not differ significantly between the two groups, and neither did TH improve the quality of life or emotional distress. The possible explanations for the negative results were firstly the very low number of hospital admissions, which did not leave enough space for further reductions as a result of a TM intervention, and secondly that changes in HR and SPO2, which are used as markers of an unstable clinical condition, are often unable to reflect changes in patient health status, leading to underestimation of AECOPDs [47].

Walker et al. [48] included 312 patients with COPD GOLD stage II or higher and a history of AECOPD, with or without hospitalization in the previous 12 months, from 5 European countries, applying the CHROMED monitoring platform for 9 months at approximately the same time each day. The platform comprised a device that measured within-breath respiratory mechanical impedance using the forced oscillation technique, a touch screen computer, and a mobile modem. When an alert was generated, a variety of actions were possible, ranging from no action to taking a course of antibiotics or corticosteroids or face-to-face assessment. There was no difference between the two groups in time to first hospitalization, number of hospitalizations, number of moderate exacerbations, or number of patients free from hospital admission. However, among patients previously hospitalized for AECOPD, there was a 53% reduction in the hospitalization rate in the treatment group compared with the control group (0.85 vs. 1.88 admissions/year; $p = 0.017$). The negative results of the study could be attributed to the low number of hospitalizations and the variation between different healthcare systems [48].

Telemonitoring requires commitment and appropriate training of the study team in order to help COPD patients and to extract safe conclusions regarding the intervention's role in preventing exacerbations. This was shown in a pilot study by Bentley et al. [49], which demonstrated a negative impact of TM when comparing to face-to-face visits. The SOC team received 6 home visits after discharge, while the intervention team used TH equipment that could monitor and transmit vital signs to the study clinicians after the third visit. The intervention lasted 8 weeks. An increase in hospital admissions (34% vs. 16%) and a higher duration of hospitalization were reported during the 8-month follow-up period. The study had serious issues, such as slow recruitment and gaps in data collection due to problems related to research team dedication (a frontline clinical team who experienced a 60% loss of staff capacity during the study) and inadequate staff training [49].

4.2. Telemedicine Involving Primarily Self-Management Techniques

Self-management supported by a digital health system did not improve exacerbation-related outcomes in the study by Farmer et al. [50]. A fully automated, Internet-linked, tablet-computer-based system for monitoring and self-management support was provided to 110 patients with moderate to very severe COPD, while 56 patients received the usual care. The intervention consisted of the monitoring of oxygen saturation and HR; a daily symptom diary with questions regarding general well-being, cough, breathlessness, sputum, and use of medications; monthly mood screening questionnaires; and training videos with inhaler techniques, pulmonary rehabilitation exercises, and self-management techniques for breathlessness. Safety thresholds for vital signs, symptoms, or psychological scores generated "alerts" and data were reviewed by a member of the respiratory team twice weekly. The study duration was 12 months. The primary outcome related to quality of life improvement was not achieved and no reduction in the number of exacerbations was seen in the intervention group. The relative risk of hospital admission for the digital health group was 0.83 (0.56–1.24, $p = 0.37$) and no reduction in the use of healthcare services was noticed, except for fewer visits to the GP practice nurses (1.5 for digital health versus 2.5 for usual care, $p = 0.03$) [50].

Lewis et al. [51] included 40 COPD GOLD stage II–III patients after completing at least 12 sessions of pulmonary rehabilitation. In the TH group, oxygen saturation, temperature, and symptoms were recorded daily for 26 weeks. There was no difference between the two groups in ED visits, hospital admissions, or hospitalization days during the monitoring period; however, in the TM group, fewer primary care contacts for chest problems ($p < 0.03$) were documented. The small size of the study, the short duration, and the fact the participants in the TM group were stabilized, since they had completed the pulmonary rehabilitation course, could have contributed to the negative results of the study [51].

Rassouli et al. [52] recruited 168 COPD patients with a mean FEV1 of 51%. Patients in the TH group completed CAT scores weekly and answered six questions focused on the detection of AECOPD daily. There was no difference in favor of the TH group regarding total number of AECOPDs, hospital admissions, or ED visits. Nevertheless, in the TH group, the rate of CAT increase was significantly reduced, more moderate AECOPDs were detected, the satisfaction with care was higher, and there was a trend towards shorter length of hospitalization and reduced COPD-related costs. The negative results regarding AECOPD outcomes resulted from the fact that the study's primary outcome was difference in weekly CAT score, so there was insufficient statistical power to show significant differences, which could be achieved by including considerably more patients [52].

In an RCT with a different approach, Sorknaes et al. [53] evaluated the effects of 7 days real-time teleconsultations between hospital-based nurses and patients discharged after hospital admission for an AECOPD. The study included a total of 266 COPD patients discharged after an AECOPD. Patients in the TM group received a video device, an oximeter, and a spirometer; they were evaluated daily for one week and received a proper teleconsultation from a nurse, initiated 24 h after discharge and with a 26-week follow-up. No significant difference in total hospital readmissions, time before first readmission, mortality, time to mortality, hospital readmissions per patient, or hospital days per patient at 4, 8, 12, or 26 weeks after discharge was observed. The negative results could be attributed to the very short duration of the intervention (7 days) and to the fact that the teleconsultation was provided only by a nurse through a checklist [53]. Table 2 summarizes the characteristics of the RCTs on TM that showed negative results.

Table 2. Telemedicine studies showing negative results.

Author (Year)	Country	Primary Objective	Secondary Objectives	COPD Severity	TM Duration	n Telemonitoring Group	n Control Group	Patient Effort Required	Telemonitoring Intervention	Telemonitoring Data	Exacerbation Outcomes	Other Study Outcomes
Lewis (2010) [51]	UK	Hospital admissions	ED visits, length of hospital admissions, GP contacts	GOLD COPD stage II–III	6 m	20	20	Mild	Telemonitoring plus e-questionnaire plus physician on demand	SPO2, TEMP, questionnaire	ED visits=; hospital admissions=; length of hospitalization=; GP contacts for chest problems=	-
Antoniades (2012) [36]	Australia	Hospital admissions, inpatient-days, HRQL	6MWT at baseline and 12 months, adherence to daily monitoring, reproducibility of the physiological measurements, and patient acceptance of RM	GOLD COPD stage II–III, at least 1 hospitalization in the last 12 m	12 m	22	22	High	Remote TM	PFTs, HR, SPO2, BP, TEMP, weight, sputum, symptoms, medication usage	Hospital admissions=; length of hospitalization=	HRQL=; 6MWT=; adherence 80%
Chau (2012) [37]	Hong Kong	Hospital readmissions, use of ED, pulmonary function, user satisfaction, HRQL	-	GOLD COPD stage II–III, at least 1 hospitalization in the last 12 m	2 m	22	18	Mild	Remote TM	SPO2, HR, RR	Hospital readmissions=; use of ED services=	User satisfaction+; HRQL=; pulmonary function=
De San Miguel (2013) [38]	Australia	ED visits, hospital admissions, hospitalization days	Costs, HRQL, satisfaction	Domiciliary oxygen	6 m	40	40	Mild	Remote TM	BP, weight, TEMP, HR, SPO2, questionnaire	ED visits=; hospital admissions=; hospitalization days=	Costs=; HRQL=, over time=; satisfaction+
Jodar-Sanchez (2013) [41]	Spain	ED visits, hospital admissions, HRQL	-	COPD GOLD stage IV, with LTOT, at least one hospitalization for respiratory illness in the previous year	4 m	24	21	High	Remote TM	PFTs, HR, SPO2, BP	ED visits=; specialist consultations=; hospital admissions=	HRQL=
Pinnock (2013) [43]	UK	TTFH	TTFH or all cause death, number and duration of hospital admissions, number of deaths at one year, number of exacerbations self-reported by participants, HRQL, anxiety and depression, number and duration of contacts with community services	Patients hospitalized for an AECOPD within the past year in the previous year	12 m	128	128	Mild	Remote telemonitoring, e-diary, telenursing and physician on demand	SPO2, symptoms	TTFH=; TTFH with an AECOPD or all cause death=; number and duration of hospital admissions with an AECOPD=; number and duration of admissions for any cause=; number of deaths at one year=; number of exacerbations self-reported by participants=	HRQL=; HADS=; number and duration of contacts with community services+

123

Table 2. Cont.

Author (Year)	Country	Primary Objective	Secondary Objectives	COPD Severity	TM Duration	n Telemonitoring Group	n Control Group	Patient Effort Required	Telemonitoring Intervention	Telemonitoring Data	Exacerbation Outcomes	Other Study Outcomes
Sorknaes (2013) [3]	Denmark	Hospitals readmissions	Mortality, time to mortality and time before first readmission, hospital readmissions per patient, and hospital days per patient	COPD GOLD stage I–IV, hospitalization for AECOPD	7 d/6 m follow-up	132	134	High	Telemonitoring plus teleconsultation	PFTs, SPO2, HR	total hospital readmissions=; time to first readmission=; mortality=; time to mortality=; hospital readmissions per patient=; hospital days per patient=	
Bentley (2014) [39]	UK	% participants readmitted to hospital with COPD, change in HRQL	% of patients requiring unscheduled healthcare support, cost-effectiveness	Between 1 and 3 admissions in the previous 12 M	2 m TM/6 m follow-up	32	31	Mild	Remote TM	SPO2, HR, BP, symptoms	hospital readmissions+	SGRQ+; costs+
Jakobsen (2015) [40]	Denmark	Readmission within 30 days after initial discharge	Mortality, need for manual or mechanical ventilation or NIMV, physiological measures, length of hospitalization, HRQL, user satisfaction, adverse events	COPD GOLD stage III–IV, had an AECOPD and who had an expected hospitalization >2 d	Intervention during home hospitalisation, 6 m follow-up	29	28	High	TM with virtual ward rounds	PFTs, HR, SPO2, TEMP, medicine administration	Non-inferiority not proven	Physiological measures=; length of hospitalizations=; HRQL=
McDowell (2015) [41]	Northern Ireland	HRQL	AECOPDs, hospital admissions, ED visits, GP contacts, satisfaction, and cost-effectiveness	GOLD COPD stage II–III, and at least two of: emergency department admissions, hospital admissions or emergency GP contacts in the 12 months before the study	6 m	55	55	Mild	Telemonitoring plus telenursing and physician on demand	BP, HR, SPO2, questionnaire	AECOPDs=; hospital admissions=; ED visits=; GP contacts =	SGRQ+; HADS anxiety score=; HADS depression score=; cost-effectiveness=

Table 2. Cont.

Author (Year)	Country	Primary Objective	Secondary Objectives	COPD Severity	TM Duration	n Telemonitoring Group	n Control Group	Patient Effort Required	Telemonitoring Intervention	Telemonitoring Data	Exacerbation Outcomes	Other Study Outcomes
Ringbaek (2015) [45]	Denmark	Hospital admissions for AECOPD	Number of all-cause hospital admissions, time to first hospital admission, time to first hospital admission caused by AECOPD, number of ED visits, number of visits to the outpatient clinic, number of AECOPD requiring treatment with systemic steroids or antibiotics but not admission to hospital, length of hospitalization, and all-cause mortality	COPD GOLD stage III–IV, hospital admission due to AECOPD within the previous 36 months and/or treated with LTOT for at least 3 months	6 m	141	140	High	Telemonitoring plus teleconsultation	PFTs, SPO2, mMRC dyspnea scale, sputum color, volume, and purulence	Hospital admissions=; AECOPDs=; all-cause hospital admissions=; time to first hospital admission=; number of ED visits=; length of hospitalizations=; number of visits to the outpatient clinic=; number of AECOPD requiring treatment with systemic steroids and/or antibiotics but not admission to hospital=; all-cause mortality=	-
Cordova (2016) [46]	USA	Composite outcome of the number of hospitalizations and deaths	Frequency and severity of AECOPD symptoms, daily PEF, dyspnea score, Duke Activity Status Index, HRQL	Patients hospitalized for an AECOPD within the past year or using supplemental O2	24 m	39	40	High	TM plus self-assessment plus phone contact	PEF, dyspnea, sputum quantity, color, and consistency, cough, wheeze, sore throat, nasal congestion, TEMP	Hospital admissions=; length of hospitalizations=; AECOPD symptoms=	HRQL=
Vianello (2016) [47]	Italy	HRQL	Number and duration of hospitalizations due to AECOPD, number of readmissions due to AECOPD, number of appointments with a pulmonary specialist, number of ED visits, number of deaths, emotional distress	COPD GOLD stage III–IV	12 m	211	104	Low	TM plus telenursing or nurse and doctor on demand	SPO2, HR	hospitalizations=; length of hospitalizations=; readmission rate due to AECOPD=; specialist visits=; ED visits=; deaths=	HRQL=; ↑HADS=

Table 2. Cont.

Author (Year)	Country	Primary Objective	Secondary Objectives	COPD Severity	TM Duration	n Telemonitoring Group	n Control Group	Patient Effort Required	Telemonitoring Intervention	Telemonitoring Data	Exacerbation Outcomes	Other Study Outcomes
Farmer (2017) [43]	UK	HRQL	Mortality, number with at least one admission, number of AECOPDs, medication adherence, smoking cessation, HRQL, change in lung function, number of GP contacts, number of nurse contacts	COPD GOLD stage II–IV	12 m	110	56	Mild	Remote TM	HR, SPO2, symptoms and anxiety/depression questionnaire	Hospital admissions=; AECOPDs=; mortality=	HRQL=; medication adherence=; smoking cessation=; change in lung function=; number of GP contacts=; number of nurse contacts=
Rose (2018) [44]	Canada	ED visits for AECOPD	Hospitalizations, number of hospitalized days at 1 year, mortality, time to first ED presentation, change in BODE index, HRQL, HADS, COPD Self-Efficacy Scale, Client Satisfaction Questionnaire-8 (CSQ8) and Caregiver Impact Scale	≥1 ED visit or hospital admission for AECOPD in the previous 12 months and ≥2 prognostically-important COPD associated comorbidities	12 m	236	234	Mild	Telehealth plus self-management	Health behavior, symptom monitoring	ED visits=; time to first ED visit=; risk for ED visit=; hospitalizations=; risk for hospital admission=; length of hospitalization=; mortality=;	BODE=; HRQL=; HADS=
Soriano (2018) [45]	Spain	Number of AECOPDs, ED visits, hospital admissions, length of hospitalization	Costs, HRQL, satisfaction	COPD GOLD stage III–IV, LTOT, ≥2 moderate or severe AECOPDs in the previous year (with or without hospitalization)	12 m	115	114	High	TM plus self-management plus teleconsultation	PFTs, SPO2, HR, BP, RR, oxygen therapy compliance	AECOPDs=; ED visits=; hospital admissions=; mortality=; length of hospitalizations=; days in ICU=	HRQL=; costs=
Walker (2018) [46]	Spain, United Kingdom, Slovenia, Estonia, and Sweden	TTFH, HRQL	Moderate exacerbation rate;rehospitalizations, CAT, PHQ-9, and MLHFQ questionnaires; and cost-utility analysis	COPD GOLD stage ≥ II and a history of AECOPD in the previous 12 months	9 m	154	158	High	Remote TM	within-breath respiratory mechanical impedance using FOT	TTFH=; hospitalizations=; moderate exacerbations=; readmission rate due to AECOPD=	HRQL=

126

Table 2. Cont.

Author (Year)	Country	Primary Objective	Secondary Objectives	COPD Severity	TM Duration	n Telemonitoring Group	n Control Group	Patient Effort Required	Telemonitoring Intervention	Telemonitoring Data	Exacerbation Outcomes	Other Study Outcomes
Boer (2019) [36]	Netherlands	Exacerbation-free time	Exacerbation-related outcomes, health status, self-efficacy, self-management behavior, healthcare utilization, and usability	≥2 AECOPDs in the previous 12 months	12 m	43	44	High	Self-management with an innovative mobile health tool	PFTs, HR, SPO2, TEMP, questionnaire concerning changes in symptoms, physical limitations, and emotions	exacerbation-free weeks=	health status=; self-efficacy=; self-management behaviors=; healthcare utilization=
Rassouli (2021) [52]	Switzerland and Germany	Difference in weekly CAT score	Number of AECOPDs and hospital admissions, length of hospitalization, treatment costs per patient and year	FEV1 51%	12 m	84	84	Mild	Telehealth plus self-management	Daily symptoms, CAT score	AECOPDs=; ED visits=; hospital admissions=; length of hospitalizations=	CAT score=; satisfaction=; Costs=

BODE: body mass index, airflow obstruction, dyspnea, and exercise capacity; CAT: COPD Assessment Tool; CSQ8: Client Satisfaction Questionnaire-8; COPD: chronic obstructive pulmonary disease; ECG: electrocardiogram; ED: emergency department; FEV1: forced expiratory volume in one second; FOT: forced oscillation technique; HRQL: health-related quality of life; HR: heart rate; HMV: home mechanical ventilation; HADS: hospital anxiety and depression scale; LTOT: long term oxygen therapy; PEF: peak expiratory flow; PHQ-9: Patient Health Questionnaire; PFTs: pulmonary function tests; RR: respiration rate; SGRQ: Saint George's Respiratory Questionnaire; SPO2: pulse arterial oxygen saturation; SES: COPD Self-Efficacy Scale; TEMP: temperature; TH: telehealth; TM: telemonitoring; TTFH: time to first hospitalization; 6MWT: six minute walking test.

5. Conclusions and the Way Forward

The goal of telemedicine is the early identification and diagnosis of AECOPDs and timely access to appropriate treatment in order to improve patient outcomes. An important issue for the effective application of telemonitoring in COPD is the parameters monitored in terms of reliable prediction of an AECOPD (e.g., FEV1, symptoms, pulse oximetry). When an algorithm is used, the design is even more crucial regarding the satisfactory sensitivity and specificity of the method. Moreover, the effort that was required from the patients was not associated with the outcomes of the studies; however, it is likely that patients would be more compliant to interventions that would require minimal effort on their end. The results of the negative studies regarding exacerbations, hospital admissions, ED visits, and total GP calls could be attributed to the short telemonitoring period and the fact that in most of them, healthcare utilization and exacerbations were not the primary endpoints. Importantly, the small number of participants may have led to negative results and may have additionally precluded the extraction of safe conclusions. Additionally, the short follow-up periods of many studies were not long enough to capture the natural history of AECOPD, and in our opinion a minimum of 12 months would be required. Moreover, adherence to inhaled medication, which is enhanced during RCTs, may additionally lead to reduced AECOPDs and hospital admissions in both intervention and usual care groups, thereby resulting in non-significant differences. The commitment and appropriate training of the study team involved in such programs is crucial for successful telehealth services, while the interruption of monitoring during weekends by healthcare interventions may have affected the results in some cases, although prevention of exacerbations was reported without active intervention by the study team, which was attributed to better disease awareness and self-management. Finally, it is unknown which patients will benefit more from telemedicine, and larger RCTs are needed with subgroup analysis to define the most appropriate population for telemonitoring interventions. These studies would need to be of a proper length and size, and following a multifactorial evaluation would need to involve the appropriate participants who will adopt these telemonitoring interventions, which ideally will require minimal patient effort, in order to maximize the engagement and potential benefits. The proposed characteristics of future studies are summarized in Table 3.

Table 3. Proposed characteristics of future studies.

- A minimum 12-month follow-up period
- AECOPDs and healthcare utilization should be the primary endpoint
- Appropriate parameters monitored in terms of reliable prediction of an AECOPD (e.g., FEV1, symptoms, pulse oximetry, heart rate, respiratory rate)
- Large number of participants
- Subgroup analysis in order to define the most appropriate population for telemonitoring intervention
- Commitment and appropriate training of the study team involved
- Telemonitoring and teleconsultation during the weekends
- Interventions that would require minimal effort on the patients' end would achieve higher compliance

Author Contributions: Conceptualization, A.K., A.G., C.K., K.I.G. and K.K.; methodology, C.K., A.G. and A.K.; software, C.K., G.N., N.G. and A.G. validation, C.K.,A.G., A.K. and K.K.; formal analysis, C.K., A.G. and G.N.; investigation, C.K. and A.G.; resources, A.K. and K.K.; data curation, C.K., A.G., A.K. and K.K.; writing—original draft preparation, C.K., A.G., G.N., N.G. and K.I.G.; writing—review and editing, A.K. and K.K.; visualization, A.G.; supervision, A.K.; project administration, K.K.; funding acquisition, A.K. All authors have read and agreed to the published version of the manuscript.

Funding: The present study was partly funded by the project entitled 'PRECURSOR: PREventing COPD URgent States Of Relapse', co-financed by the European Union and Greek national funds through the Operational Program for Research and Innovation Smart Specialization Strategy (RIS3) of Ipeiros (Project Code: ΗΠ1ΑΒ-0028176).

Institutional Review Board Statement: Not applicable.

Informed Consent Statement: Not applicable.

Data Availability Statement: All data generated or analyzed during this study are included in this published article. Anonymized data will be shared upon request from any qualified investigator.

Conflicts of Interest: The authors declare no conflict of interest.

Abbreviations

BODE	body mass index, airflow obstruction, dyspnea, and exercise capacity
CAT	COPD Assessment Tool
CSQ8	Client Satisfaction Questionnaire-8
COPD	Chronic Obstructive Pulmonary Disease
ECG	electrocardiogram
ED	emergency department
FEV1	forced expiratory volume in one second
FOT	forced oscillation technique
GP	general practitioner
HRQL	health-related quality of life
HR	heart rate
HMV	home mechanical ventilation
HADS	hospital anxiety and depression scale
LTOT	long term oxygen therapy
PEF	peak expiratory flow
PHQ-9	Patient Health Questionnaire
PFTs	pulmonary function tests
RR	respiratory rate
SES	COPD Self-Efficacy Scale
SGRQ	Saint George's Respiratory Questionnaire
SOC	standard of care
SPO2	pulse arterial oxygen saturation
TEMP	temperature
TH	telehealth
TM	telemonitoring
TTFH	time to first hospitalization

References

1. Adeloye, D.; Chua, S.; Lee, C.; Basquill, C.; Papana, A.; Theodoratou, E.; Nair, H.; Gasevic, D.; Sridhar, D.; Campbell, H.; et al. Global and Regional Estimates of COPD Prevalence: Systematic Review and Meta-Analysis. *J. Glob. Health* **2015**, *5*, 020415. [CrossRef] [PubMed]
2. World Health Organization. 2020. Available online: https://www.who.int/news-room/fact-sheets/detail/the-top-10-causes-of-death (accessed on 12 December 2021).
3. 2021 GOLD Reports. Available online: https://goldcopd.org/2021-gold-reports (accessed on 14 December 2021).
4. Galani, M.; Kyriakoudi, A.; Filiou, E.; Kompoti, M.; Lazos, G.; Gennimata, S.; Vasileiadis, I.; Daganou, M.; Koutsoukou, A.; Rovina, N. Older Age, Disease Severity and Co-Morbidities Independently Predict Mortality in Critically Ill Patients with COPD Exacerbation. *Pneumon* **2021**, *34*, 1–10. [CrossRef]

5. Anzueto, A. Impact of Exacerbations on COPD. *Eur. Respir. Rev.* **2010**, *19*, 113–118. [CrossRef] [PubMed]
6. Papaioannou, A.; Bartziokas, K.; Loukides, S.; Papiris, S.; Kostikas, K. "Get Well Soon!" Why Fast Recovery from a COPD Exacerbation Matters. *Pneumon* **2016**, *29*, 238–239.
7. Vitacca, M.; Montini, A.; Comini, L. How Will Telemedicine Change Clinical Practice in Chronic Obstructive Pulmonary Disease? *Ther. Adv. Respir. Dis.* **2018**, *12*, 1753465818754778. [CrossRef]
8. Strehle, E.M.; Shabde, N. One Hundred Years of Telemedicine: Does This New Technology Have a Place in Paediatrics? *Arch. Dis. Child.* **2006**, *91*, 956–959. [CrossRef]
9. Hjelm, N.M.; Julius, H.W. Centenary of Tele-Electrocardiography and Telephonocardiography. *J. Telemed. Telecare* **2005**, *11*, 336–338. [CrossRef] [PubMed]
10. Gaveikaite, V.; Fischer, C.; Schonenberg, H.; Pauws, S.; Kitsiou, S.; Chouvarda, I.; Maglaveras, N.; Roca, J. Telehealth for Patients with Chronic Obstructive Pulmonary Disease (COPD): A Systematic Review and Meta-Analysis Protocol. *BMJ Open* **2018**, *8*, e021865. [CrossRef]
11. Bourbeau, J.; Farias, R. Making Sense of Telemedicine in the Management of COPD. *Eur. Respir. J.* **2018**, *51*, 1800851. [CrossRef]
12. Polisena, J.; Tran, K.; Cimon, K.; Hutton, B.; McGill, S.; Palmer, K.; Scott, R.E. Home Telehealth for Chronic Obstructive Pulmonary Disease: A Systematic Review and Meta-Analysis. *J. Telemed. Telecare* **2010**, *16*, 120–127. [CrossRef]
13. Lundell, S.; Holmner, Å.; Rehn, B.; Nyberg, A.; Wadell, K. Telehealthcare in COPD: A Systematic Review and Meta-Analysis on Physical Outcomes and Dyspnea. *Respir. Med.* **2015**, *109*, 11–26. [CrossRef]
14. McLean, S.; Nurmatov, U.; Liu, J.L.; Pagliari, C.; Car, J.; Sheikh, A. Telehealthcare for Chronic Obstructive Pulmonary Disease. *Cochrane Database Syst. Rev.* **2011**, *7*, CD007718. [CrossRef]
15. Pedone, C.; Lelli, D. Systematic Review of Telemonitoring in COPD: An Update. *Pneumonol. I Alergol. Pol.* **2015**, *83*, 476–484. [CrossRef]
16. Kitsiou, S.; Paré, G.; Jaana, M. Systematic Reviews and Meta-Analyses of Home Telemonitoring Interventions for Patients with Chronic Diseases: A Critical Assessment of Their Methodological Quality. *J. Med. Internet Res.* **2013**, *15*, e150. [CrossRef]
17. Barbosa, M.T.; Sousa, C.S.; Morais-Almeida, M.; Simões, M.J.; Mendes, P. Telemedicine in COPD: An Overview by Topics. *COPD* **2020**, *17*, 601–617. [CrossRef] [PubMed]
18. Jang, S.; Kim, Y.; Cho, W.-K. A Systematic Review and Meta-Analysis of Telemonitoring Interventions on Severe COPD Exacerbations. *Int. J. Environ. Res. Public Health* **2021**, *18*, 6757. [CrossRef] [PubMed]
19. Ho, T.-W.; Huang, C.-T.; Chiu, H.-C.; Ruan, S.-Y.; Tsai, Y.-J.; Yu, C.-J.; Lai, F. HINT Study Group Effectiveness of Telemonitoring in Patients with Chronic Obstructive Pulmonary Disease in Taiwan—A Randomized Controlled Trial. *Sci. Rep.* **2016**, *6*, 23797. [CrossRef]
20. Kessler, R.; Casan-Clara, P.; Koehler, D.; Tognella, S.; Viejo, J.L.; Dal Negro, R.W.; Díaz-Lobato, S.; Reissig, K.; Rodríguez González-Moro, J.M.; Devouassoux, G.; et al. COMET: A Multicomponent Home-Based Disease-Management Programme Routine Care in Severe COPD. *Eur. Respir. J.* **2018**, *51*, 1701612. [CrossRef] [PubMed]
21. Koff, P.B.; Jones, R.H.; Cashman, J.M.; Voelkel, N.F.; Vandivier, R.W. Proactive Integrated Care Improves Quality of Life in Patients with COPD. *Eur. Respir. J.* **2009**, *33*, 1031–1038. [CrossRef]
22. Pedone, C.; Chiurco, D.; Scarlata, S.; Incalzi, R.A. Efficacy of MultiparametricTelemonitoring on Respiratory Outcomes in Elderly People with COPD: A Randomized Controlled Trial. *BMC Health Serv. Res.* **2013**, *13*, 1–7. [CrossRef]
23. SegrellesCalvo, G.; Gómez-Suárez, C.; Soriano, J.B.; Zamora, E.; Gónzalez-Gamarra, A.; González-Béjar, M.; Jordán, A.; Tadeo, E.; Sebastián, A.; Fernández, G.; et al. A Home Telehealth Program for Patients with Severe COPD: The PROMETE Study. *Respir. Med.* **2014**, *108*, 453–462. [CrossRef] [PubMed]
24. Shany, T.; Hession, M.; Pryce, D.; Roberts, M.; Basilakis, J.; Redmond, S.; Lovell, N.; Schreier, G. A Small-Scale Randomised Controlled Trial of Home Telemonitoring in Patients with Severe Chronic Obstructive Pulmonary Disease. *J. Telemed. Telecare* **2017**, *23*, 650–656. [CrossRef] [PubMed]
25. Sink, E.; Patel, K.; Groenendyk, J.; Peters, R.; Som, A.; Kim, E.; Xing, M.; Blanchard, M.; Ross, W. Effectiveness of a Novel, Automated Telephone Intervention on Time to Hospitalisation in Patients with COPD: A Randomised Controlled Trial. *J. Telemed. Telecare* **2020**, *26*, 132–139. [CrossRef] [PubMed]
26. Vitacca, M.; Bianchi, L.; Guerra, A.; Fracchia, C.; Spanevello, A.; Balbi, B.; Scalvini, S. Tele-Assistance in Chronic Respiratory Failure Patients: A Randomised Clinical Trial. *Eur. Respir. J.* **2009**, *33*, 411–418. [CrossRef]
27. Mínguez Clemente, P.; Pascual-Carrasco, M.; Mata Hernández, C.; Malo de Molina, R.; Arvelo, L.A.; Cadavid, B.; López, F.; Sánchez-Madariaga, R.; Sam, A.; Trisan Alonso, A.; et al. Follow-up with Telemedicine in Early Discharge for COPD Exacerbations: Randomized Clinical Trial (TELEMEDCOPD-Trial). *COPD* **2021**, *18*, 62–69. [CrossRef] [PubMed]
28. De Toledo, P.; Jiménez, S.; del Pozo, F.; Roca, J.; Alonso, A.; Hernandez, C. Telemedicine Experience for Chronic Care in COPD. *IEEE Trans. Inf. Technol. Biomed.* **2006**, *10*, 567–573. [CrossRef]
29. Casas, A.; Troosters, T.; Garcia-Aymerich, J.; Roca, J.; Hernández, C.; Alonso, A.; del Pozo, F.; de Toledo, P.; Antó, J.M.; Rodríguez-Roisín, R.; et al. Integrated Care Prevents Hospitalisations for Exacerbations in COPD Patients. *Eur. Respir. J.* **2006**, *28*, 123–130. [CrossRef]
30. Jehn, M.; Donaldson, G.; Kiran, B.; Liebers, U.; Mueller, K.; Scherer, D.; Endlicher, W.; Witt, C. Tele-Monitoring Reduces Exacerbation of COPD in the Context of Climate Change—A Randomized Controlled Trial. *Environ. Health* **2013**, *12*, 1–8. [CrossRef]

31. Paré, G.; Poba-Nzaou, P.; Sicotte, C.; Beaupré, A.; Lefrançois, É.; Nault, D.; Saint-Jules, D. Comparing the Costs of Home Telemonitoring and Usual Care of Chronic Obstructive Pulmonary Disease Patients: A Randomized Controlled Trial. *Eur. Res. Telemed.* **2013**, *2*, 35–47. [CrossRef]
32. Dinesen, B.; Haesum, L.K.E.; Soerensen, N.; Nielsen, C.; Grann, O.; Hejlesen, O.; Toft, E.; Ehlers, L. Using Preventive Home Monitoring to Reduce Hospital Admission Rates and Reduce Costs: A Case Study of Telehealth among Chronic Obstructive Pulmonary Disease Patients. *J. Telemed. Telecare* **2012**, *18*, 221–225. [CrossRef]
33. Tabak, M.; Brusse-Keizer, M.; van der Valk, P.; Hermens, H.; Vollenbroek-Hutten, M. A Telehealth Program for Self-Management of COPD Exacerbations and Promotion of an Active Lifestyle: A Pilot Randomized Controlled Trial. *Int. J. Chron. Obstruct. Pulmon. Dis.* **2014**, *9*, 935–944. [CrossRef]
34. Vasilopoulou, M.; Papaioannou, A.I.; Kaltsakas, G.; Louvaris, Z.; Chynkiamis, N.; Spetsioti, S.; Kortianou, E.; Genimata, S.A.; Palamidas, A.; Kostikas, K.; et al. Home-Based Maintenance Tele-Rehabilitation Reduces the Risk for Acute Exacerbations of COPD, Hospitalisations and Emergency Department Visits. *Eur. Respir. J.* **2017**, *49*, 1602129. [CrossRef]
35. Antoniades, N.C.; Rochford, P.D.; Pretto, J.J.; Pierce, R.J.; Gogler, J.; Steinkrug, J.; Sharpe, K.; McDonald, C.F. Pilot Study of Remote Telemonitoring in COPD. *Telemed. J. E. Health* **2012**, *18*, 634–640. [CrossRef]
36. Boer, L.; Bischoff, E.; van der Heijden, M.; Lucas, P.; Akkermans, R.; Vercoulen, J.; Heijdra, Y.; Assendelft, W.; Schermer, T. A Smart Mobile Health Tool Versus a Paper Action Plan to Support Self-Management of Chronic Obstructive Pulmonary Disease Exacerbations: Randomized Controlled Trial. *JMIR MhealthUhealth* **2019**, *7*, e14408. [CrossRef]
37. Chau, J.P.-C.; Lee, D.T.-F.; Yu, D.S.-F.; Chow, A.Y.-M.; Yu, W.-C.; Chair, S.-Y.; Lai, A.S.F.; Chick, Y.-L. A Feasibility Study to Investigate the Acceptability and Potential Effectiveness of a Telecare Service for Older People with Chronic Obstructive Pulmonary Disease. *Int. J. Med. Inform.* **2012**, *81*, 674–682. [CrossRef]
38. Cordova, F.C.; Ciccolella, D.; Grabianowski, C.; Gaughan, J.; Brennan, K.; Goldstein, F.; Jacobs, M.R.; Criner, G.J. A Telemedicine-Based Intervention Reduces the Frequency and Severity of COPD Exacerbation Symptoms: A Randomized, Controlled Trial. *Telemed. J. E. Health* **2016**, *22*, 114–122. [CrossRef]
39. De San Miguel, K.; Smith, J.; Lewin, G. Telehealth Remote Monitoring for Community-Dwelling Older Adults with Chronic Obstructive Pulmonary Disease. *Telemed. J. E. Health* **2013**, *19*, 652–657. [CrossRef]
40. Jakobsen, A.S.; Laursen, L.C.; Rydahl-Hansen, S.; Østergaard, B.; Gerds, T.A.; Emme, C.; Schou, L.; Phanareth, K. Home-Based Telehealth Hospitalization for Exacerbation of Chronic Obstructive Pulmonary Disease: Findings from "the Virtual Hospital" Trial. *Telemed. J. E Health* **2015**, *21*, 364–373. [CrossRef]
41. Jódar-Sánchez, F.; Ortega, F.; Parra, C.; Gómez-Suárez, C.; Jordán, A.; Pérez, P.; Bonachela, P.; Leal, S.; Barrot, E. Implementation of a TelehealthProgramme for Patients with Severe Chronic Obstructive Pulmonary Disease Treated with Long-Term Oxygen Therapy. *J. Telemed. Telecare* **2013**, *19*, 11–17. [CrossRef]
42. McDowell, J.E.; McClean, S.; FitzGibbon, F.; Tate, S. A Randomised Clinical Trial of the Effectiveness of Home-Based Health Care with Telemonitoring in Patients with COPD. *J. Telemed. Telecare* **2015**, *21*, 80–87. [CrossRef]
43. Pinnock, H.; Hanley, J.; McCloughan, L.; Todd, A.; Krishan, A.; Lewis, S.; Stoddart, A.; van der Pol, M.; MacNee, W.; Sheikh, A.; et al. Effectiveness of Telemonitoring Integrated into Existing Clinical Services on Hospital Admission for Exacerbation of Chronic Obstructive Pulmonary Disease: Researcher Blind, Multicentre, Randomised Controlled Trial. *BMJ* **2013**, *347*, f6070. [CrossRef]
44. Rose, L.; Istanboulian, L.; Carriere, L.; Thomas, A.; Lee, H.-B.; Rezaie, S.; Shafai, R.; Fraser, I. Program of Integrated Care for Patients with Chronic Obstructive Pulmonary Disease and Multiple Comorbidities (PIC COPD): A Randomised Controlled Trial. *Eur. Respir. J.* **2018**, *51*, 1701567. [CrossRef]
45. Ringbæk, T.; Green, A.; Laursen, L.C.; Frausing, E.; Brøndum, E.; Ulrik, C.S. Effect of Tele Health Care on Exacerbations and Hospital Admissions in Patients with Chronic Obstructive Pulmonary Disease: A Randomized Clinical Trial. *Int. J. Chron. Obstruct. Pulmon. Dis.* **2015**, *10*, 1801–1808. [CrossRef]
46. Soriano, J.B.; García-Río, F.; Vázquez-Espinosa, E.; Conforto, J.I.; Hernando-Sanz, A.; López-Yepes, L.; Galera-Martínez, R.; Peces-Barba, G.; Gotera-Rivera, C.M.; Pérez-Warnisher, M.T.; et al. A Multicentre, Randomized Controlled Trial of Telehealth for the Management of COPD. *Respir. Med.* **2018**, *144*, 74–81. [CrossRef]
47. Vianello, A.; Fusello, M.; Gubian, L.; Rinaldo, C.; Dario, C.; Concas, A.; Saccavini, C.; Battistella, L.; Pellizzon, G.; Zanardi, G.; et al. Home Telemonitoring for Patients with Acute Exacerbation of Chronic Obstructive Pulmonary Disease: A Randomized Controlled Trial. *BMC Pulm. Med.* **2016**, *16*, 157. [CrossRef]
48. Walker, P.P.; Pompilio, P.P.; Zanaboni, P.; Bergmo, T.S.; Prikk, K.; Malinovschi, A.; Montserrat, J.M.; Middlemass, J.; Šonc, S.; Munaro, G.; et al. Telemonitoring in Chronic Obstructive Pulmonary Disease (CHROMED). A Randomized Clinical Trial. *Am. J. Respir. Crit. Care Med.* **2018**, *198*, 620–628. [CrossRef]
49. Bentley, C.L.; Mountain, G.A.; Thompson, J.; Fitzsimmons, D.A.; Lowrie, K.; Parker, S.G.; Hawley, M.S. A Pilot Randomised Controlled Trial of a Telehealth Intervention in Patients with Chronic Obstructive Pulmonary Disease: Challenges of Clinician-Led Data Collection. *Trials* **2014**, *15*, 313. [CrossRef]
50. Farmer, A.; Williams, V.; Velardo, C.; Shah, S.A.; Yu, L.-M.; Rutter, H.; Jones, L.; Williams, N.; Heneghan, C.; Price, J.; et al. Self-Management Support Using a Digital Health System Compared With Usual Care for Chronic Obstructive Pulmonary Disease: Randomized Controlled Trial. *J. Med. Internet Res.* **2017**, *19*, e7116. [CrossRef]

51. Lewis, K.E.; Annandale, J.A.; Warm, D.L.; Rees, S.E.; Hurlin, C.; Blyth, H.; Syed, Y.; Lewis, L. Does Home Telemonitoring after Pulmonary Rehabilitation Reduce Healthcare Use in Optimized COPD? A Pilot Randomized Trial. *COPD* **2010**, *7*, 44–50. [CrossRef]
52. Rassouli, F.; Germann, A.; Baty, F.; Kohler, M.; Stolz, D.; Thurnheer, R.; Brack, T.; Kähler, C.; Widmer, S.; Tschirren, U.; et al. Telehealth Mitigates COPD Disease Progression Compared to Standard of Care: A Randomized Controlled Crossover Trial. *J. Intern. Med.* **2021**, *289*, 404–410. [CrossRef]
53. Sorknaes, A.D.; Bech, M.; Madsen, H.; Titlestad, I.L.; Hounsgaard, L.; Hansen-Nord, M.; Jest, P.; Olesen, F.; Lauridsen, J.; Østergaard, B. The Effect of Real-Time Teleconsultations between Hospital-Based Nurses and Patients with Severe COPD Discharged after an Exacerbation. *J. Telemed. Telecare* **2013**, *19*, 466–474. [CrossRef] [PubMed]

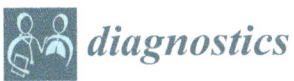

Article

COPD Guidelines in the Asia-Pacific Regions: Similarities and Differences

Shih-Lung Cheng [1,2,*] and Ching-Hsiung Lin [3,4,5]

1. Department of Internal Medicine, Far Eastern Memorial Hospital, Taipei 22060, Taiwan
2. Department of Chemical Engineering and Materials Science, Yuan Ze University, Zhongli District, Taoyuan 320315, Taiwan
3. Division of Chest Medicine, Department of Internal Medicine, Changhua Christian Hospital, Changhua 50006, Taiwan; teddy@cch.org.tw
4. Institute of Genomics and Bioinformatics, National Chung Hsing University, Taichung 40227, Taiwan
5. Department of Recreation and Holistic Wellness, MingDao University, Changhua 50006, Taiwan
* Correspondence: shihlungcheng@gmail.com; Tel: +886-2-8966-7000 (ext. 2160); Fax: +886-2-7738-0708

Abstract: Chronic obstructive pulmonary disease (COPD) is a preventable and treatable disease that is associated with significant morbidity and mortality, giving rise to an enormous social and economic burden. The Global Strategy for the Diagnosis, Management and Prevention of Chronic Obstructive Pulmonary Disease (GOLD) report is one of the most frequently used documents for managing COPD patients worldwide. A survey was conducted across country-level members of Asia-Pacific Society of Respiratory (APSR) for collecting an updated version of local COPD guidelines, which were implemented in each country. This is the first report to summarize the similarities and differences among the COPD guidelines across the Asia-Pacific region. The degree of airflow limitation, assessment of COPD severity, management, and pharmacologic therapy of stable COPD will be reviewed in this report.

Keywords: COPD guideline; Asia

Citation: Cheng, S.-L.; Lin, C.-H. COPD Guidelines in the Asia-Pacific Regions: Similarities and Differences. Diagnostics 2021, 11, 1153. https://doi.org/10.3390/diagnostics11071153

Academic Editor: Koichi Nishimura

Received: 1 June 2021
Accepted: 21 June 2021
Published: 24 June 2021

Publisher's Note: MDPI stays neutral with regard to jurisdictional claims in published maps and institutional affiliations.

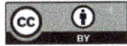

Copyright: © 2021 by the authors. Licensee MDPI, Basel, Switzerland. This article is an open access article distributed under the terms and conditions of the Creative Commons Attribution (CC BY) license (https://creativecommons.org/licenses/by/4.0/).

1. Introduction

Although chronic obstructive pulmonary disease (COPD) is a preventable and treatable disease, it is associated with significant morbidity and mortality, giving rise to an enormous social and economic burden. The results from the Epidemiology and Impact of COPD (EPIC) Asia population-based survey suggest a high prevalence of COPD in the participating Asia-Pacific territories [1] and indicate a substantial socioeconomic burden of the disease in this region. Individuals with the disease reported substantial limitations in their daily activities and loss in work productivity. To address this situation and influence the behavior of healthcare providers and health policy makers and payers, numerous organizations have developed clinical practice guidelines (CPG) to assist in the diagnosis and treatment of COPD. In such an environment, CPG development often relies upon expert opinion. Conflicting interpretations of the literature regarding COPD management may result in disparities across guidelines. Local factors, such as the availability of certain health care services or the cost impact of an intervention, may also influence how local experts view and apply the published literature during guideline development.

The Global Strategy for the Diagnosis, Management and Prevention of Chronic Obstructive Pulmonary Disease (GOLD) report is one of the most frequently used documents for managing COPD patients worldwide [2,3]. It was developed by using an evidence-based methodology and expert opinion consensus and is considered the most up-to-date, comprehensive reference for COPD diagnosis and management. However, a major gap is that its focus is only in the application of the recommended GOLD strategies for pharmacological treatment of COPD based on the A, B, C, and D groups. Here, our focus of this survey is to determine the degree of consensus in the Asian Pacific region's practice guidelines for COPD regarding the diagnosis and management of COPD.

Estimated Prevalence

The prevalence of COPD in the Asia-Pacific countries is estimated at 14.5% in Australia [4], 4.4% to 16.7% in China [5–7], and 5.6% in Indonesia [1]; the prevalence of Air Flow Limitation (FEV1/FVC < 70%) was reported at 10.9% and COPD (after excluding asthmatics) was 8.6% in Japan [8], 13.4% in Korea [9], 4.7% in Malaysia [1], 5.4% to 6.1% in Taiwan [1,10], 3.7% to 6.8% in Thailand [11], 3.5% to 20.8% in Philippines [1,12], and 6.7% in Vietnam [1], respectively (Table 1).

Table 1. Publication year of current and last version of Asia Pacific (APAC) guidelines, and COPD prevalence in the reviewed APAC countries.

	Australia/New Zealand *	China	Indonesia	Japan	Korea	Malaysia	Taiwan	Thailand	Philippines	Vietnam
Current version	2020	2017	2011	2018	2018	2009	2020	2010	2009	2009
Last version	2013	2007	NA	2009	2014	1998	2011	NA	2003	2009
Planned next version	NA	NA	NA	NA	NA	NA	2023	2016	NA	2018
COPD prevalence	14.5%	4.4–16.7%	5.6%	8.6–10.9%	13.4%	4.7%	5.4–6.1%	3.7–6.8%	3.5–20.8%	6.7%

* Stepwise management table of COPD was published in 2017; Concise Guide for Primary Care (COPD-X plan) was published in 2017.

2. Method

A survey was conducted across country-level members of the Asia-Pacific Society of Respiratory (APSR) for collecting an updated version of COPD guidelines which were implemented in each country. The APSR sent a questionnaire to members, who were asked to provide the current local guideline and comparative review of the collected guidelines. Ten guidelines were reviewed, including those of Australia/New Zealand, China, Indonesia, Japan, Korea, Malaysia, Taiwan, Thailand, Philippines, and Vietnam, in either English or national language. The key disease management graphs, flowcharts, and algorithms were translated into English language for review. Detailed information was completely collected, including the definition, the approach to diagnosis, severity classification of staging, pharmacotherapy for stable COPD, and other recommendations. In the Asia-Pacific available COPD guidelines, Australia, Japan, Korea, Taiwan, and China have revised and updated guidelines during the period of 2013 to 2020 (Table 1). Guidelines in the other countries were not revised in the recent three years. We compared the similarities and differences between these guidelines.

The different methods used to estimate disease prevalence including expert opinion, patient-reported diagnosis, and symptom-based or spirometry-based methods may affect the results. In the People's Republic of China, COPD is one of the most common chronic diseases in the population older than 40 years of age, with a prevalence of 8.2% in 2007 and increased to 13.6% in 2015 using spirometry-based survey. [5,7] Comparatively higher prevalence with 13.7% to 13.4% was noted in Korea using spirometry-based survey [9,13]. Another study in the Asia-Pacific region, EPIC Asia population-based survey [1] based on face-to-face or fixed-line telephone interviews, revealed that the prevalence of COPD is between 6.2% and 19.1%. Regarding the estimated prevalence rate of COPD in each country, there is no appropriate method to do this in current status.

3. Results

COPD diagnosis, classification, and treatment recommendation from Taiwan and China were similar to the GOLD guidelines. The degree of airflow limitation, assessment of COPD severity, management, and pharmacologic therapy of stable COPD were based on the GOLD principles. Australia, Japan, and Korea guidelines display some differences regarding classification and management strategy of stable COPD compared with the GOLD (Table 2). Besides, Taiwan guidelines have been written based on GRADE (Grading of Recommendations, Assessment, Development and Evaluations)'s recommendation, which is the most widely adopted tool for grading the quality of evidence and for making recommendations.

Table 2. Comparison of GOLD 2015 and APAC guidelines with current version updated after 2011.

	Disease Classification and Management Recommendation Same as GOLD	Major Difference in COPD Diagnosis Classification	Major Difference in COPD Treatment Recommendation
Australia	No	(1) Typical symptoms and lung function assessed in parallel for COPD severity classification (2) FEV1 40%, 60% and 80% predicted as the cut points of COPD severity (3) No specified cut points of mMRC and CAT for symptom evaluation	(1) Stepwise management of stable COPD; therapeutic choices appropriately fully aligned with disease severity.
China	Yes		
Japan	No	(1) Typical symptoms and lung function assessed in parallel for COPD severity classification (2) No specified cut points of mMRC and CAT for symptom evaluation	(1) Stepwise management of stable COPD; therapeutic choices not fully aligned with disease severity.
Korea	No	(1) FEV1 60% predicted as the cut point of high- and low-risk class. (2) Combined GOLD C and GOLD D into one group (Korean group 'da')	(1) Specified criteria, the occurrence of exacerbation or mMRC ≥ 2 despite of current treatment, for add up treatment from first therapeutic choice. (2) Mixed treatment recommendation of GOLD C and D for group 'da.'
Taiwan	Yes		

3.1. Combined COPD Assessment

The Korean COPD guideline categorizes severity into three groups, Group ga (GOLD Group A), Group na (GOLD Group B), and Group da (GOLD Group C and D) [13] (Figure 1). The spirometric cutoff point of FEV1 is 60% predicted to distinct Group ga, na from Group da. They further divide Group da into two groups with FEV1 < 60% predicted, but >=50% predicted, or FEV1 < 50% predicted. [14]. Assessment of symptoms and exacerbation is similar as described in GOLD. In Australia, COPD-X concise guide [15] for primary care categorizes the severity of COPD into mild (FEV1: 60–80% of predicted), moderate (FEV1: 40–59% of predicted), and severe (FEV1: <40% of predicted) accompanied with typical symptoms of varying degree of dyspnea, cough, and limitation of daily activity (Figure 2) [16]. The rationale was that regular treatment with inhaled corticosteroid (ICS) can improve symptoms, lung function, quality of life, and reduce the frequency of exacerbation for patients with FEV1 < 50% predicted and a history of frequent exacerbations, observed in several clinical studies [16–18].

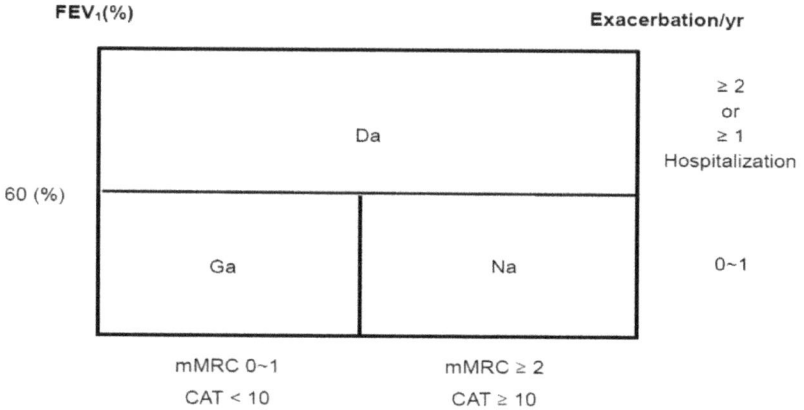

Figure 1. Korean COPD classification system and GOLD classification system.

Based on COPD-X Plan: Australian and new Zeeland Guidelines for the Management of COPD; Australian Therapeutic Guidelines

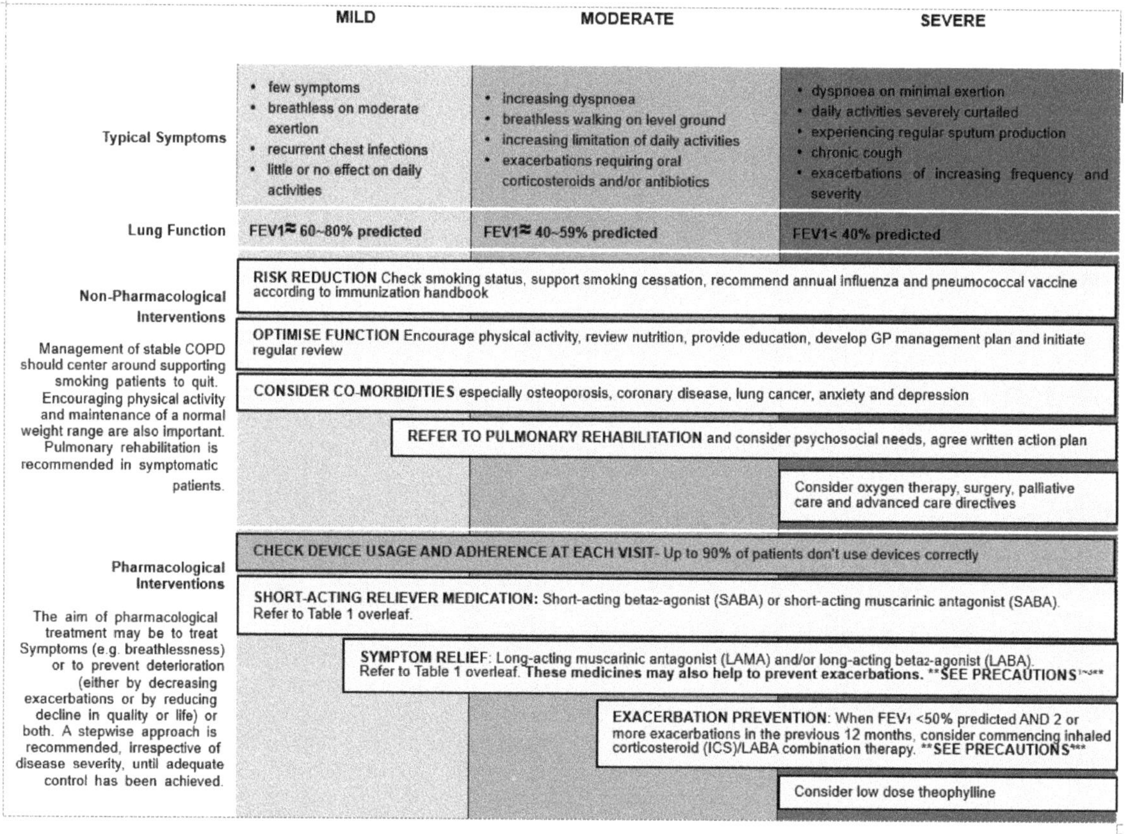

Figure 2. Stepwise management of stable COPD guidelines in Australia and New Zealand.

3.2. Pharmacologic Management of Stable Disease

In the GOLD guideline, the initial pharmacological management of COPD is according to patient group which has different recommended treatments. In the guidelines of Australia, Japan, and Korea (Figure 2 [15], Figure 3 [19], and Figure 4 [14]), a stepwise approach of optimized pharmacotherapy for stable COPD is used which recommends a gradual increase of bronchodilators, inhaled corticosteroids, or other drugs based on a comprehensive evaluation of symptoms, airflow obstruction, and exacerbation. In Japan's 2018 guideline, ICS positioning for COPD treatment had been revised from the previous criteria of FEV1 < 50% of predicted, frequent exacerbation, and concomitant asthma to only the concomitant asthma (ACO) criterion.

3.3. Non-Pharmacologic Management

Most guidelines had emphasized the importance of pulmonary rehabilitation, long-term oxygen therapy, and self-management plan including smoking cessation and vaccination. Particularly, Japan's guideline (fifth edition) discussed the nutrition management including nutritional impairment, evaluation, therapy, and diet education [19]. COPD patients whose BMI is less than 90% are suspected to have a nutrition disorder and nutrition therapy may be indicated. Nutritionists, physician, and nurses should form a team to provide nutritional guidance.

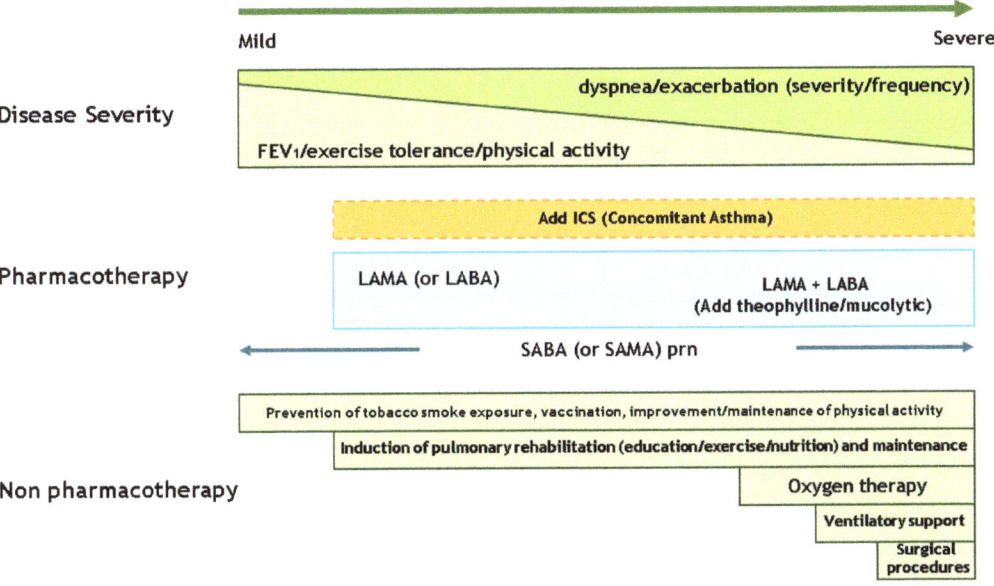

- The severity of COPD should be comprehensively assessed on the basis of not only the degree of decrease of FEV_1 (clinical stage), but also the degree of impairment of exercise tolerance/physical activity, intensity of dyspnea, and frequency/severity of exacerbation.
- FEV_1, exercise tolerance, and physical activity usually decrease in accordance with increased severity of COPD, and increased dyspnea and more frequent exacerbation are noted. However, when there is a gap between the degree of FEV_1 and other factors, attention should be paid to presence of comorbidities such as cardiac diseases.
- Treatment with medication and non-medication therapies should be given. When medication with a single drug is not sufficiently successful, LAMA and LABA should be used in combination (use of LAMA/LABA combinations is also allowed).
- ICS should be used in cases with possible concomitant asthmatic conditions. LABA/ICS combinations are also allowed.

Figure 3. Stepwise approach recommended by the fifth edition of Japanese Respiratory Society COPD guidelines.

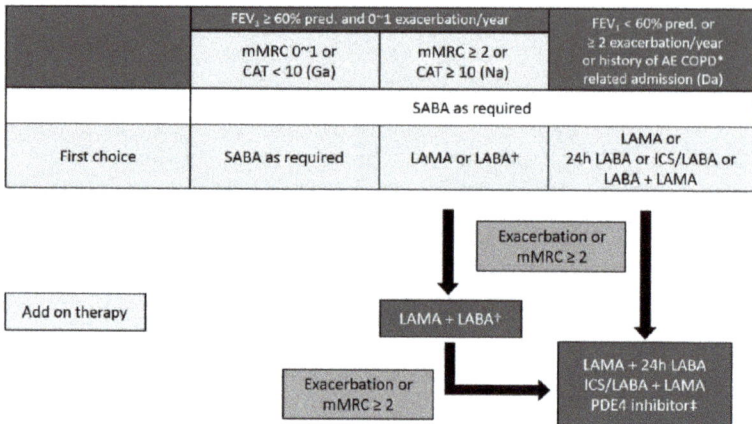

*AE COPD: Acute exacerbation of COPD

†Including 24h LABA

‡FEV1 < 50%, chronic bronchitis, and history of exacerbation

SABA: Short Acting Beta Agonist

LABA: Long Acting Beta Agonist

LAMA: Long Acting Muscarinic antagonist

Figure 4. Algorithm of pharmacologic treatment in patients with stable COPD in Korea.

3.4. Coexisting Asthma and COPD

Coexisting asthma and COPD are only defined and described in Australia and Japan guidelines. This Australia guideline recommends that an FEV1 increase over 12% and 200 mL constitutes a positive bronchodilator response. An FEV1 increase >400 mL strongly suggests underlying asthma or coexisting asthma and COPD diagnosis. Besides, the diagnosis of asthma–COPD overlap (ACO) has both characteristics of COPD and asthma (Figure 5).

3.5. End-of-Life ISSUES

GOLD 2013, for the first time, proposed that palliative care may be applied in advanced severe COPD patients. Among these guidelines in the Asia-Pacific region, Taiwan, Japan, China [20], and Australia [15] may already have their policies about end-of-life care. Improving quality of life, optimizing function, helping with decision-making about end-of-life care, and providing emotional and spiritual support to patients and family are the main goals. In Taiwan, the National Health Insurance Administration Ministry of Health and Welfare had programmed hospice-care plans in 2011 and provided in-hospital critical care facilities for patients with advanced diseases and poor response to regular treatments instead of home or hospice ward care.

Fundamentals	
40 years of age or older, Chronic airway inflammation: post-bronchodilator $FEV_1/FVC < 70\%$	
[Characteristics of COPD] One of item (1), (2), and (3)	[Characteristics of Asthma] Two of item (1), (2), and (3) / One of item (1), (2), and (3) with two or more of item (4)
(1) At least 10 pack-years of tobacco smoking or equivalent air pollution exposure	(1) Variable (over the course of one day, from day to day, seasonal) or paroxysmal respiratory symptoms (cough, sputum, and dyspnea)
(2) Present low attenuation area denoting emphysematous change on chest CT scan	(2) History of asthma before 40 years of age
	(3) FeNO > 35ppb
(3) Abnormal pulmonary diffusing capacity ($\%D_{LCO} < 80\%$ or $\%D_{LCO}/V_A < 80\%$)	(4)-1. Comorbidity of perennial allergic rhinitis -2. Bronchodilator reversibility (increase in FEV_1 >12% and > 200mL from baseline) -3. Peripheral blood eosinophil counts of >5% or 300/μL -4. Higher IgE (total IgE or specific IgE sensitized to perennial inhalation antigen)

1. The diagnostic criteria of ACO are having both characteristics of COPD and asthma. (Characteristics of COPD; One of item (1), (2), and (3) of [Characteristics of COPD.] Characteristics of asthma; Two of item (1), (2), and (3) of [characteristics of asthma] / one of items (1), (2), (3) with two or more of item (4) of [characteristics of asthma.])
2. Diagnosed as COPD when the patient match only characteristics of COPD. And diagnosed as asthma with the remodeling when the patient match only characteristics of asthma.
3. If you can not determine the characteristics of asthma when diagnosing ACO, it is important to observe the progress of the presence or absence of features of asthma.
4. Perennial inhalation antigens are house dust, mite, molds, animal scales, feathers, etc. Seasonal inhalation antigens are pollen of tree, plant, and weed, etc.

Figure 5. Diagnostic criteria of asthma–COPD overlap in Japanese ACO guideline 2018.

4. Discussion

There are several studies evaluating and validating the new GOLD assessment system; however, uneven distribution of COPD patients and limited data on the clinical outcomes are noticed under these combined assessments. [21–24] The degree of the COPD Assessment Test (CAT) score of ≥10 might not be equivalent to that of the mMRC score of ≥2 for categorizing patients' symptoms. [25–28] Neither the 2007 GOLD nor the 2011 classification scheme has sufficient discriminatory power to be used clinically for risk classification to predict total mortality at the individual level. [29] Accordingly, some countries have developed COPD guidelines to build up appropriate strategies for diagnosis, assessment, pharmacotherapy, and prediction of acute exacerbation and mortality based on evidence and real-world clinical practice.

The Korean and Australia guidelines stratified the lung function severity and exacerbation risk with FEV1 < 60% or ≥ 60% of predicted value. From the validation study in Korea, it was found that there were many patients (15.3% to 16%) who experienced exacerbation with FEV1 between 50% and 60% of predicted value. [14] The cutoff point of an FEV1 50% predicted does not address the heterogeneity in the GOLD Stage II (50%–80% predicted). Patients with limited airflow around FEV1 50% to 60% predicted had a more rapid decline in lung function than patients with FEV1 < 50% in the TORCH study [30,31]. A recent study showed that parameters related to volume, diffusing capacity, and reactance showed break-points around 65% of FEV1 which may have an impact on patients' management plan.

The strategy for stable COPD management was based on lung function severity before GOLD 2011. A refinement of the ABCD assessment tool had been separated from spirometric grade from "ABCD" groups in GOLD 2020. A stepwise approach policy is currently presented in the Japan and Australia guidelines. The management strategy is similar in the Korea and GOLD guidelines including for symptoms severity and exacerbation frequency. Moreover, a phenotype-guided treatment policy has been shown in the Spanish and Czech guidelines. [32,33] Which strategies are optimal in clinical practice guidelines for COPD management? There were several strategies including lung function-guided, stepwise approach-guided, GOLD A–D-guided, and phenotype-guided strategies. The optimal treatment of COPD patients requires an individualized, multidisciplinary approach to the lung function severity, patient's symptoms, clinical phenotypes, biomarkers, comorbidity evaluation, and needs.

The treatment of patients with COPD in a more personalized way must address diverse aspects not only related with the disease, but also with its comorbidities, and current schemes do not offer such personalized medical treatment. Comorbidity evaluation and management were all mentioned in each Asia country CPG. In the JRS guideline [19], the comorbidities included systemic inflammation, osteoporosis, musculoskeletal defect, cardiovascular disorders, gastro-intestinal dysfunction, depression, metabolic disorders, and obstructive sleep apnea. Additionally, the variability of the clinical presentation interacts with comorbidities to form a complex clinical scenario for clinicians. Different comorbidities have different evaluation and management policies. Consequently, the CPG or consensus should be reached over a practical approach for combining comorbidities and disease presentation markers in the therapeutic algorithm, in order to improve the quality of clinical care.

In a previous study, the increased total health expenditure was shown as share GDP $\geq 7\%$ in Korea, Japan, and Australia in 2007. [34] In Japan, major reforms are needed to reduce waste and enhance cost-effectiveness. Moreover, a national system to accredit training programs, including for general practice, has been introduced. [35] The challenges of the healthcare system in Korea include over-consumption and excessively high frequency of specialist consultation, which are major problems for the medical system. The government and the primary care group seek to strengthen primary care, but this is opposed by the medical society governed by the specialist group. [35] In Australia, some provider payment methods were performed such as case payment, diagnostic-related groups, etc. [34]. We think that guideline differences are driven by the disparities in diagnosis modalities or by the treatment variations in different healthcare systems and the socioeconomic burden in each country.

Additionally, diagnosis tools and management of COPD were among the lower guideline-recommended levels in most of the regions investigated among primary care physicians or general practitioners (GPs). [36] The survey demonstrated that the GPs' understanding of COPD was variable and large numbers of GPs have very limited knowledge of COPD and its management in Asia countries. The percentage for COPD management by guideline is as follows: Australia 64%, Japan 74%, Korea 54%, and Taiwan 70%. In China, only 50% of patients with COPD have ever had spirometry tests in tertiary hospitals, and only 18% had in primary or secondary hospitals. [37] Therefore, from the education system, clinical practice, and medical impact, there appears to be an optimal strategy developed to simplify the guidelines for daily practice in each country.

Research evidence has raised concerns that hospital death may be preceded by potentially burdensome and inappropriate hospital admission and aggressive treatments shortly before death, which could be a threat to better end-of-life care and death. [38–41] On the other hand, enabling people to have end-of-life care at home compared with end-of-life care in hospital may incur a potential cost saving. [42,43] The concepts of palliative and hospice care should be established gradually in regards to diseases with an advanced stage.

APSR Recommendations for COPD Diagnosis and Treatment

1. COPD is characterized by persistent respiratory symptoms and airflow limitation. Spirometry is required to make the diagnosis.
2. The severity of COPD should be comprehensively assessed on the basis of the degree of obstruction severity (FEV1, GOLD stage), impairment of exercise tolerance/physical activity, intensity of dyspnea, and frequency/ severity of exacerbation.
3. The goal of pharmacological treatment should be to treat the symptoms (e.g., breathlessness) or to prevent deterioration (either by decreasing exacerbations or by reducing the decline in lung function and quality of life) or both. A stepwise approach is recommended, irrespective of disease severity, until adequate control has been achieved.

4. Management of non-pharmacological strategies for stable COPD should center around supporting smoking patients to quit. Encouraging physical activity and maintenance of a normal weight range are also important. Pulmonary rehabilitation is recommended in all symptomatic patients.
5. Stepwise management of optimized pharmacotherapy for stable COPD which recommends gradual increase of bronchodilators, inhaled corticosteroids, or other drugs based on clinical symptoms, airflow obstruction severity, and exacerbation history.
6. ICS should be used in cases with concomitant asthmatic conditions and/or 2 or more exacerbations in the previous 12 months. LABA/ICS combinations are also allowed.
7. In the end-of-life care, improving quality of life and providing emotional and spiritual support to COPD patients and their family are the main goals.

5. Conclusions

This is the first report to summarize the similarities and differences among the COPD guidelines across the Asia-Pacific region. The guideline developed in each country would be based on clinical evidence, experts' consensus, healthcare insurance, reality of clinical practice, and the best interests of patients. We hope, through collaboration of research, that the guidelines will evolve positively and that differences or gaps will diminish with time.

Author Contributions: S.-L.C. and C.-H.L.; methodology, validation, and formal analysis; S.-L.C.; writing—original draft preparation, S.-L.C.; writing—review and editing, C.-H.L. Both authors have read and agreed to the published version of the manuscript.

Funding: This research received no external funding.

Institutional Review Board Statement: Not applicable.

Informed Consent Statement: Not applicable.

Data Availability Statement: Not applicable.

Acknowledgments: Thanks to the professors for finishing this work including: Kazuto Matsunaga (Japan); Chin Kook Rhee (Korea); Diahn-Warng Perng (Taiwan).

Conflicts of Interest: The authors declare no conflict of interest.

References

1. Lim, S.; Lam, D.C.-L.; Muttalif, A.R.; Yunus, F.; Wongtim, S.; Lan, L.T.T.; Shetty, V.; Chu, R.; Zheng, J.; Perng, D.-W.; et al. Impact of chronic obstructive pulmonary disease (COPD) in the Asia-Pacific region: The EPIC Asia population-based survey. *Asia Pac. Fam. Med.* **2015**, *14*, 1–11. [CrossRef]
2. Vogelmeier, C.F.; Criner, G.J.; Martinez, F.J.; Anzueto, A.; Barnes, P.J.; Bourbeau, J.; Celli, B.R.; Chen, R.; Decramer, M.; Fabbri, L.M.; et al. Global strategy for the diagnosis, management, and prevention of chronic obstructive pulmonary disease: GOLD executive summary. *Am. J. Respir. Crit. Care Med.* **2017**, *195*, 557–582. [CrossRef]
3. Global Initiative for Chronic Obstructive Lung Disease (GOLD). Global Strategy for the Diagnosis, Management and Prevention of Chronic Obstructive Pulmonary Disease. GOLD. 2015. Available online: http://www.goldcopd.org/uploads/users/files/GOLD_Report_2015_Feb18.pdf. (accessed on 27 March 2015).
4. Cooksley, N.A.; Atkinson, D.; Marks, G.B.; Toelle, B.G.; Reeve, D.; Johns, D.P.; Abramson, M.; Burton, D.L.; James, A.L.; Wood-Baker, R.; et al. Prevalence of airflow obstruction and reduced forced vital capacity in an Aboriginal Australian population: The cross-sectional BOLD study. *Respirology* **2015**, *20*, 766–774. [CrossRef] [PubMed]
5. Zhong, N.; Wang, C.; Yao, W.; Chen, P.; Kang, J.; Huang, S.; Wang, C.; Ni, D.; Zhou, Y.; Liu, S.; et al. Prevalence of chronic obstructive pulmonary disease in China: A large, population-based survey. *Am. J. Respir. Crit Care Med.* **2007**, *176*, 753–760. [CrossRef] [PubMed]
6. Fang, X.; Wang, X.; Bai, C. COPD in China: The burden and importance of proper management. *Chest* **2011**, *139*, 920–929. [CrossRef] [PubMed]
7. Fang, L.; Gao, P.; Bao, H.; Tang, X.; Wang, B.; Feng, Y.; Cong, S.; Juan, J.; Fan, J.; Lu, K.; et al. Chronic obstructive pulmonary disease in China: A nationwide prevalence study. *Lancet Respir. Med.* **2018**, *6*, 421–430. [CrossRef]
8. Fukuchi, Y.; Nishimura, M.; Ichinose, M.; Adachi, M.; Nagai, A.; Kuriyama, T.; Takahashi, K.; Nishimura, K.; Ishioka, S.; Aizawa, H.; et al. COPD in Japan: The Nippon COPD Epidemiology study. *Respirology* **2004**, *9*, 458–465. [CrossRef] [PubMed]
9. Hwang, Y.I.; Park, Y.B.; Yoo, K.H. Recent Trends in the Prevalence of Chronic Obstructive Pulmonary Disease in Korea. *Tuberc. Respir. Dis.* **2017**, *80*, 226–229. [CrossRef]

10. Yu, C.-J.; Cheng, S.-L.; Chan, M.-C.; Wang, C.-C.; Lin, C.-H.; Wang, H.-C.; Hsu, J.-Y.; Hang, L.-W.; Chang, C.-J.; Perng, S.D.-W. COPD in Taiwan: A National Epidemiology Survey. *Int. J. Chronic Obstr. Pulm. Dis.* **2015**, *10*, 2459–2467. [CrossRef]
11. Pothirat, C.; Chaiwong, W.; Phetsuk, N.; Pisalthanapuna, S.; Chetsadaphan, N.; Inchai, J. A comparative study of COPD burden between urban vs rural communities in northern Thailand. *Int. J. Chronic Obstr. Pulm. Dis.* **2015**, *10*, 1035–1042. [CrossRef]
12. Idolor, L.F.; Guia, T.S.D.E.; Francisco, N.A.; Roa, C.C.; Ayuyao, F.G.; Tady, C.Z.; Tan, D.T.; Banal-Yang, S.; Balanag, V.M., Jr.; Reyes, M.T.N.; et al. Burden of obstructive lung disease in a rural setting in the philippines. *Respirology* **2011**, *16*, 1111–1118. [CrossRef]
13. Park, H.; Jung, S.Y.; Lee, K.; Bae, W.K.; Lee, K.; Han, J.-S.; Kim, S.; Choo, S.; Jeong, J.-M.; Kim, H.-R.; et al. Prevalence of Chronic Obstructive Lung Disease in Korea Using Data from the Fifth Korea National Health and Nutrition Examination Survey. *Korean J. Fam. Med.* **2015**, *36*, 128–134. [CrossRef] [PubMed]
14. Park, Y.-B.; Rhee, C.K.; Yoon, H.K.; Oh, Y.-M.; Lim, S.Y.; Lee, J.H.; Yoo, K.-H.; Ahn, J.H. on behalf of the Committee of the Korean COPD Guideline 2018 Revised (2018) COPD Clinical Practice Guideline of the Korean Academy of Tuberculosis and Respiratory Disease: A Summary. *Tuberc. Respir. Dis.* **2018**, *81*, 261–273. [CrossRef]
15. Yang, I.A.; Dabscheck, E.; Johnson George, J.; Jenkins, S.; Christine McDonald, A.M.; McDonald, V.; Smith, B.; Zwar, N.; Brown, J.L.; O'Brien, M.; et al. The COPD-X Plan: Australian and New Zealand Guidelines for the management of Chronic Obstructive Pulmonary Disease 2020. In *COPD-X Guidelines–Version 2.62 (October 2020)*; Lung Foundation Australia: Milton, Australia, 2020.
16. Jung, K.S.; Park, H.Y.; Park, S.Y.; Kim, S.K.; Kim, Y.-K.; Shim, J.-J.; Moon, H.S.; Lee, K.H.; Yoo, J.-H.; Lee, S.D. Comparison of tiotropium plus fluticasone propionate/salmeterol with tiotropium in COPD: A randomized controlled study. *Respir. Med.* **2012**, *106*, 382–389. [CrossRef] [PubMed]
17. Calverley, P.; Pauwels, R.; Vestbo, J.; Jones, P.; Pride, N.; Gulsvik, A.; Anderson, J.; Maden, C.; TRial of Inhaled STeroids and Long-Acting beta2 Agonists Study Group. Combined salmeterol and fluticasone in the treatment of chronic obstructive pulmonary disease: A randomised controlled trial. *Lancet* **2003**, *361*, 449–456. [CrossRef]
18. Calverley, P.M.; Anderson, J.A.; Celli, B.R.; Ferguson, G.T.; Jenkins, C.R.; Jones, P.W.; Yates, J.C.; Vestbo, J. Salmeterol and Fluticasone Propionate and Survival in Chronic Obstructive Pulmonary Disease. *N. Engl. J. Med.* **2007**, *356*, 775–789. [CrossRef]
19. Japanese Respiratory Society. *Guidelines for the Diagnosis and Treatment of COPD*, 5th ed.; Japanese Respiratory Society: Tokyo, Japan, 2018; Available online: https://www.jrs.or.jp/modules/guidelines/index.php?content_id=1 (accessed on 19 April 2013).
20. Zhang, J.; Cai, B.-Q.; Cai, S.-X.; Chen, R.-C.; Cui, L.-Y.; Feng, Y.-L.; Gu, Y.-T.; Huang, S.-G.; Liu, R.-Y.; Liu, G.-N.; et al. Expert consensus on acute exacerbation of chronic obstructive pulmonary disease in the People's Republic of China. *Int. J. Chronic Obstr. Pulm. Dis.* **2014**, *9*, 381–395. [CrossRef]
21. Han, M.K.; Müllerová, H.; Curran-Everett, D.; Dransfield, M.T.; Washko, G.R.; Regan, E.A.; Bowler, R.P.; Beaty, T.H.; Hokanson, J.E.; Lynch, D.A.; et al. GOLD 2011 disease severity classification in COPDGene: A prospective cohort study. *Lancet Respir. Med.* **2013**, *1*, 43–50. [CrossRef]
22. Lange, P.; Marott, J.L.; Vestbo, J.; Olsen, K.R.; Ingebrigtsen, T.S.; Dahl, M.; Nordestgaard, B.G. Prediction of the clinical course of chronic obstructive pul¬monary disease, using the new GOLD classification: A study of the gen¬eral population. *Am. J. Respir. Crit. Care Med.* **2012**, *186*, 975–981. [CrossRef]
23. Soriano, J.B.; Alfageme, I.; Almagro, P.; Casanova, C.; Esteban, C.; Soler-Cataluña, J.J.; De Torres, J.P.; Martínez-Camblor, P.; Miravitlles, M.; Celli, B.R.; et al. Distribution and Prognostic Validity of the New Global Initiative for Chronic Obstructive Lung Disease Grading Classification. *Chest* **2013**, *143*, 694–702. [CrossRef]
24. Johannessen, A.; Nilsen, R.M.; Storebø, M.; Gulsvik, A.; Eagan, T.; Bakke, P. Comparison of 2011 and 2007 Global Initiative for Chronic Obstructive Lung Disease Guidelines for Predicting Mortality and Hospitalization. *Am. J. Respir. Crit. Care Med.* **2013**, *188*, 51–59. [CrossRef] [PubMed]
25. Jones, P.W.; Adamek, L.; Nadeau, G.; Banik, N. Comparisons of health status scores with MRC grades in COPD: Implications for the GOLD 2011 classification. *Eur. Respir. J.* **2013**, *42*, 647–654. [CrossRef] [PubMed]
26. Kim, S.; Oh, J.; Kim, Y.-I.; Ban, H.-J.; Kwon, Y.-S.; Oh, I.-J.; Kim, K.-S.; Kim, Y.-C.; Lim, S.-C. Differences in classification of COPD group using COPD assessment test (CAT) or modified Medical Research Council (mMRC) dyspnea scores: A cross-sectional analyses. *BMC Pulm. Med.* **2013**, *13*, 35. [CrossRef]
27. Zogg, S.; Dürr, S.; Miedinger, D.; Steveling, E.H.; Maier, S.; Leuppi, J.D. Differences in classification of COPD patients into risk groups A-D: A cross-sectional study. *BMC Res. Notes* **2014**, *7*, 562. [CrossRef] [PubMed]
28. Rhee, C.K.; Kim, J.W.; Hwang, Y.I.; Lee, J.H.; Jung, K.-S.; Lee, M.G.; Yoo, K.H.; Lee, S.H.; Shin, K.-C.; Yoon, H.K. Discrepancies between modified Medical Research Council dyspnea score and COPD assessment test score in patients with COPD. *Int. J. Chronic Obstr. Pulm. Dis.* **2015**, *10*, 1623–1631. [CrossRef]
29. Soriano, J.B.; Lamprecht, B.; Ramírez, A.S.; Martinez-Camblor, P.; Kaiser, B.; Alfageme, I.; Almagro, P.; Casanova, C.; Esteban, C.; Soler-Cataluña, J.J.; et al. Mortality prediction in chronic obstructive pulmonary disease comparing the GOLD 2007 and 2011 staging systems: A pooled analysis of individual patient data. *Lancet Respir. Med.* **2015**, *3*, 443–450. [CrossRef]
30. Celli, B.R.; Thomas, N.E.; Anderson, J.A.; Ferguson, G.T.; Jenkins, C.R.; Jones, P.W.; Vestbo, J.; Knobil, K.; Yates, J.C.; Calverle, P.M.A. Effect of pharmacotherapy on rate of decline of lung function in chronic obstructive pulmonary disease: Results from the TORCH study. *Am. J. Respir. Crit Care Med.* **2008**, *178*, 332–338. [CrossRef] [PubMed]
31. Jenkins, C.R.; Jones, P.W.; Calverley, P.M.A.; Celli, B.; Anderson, J.A.; Ferguson, G.T.; Yates, J.C.; Willits, L.R.; Vestbo, J. Efficacy of salmeterol/fluticasone propionate by GOLD stage of chronic obstructive pulmonary disease: Analysis from the randomised, placebo-controlled TORCH study. *Respir. Res.* **2009**, *10*, 59. [CrossRef] [PubMed]

32. Koblizek, V.; Chlumsky, J.; Zindr, V.; Neumannova, K.; Zatloukal, J.; Zak, J.; Sedlák, V.; Kocianova, J.; Zatloukal, J.; Hejduk, K.; et al. Chronic Obstructive Pulmonary Disease: Official diagnosis and treatment guidelines of the Czech Pneumological and Phthisiological Society; a novel phenotypic approach to COPD with patient-oriented care. *Biomed. Pap.* **2013**, *157*, 189–201. [CrossRef] [PubMed]
33. Miravitlles, M.; Soler-Cataluña, J.J.; Calle, M.; Molina, J.; Almagro, P.; Quintano, J.A.; Riesco, J.A.; Trigueros, J.A.; Piñera, P.; Simón, A.; et al. Spanish Guideline for COPD (GesEPOC). Update 2014. *Arch. Bronconeumol.* **2014**, *50* (Suppl. 1), 1–16. [CrossRef]
34. WHO. *Health Financing Strategy for Asia Pacific Region (2010–2015)*; WHO: Geneva, Switzerland, 2009; NLM Classification: WA 525; ISBN 978-92-9061-458-6.
35. Van Weel, C.; Kassai, R.; Tsoi, G.W.; Hwang, S.-J.; Cho, K.; Wong, S.Y.-S.; Phui-Nah, C.; Jiang, S.; Ii, M.; Goodyear-Smith, F. Evolving health policy for primary care in the Asia Pacific region. *Br. J. Gen. Pract.* **2016**, *66*, e451–e453. [CrossRef]
36. Aisanov, Z.; Bai, C.; Bauerle, O.; Colodenco, F.D.; Feldman, C.; Hashimoto, S.; Jardim, J.; Lai, C.K.W.; Laniado-Laborin, R.; Nadeau, G.; et al. Primary care physician perceptions on the diagnosis and management of chronic obstructive pulmonary disease in diverse regions of the world. *Int. J. Chronic Obstr. Pulm. Dis.* **2012**, *7*, 271–282. [CrossRef]
37. Shen, N.; He, B. Is the new GOLD classification applicable in China? *Lancet Glob. Health* **2013**, *1*, e247–e248. [CrossRef]
38. Teno, J.M.; Gozalo, P.L.; Bynum, J.P.W.; Leland, N.E.; Miller, S.C.; Morden, N.E.; Scupp, T.; Goodman, D.C.; Mor, V. Change in end-of-life care for Medicare beneficiaries: Site of death, place of care, and health care transitions in 2000, 2005, and 2009. *JAMA* **2013**, *309*, 470–477. [CrossRef] [PubMed]
39. Block, L.V.D.; Deschepper, R.; Drieskens, K.; Bauwens, S.; Bilsen, J.; Bossuyt, N.; Deliens, L. Hospitalisations at the end of life: Using a sentinel surveillance network to study hospital use and associated patient, disease and healthcare factors. *BMC Health Serv. Res.* **2007**, *7*, 69. [CrossRef]
40. Willard, C.; Luker, K. Challenges to end of life care in the acute hospital setting. *Palliat. Med.* **2006**, *20*, 611–615. [CrossRef] [PubMed]
41. Wright, A.A.; Keating, N.L.; Balboni, T.A.; Matulonis, U.A.; Block, S.D.; Prigerson, H.G. Place of Death: Correlations With Quality of Life of Patients With Cancer and Predictors of Bereaved Caregivers' Mental Health. *J. Clin. Oncol.* **2010**, *28*, 4457–4464. [CrossRef]
42. Hatziandreu, E.; Archontakis, F.; Daly, A. The Potential Cost Savings of Greater Use of Home- and Hospice- Based End of Life Care in England. 2008. Available online: http://www.rand.org/pubs/technical_reports/TR642.html (accessed on 25 January 2014).
43. Marie Curie Cancer Care. Understanding the Cost of End of Life Care in Different Settings. 2012. Available online: https://www.mariecurie.org.uk/globalassets/media/documents/commissioning-our-services/publications/understanding-cost-end-life-care-different-settingspdf (accessed on 25 January 2014).

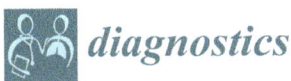

Article

Is Blood Eosinophil Count a Biomarker for Chronic Obstructive Pulmonary Disease in a Real-World Clinical Setting? Predictive Property and Longitudinal Stability in Japanese Patients

Koichi Nishimura [1,*], Masaaki Kusunose [1], Ryo Sanda [1], Mio Mori [1], Ayumi Shibayama [2] and Kazuhito Nakayasu [3]

1. Department of Respiratory Medicine, National Center for Geriatrics and Gerontology, Obu 474-8511, Japan; kusunose@ncgg.go.jp (M.K.); ryo-sand@ncgg.go.jp (R.S.); mio-mori@ncgg.go.jp (M.M.)
2. Department of Nursing, National Center for Geriatrics and Gerontology, Obu 474-8511, Japan; ayuminarita3@ncgg.go.jp
3. Data Research Section, Kondo Photo Process Co., Ltd., Osaka 543-0011, Japan; nakayasu@mydo-kond.co.jp
* Correspondence: koichi-nishimura@nifty.com; Tel.: +81-562-46-2311

Abstract: The authors examined predictive properties and the longitudinal stability of blood eosinophil count (BEC) or three strata (<100 cells/mm^3, 100–299 cells/mm^3 and ≥300 cells/mm^3) in patients with chronic obstructive pulmonary disease (COPD) for up to six and a half years as part of a hospital-based cohort study. Of the 135 patients enrolled, 21 (15.6%) were confirmed to have died during the follow-up period. Episodes of acute exacerbation of COPD (AECOPD) were identified in 74 out of 130 available patients (56.9%), and admission due to AECOPD in 35 out of 132 (26.5%). Univariate Cox proportional hazards analyses revealed that almost all the age, forced expiratory volume in 1 s (FEV$_1$) and health status measures using St. George's Respiratory Questionnaire (SGRQ) Total and COPD Assessment Test (CAT) Score were significantly related to these types of events, but the relationship between age and AECOPD did not reach statistical significance ($p = 0.05$). Neither BEC nor the three different groups stratified by BEC were significant predictors of any subsequent events. There were no significant differences in the BEC between Visits 1–3 ($p = 0.127$, Friedman test). The ICC value was 0.755 using log-transformed data, indicating excellent repeatability. In the case of assigning to strata, Fleiss' kappa was calculated to be 0.464, indicating moderate agreement. The predictive properties of BEC may be limited in a real-world Japanese clinical setting. Attention must be paid to the fact that the longitudinal stability of the three strata is regarded as moderate.

Keywords: inhaled corticosteroids (ICS); chronic obstructive pulmonary disease (COPD); blood eosinophil count (BEC); eosinophil; the Global Initiative for Chronic Obstructive Lung Disease (GOLD); acute exacerbation of COPD (AECOPD)

Citation: Nishimura, K.; Kusunose, M.; Sanda, R.; Mori, M.; Shibayama, A.; Nakayasu, K. Is Blood Eosinophil Count a Biomarker for Chronic Obstructive Pulmonary Disease in a Real-World Clinical Setting? Predictive Property and Longitudinal Stability in Japanese Patients. *Diagnostics* **2021**, *11*, 404. https://doi.org/10.3390/diagnostics11030404

Academic Editor: Philippe A. Grenier

Received: 14 February 2021
Accepted: 23 February 2021
Published: 27 February 2021

Publisher's Note: MDPI stays neutral with regard to jurisdictional claims in published maps and institutional affiliations.

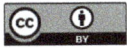

Copyright: © 2021 by the authors. Licensee MDPI, Basel, Switzerland. This article is an open access article distributed under the terms and conditions of the Creative Commons Attribution (CC BY) license (https://creativecommons.org/licenses/by/4.0/).

1. Introduction

The question of whether inhaled corticosteroids (ICS) should be administered to patients with chronic obstructive pulmonary disease (COPD) has been debated for over three decades [1–4]. It could not have been expected that blood eosinophil count (BEC) would emerge at the heart of this debate. Some post-hoc analyses of relatively large-scale clinical trials for studying ICS-containing regimens in patients with moderate and severe COPD have reported that the BEC is significantly able to predict the response to ICS since this medication was most efficacious in the prevention of exacerbation in patients with higher baseline BEC [5–7]. This hypothesis was subsequently investigated in the development procedures of the single-inhaler triple therapy and the BEC was thus established as a prognostic biomarker [8–10]. The Global Initiative for Chronic Obstructive Lung Disease (GOLD) document has changed to reflect these new findings, especially in Group D, and currently reports that ICS-containing regimens have little or no effect at a blood eosinophil count of <100 cells/mm^3, and that a threshold blood eosinophil count of ≥300 cells/mm^3 or frequent exacerbation with a threshold blood eosinophil count of ≥100 cells/mm^3 can be used to identify patients with the greatest likelihood of treatment benefit with ICS [11].

However, the health indicators including biomarkers should be discussed from the following three different perspectives. First, they can differentiate between people who have better health and those with worse health (a discriminative property). Second, they can measure how much the health condition changes (an evaluative property). Third, they can predict the future outcomes of patients (a predictive property). Therefore, to determine whether or not the BEC can be regarded as a biomarker in COPD, multifaceted analysis and evaluation as an outcome marker will be required.

Compared with western countries, ICS may have been less preferably prescribed for patients with COPD in Japan. In the 5th version of the Japanese guidelines published by The Japanese Respiratory Society in 2018, the description reads that ICS should be given only in patients with asthma-complicated COPD or Asthma and COPD Overlap (ACO) [12]. It is reported that the blood eosinophil data from global studies are of relevance in Japan although there was a slightly lower median eosinophil count for Japanese patients within multi-country studies [13]. One of the opposing views is that BEC may be liable to variation and considered to be unreliable as a biomarker [14–24]. The accuracy and diagnostic value of the BEC may be critical to the selection of appropriate ICS-containing treatments and should continue to be studied also in Japan.

The authors hypothesized that BEC could predict exacerbation or other subsequent events even in real-world clinical practice since it has been reported that possible reduction of the future acute exacerbation of COPD (AECOPD) by ICS is related to the blood eosinophil count. In addition to analysis of the absolute number of the BEC, the counts are divided into the following three groups according to GOLD 2019 thresholds: non-eosinophilic, intermediate and eosinophilic defined as BEC <100 cells/mm^3, 100–299 cells/mm^3 and ≥300 cells/mm^3, respectively. We aimed to investigate how BEC, or the three strata are cross-sectionally related to other clinical measures at baseline and to examine predictive properties of the baseline values regarding mortality, AECOPD and admission due to AECOPD. As a secondary purpose of the present study, it was our objective to determine the longitudinal stability of their counts. We analysed the longitudinal stability of the three strata described above from the first to the second visit and from the second to the third visit.

2. Materials and Methods

2.1. Participants

Participants were recruited between April 2013 and August 2019 from our outpatient clinic, and they were prospectively followed up until May 2020 as part of a hospital-based cohort study [25]. The criteria for inclusion were (1) a diagnosis of stable COPD; (2) age over 50 years; (2) current or former smokers with a smoking history of more than 10 pack-years; (3) chronic fixed airflow limitation defined by fixed ratio, or forced expiratory volume in 1 s (FEV_1) to forced vital capacity (FVC) of less than 0.7 according to the Global Initiative for Chronic Obstructive Lung Disease (GOLD); (4) regular attendance at the authors' clinic for more than 6 months to avoid any subsequent changes caused by new medical interventions; and (5) no changes in treatment regimen during the preceding four weeks. Eligible COPD patients had their clinical measures including pulmonary function as well as patient-reported outcomes (PROs) evaluated at entry, and every 6 months thereafter over a 5-year period. When an exacerbation of COPD requiring a change in treatment occurred within 4 weeks of a reassessment day, the evaluation was postponed for at least 8 weeks until the patient recovered. Written informed consent was obtained from all participants.

2.2. Measurement

All eligible patients completed the following examinations on the same day. They underwent a routine blood test and pulmonary function tests while sitting including post-bronchodilator spirometry (CHESTAC-8800; Chest, Tokyo, Japan), residual volume (RV) measured by the closed-circuit helium method, and diffusing capacity for carbon monoxide (DL_{CO}) measured by the single-breath technique in accordance with guidelines published by the American Thoracic Society and European Respiratory Society Task Force in 2005 [26]. The predicted values for FEV_1 and vital capacity were calculated according to the proposal from the Japanese Respiratory Society [27]. Participants were also asked to complete the previously validated Japanese versions of the COPD Assessment Test (CAT) [28,29], St. George's Respiratory Questionnaire (SGRQ) (version 2) [30,31], Hyland Scale and Dyspnoea-12 (D-12) [32–34]. They were self-administered under site supervision in the aforementioned order (in a booklet form). Disease-specific health status was assessed using CAT and SGRQ, global health by Hyland Scale and the severity of dyspnoea by D-12.

Outcomes were continuously monitored, and the survival status of all enrolled patients was assessed up until May 2020. The period from entry to the last attendance or death was recorded for the analysis. Acute exacerbation of chronic obstructive pulmonary disease (AECOPD) defined as a worsening of respiratory symptoms that required treatment with oral corticosteroids or antibiotics, or both, and admission due to AECOPD was also recorded throughout the individual follow-up periods. The predictive properties of observational parameters obtained at baseline were analysed in regard to the potential future events of mortality, AECOPD and admission due to AECOPD. To examine the predictive properties, FEV_1 and the SGRQ Total and CAT scores were also analysed as control indicators [35–38].

On the other hand, to examine the longitudinal stability of BEC, we included all the patients in whom a differential blood cell count was available at all the study visits 1–3 and analysed a sequence of data obtained three times in a row at intervals of 6 to 9 months. The BEC data obtained from participants who missed a visit were excluded from the analysis of longitudinal stability.

2.3. Statistical Methods

All results are expressed as mean ± standard deviation (SD) or using median and interquartile range (IQR). A p value of less than 0.05 was considered to be statistically significant. Relationships between two sets of data were analysed by Spearman's rank correlation tests. The significance of between-group differences among non-eosinophilic, intermediate, and eosinophilic groups was determined by Steel–Dwass test and Kruskal–Wallis test. Univariate Cox proportional hazards analyses were performed to investigate the relationships between the clinical measurements at baseline and subsequent events. Results of regression analyses are presented in terms of hazard ratio (HR) with corresponding 95% confidence intervals (CI). Longitudinal stability of BEC was analysed by Friedman test, intraclass correlation coefficient (ICC) and Fleiss' kappa. ICC values were calculated using both log-transformed and raw data, and interpreted as excellent (≥ 0.75), good (≥ 0.60 to <0.75), fair (≥ 0.40 to <0.60) or poor (<0.40) [39], and Fleiss' kappa for categorized data as almost perfect (0.81 to 1.00), substantial (0.61 to 0.80), moderate (0.41 to 0.60), fair (0.21 to 0.40) or slight (0.01 to 0.20) [40].

3. Results

3.1. Cross-Sectional Observation at Baseline

Baseline characteristics of the 135 consecutive patients (123 males) are presented in Table 1. The average age and FEV_1 were 74.9 ± 6.7 years and 1.70 ± 0.54 L, and 31 patients were current smokers. Eighty-three patients were treated with multiple-inhaler triple therapy, that is, a combination of long-acting muscarinic antagonist (LAMA) and beta2-agonist (LABA) and inhaled corticosteroid (ICS), 33 patients with tiotropium bromide alone, 13 patients with ICS/LABA and 6 patients with no long-acting bronchodilators. While 96 (71.1%) patients were receiving the regimen for treatment including:

Table 1. Baseline characteristics in 135 patients with chronic obstructive pulmonary disease (COPD) and Spearman's rank correlation coefficients with the blood eosinophil count (BEC).

					Correlations	
					With BEC	
	Median	IQR	Max	Min	rs	p Value
		147				

ICS at baseline, the BEC was not statistically different between patients taking ICS and those not taking ICS, and some of the other measures were worse in patients with ICS (Appendix A. Table A1).

Spearman's rank correlation coefficients were obtained to investigate relationships between the BEC at baseline and various factors as shown in Table 1. The BEC was not significantly correlated with clinical, physiological, or patient-reported measures except residual volume (rs = 0.172, p = 0.047). In pairwise comparisons of the three groups stratified by BEC (Table 2), there were no significant differences in the measures among non-eosinophilic, intermediate and eosinophilic groups except that for residual volume between the intermediate and eosinophilic groups (p = 0.036, Steel–Dwass test). Although the Kruskal–Wallis test was also performed here, there were no significant differences among the three groups.

3.2. Predictive Properties of BEC

Of the 135 patients enrolled, 21 patients (15.6%) were confirmed to have died during the follow-up period, which was an average of 41.9 ± 21.8 months, ranging from 3 to 80. The first episodes of AECOPD were identified in 74 out of 130 available patients (56.9%). The duration from entry to the last attendance or the first episode of AECOPD averaged 22.3 ± 19.5 months, ranging from 0 to 79. Thirty-five out of 132 available patients (26.5%) were hospitalized due to AECOPD at least once during the follow-up period of average 31.8 ± 22.6 months, ranging from 2 to 79. Table 3 shows the results from the univariate Cox proportional hazards model in analysing the relationship of the BEC, the three different groups stratified by BEC and the other major clinical measures with mortality, AECOPD and admission due to AECOPD. Almost all the age, FEV_1, SGRQ Total and CAT Score were significantly strongly related to these types of events but the predictive relationship between age and AECOPD did not reach statistical significance. Neither the BEC nor the three different groups stratified by BEC were significant predictors of subsequent events. A Kaplan–Meier plot for the three different groups stratified by the BEC associated with patient survival is shown in Figure 1.

Table 2. Comparison of clinical indices between eosinophilic, intermediate and non-eosinophilic groups classified by BEC.

		Non-Eosinophilic Group		Intermediate Group		Eosinophilic Group	
		$n = 37$		$n = 69$		$n = 29$	
Blood Eosinophil Count (/mm^3)		<100		≥100 and <300		≥300	
Age	years	74.0	(72.0–80.0)	74.0	(72.0–80.0)	73.0	(69.0–79.0)
BMI	kg/m^2	22.6	(19.5–24.2)	22.8	(20.8–24.9)	21.8	(20.5–23.8)
Cumulative Smoking	pack-years	54.0	(37.5–78.8)	51.0	(38.0–63.0)	50.0	(40.0–71.8)
FVC	% pred.	100.4	(87.2–108.5)	97.4	(82.2–109.8)	91.8	(78.0–104.3)
FEV$_1$	Liters	1.62	(1.38–1.98)	1.71	(1.38–2.10)	1.62	(1.21–2.07)
FEV$_1$/FVC	%	59.1	(48.4–66.7)	60.8	(51.6–64.4)	55.8	(43.8–63.4)
RV §	% pred.	123.9	(93.1–137.2)	109.7	(91.7–137.5)	121.9	(115.4–147.7) ***
RV/TLC §	%	44.4	(39.8–49.7)	43.3	(37.6–50.6) ‡‡	44.9	(41.0–56.0) ***
DLco ¶	% pred.	48.5	(39.3–59.2)	55.3	(41.1–66.8) **	46.7	(33.7–64.3) ***
PaO$_2$ $^{(1)}$	mmHg	79.3	(72.8–87.1)	77.2	(70.7–81.8)	75.8	(70.8–82.1)
BNP $^{(2)}$	pg/mL	27.8	(10.6–46.4)	25.1	(14.1–49.9)	20.4	(8.4–46.7)
SGRQ Total Score	(0–100)	19.7	(9.4–28.5)	21.5	(8.9–34.8)	25.3	(16.3–40.8)
CAT Score	(0–40)	8.0	(3.0–12.0)	8.0	(4.0–12.0)	9.0	(5.0–15.0)
Hyland Scale Score	(0–100)	65.0	(60.0–75.0)	70.0	(65.0–80.0)	65.0	(50.0–75.0)
D-12 Total Score §	(0–36)	0.5	(0.0–2.0) *	0.0	(0.0–1.0)	1.0	(0.0–2.0)

Data are presented as median (IQR). ‡‡ $p < 0.05$ versus eosinophilic group (Steel–Dwass test). No significant difference among three groups with the Kruskal–Wallis test. $^{(1)}$ One patient receiving oxygen, $^{(2)}$ < 5.8 pg/mL considered as 5.7 pg/mL in ten patients, § $n = 134$, ¶ $n = 133$, * $n = 36$, ** $n = 68$, *** $n = 28$. IQR, interquartile range; SGRQ, the St. George's Respiratory Questionnaire; CAT, the COPD Assessment Test; D-12, Dyspnoea-12. The numbers in parentheses denote possible score range.

Table 3. Univariate Cox proportional hazards analyses on the relationship between major clinical measurements and future events.

		All Deaths ($n = 135$)		AECOPD ($n = 130$)		Admission Due to AECOPD ($n = 132$)	
		Hazard Ratio (95% CI)	p Value	Hazard Ratio (95% CI)	p Value	Hazard Ratio (95% CI)	p Value
Blood eosinophil count	/mm^3	0.999 (0.995–1.002)	0.352	1.000 (0.999–1.001)	0.915	1.000 (0.998–1.002)	0.869
Three different groups of blood eosinophil count	<100/mm^3 (Ref.)	1		1		1	
	≥100/mm^3 and <300/mm^3	0.849 (0.329–2.192)	0.735	1.285 (0.735–2.247)	0.379	1.289 (0.564–2.946)	0.547
	≥300/mm^3	0.461 (0.118–1.803)	0.266	1.503 (0.773–2.921)	0.230	1.445 (0.542–3.854)	0.462
Age	years	1.098 (1.025–1.176)	0.007	1.040 (1.000–1.081)	0.050	1.091 (1.027–1.158)	0.005
FEV$_1$	Litres	0.293 (0.126–0.679)	0.004	0.318 (0.195–0.519)	<0.001	0.127 (0.061–0.263)	<0.001
SGRQ Total Score	(0–100)	1.023 (1.001–1.047)	0.043	1.028 (1.014–1.043)	<0.001	1.047 (1.027–1.067)	<0.001
CAT Score	(0–40)	1.067 (1.013–1.125)	0.015	1.066 (1.030–1.103)	<0.001	1.144 (1.089–1.203)	<0.001

AECOPD, acute exacerbation of COPD; SGRQ, the St. George's Respiratory Questionnaire; CAT, the COPD Assessment test.

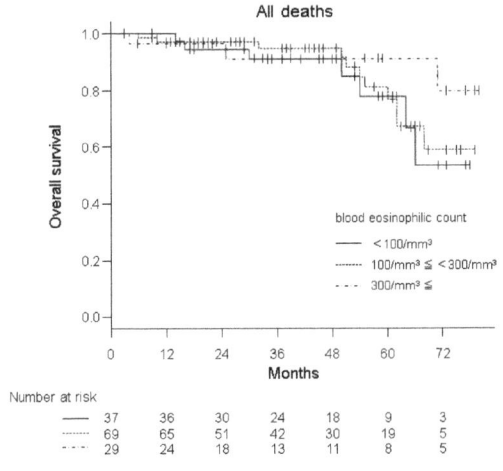

Figure 1. Kaplan–Meier survival curves based on three strata (non-eosinophilic, intermediate and eosinophilic groups) defined by BEC at baseline.

3.3. Longitudinal Stability of BEC

The mean BEC count was $207 \pm 151/mm^3$ at Visit 1 (baseline), $202 \pm 125/mm^3$ at Visit 2 and $210 \pm 173/mm^3$ at Visit 3 in 86 patients whose counts were available for all three visits (Appendix B. Table A2). There were no significant differences between them ($p = 0.127$, Friedman test). The ICC value was 0.755 (95%CI: 0.647–0.833) using log-transformed data, indicating excellent repeatability while it was 0.596 (95%CI: 0.482–0.698) using raw data, suggesting it was fair. To assess the reliability of agreement between three consecutive measures when assigning to strata, Fleiss' kappa was calculated to be 0.464, indicating moderate agreement.

At Visit 1 the number of patients in the non-eosinophilic, intermediate, and eosinophilic groups were 20 (23.3%), 48 (55.8%) and 18 (20.9%), respectively (Appendix B. Table A2). The changes between strata over consecutive visits and the resulting distributions are shown in Figure 2. Eleven patients (13%) were persistently non-eosinophilic at all three study visits, but only eight of the patients (9%) were continuously eosinophilic. On the other hand, 26 (30%) patients remained intermediate throughout the period.

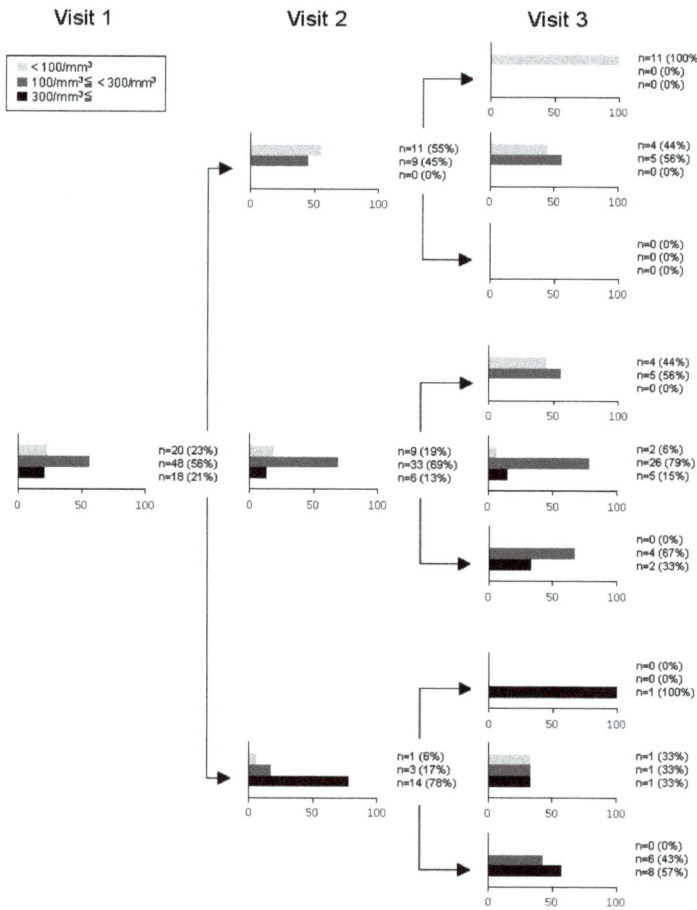

Figure 2. The number and percentage of patients according to three strata (non-eosinophilic, intermediate and eosinophilic groups) defined by BEC at Visits 1, 2 and 3. The proportions of patients at Visit 1 are sequentially subdivided according to their BEC at Visit 2, and the proportions of patients at Visit 2 are sequentially subdivided according to their BEC at Visit 3.

4. Discussion

In the present study, the predictive properties of BEC were examined for mortality, AECOPD and admission due to AECOPD using univariate Cox proportional hazards analysis. Although it was clearly demonstrated that typical outcome measures such as FEV_1 as well as health status measure could predict the future event, the BEC was shown to be a poor predictor. Furthermore, since the cross-sectional relationship of BEC with clinical, physiological outcome markers was also interpreted as almost negative, the discriminative properties of BEC have also not been confirmed. These negative results might give contradictory findings that BEC is a poor predictive biomarker for the response to ICS in the prevention of AECOPD. Although the association of relative eosinophilia with exacerbations in clinical trials may be population or circumstance specific, attention should be paid to the universal fact that BEC is generally considered to be a biomarker for COPD.

To our knowledge, eosinophilic predictor properties of mortality have been examined in a few cohort studies though the findings have been equivocal [16,41–43]. The prognostic value was reported to be positive in the CHAIN cohort, the BODE cohort [41] and in two studies including the Korean Obstructive Lung Disease (KOLD) cohort [16,42], all showing all-cause mortality was lower in patients with high eosinophil counts compared with those with values <300 cells/mm^3. Conversely, the findings were negative in the Initiatives BPCO French cohort which was in agreement with our own results (Table 4) [43].

Most cohort studies have continued to pay attention to the association between BEC and AECOPD [21], but they have also provided inconsistent results. While some have reported a positive association between BEC with COPD exacerbation frequency [18,44–46], other cohort studies have reported that there was no evidence of such an association (Table 4) [20,41,43,47]. Although most previous studies were designed to statistically compare the frequency of AECOPD between groups, the period from baseline to the first exacerbation is intended to be analysed using the univariate Cox proportional hazards model. Although the present study had the smallest sample size and thus be a potential weak point (Table 4), the following differences among the studies may also have both positive and negative influences on the results; cut-off levels of the BEC, methods of comparison, a definition of the AECOPD and study periods. Thus, it is not easy to compare the results obtained from different studies, and the relationship between BEC and AECOPD has not been established even in the literature.

On the other hand, some baseline clinical characteristics of COPD according to eosinophil levels have also been reported. Recent meta-analysis revealed that men, ex-smokers, individuals with a history of ischemic heart disease, and individuals with a higher body mass index (BMI) were at higher risk of eosinophilic COPD [48]. Regarding more COPD-specific health outcome measures, the findings of the SPIROMICS cohort showed that at baseline, the high blood eosinophil group had slightly increased airway wall thickness, higher SGRQ Symptom scores, and increased wheezing, but no evidence of an association with the other indices of COPD severity, such as emphysema measured by CT density or the CAT [47]. However, the Initiatives BPCO French cohort group reported that SGRQ Total score was more impaired in lower eosinophilic categories [43]. Korean investigators found that the high group had a longer six-minute walk distance, higher body mass index, lower emphysema index measured by CT and higher inspiratory capacity/total lung capacity ratio (IC/TLC) [42]. In the present study, from cross-sectional observation at baseline, the relationship between baseline characteristics and the BEC was negative and comparison of clinical indices between eosinophilic, intermediate and non-eosinophilic groups classified by BEC was not significantly different except for residual volume, a result that may be related to the Korean findings regarding IC/TLC.

Table 4. The predictive properties of blood eosinophil count in subjects with COPD in the literature.

Publication Year	Reference	First Author	The Name of the Cohort or Database	Association with Mortality	Association with AECOPD
2016	#45	Vedel-Krogh S	the Copenhagen General Population Study (n = 4.303)	N.A.	positive
2017	#41	Casanova C	the CHAIN cohort (n = 424) and BODE cohort (n = 308)	positive	negative
2017	#47	Hastie AT	the SPIROMICS cohort (n = 2.499)	N.A.	negative
2017	#43	Zysman M	Initiatives BPCO French cohort (n = 458)	negative	negative
2018	#16	Shin SH	the Korean Obstructive Lung Disease cohort (n = 299)	positive	N.A.
2018	#42	Oh YM	the Korean Obstructive Lung Disease cohort (n = 395) and COPD in Dusty Area cohort of Kangwon University Hospital (n = 234)	positive	N.A.
2018	#18	Yun JH	the COPDGene (n = 1.553) and ECLIPSE (n = 1.895) studies	N.A.	positive
2019	#46	Vogelmeier CF	the UK Clinical Practice Research Datalink (n = 15,364) and US Optum Clinformatics™ Data Mart databases (n = 139,465)	N.A.	positive
2020	#20	Miravitlles M	a primary care electronic medical record database in Catalonia, Spain (n = 57,209)	N.A.	negative
2020	#44	Tashiro H	retrospective medical records at the Saga University Hospital (n = 481)	N.A.	positive
The present study		Nishimura K	the hospital-based cohort at NCGG, Japan (n = 135)	negative	negative

AECOPD, acute exacerbation of COPD; n, the number of patients with COPD; N.A., not available.

While it has been reported that BEC is a consistently positive predictor of ICS response, both discriminative and predictive properties were all non-significant' in the present study. Our result may lead to doubts about the utility of BEC as a COPD biomarker. However, a couple of cohort studies have reported the same findings although there has been some inconsistency. Some recent review articles have suggested a possible reason in that randomized controlled trials focus more on frequent exacerbators than cohort studies including patients with no prior exacerbation history, and that differences in the included participants may produce the inconsistent results.

The longitudinal stability of BEC with a Fleiss' kappa of 0.464 and an ICC of 0.755 using log-transformed data was considered to be moderate or excellent, showing similar findings to previous studies. While Fleiss' kappa has not been reported, ICC has been reported to be 0.87–0.89 by Southworth et al. [17], 0.84 by Long et al. [19], 0.57 by Yun et al. [18] and 0.55 by Yoon et al. [23]. Although it is reported that log-transformed data were used to calculate ICC in the former two studies, this was not the case in the latter two manuscripts. The recent GOLD documents state that a threshold BEC of $\geq$300 /mm^3 can be used to identify patients with the greatest likelihood of treatment benefit with ICS. In the present study nearly 20% of patients were assigned to this eosinophilic group at every visit, but only 9% were continuously eosinophilic over three visits. Of 18 patients assigned to the eosinophilic group at Visit 1, one was changed to the non-eosinophilic group at Visit 2 and another one at Visit 3. This might suggest that 5–6 % of the eosinophilic group can be subsequently subject to change to the non-eosinophilic group. On the hand, almost a quarter were assigned to the non-eosinophilic group at Visit 1, but 13% remained in the non-eosinophilic throughout all visits. Of 20 patients assigned to the non-eosinophilic group at Visit 1, none were subsequently changed to the eosinophilic group at Visits 2 and 3.

Greulich T et al. also reported the absolute number and percentage of patients according to three groups defined by different thresholds (150 and 300 cells/mm^3) at Visits 1, 2 and 3 [24]. They reported that nearly 5% were continuously eosinophilic defined by $\geq$300 cells/mm^3 over three visits, but 26% remained non-eosinophilic defined by <150 cells/mm^3 throughout all visits. It may not be easy to compare the results between studies due to different thresholds. Therefore, in the use of BEC as a biomarker to guide the use of ICS therapy for exacerbation prevention, although the treatment choice should not be based on a one-off BEC measure, the first categorization may often be correct. Of course, the measurement should be repeated even after the determination of the ICS.

Some limitations of the present study should be mentioned. Most of the issues are related to the study design. First, the present study was limited by the small sample size and distinct male preponderance of the participants. Although the latter is typically observed in patients with COPD in Japan, generalization of these results to women with COPD may be uncertain. This study design might exhibit selection bias because we recruited only patients who could attend our outpatient clinic on a regular basis. It is likely that we did not include enough of those patients without any subjective symptoms who were unaware of having COPD, or patients who could not regularly attend our clinic due to the heavy physical burden. A small proportion of patients with severe or very severe COPD in the present single-centre study might cause a bias. Furthermore, Mathioudakis AG et al. recently conducted a post hoc analysis of ISOLDE and found that the BEC change after ICS administration may predict clinical response to ICS therapy [49]. This hypothesis may need validation in prospectively designed studies but is inconsistent with the present study which found that the BEC was not statistically different between patients taking ICS and those not taking ICS.

5. Conclusions

Previous cohort studies evaluating BEC as a mortality or exacerbation predictor have provided inconsistent results. Although most studies were designed to statistically compare the frequency of AECOPD between groups, the period from baseline to death, the first exacerbation and admission due to AECOPD are intended to be analysed using univariate Cox proportional hazards model in a hospital-based cohort study. Almost all the age, FEV_1, SGRQ Total and CAT Score were significantly strongly related to these types of events, but the predictive relationship between age and AECOPD did not reach statistical significance. Neither BEC nor the three different groups stratified by BEC were significant predictors of subsequent events. As for longitudinal stability, the ICC value was 0.755 using log-transformed data, suggesting excellent, and in the case of assigning with strata, Fleiss' kappa was calculated to be 0.464, indicating moderate agreement. The predictive properties of BEC may be limited in a real-world Japanese clinical setting. Attention must be paid to the fact that the longitudinal stability of the three strata is regarded as moderate.

Author Contributions: K.N. (Koichi Nishimura) contributed, as the principal investigator, to the study concept and design, analysis of the results and writing of the manuscript. M.K., R.S., M.M. and A.S. facilitated the conduct of the study and collection of data. K.N. (Kazuhito Nakayasu) contributed to statistical analysis. All authors have read and agreed to the published version of the manuscript.

Funding: Partial funding was provided by the Research Funding for Longevity Sciences (30-24) from the National Center for Geriatrics and Gerontology (NCGG), Japan.

Conflicts of Interest: The authors declare no conflict of interest.

Ethics Approval: Ethics approval for this study was granted by the Institutional Ethics Committee of the National Center for Geriatrics and Gerontology (No. 1138) (dated 18 May 2018).

Appendix A

Table A1. Comparison between ICS administered and unadministered patients.

		ICS Administered	ICS Unadministered	Mann–Whitney's U Test
		$n = 96$	$n = 39$	p-Value
Blood eosinophil count	/mm^3	220 ± 174	178 ± 124	0.306
FEV_1	Litres	1.53 ± 0.48	2.12 ± 0.46	<0.001
FEV_1	% pred.	64.2 ± 20.1	79.9 ± 16.4	<0.001
SGRQ Total Score	(0–100)	27.5 ± 17.1	16.3 ± 11.8	<0.001
CAT Score	(0–40)	11.0 ± 7.0	5.6 ± 4.6	<0.001

Data are presented as mean ± SD. ICS, inhaled corticosteroids; SGRQ, the St. George's Respiratory Questionnaire; CAT, the COPD Assessment Test. The numbers in parentheses denote possible score range.

Appendix B

Table A2. The distribution or f blood eosinophil count in 86 patients with COPD at Visits 1, 2 and 3.

	Mean (*)	SD (*)	Median (*)	Max (*)	Min (*)	75th Percentile (*)	25th Percentile (*)	Non-Eosinophilic Group	Intermediate Group	Eosinophilic Group
Visit 1	207	151	169	929	11	271	109	$n = 20$ (23.3%)	$n = 48$ (55.8%)	$n = 18$ (20.9%)
Visit 2	202	125	162	552	9	281	109	$n = 21$ (24.4%)	$n = 45$ (52.3%)	$n = 20$ (23.3%)
Visit 3	210	173	166	971	7	270	99	$n = 22$ (25.6%)	$n = 47$ (54.7%)	$n = 17$ (19.8%)

*: Unit is $/mm^3$

References

1. Barnes, P.J. Inhaled Corticosteroids Are Not Beneficial in Chronic Obstructive Pulmonary Disease. *Am. J. Respir. Crit. Care Med.* **2000**, *161*, 342–344. [CrossRef] [PubMed]
2. Calverley, P.M. Inhaled Corticosteroids Are Beneficial in Chronic Obstructive Pulmonary Disease. *Am. J. Respir. Crit. Care Med.* **2000**, *161*, 341–342. [CrossRef]
3. Postma, D.S.; Calverley, P. Inhaled corticosteroids in COPD: A case in favour. *Eur. Respir. J.* **2009**, *34*, 10–12. [CrossRef] [PubMed]
4. Suissa, S.; Barnes, P.J. Inhaled corticosteroids in COPD: The case against. *Eur. Respir. J.* **2009**, *34*, 13–16. [CrossRef] [PubMed]
5. Pascoe, S.; Locantore, N.; Dransfield, M.T.; Barnes, N.C.; Pavord, I.D. Blood eosinophil counts, exacerbations, and response to the addition of inhaled fluticasone furoate to vilanterol in patients with chronic obstructive pulmonary disease: A secondary analysis of data from two parallel randomised controlled trials. *Lancet Respir. Med.* **2015**, *3*, 435–442. [CrossRef]
6. Siddiqui, S.H.; Guasconi, A.; Vestbo, J.; Jones, P.; Agusti, A.; Paggiaro, P.; Wedzicha, J.A.; Singh, D. Blood Eosinophils: A Biomarker of Response to Extrafine Beclomethasone/Formoterol in Chronic Obstructive Pulmonary Disease. *Am. J. Respir. Crit. Care Med.* **2015**, *192*, 523–525. [CrossRef] [PubMed]
7. Bafadhel, M.; Peterson, S.; De Blas, M.A.; Calverley, P.M.; Rennard, S.I.; Richter, K.; Fagerås, M. Predictors of exacerbation risk and response to budesonide in patients with chronic obstructive pulmonary disease: A post-hoc analysis of three randomised trials. *Lancet Respir. Med.* **2018**, *6*, 117–126. [CrossRef]
8. Vestbo, J.; Papi, A.; Corradi, M.; Blazhko, V.; Montagna, I.; Francisco, C.; Cohuet, G.; Vezzoli, S.; Scuri, M.; Singh, D. Single inhaler extrafine triple therapy versus long-acting muscarinic antagonist therapy for chronic obstructive pulmonary disease (TRINITY): A double-blind, parallel group, randomised controlled trial. *Lancet* **2017**, *389*, 1919–1929. [CrossRef]
9. Lipson, D.A.; Barnhart, F.; Brealey, N.; Brooks, J.; Criner, G.J.; Day, N.C.; Dransfield, M.T.; Halpin, D.M.; Han, M.K.; Jones, C.E.; et al. Once-Daily Single-Inhaler Triple versus Dual Therapy in Patients with COPD. *N. Engl. J. Med.* **2018**, *378*, 1671–1680. [CrossRef]
10. Papi, A.; Vestbo, J.; Fabbri, L.; Corradi, M.; Prunier, H.; Cohuet, G.; Guasconi, A.; Montagna, I.; Vezzoli, S.; Petruzzelli, S.; et al. Extrafine inhaled triple therapy versus dual bronchodilator therapy in chronic obstructive pulmonary disease (TRIBUTE): A double-blind, parallel group, randomised controlled trial. *Lancet* **2018**, *391*, 1076–1084. [CrossRef]
11. Pascoe, S.; Barnes, N.; Brusselle, G.; Compton, C.; Criner, G.J.; Dransfield, M.T.; Halpin, D.M.G.; Han, M.K.; Hartley, B.; Lange, P.; et al. Blood eosinophils and treatment response with triple and dual combination therapy in chronic obstructive pulmonary disease: Analysis of the IMPACT trial. *Lancet Respir. Med.* **2019**, *7*, 745–756. [CrossRef]
12. The Japanese Respiratory Society. *The JRS Guidelines for the Management of Chronic Obstructive Pulmonary Disease*; The Japanese Respiratory Society location: Tokyo, Japan, 2018.
13. Barnes, N.; Ishii, T.; Hizawa, N.; Midwinter, D.; James, M.; Hilton, E.; Jones, P.W. The distribution of blood eosinophil levels in a Japanese COPD clinical trial database and in the rest of the world. *Int. J. Chronic Obstr. Pulm. Dis.* **2018**, *13*, 433–440. [CrossRef]
14. Landis, S.H.; Suruki, R.; Hilton, E.; Compton, C.; Galwey, N.W. Stability of Blood Eosinophil Count in Patients with COPD in the UK Clinical Practice Research Datalink. *COPD: J. Chronic Obstr. Pulm. Dis.* **2017**, *14*, 382–388. [CrossRef] [PubMed]
15. Oshagbemi, O.A.; Burden, A.M.; Braeken, D.C.W.; Henskens, Y.; Wouters, E.F.M.; Driessen, J.H.M.; Der Zee, A.H.M.-V.; De Vries, F.; Franssen, F.M.E. Stability of Blood Eosinophils in Patients with Chronic Obstructive Pulmonary Disease and in Control Subjects, and the Impact of Sex, Age, Smoking, and Baseline Counts. *Am. J. Respir. Crit. Care Med.* **2017**, *195*, 1402–1404. [CrossRef] [PubMed]
16. Shin, S.H.; KOLD Study Group; Park, H.Y.; Kang, D.; Cho, J.; Kwon, S.O.; Park, J.H.; Lee, J.S.; Oh, Y.-M.; Sin, D.D.; et al. Serial blood eosinophils and clinical outcome in patients with chronic obstructive pulmonary disease. *Respir. Res.* **2018**, *19*, 1–9. [CrossRef] [PubMed]
17. Southworth, T.; Beech, G.; Foden, P.; Kolsum, U.; Singh, D. The reproducibility of COPD blood eosinophil counts. *Eur. Respir. J.* **2018**, *52*, 1800427. [CrossRef]
18. Yun, J.H.; Lamb, A.; Chase, R.; Singh, D.; Parker, M.M.; Saferali, A.; Vestbo, J.; Tal-Singer, R.; Castaldi, P.J.; Silverman, E.K.; et al. Blood eosinophil count thresholds and exacerbations in patients with chronic obstructive pulmonary disease. *J. Allergy Clin. Immunol.* **2018**, *141*, 2037–2047.e10. [CrossRef] [PubMed]
19. Long, G.H.; Southworth, T.; Kolsum, U.; Donaldson, G.C.; Wedzicha, J.A.; Brightling, C.E.; Singh, D. The stability of blood Eosinophils in chronic obstructive pulmonary disease. *Respir. Res.* **2020**, *21*, 15. [CrossRef] [PubMed]

20. Miravitlles, M.; Monteagudo, M.; Solntseva, I.; Alcazar, B. Blood Eosinophil Counts and Their Variability and Risk of Exacerbations in COPD: A Population-Based Study. *Arch. Bronconeumol.* **2021**, *57*, 13–20. [CrossRef]
21. Singh, D.; Bafadhel, M.; Brightling, C.E.; Sciurba, F.C.; Curtis, J.L.; Martinez, F.J.; Pasquale, C.B.; Merrill, D.D.; Metzdorf, N.; Petruzzelli, S.; et al. Blood Eosinophil Counts in Clinical Trials for Chronic Obstructive Pulmonary Disease. *Am. J. Respir. Crit. Care Med.* **2020**, *202*, 660–671. [CrossRef] [PubMed]
22. Van Rossem, I.; Vandevoorde, J.; Hanon, S.; DeRidder, S.; Vanderhelst, E. The stability of blood eosinophils in stable chronic obstructive pulmonary disease: A retrospective study in Belgian primary care. *BMC Pulm. Med.* **2020**, *20*, 200. [CrossRef]
23. Yoon, J.-K.; Lee, J.-K.; Lee, C.-H.; Hwang, Y.I.; Kim, H.; Park, D.; Hwang, K.-E.; Kim, S.-H.; Jung, K.-S.; Yoo, K.H.; et al. The Association Between Eosinophil Variability Patterns and the Efficacy of Inhaled Corticosteroids in Stable COPD Patients. *Int. J. Chronic Obstr. Pulm. Dis.* **2020**, *15*, 2061–2070. [CrossRef] [PubMed]
24. Greulich, T.; Mager, S.; Lucke, T.; Koczulla, A.R.; Bals, R.; Fähndrich, S.; Jörres, R.A.; Alter, P.; Kirsten, A.-M.; Vogelmeier, C.F.; et al. Longitudinal stability of blood eosinophil count strata in the COPD COSYCONET cohort. *Int. J. Chronic Obstr. Pulm. Dis.* **2018**, *13*, 2999–3002. [CrossRef]
25. Kusunose, M.; Oga, T.; Nakamura, S.; Hasegawa, Y.; Nishimura, K. Frailty and patient-reported outcomes in subjects with chronic obstructive pulmonary disease: Are they independent entities? *BMJ Open Respir. Res.* **2017**, *4*, e000196. [CrossRef] [PubMed]
26. Miller, M.R.; Hankinson, J.; Brusasco, V.; Burgos, F.; Casaburi, R.; Coates, A.; Crapo, R.; Enright, P.; Van Der Grinten, C.P.M.; Gustafsson, P.; et al. Standardisation of spirometry. *Eur. Respir. J.* **2005**, *26*, 319–338. [CrossRef] [PubMed]
27. Sasaki, H.; Nakamura, M.; Kida, K.; Kambe, M.; Takahashi, K.; Fujimura, M. Reference values for spirogram and blood gas analysis in Japanese adults. *J. Jpn. Respir. Soc.* **2001**, *39*, S1–S17.
28. Jones, P.W.; Harding, G.; Berry, P.; Wiklund, I.; Chen, W.H.; Leidy, N.K. Development and first validation of the COPD Assessment Test. *Eur. Respir. J.* **2009**, *34*, 648–654. [CrossRef]
29. Tsuda, T.; Suematsu, R.; Kamohara, K.; Kurose, M.; Arakawa, I.; Tomioka, R.; Kawayama, T.; Hoshino, T.; Aizawa, H. Development of the Japanese version of the COPD Assessment Test. *Respir. Investig.* **2012**, *50*, 34–39. [CrossRef]
30. Jones, P.W.; Quirk, F.H.; Baveystock, C.M.; Littlejohns, P. A Self-complete Measure of Health Status for Chronic Airflow Limitation: The St. George's Respiratory Questionnaire. *Am. Rev. Respir. Dis.* **1992**, *145*, 1321–1327. [CrossRef]
31. Hajiro, T.; Nishimura, K.; Tsukino, M.; Ikeda, A.; Koyama, H.; Izumi, T. Comparison of Discriminative Properties among Disease-specific Questionnaires for Measuring Health-related Quality of Life in Patients with Chronic Obstructive Pulmonary Disease. *Am. J. Respir. Crit. Care Med.* **1998**, *157*, 785–790. [CrossRef]
32. Hyland, M.E.; Sodergren, S.C. Development of a new type of global quality of life scale, and comparison of performance and preference for 12 global scales. *Qual. Life Res.* **1996**, *5*, 469–480. [CrossRef] [PubMed]
33. Nishimura, K.; Oga, T.; Ikeda, A.; Hajiro, T.; Tsukino, M.; Koyama, H. Comparison of Health-Related Quality of Life Measurements Using a Single Value in Patients with Asthma and Chronic Obstructive Pulmonary Disease. *J. Asthma* **2008**, *45*, 615–620. [CrossRef]
34. Yorke, J.; Moosavi, S.H.; Shuldham, C.; Jones, P.W. Quantification of dyspnoea using descriptors: Development and initial testing of the Dyspnoea-12. *Thorax* **2009**, *65*, 21–26. [CrossRef]
35. Anthonisen, N.R.; Wright, E.C.; Hodgkin, J.E. Prognosis in Chronic Obstructive Pulmonary Disease 1–3. *Am. Rev. Respir. Dis.* **1986**, *133*, 14–20. [CrossRef]
36. Gupta, N.; Pinto, L.; Aaron, S.D.; Marciniuk, D.D.; O'Donnell, D.E.; Walker, B.L.; Fitzgerald, J.M.; Sin, D.; Marciniuk, D.; O'Donnell, D.; et al. The COPD Assessment Test. *Chest* **2016**, *150*, 1069–1079. [CrossRef]
37. Oga, T.; Nishimura, K.; Tsukino, M.; Sato, S.; Hajiro, T. Analysis of the Factors Related to Mortality in Chronic Obstructive Pulmonary Disease. *Am. J. Respir. Crit. Care Med.* **2003**, *167*, 544–549. [CrossRef]
38. Bikov, A.; Lange, P.; Anderson, J.A.; Brook, R.D.; Calverley, P.M.A.; Celli, B.R.; Cowans, N.J.; Crim, C.; Dixon, I.J.; Martinez, F.J.; et al. FEV1 is a stronger mortality predictor than FVC in patients with moderate COPD and with an increased risk for cardiovascular disease. *Int. J. Chronic Obstr. Pulm. Dis.* **2020**, *15*, 1135–1142. [CrossRef] [PubMed]
39. Cicchetti, D.V. Guidelines, criteria, and rules of thumb for evaluating normed and standardized assessment instruments in psychology. *Psychol. Assess.* **1994**, *6*, 284. [CrossRef]
40. Landis, J.R.; Koch, G.G. The Measurement of Observer Agreement for Categorical Data. *Biometrics* **1977**, *33*, 159. [CrossRef] [PubMed]
41. Casanova, C.; Celli, B.R.; De-Torres, J.P.; Martínez-Gonzalez, C.; Cosio, B.G.; Pinto-Plata, V.; De Lucas-Ramos, P.; Divo, M.; Fuster, A.; Peces-Barba, G.; et al. Prevalence of persistent blood eosinophilia: Relation to outcomes in patients with COPD. *Eur. Respir. J.* **2017**, *50*, 1701162. [CrossRef] [PubMed]
42. Oh, Y.-M.; Lee, K.S.; Hong, Y.; Hwang, S.C.; Kim, J.Y.; Kim, D.K.; Yoo, K.H.; Lee, J.-H.; Kim, T.-H.; Lim, S.Y.; et al. Blood eosinophil count as a prognostic biomarker in COPD. *Int. J. Chronic Obstr. Pulm. Dis.* **2018**, *13*, 3589–3596. [CrossRef] [PubMed]
43. Zysman, M.; Deslee, G.; Caillaud, D.; Chanez, P.; Escamilla, R.; Court-Fortune, I.; Nesme-Meyer, P.; Perez, T.; Paillasseur, J.-L.; Pinet, C.; et al. Relationship between blood eosinophils, clinical characteristics, and mortality in patients with COPD. *Int. J. Chronic Obstr. Pulm. Dis.* **2017**, *12*, 1819–1824. [CrossRef]
44. Tashiro, H.; Kurihara, Y.; Takahashi, K.; Sadamatsu, H.; Haraguchi, T.; Tajiri, R.; Takamori, A.; Kimura, S.; Sueoka-Aragane, N. Clinical features of Japanese patients with exacerbations of chronic obstructive pulmonary disease. *BMC Pulm. Med.* **2020**, *20*, 318. [CrossRef] [PubMed]

45. Vedel-Krogh, S.; Nielsen, S.F.; Lange, P.; Vestbo, J.; Nordestgaard, B.G. Blood Eosinophils and Exacerbations in Chronic Obstructive Pulmonary Disease. The Copenhagen General Population Study. *Am. J. Respir. Crit. Care Med.* **2016**, *193*, 965–974. [CrossRef] [PubMed]
46. Vogelmeier, C.F.; Kostikas, K.; Fang, J.; Tian, H.; Jones, B.; Morgan, C.L.; Fogel, R.; Gutzwiller, F.S.; Cao, H. Evaluation of exacerbations and blood eosinophils in UK and US COPD populations. *Respir. Res.* **2019**, *20*, 1–10. [CrossRef] [PubMed]
47. Hastie, A.T.; Martinez, F.J.; Curtis, J.L.; Doerschuk, C.M.; Hansel, N.N.; Christenson, S.; Putcha, N.; Ortega, V.E.; Li, X.; Barr, R.G.; et al. Association of sputum and blood eosinophil concentrations with clinical measures of COPD severity: An analysis of the SPIROMICS cohort. *Lancet Respir. Med.* **2017**, *5*, 956–967. [CrossRef]
48. Wu, H.-X.; Zhuo, K.-Q.; Cheng, D.-Y. Prevalence and Baseline Clinical Characteristics of Eosinophilic Chronic Obstructive Pulmonary Disease: A Meta-Analysis and Systematic Review. *Front. Med.* **2019**, *6*, 282. [CrossRef]
49. Mathioudakis, A.G.; Bikov, A.; Foden, P.; LaHousse, L.; Brusselle, G.; Singh, D.; Vestbo, J. Change in blood eosinophils following treatment with inhaled corticosteroids may predict long-term clinical response in COPD. *Eur. Respir. J.* **2020**, *55*, 1902119. [CrossRef] [PubMed]

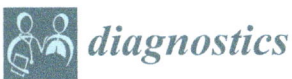

Article

Are Fatigue and Pain Overlooked in Subjects with Stable Chronic Obstructive Pulmonary Disease?

Koichi Nishimura [1,*], Kazuhito Nakayasu [2], Mio Mori [1], Ryo Sanda [1], Ayumi Shibayama [3] and Masaaki Kusunose [1]

1. Department of Respiratory Medicine, National Center for Geriatrics and Gerontology, Obu 474-8511, Japan; mio-mori@ncgg.go.jp (M.M.); ryo-sand@ncgg.go.jp (R.S.); kusunose@ncgg.go.jp (M.K.)
2. Data Research Section, Kondo Photo Process Co., Ltd., Osaka 543-0011, Japan; nakayasu@mydo-kond.co.jp
3. Department of Nursing, National Center for Geriatrics and Gerontology, Obu 474-8511, Japan; ayuminarita3@ncgg.go.jp
* Correspondence: koichi-nishimura@nifty.com; Tel.: +81-562-46-2311

Abstract: Although there have been many published reports on fatigue and pain in patients with chronic obstructive pulmonary disease (COPD), it is considered that these symptoms are seldom, if ever, asked about during consultations in Japanese clinical practice. To bridge this gap between the literature and daily clinical experience, the authors attempted to gain a better understanding of fatigue and pain in Japanese subjects with COPD. The Brief Fatigue Inventory (BFI) to analyse and quantify the degree of fatigue, the revised Short–Form McGill Pain Questionnaire 2 (SF-MPQ-2) for measuring pain and the Kihon Checklist to judge whether a participant is frail and elderly were administered to 89 subjects with stable COPD. The median BFI and SF-MPQ-2 Total scores were 1.00 [IQR: 0.11–2.78] and 0.00 [IQR: 0.00–0.27], respectively. They were all skewed toward the milder end of the respective scales. A floor effect was noted in around a quarter on the BFI and over half on the SF-MPQ-2. The BFI scores were significantly different between groups regarding frailty determined by the Kihon Checklist but not between groups classified by the severity of airflow limitation. Compared to the literature, neither fatigue nor pain are considered to be frequent, important problems in a real-world Japanese clinical setting, especially among subjects with mild to moderate COPD. In addition, our results might suggest that fatigue is more closely related to frailty than COPD.

Keywords: chronic obstructive pulmonary disease (COPD); the Brief Fatigue Inventory (BFI); the revised Short–Form McGill Pain Questionnaire 2 (SF-MPQ-2); the Kihon Checklist; fatigue; pain

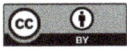

1. Introduction

Breathlessness is undoubtedly believed to be one of the most important perceptions experienced in subjects with chronic obstructive pulmonary disease (COPD). This is likely followed by coughing, as well as sputum production, symptoms which are described in most of the clinical practice guidelines [1]. Antoniu et al. has stated that the most prevalent, clinically significant extra-respiratory symptom was fatigue, which was reported in 95.7%, followed by pain in 74.5%, of patients hospitalized for a COPD exacerbation [2]. Upon closer examination of the published ranking lists of symptoms in subjects with stable COPD, Walke et al. reported that shortness of breath was followed by physical discomfort, fatigue, problems with appetite, anxiety, and pain [3]. Blinderman et al. found that lack of energy was in second place, while dry mouth was third, other pain (non-chest) was eighth, and chest pain twelfth [4]. Peters et al. also found that around half of patients with COPD had abnormal fatigue [5]. Guyatt et al. stipulated that one of the four domains should be named as fatigue during the development of the Chronic Respiratory Disease Questionnaire (CRQ), the first disease-specific tool for measuring quality of life globally [6]. Thus, although fatigue may be the second most frequent symptom that is reported after dyspnoea by subjects with COPD, it is a frequently ignored symptom in daily clinical practice [7].

Prevalence rates for pain have also been reported to be surprisingly high in subjects with COPD over the last decade [8–17]. In a systematic review published in 2015, Lee et al. reported that the pooled prevalence of pain in moderate to very severe COPD was 66% (95% CI, 44–85%) [18]. Despite these findings, we were unsure of their applicability to Japanese COPD patients as pain is seldom, if ever, asked about during consultations in this country; neither has it been included as a primary or secondary endpoint in most clinical trials. Notwithstanding, a recent review has stated that chronic pain warrants consideration within clinical practice guidelines for COPD [19].

When interviewing a candidate suspected of COPD, we often ask about breathlessness, cough, sputum and wheezing but not fatigue or pain. We are aware of only a small number of chest physicians in Japan who are of the opinion that these symptoms should be asked about in the consulting room. Although many published reports have studied fatigue and pain, it is unclear whether they should be checked during every examination. The aim of this study was to bridge the gap between the literature and daily clinical experience by gaining a better understanding of fatigue and pain in subjects with COPD. COPD is occasionally considered to be an accelerated aging disease since it is well known that aging of the lungs and COPD have many similarities and are sometimes difficult to distinguish from each other [20]. The frequency of fatigue, as well as breathlessness, is also thought to increase progressively with advancing years [21–25]. Since the age of patients with COPD is considered to be much older in Japan than in western countries [26], we hypothesized that aging could play a role in the appearance of symptoms such as fatigue and pain. Hence, the secondary purpose of the present study was to examine the prevalence of the above symptoms and their relationship with frailty in subjects with stable COPD [27,28].

2. Materials and Methods

2.1. Participants

We recruited 89 consecutive patients with stable COPD who attended the outpatient clinic at the Department of Respiratory Medicine of the National Center for Geriatrics and Gerontology (NCGG) from August 2018 to August 2020. The inclusion criteria were: (1) age more than 50 years; (2) smoking history exceeding 10 pack-years; (3) chronic fixed airflow limitation; (4) regular clinic attendance for more than half a year to avoid any changes induced by new medical interventions; (5) no uncontrolled co-morbidities and (6) no variation in treatment in the preceding four weeks. Chronic fixed airflow limitation was defined as a maximal ratio of forced expiratory volume in 1 s (FEV_1) to forced vital capacity (FVC) of under 0.7. All participants gave written informed consent.

2.2. Measurements

Baseline measurements of the participants' pulmonary function were taken in a single day. These comprised post-bronchodilator spirometry (CHESTAC-8800; Chest, Tokyo, Japan), residual volume (RV) using the closed-circuit helium method, and diffusing capacity for carbon monoxide (DL_{CO}) measured by the single-breath technique as reported by the American Thoracic Society and European Respiratory Society Task Force in 2005 [29]. Calculations of the predicted values for FEV_1 and vital capacity were performed as recommended by the Japan Respiratory Society [30].

2.3. Assessment of Fatigue, Pain, Breathlessness and Frailty

Validated Japanese versions of the following patient-reported outcome measurement tools were used in the present study; the Brief Fatigue Inventory (BFI) to analyse and quantify the degree of fatigue, the revised Short-Form McGill Pain Questionnaire (SF-MPQ-2) for measuring pain, the Dyspnoea-12 (D-12) to assess the severity of breathlessness and the Kihon Checklist to judge whether a participant is a frail elderly person. Participants were asked to complete these self-administered questionnaires under supervision in the aforementioned order (in a booklet form).

The BFI is a questionnaire originally designed to assess fatigue in cancer patients [31], but it has also been administered in subjects with COPD [13,32,33]. It consists of 9 numerical scales ranging from 0 to 10. The first three items in the BFI ask patients to rate the severity on an eleven-point rating scale with "0" being "no fatigue," and "10" being "fatigue as bad as you can imagine." An additional six items assess how greatly fatigue interferes with different aspects of daily activities. Each interference item is also scored on an eleven-point rating scale from "0" (does not interfere) to "10" (completely interferes). A mean BFI score is calculated as the mean of the intensity and interference items. The reliability of the Japanese version of the BFI was assessed by Okuyama et al. in the outpatient clinics of 6 oncology divisions and yielded a Cronbach's alpha value of 0.96 [34]. Furthermore, using the same tool, they reported that fatigue severity should be categorized as mild (1–3), moderate (4–6), and severe (7–10).

Although the Short Form McGill Pain Questionnaire (SF-MPQ) has been reported to be successfully administered in subjects with stable or exacerbated COPD to quantify the degree of pain [15], it was revised to the SF-MPQ-2 by adding symptoms relevant to neuropathic pain and by modifying the response format. It has thus become a tool for measuring both neuropathic and non–neuropathic pain [35,36]. The SF-MPQ-2 comprises 22 items investigating 4 dimensions: 6 items in Continuous pain, 6 in Intermittent pain, 6 in Neuropathic pain and 4 in Affective descriptors. Each item has an eleven-point numerical rating scale from 0 to 10. A lower score indicates less severe pain. For each of dimensions, scores are calculated by taking the mean of the item ratings included in the scale. The total score is calculated to be the mean of all SF-MPQ-2 item ratings. The internal consistency, or Cronbach's alpha coefficient, of the Japanese version of the SF-MPQ-2 has been reported to be 0.907 of the total score [36].

To assess the severity of dyspnoea, we used the D-12, which consists of twelve items (seven physical and five affective), each with a four-point grading scale (0–3), producing a Total Score (range 0–36, with higher scores representing more severe breathlessness) [37,38].

The authors also administered the Kihon Checklist to judge whether a participant is a frail elderly person [27,28,39,40]. This is a self-administered questionnaire comprising 25 items in a yes/no question format dealing with instrumental (3 items) and social activities of daily living (4 items), physical strength (5 items), nutritional status (2 items), oral function (3 items), cognitive status (3 items), and depression risk (5 items) [39,40]. One question concerns body mass index (BMI) and is usually self-scored but we calculated this using data collected at the same time as the pulmonary function tests. The Kihon Checklist total score, which is a sum of 25 answers, ranges from 0 (no frailty) to 25 (severe frailty) and patients' frailty status was classified as robust (0–3), pre-frail (4–7) and frail (8–25), as reported in the literature [28,39,40].

2.4. Statistical Methods

Cronbach's coefficient alpha was used to assess internal consistency. Score distributions of the tools were evaluated with the Shapiro-Wilk test and by inspection of histograms. Spearman's rank correlation tests were used to examine relationships between two sets of data and differences between groups were assessed by the Steel-Dwass test. All *p* values less than 0.05 were deemed to be statistically significant. The results are expressed as mean ± standard deviation (SD) with some exceptions in the tables.

3. Results

3.1. Characteristics of the Study Subjects

A total of 89 consecutive patients (83 men) with COPD, and a wide range of FEV_1 (69.8 ± 21.0%pred) were studied. Seventy-six subjects were former smokers while 13 were current smokers. Their demographic details, as well as the results of pulmonary function tests, are shown in Table 1. Using the classification of severity of airflow limitation of the

Global Initiative for Chronic Obstructive Lung Disease (GOLD) criteria [1], 30 subjects (33.7%) were in GOLD 1 (defined as $FEV_1 \geq 80\%$ predicted), 46 (51.7%) in GOLD 2 ($50\% \leq FEV_1 < 80\%$ predicted), 9 (10.1%) in GOLD 3 ($30\% \leq FEV_1 < 50\%$ predicted) and 4 (4.5%) in GOLD 4 ($FEV_1 < 30\%$ predicted).

Table 1. Baseline characteristics in 89 subjects with COPD and Spearman's rank correlation coefficients with Brief Fatigue Inventory (BFI) and Short-form McGill Pain Questionnaire (SF-MPQ)-2 Total scores.

		Median	IQR	Correlation Coefficients (Rs) with	
				BFI Score	SF-MPQ-2 Total Score
Age	years	78.0	74.0–82.0	0.165	0.162
BMI	kg/m^2	22.6	20.9–24.4	0.036	0.121
Cumulative Smoking	pack-years	60.0	39.0–79.5	0.152	0.112
SVC	Liters	3.22	2.54–3.62	−0.247 *	0.089
FEV_1	Liters	1.69	1.31–2.03	−0.305 **	0.062
FEV_1/FVC	%	58.9	48.6–64.2	−0.242 *	0.015
RV/TLC [1]	%	42.0	35.3–50.2	0.240 *	−0.039
DLco [2]	mL/min/mmHg	10.86	6.83–13.55	−0.260 *	0.116
PaO_2 [3]	mmHg	78.1	71.9–86.6	−0.171	−0.088
Kihon Checklist Total score	(0–25)	5	2–9	0.531 ***	0.293 **
BFI score	(0–10)	1.00	0.11–2.78	N.A.	0.233 *
SF-MPQ-2 Total score	(0–10)	0.00	0.00–0.27	0.233 *	N.A.
Continuous pain	(0–10)	0.00	0.00–0.00	0.226 *	0.753 ***
Intermittent pain	(0–10)	0.00	0.00–0.00	0.165	0.600 ***
Neuropathic pain	(0–10)	0.00	0.00–0.50	0.280 **	0.906 ***
Affective descriptors	(0–10)	0.00	0.00–0.00	0.401 ***	0.556 ***
D-12 Total score	(0–36)	0	0–1	0.319 **	0.045
D-12 Physical score	(0–21)	0	0–1	0.308 **	0.049
D-12 Affect score	(0–15)	0	0–0	0.409 ***	−0.005

***: $p < 0.001$, **: $p < 0.01$, *: $p < 0.05$, [1] $n = 88$, [2] $n = 86$, [3] two patients receiving oxygen; IQR, interquartile range; BFI, Brief Fatigue Inventory; SF-MPQ-2, Short-form McGill Pain Questionnaire 2; D-12, Dyspnoea-12. The numbers in parentheses denote possible score range.

3.2. Internal Consistency and Distribution of Scores

The internal consistency of the BFI, SF-MPQ-2 Total, and D-12 Total scores as assessed by Cronbach's coefficient alpha was excellent (alpha over 0.9) except for three subscales of the SF-MPQ-2, which ranged from 0.773 (both Continuous and Neuropathic pain) to 0.877 (Affective descriptors) (Table 2). Frequency distribution histograms of the scores obtained from the BFI, SF-MPQ-2 Total, and D-12 Total scores are shown in Figure 1 (Shapiro-Wilk test; $p < 0.001$, all). They were all skewed toward the milder end of the respective scales. A floor effect was noted in 22 subjects (24.7%) on the BFI, in 45 subjects (50.6%) on the SF-MPQ-2 and in 46 subjects (51.7%) on the D-12 Total (Table 2). According to Okayama's proposal, the BFI score was 1.00 or more, that is more than mild fatigue, in 47 (52.8%) out of the 89 subjects.

Table 2. The internal consistency and the score distribution in the questionnaires.

Patient-Reported Outcomes	Possible Score Range	Items (n)	Cronbach's α Coefficient	Score Distribution						Floor Effect	Ceiling Effect
				Mean	SD	Median	Max	Min	IQR		
BFI score	0–10	9	0.975	1.70	1.92	1.00	6.78	0.00	0.11–2.78	24.7%	0.0%
SF-MPQ-2 Total score	0–10	22	0.934	0.34	0.77	0.00	4.41	0.00	0.00–0.27	50.6%	0.0%
Continuous pain	0–10	6	0.733	0.35	0.81	0.00	3.50	0.00	0.00–0.00	76.4%	0.0%
Intermittent pain	0–10	6	0.906	0.23	0.75	0.00	5.00	0.00	0.00–0.00	83.1%	0.0%
Neuropathic pain	0–10	6	0.733	0.49	0.91	0.00	4.33	0.00	0.00–0.50	56.2%	0.0%
Affective descriptors	0–10	4	0.877	0.26	0.97	0.00	6.00	0.00	0.00–0.00	85.4%	0.0%
D-12 Total score	0–36	12	0.960	2.2	4.8	0	25	0	0–1	51.7%	0.0%
D-12 Physical score	0–21	7	0.925	1.6	3.0	0	15	0	0–1	51.7%	0.0%
D-12 Affect score	0–15	5	0.964	0.6	1.9	0	10	0	0–0	86.5%	0.0%

IQR, interquartile range; BFI, Brief Fatigue Inventory; SF-MPQ-2, Short-form McGill Pain Questionnaire 2; D-12, Dyspnoea-12.

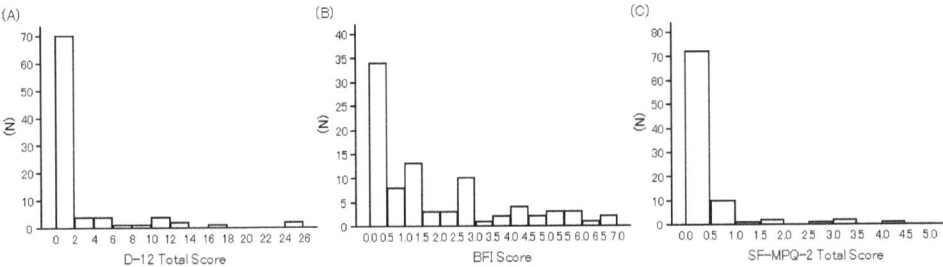

Figure 1. Frequency distribution histograms of the Dyspnoea-12 (D-12) Total Score (**A**), the Brief Fatigue Inventory (BFI) Score (**B**) and revised Short–Form McGill Pain Questionnaire 2 (SF-MPQ-2) Total Score (**C**) in 89 subjects with COPD. The D-12 is designed for measuring dyspnoea, BFI for fatigue and SF-MPQ-2 for pain. Higher scores in all the tools included herein indicate more severe impairment. The scores were all skewed toward the milder end of the respective scales.

3.3. Relationship between Fatigue and Physiological or Clinical Factors

Spearman's rank correlation coefficients (Rs) between the BFI score and physiological or clinical factors are shown in Table 1. The BFI score may be marginally characterized by negative correlations with airflow limitation as well as diffusion capacity and by a positive association with hyperinflation (absolute value of Rs = 0.240 to 0.305). The Kihon Checklist Total score correlated most strongly with the BFI score (Rs = 0.531). In a comparison between groups stratified by airflow limitation severity, the BFI score was significantly different between GOLD1 and GOLD 3+4 ($p < 0.05$, Steel-Dwass test) but not between GOLD 1 and 2 nor between GOLD 2 and 3+4 (Table 3). As categorized by the Kihon Checklist total score, there were significant differences in the BFI scores between groups with and without frailty (Table 4).

3.4. Relationship between Pain and Physiological or Clinical Factors

There were no statistically significant correlations between the SF-MPQ-2 Total scores and clinical and physiological factors (Table 1). However, there was a significant correlation between the SF-MPQ-2 Total scores and both the Kihon Checklist Total and BFI scores (Rs = 0.293 and 0.233, respectively). There were no significant differences between the scores obtained for the SF-MPQ-2 Total and its four subscales and the GOLD criteria (Table 3). In addition, the SF-MPQ-2 Total, Neuropathic pain and Affective descriptors' scores were significantly different between the robust and frail groups (Table 4).

3.5. Relationship between Dyspnoea and Physiological or Clinical Factors

The D-12 Total, Physical and Affect scores were significantly different between GOLD1 and GOLD3+4 and between GOLD2 and GOLD3+4 (Table 3), but there were no significant differences among the robust, pre-frail and frail groups (Table 4).

Table 3. Comparison of clinical indices and scores obtained from fatigue, pain and dyspnoea.

		GOLD 1 (n = 30)		GOLD 2 (n = 46)		GOLD 3+4 (n = 13)	
		Median	IQR	Median	IQR	Median	IQR
Age	years	77.0	71.0–82.0	78.0	74.0–84.0	77.0	73.0–80.0
BMI	kg/m^2	22.9	21.1–24.2	22.9	21.0–25.1	21.8	18.3–23.4
Cumulative Smoking	pack-years	46.5 **	30.0–61.0	66.5	50.0–86.0	50.0	40.0–75.0
SVC	Liters	3.50 **	3.22–4.05	3.08 §	2.44–3.57	2.39 ¶¶	2.14–2.61
FEV$_1$	Liters	2.18 ***	1.98–2.45	1.59 §§§	1.39–1.83	0.85 ¶¶	0.68–1.03
FEV$_1$/FVC	%	64.3 ***	59.8–66.5	56.8 §§§	48.8–62.5	35.2 ¶¶	33.1–40.8
RV/TLC [1]	%	35.4 **	32.4–43.5	43.4 §	37.6–49.3	52.4 ¶¶	50.2–55.9
DLco [2]	mL/min/mmHg	12.34	9.52–14.51	10.25	6.72–13.54	8.38 ¶	5.94–10.59
PaO$_2$ [3]	mmHg	79.0	76.0–87.8	80.4 §§	72.4–87.7	70.9 ¶¶	64.8–72.3
Kihon Checklist Total score	(0–25)	3	1–6	6	2–10	6	3–15
BFI score	(0–10)	0.44	0.00–1.89	1.00	0.00–2.78	2.89 ¶	1.00–5.67
SF-MPQ-2 Total score	(0–10)	0.02	0.00–0.45	0.05	0.00–0.27	0.00	0.00–0.23
Continuous pain	(0–10)	0.00	0.00–0.50	0.00	0.00–0.00	0.00	0.00–0.00
Intermittent pain	(0–10)	0.00	0.00–0.00	0.00	0.00–0.00	0.00	0.00–0.00
Neuropathic pain	(0–10)	0.00	0.00–0.50	0.00	0.00–0.67	0.00	0.00–0.33
Affective descriptors	(0–10)	0.00	0.00–0.00	0.00	0.00–0.00	0.00	0.00–0.00
D-12 Total score	(0–36)	0	0–1	1 §§	0–1	8 ¶¶	1–12
D-12 Physical score	(0–21)	0	0–1	1 §§	0–1	7 ¶¶	1–8
D-12 Affect score	(0–15)	0	0–0	0 §§	0–0	0 ¶¶	0–5

In comparison between GOLD1 and GOLD2 (Steel-Dwass test), ***: $p < 0.001$, **: $p < 0.01$. In comparison between GOLD1 and GOLD3+4 (Steel-Dwass test), §§§: $p < 0.001$, §§: $p < 0.01$, §: $p < 0.05$. In comparison between GOLD2 and GOLD3+4 (Steel-Dwass test), ¶¶: $p < 0.001$, ¶: $p < 0.01$, ¶: $p < 0.05$. [1] $n = 88$, [2] $n = 86$, [3] two patients receiving oxygen. IQR, interquartile range; BFI, Brief Fatigue Inventory; SF-MPQ-2, Short-form McGill Pain Questionnaire 2; D-12, Dyspnoea-12. The numbers in parentheses denote possible score range.

Table 4. Comparison of clinical indices and scores obtained from fatigue, pain and dyspnoea measurement tools between robust, pre-frail and frail groups classified by the Kihon Checklist in 89 subjects with COPD.

		Robust (n = 37)		Pre-Frail (n = 23)		Frail (n = 29)	
		Median	IQR	Median	IQR	Median	IQR
Age	years	75.0	69.0–80.0	77.0	75.0–82.0	79.0 ¶	76.0–85.0
BMI	kg/m²	22.7	21.1–24.2	21.7	19.6–24.2	23.0	21.1–24.8
Cumulative Smoking	pack-years	50.0	37.0–61.0	56.0	38.0–80.0	71.8 ¶	50.0–80.0
SVC	Liters	3.39	3.00–3.75	3.03	2.47–3.33	2.77 ¶	2.32–3.57
FEV$_1$	Liters	2.01	1.51–2.30	1.67	1.39–1.99	1.49 ¶¶	1.03–1.87
FEV$_1$/FVC	%	63.0	53.8–65.0	58.5	46.7–64.6	57.5	42.5–62.5
RV/TLC [1]	%	38.9 *	33.1–45.0	45.2	37.0–51.0	47.0 ¶	36.5–52.4
DLco [2]	mL/min/mmHg	12.92 **	10.93–15.01	8.85	6.34–11.97	9.52 ¶	5.04–12.55
PaO$_2$ [3]	mmHg	79.0	75.2–88.0	81.3 §	72.8–92.8	73.5 ¶	69.4–79.5
Kihon Checklist Total score	(0–25)	2 ***	1–2	5 §§§	5–6	11 ¶¶¶	9–15
BFI score	(0–10)	0.22 *	0.00–1.00	1.89 §	0.11–2.78	2.89 ¶¶¶	1.11–5.44
SF-MPQ-2 Total score	(0–10)	0.00	0.00–0.14	0.05	0.00–0.23	0.23 ¶	0.00–0.59
Continuous pain	(0–10)	0.00	0.00–0.00	0.00	0.00–0.00	0.00	0.00–0.83
Intermittent pain	(0–10)	0.00	0.00–0.00	0.00	0.00–0.17	0.00	0.00–0.00
Neuropathic pain	(0–10)	0.00	0.00–0.17	0.00	0.00–0.83	0.33 ¶	0.00–1.33
Affective descriptors	(0–10)	0.00	0.00–0.00	0.00	0.00–0.00	0.00 ¶	0.00–0.75
D-12 Total score	(0–36)	0	0–1	1	0–1	1	0–5
D-12 Physical score	(0–21)	0	0–1	1	0–1	1	0–5
D-12 Affect score	(0–15)	0	0–0	0	0–0	0	0–0

In comparison between robust and pre-frail (Steel-Dwass test), ***: $p < 0.001$, **: $p < 0.01$, *: $p < 0.05$. In comparison between pre-frail and frail (Steel-Dwass test), §§§: $p < 0.001$, §: $p < 0.05$. In comparison between robust and frail (Steel-Dwass test), ¶¶¶: $p < 0.001$, ¶¶: $p < 0.01$, ¶: $p < 0.05$. [1] $n = 88$, [2] $n = 86$, [3] two patients receiving oxygen. IQR, interquartile range; BFI, Brief Fatigue Inventory; SF-MPQ-2, Short-form McGill Pain Questionnaire 2; D-12, Dyspnoea-12. The numbers in parentheses denote possible score range.

4. Discussion

Despite many published reports that fatigue and pain are frequently observed, important symptoms in subjects with stable COPD, our findings could provide little support for these assertions. Since the BFI and SF-MPQ-2 Total scores were remarkably skewed toward the milder end of the scales and high floor effects were observed, we could not clearly establish whether fatigue and pain were common problems in the participants. However, the findings deserve careful and thoughtful consideration since the D-12 scores were also skewed toward the milder end despite dyspnoea being considered one of the COPD-specific symptoms. Although the authors carefully selected validated Japanese versions of PRO measurement tools with a history of use in COPD [10,15,33,34,36], there is the possibility that neither the BFI nor the SF-MPQ-2 performed adequately in the present study. Another possible reason for the differences with previously reported findings may be the fact that there were considerable numbers of subjects with relatively mild to moderate COPD as mean FEV_1 was 69.8 (21.0) %predicted. If more patients with severe COPD were enrolled, it is possible that the scores might have been more normally distributed.

The BFI scores were significantly different between groups as determined by frailty but not between groups classified by the severity of airflow limitation. This might suggest that fatigue is more closely related to frailty than COPD. Since it has been reported that fatigue is more frequently complained of in elderly people, frailty may lead to frequent development of fatigue in subjects with COPD as previously reported [21,22,24]. On the other hand, since dyspnoea was different between airflow limitation-based groups but not between frail and robust subjects, dyspnoea appears to be closely associated with COPD but only distantly with frailty.

To discuss the prevalence of fatigue as well as pain, standardized tools which have been psychometrically validated and reproducible should be used. Single, closed questions with a yes or no answer format are not recommended since they may lead to measurement errors such as overestimation of the specific symptoms. In addition to standardized instruments, reference scores for the general population or healthy non-smoking subjects are necessary to compare the prevalence between different groups. Although the authors performed a search for BFI reference scores, the knowledge and information obtained by preceding studies have been limited. Chen et al. first reported the reliability and validity of the BFI in subjects with COPD in 2016 [33]. They noted that the BFI score was 3.92 (2.51) at first administration and 3.66 (2.43) at the second in all COPD subjects. Furthermore, it was 3.53 (2.51) in 6 patients with mild COPD and there was no significant difference between groups classified by COPD severity. Chen et al. subsequently reported in 2018 that the BFI score was 4.3 (2.0) in subjects with COPD and that the prevalence of fatigue was 77% [13], but information on cut-off scores was not provided [41]. We found the prevalence of more than mild fatigue to be 52.8% but since this threshold of the BFI was originally developed by Okuyama et al. with results from cancer patients, our finding should be treated with caution [34]. The BFI score was 1.70 (1.92) across all subjects with COPD in the present study and we are unable to explain the wide variation in published findings. There is a wide range of reported prevalence of pain in the published literature. Maignan et al. reported that, in 50 subjects, the median SF-MPQ score (not SF-MPQ-2) was 29.7 [IQR: 13.6–38.2] at the AECOPD phase and 1.4 [0.0–11.2] at the stable phase, and 46 (92%) patients reported pain during AECOPD compared to 29 (58%) in the stable phase [15]. As in other reports, information on cut-off scores was not provided [15]. In the present study, the SF-MPQ-2 Total and subscale scores were likely to be very low in almost all subjects with COPD and the skewed distribution was quite pronounced. Although there have been some reports of concurrent pain and dyspnoea in subjects with COPD [13,42], the SF-MPQ-2 Total score was not significantly correlated with D-12 scores nor COPD severity in the present study. Therefore, we have formed the impression that chronic pain might be sporadically reported in some patients. We also note the possible role of coexisting illness although major comorbidity was excluded from the study.

Why do subjects with COPD experience fatigue or pain? Although an association between fatigue or pain and COPD has been frequently reported in the literature, only a few studies have explored the underlying mechanism of this association. It is considered that COPD is associated with systemic manifestations and comorbidities. One of the most important possible mechanisms is mediated by elevated levels of nonspecific inflammatory cytokines, which can derive from the lung and enter systemic circulation [43,44]. This 'overspill' hypothesis may include not only comorbidities such as skeletal muscle dysfunction, cardiovascular disease, osteoporosis, and diabetes but also fatigue and pain. The relationship with inflammatory markers requires further study. In addition, from the point of view of the 'overspill' hypothesis, comorbidities may have been one of the important outcomes. Since "no uncontrolled co-morbidities" was one of the inclusion criteria, most subjects with comorbidities were excluded from the present study. Data on comorbidities should have been collected in a quantitative way using the Charlson comorbidity index and this was a particular limitation of our study. Although it is reported that fibromyalgia should be distinguished from similar symptoms in subjects with severe asthma complaining of pain as well as extra-pulmonary asthma symptoms [45,46], it is believed that such patients were not included.

Some other limitations of the present study should be mentioned. First, frailty is considered to be one of the defining characteristics of aging and the developments of several concise measurement tools have consequently been reported in the literature. The Cardiovascular Health Study Index developed by Fried et al. has been the most widely used to assess this biological syndrome [27]. Other tools have also been validated, such as the Frailty Index and Clinical Frailty Scale using the cumulative deficit approach [47–49]. Although we used the Kihon Checklist to assess frailty status, variations in the classification of frailty between these screening tools might exist [50]. Second, there is the possibility of selection bias and care should be taken with any generalization of our results. Only patients who could regularly attend our outpatient clinic were recruited. Patients without any subjective symptoms and thus unaware of having COPD were not represented. Others who were unable to regularly attend our clinic due to the great physical effort involved would also have been excluded. This single-center study was also limited by its small sample size and the fact that most of the subjects were male, even though it includes most of the stable COPD patients who attended our hospital during the study period. The participants were overwhelmingly male because there were relatively few female COPD patients in Japan at the time. The study sample therefore reflects the reality of clinical COPD in our population.

5. Conclusions

In conclusion, the median BFI and SF-MPQ-2 Total scores were 1.00 [IQR: 0.11–2.78] and 0.00 [IQR: 0.00–0.27], respectively. They were all skewed toward the milder end of the respective scales. A floor effect was noted in around a quarter on the BFI and over half on the SF-MPQ-2. The BFI scores were significantly different between groups regarding frailty determined by the Kihon Checklist, but not between groups classified by the severity of airflow limitation. Compared to the literature, neither fatigue nor pain are considered to be frequent important problems in a real-world Japanese clinical setting, especially among subjects with mild to moderate COPD. In addition, our results might suggest that fatigue is more closely related to frailty than COPD.

Author Contributions: K.N. (Koichi Nishimura) contributed, as the principal investigator, to the study concept and design, analysis of the results, and writing of the manuscript. K.N. (Kazuhito Nakayasu) contributed to statistical analysis. M.M., R.S., A.S. and M.K. contributed to acquisition of data. All authors have read and agreed to the published version of the manuscript.

Funding: This study was partly supported by the Research Funding for Longevity Sciences (21-29) from the National Center for Geriatrics and Gerontology (NCGG), Japan.

Institutional Review Board Statement: The study was conducted according to the guidelines of the Declaration of Helsinki, and approved by the Institutional Ethics Committee of the National Center for Geriatrics and Gerontology (protocol code 1138-3 and 7 December 2020).

Informed Consent Statement: Committee of the National Center for Geriatrics and Gerontology (No. 1138-2). Informed consent was obtained from all subjects involved in the study.

Data Availability Statement: The datasets generated during and/or analyzed during the current study are available from the corresponding author on reasonable request.

Conflicts of Interest: The authors declare no conflict of interest.

References

1. Singh, D.; Agusti, A.; Anzueto, A.; Barnes, P.J.; Bourbeau, J.; Celli, B.R.; Criner, G.J.; Frith, P.; Halpin, D.M.G.; Han, M.; et al. Global Strategy for the Diagnosis, Management, and Prevention of Chronic Obstructive Lung Disease: The GOLD science committee report 2019. *Eur. Respir. J.* **2019**, *53*, 1900164. [CrossRef] [PubMed]
2. Antoniu, S.A.; Apostol, A.; Boiculese, L.V. Extra-respiratory symptoms in patients hospitalized for a COPD exacerbation: Prevalence, clinical burden and their impact on functional status. *Clin. Respir. J.* **2019**, *13*, 735–740. [CrossRef]
3. Walke, L.M.; Byers, A.L.; Tinetti, M.E.; Dubin, J.A.; McCorkle, R.; Fried, T.R. Range and severity of symptoms over time among older adults with chronic obstructive pulmonary disease and heart failure. *Arch. Intern. Med.* **2007**, *167*, 2503–2508. [CrossRef] [PubMed]
4. Blinderman, C.D.; Homel, P.; Billings, J.A.; Tennstedt, S.; Portenoy, R.K. Symptom distress and quality of life in patients with advanced chronic obstructive pulmonary disease. *J. Pain Symptom. Manag.* **2009**, *38*, 115–123. [CrossRef]
5. Peters, J.B.; Heijdra, Y.F.; Daudey, L.; Boer, L.M.; Molema, J.; Dekhuijzen, P.N.; Schermer, T.R.; Vercoulen, J.H. Course of normal and abnormal fatigue in patients with chronic obstructive pulmonary disease, and its relationship with domains of health status. *Patient Educ. Couns.* **2011**, *85*, 281–285. [CrossRef]
6. Guyatt, G.H.; Berman, L.B.; Townsend, M.; Pugsley, S.O.; Chambers, L.W. A measure of quality of life for clinical trials in chronic lung disease. *Thorax* **1987**, *42*, 773–778. [CrossRef]
7. Spruit, M.A.; Vercoulen, J.H.; Sprangers, M.A.G.; Wouters, E.F.M.; Consortium, F.A. Fatigue in COPD: An important yet ignored symptom. *Lancet Respir. Med.* **2017**, *5*, 542–544. [CrossRef]
8. Roberts, M.H.; Mapel, D.W.; Hartry, A.; Von Worley, A.; Thomson, H. Chronic pain and pain medication use in chronic obstructive pulmonary disease. A cross-sectional study. *Ann. Am. Thorac. Soc.* **2013**, *10*, 290–298. [CrossRef] [PubMed]
9. Janssen, D.J.; Wouters, E.F.; Parra, Y.L.; Stakenborg, K.; Franssen, F.M. Prevalence of thoracic pain in patients with chronic obstructive pulmonary disease and relationship with patient characteristics: A cross-sectional observational study. *BMC Pulm. Med.* **2016**, *16*, 47. [CrossRef] [PubMed]
10. Chen, Y.W.; Camp, P.G.; Coxson, H.O.; Road, J.D.; Guenette, J.A.; Hunt, M.A.; Reid, W.D. Comorbidities That Cause Pain and the Contributors to Pain in Individuals With Chronic Obstructive Pulmonary Disease. *Arch. Phys. Med. Rehabil.* **2017**, *98*, 1535–1543. [CrossRef] [PubMed]
11. Andenaes, R.; Momyr, A.; Brekke, I. Reporting of pain by people with chronic obstructive pulmonary disease (COPD): Comparative results from the HUNT3 population-based survey. *BMC Public Health* **2018**, *18*, 181. [CrossRef] [PubMed]
12. Bentsen, S.B.; Miaskowski, C.; Cooper, B.A.; Christensen, V.L.; Henriksen, A.H.; Holm, A.M.; Rustoen, T. Distinct pain profiles in patients with chronic obstructive pulmonary disease. *Int. J. Chron. Obstruct. Pulmon. Dis.* **2018**, *13*, 801–811. [CrossRef] [PubMed]
13. Chen, Y.W.; Camp, P.G.; Coxson, H.O.; Road, J.D.; Guenette, J.A.; Hunt, M.A.; Reid, W.D. A Comparison of Pain, Fatigue, Dyspnea and their Impact on Quality of Life in Pulmonary Rehabilitation Participants with Chronic Obstructive Pulmonary Disease. *COPD* **2018**, *15*, 65–72. [CrossRef] [PubMed]
14. De Miguel-Diez, J.; Lopez-de-Andres, A.; Hernandez-Barrera, V.; Jimenez-Trujillo, I.; Del Barrio, J.L.; Puente-Maestu, L.; Martinez-Huedo, M.A.; Jimenez-Garcia, R. Prevalence of Pain in COPD Patients and Associated Factors: Report From a Population-based Study. *Clin. J. Pain* **2018**, *34*, 787–794. [CrossRef]
15. Maignan, M.; Chauny, J.M.; Daoust, R.; Duc, L.; Mabiala-Makele, P.; Collomb-Muret, R.; Roustit, M.; Maindet, C.; Pepin, J.L.; Viglino, D. Pain during exacerbation of chronic obstructive pulmonary disease: A prospective cohort study. *PLoS ONE* **2019**, *14*, e0217370. [CrossRef]
16. Hansen, J.; Molsted, S.; Ekholm, O.; Hansen, H. Pain Prevalence, Localization, and Intensity in Adults with and without COPD: Results from the Danish Health and Morbidity Survey (a Self-reported Survey). *Int. J. Chron. Obstruct. Pulmon. Dis.* **2020**, *15*, 3303–3311. [CrossRef]
17. Raphaely, R.A.; Mongiardo, M.A.; Goldstein, R.L.; Robinson, S.A.; Wan, E.S.; Moy, M.L. Pain in Veterans with COPD: Relationship with physical activity and exercise capacity. *BMC Pulm. Med.* **2021**, *21*, 238. [CrossRef] [PubMed]
18. Lee, A.L.; Harrison, S.L.; Goldstein, R.S.; Brooks, D. Pain and its clinical associations in individuals with COPD: A systematic review. *Chest* **2015**, *147*, 1246–1258. [CrossRef]
19. Lewthwaite, H.; Williams, G.; Baldock, K.L.; Williams, M.T. Systematic Review of Pain in Clinical Practice Guidelines for Management of COPD: A Case for Including Chronic Pain? *Healthcare* **2019**, *7*, 15. [CrossRef] [PubMed]

20. MacNee, W. Is Chronic Obstructive Pulmonary Disease an Accelerated Aging Disease? *Ann. Am. Thorac. Soc.* **2016**, *13*, S429–S437. [CrossRef]
21. Liao, S.; Ferrell, B.A. Fatigue in an older population. *J. Am. Geriatr. Soc.* **2000**, *48*, 426–430. [CrossRef]
22. Toye, C.; White, K.; Rooksby, K. Fatigue in frail elderly people. *Int. J. Palliat. Nurs.* **2006**, *12*, 202–208. [CrossRef]
23. Bowden, J.A.; To, T.H.; Abernethy, A.P.; Currow, D.C. Predictors of chronic breathlessness: A large population study. *BMC Public Health* **2011**, *11*, 33. [CrossRef]
24. Zengarini, E.; Ruggiero, C.; Perez-Zepeda, M.U.; Hoogendijk, E.O.; Vellas, B.; Mecocci, P.; Cesari, M. Fatigue: Relevance and implications in the aging population. *Exp. Gerontol.* **2015**, *70*, 78–83. [CrossRef] [PubMed]
25. Smith, A.K.; Currow, D.C.; Abernethy, A.P.; Johnson, M.J.; Miao, Y.; Boscardin, W.J.; Ritchie, C.S. Prevalence and Outcomes of Breathlessness in Older Adults: A National Population Study. *J. Am. Geriatr. Soc.* **2016**, *64*, 2035–2041. [CrossRef]
26. Fukuchi, Y.; Nishimura, M.; Ichinose, M.; Adachi, M.; Nagai, A.; Kuriyama, T.; Takahashi, K.; Nishimura, K.; Ishioka, S.; Aizawa, H.; et al. COPD in Japan: The Nippon COPD Epidemiology study. *Respirology* **2004**, *9*, 458–465. [CrossRef]
27. Fried, L.P.; Tangen, C.M.; Walston, J.; Newman, A.B.; Hirsch, C.; Gottdiener, J.; Seeman, T.; Tracy, R.; Kop, W.J.; Burke, G.; et al. Frailty in older adults: Evidence for a phenotype. *J. Gerontol. A Biol. Sci. Med. Sci.* **2001**, *56*, M146–M156. [CrossRef]
28. Kusunose, M.; Oga, T.; Nakamura, S.; Hasegawa, Y.; Nishimura, K. Frailty and patient-reported outcomes in subjects with chronic obstructive pulmonary disease: Are they independent entities? *BMJ Open Respir. Res.* **2017**, *4*, e000196. [CrossRef] [PubMed]
29. Miller, M.R.; Hankinson, J.; Brusasco, V.; Burgos, F.; Casaburi, R.; Coates, A.; Crapo, R.; Enright, P.; van der Grinten, C.P.; Gustafsson, P.; et al. Standardisation of spirometry. *Eur. Respir. J.* **2005**, *26*, 319–338. [CrossRef] [PubMed]
30. Sasaki, H.; Nakamura, M.; Kida, K.; Kambe, M.; Takahashi, K.; Fujimura, M. Reference values for spirogram and blood gas analysis in Japanese adults. *J. Jpn. Respir. Soc.* **2001**, *39*, S1–S17.
31. Mendoza, T.R.; Wang, X.S.; Cleeland, C.S.; Morrissey, M.; Johnson, B.A.; Wendt, J.K.; Huber, S.L. The rapid assessment of fatigue severity in cancer patients: Use of the Brief Fatigue Inventory. *Cancer* **1999**, *85*, 1186–1196. [CrossRef]
32. Doyle, T.; Palmer, S.; Johnson, J.; Babyak, M.A.; Smith, P.; Mabe, S.; Welty-Wolf, K.; Martinu, T.; Blumenthal, J.A. Association of anxiety and depression with pulmonary-specific symptoms in chronic obstructive pulmonary disease. *Int. J. Psychiatry Med.* **2013**, *45*, 189–202. [CrossRef]
33. Chen, Y.W.; Coxson, H.O.; Reid, W.D. Reliability and Validity of the Brief Fatigue Inventory and Dyspnea Inventory in People With Chronic Obstructive Pulmonary Disease. *J. Pain Symptom. Manag.* **2016**, *52*, 298–304. [CrossRef] [PubMed]
34. Okuyama, T.; Wang, X.S.; Akechi, T.; Mendoza, T.R.; Hosaka, T.; Cleeland, C.S.; Uchitomi, Y. Validation study of the Japanese version of the brief fatigue inventory. *J. Pain Symptom Manag.* **2003**, *25*, 106–117. [CrossRef]
35. Dworkin, R.H.; Turk, D.C.; Revicki, D.A.; Harding, G.; Coyne, K.S.; Peirce-Sandner, S.; Bhagwat, D.; Everton, D.; Burke, L.B.; Cowan, P.; et al. Development and initial validation of an expanded and revised version of the Short-form McGill Pain Questionnaire (SF-MPQ-2). *Pain* **2009**, *144*, 35–42. [CrossRef] [PubMed]
36. Maruo, T.; Nakae, A.; Maeda, L.; Kenrin, S.; Takahashi, K.; Morris, S.; Hosomi, K.; Kanatani, H.; Matsuzaki, T.; Saitoh, Y. Validity, reliability, and assessment sensitivity of the Japanese version of the short-form McGill pain questionnaire 2 in Japanese patients with neuropathic and non-neuropathic pain. *Pain Med.* **2014**, *15*, 1930–1937. [CrossRef] [PubMed]
37. Yorke, J.; Moosavi, S.H.; Shuldham, C.; Jones, P.W. Quantification of dyspnoea using descriptors: Development and initial testing of the Dyspnoea-12. *Thorax* **2010**, *65*, 21–26. [CrossRef]
38. Nishimura, K.; Oga, T.; Nakayasu, K.; Taniguchi, H.; Ogawa, T.; Watanabe, F.; Arizono, S.; Kusunose, M.; Sanda, R.; Shibayama, A.; et al. Comparison between tools for measuring breathlessness: Cross-sectional validation of the Japanese version of the Dyspnoea-12. *Clin. Respir. J.* **2021**, *65*, 21–26. [CrossRef]
39. Arai, H.; Satake, S. English translation of the Kihon Checklist. *Geriatr. Gerontol. Int.* **2015**, *15*, 518–519. [CrossRef] [PubMed]
40. Satake, S.; Senda, K.; Hong, Y.J.; Miura, H.; Endo, H.; Sakurai, T.; Kondo, I.; Toba, K. Validity of the Kihon Checklist for assessing frailty status. *Geriatr. Gerontol. Int.* **2016**, *16*, 709–715. [CrossRef]
41. Ebadi, Z.; Goertz, Y.M.J.; Van Herck, M.; Janssen, D.J.A.; Spruit, M.A.; Burtin, C.; Thong, M.S.Y.; Muris, J.; Otker, J.; Looijmans, M.; et al. The prevalence and related factors of fatigue in patients with COPD: A systematic review. *Eur. Respir. Rev.* **2021**, *30*, 200298. [CrossRef] [PubMed]
42. Moy, M.L.; Daniel, R.A.; Cruz Rivera, P.N.; Mongiardo, M.A.; Goldstein, R.L.; Higgins, D.M.; Salat, D.H. Co-occurrence of pain and dyspnea in Veterans with COPD: Relationship to functional status and a pilot study of neural correlates using structural and functional magnetic resonance imaging. *PLoS ONE* **2021**, *16*, e0254653. [CrossRef]
43. Barnes, P.J. Chronic obstructive pulmonary disease: Effects beyond the lungs. *PLoS Med.* **2010**, *7*, e1000220. [CrossRef] [PubMed]
44. Sinden, N.J.; Stockley, R.A. Systemic inflammation and comorbidity in COPD: A result of 'overspill' of inflammatory mediators from the lungs? Review of the evidence. *Thorax* **2010**, *65*, 930–936. [CrossRef]
45. Martinez-Moragon, E.; Plaza, V.; Torres, I.; Rosado, A.; Urrutia, I.; Casas, X.; Hinojosa, B.; Blanco-Aparicio, M.; Delgado, J.; Quirce, S. Fibromyalgia as a cause of uncontrolled asthma: A case–control multicenter study. *Curr. Med. Res. Opin.* **2017**, *33*, 2181–2186. [CrossRef]
46. Hyland, M.E.; Lanario, J.W.; Wei, Y.; Jones, R.C.; Masoli, M. Evidence for similarity in symptoms and mechanism: The extra-pulmonary symptoms of severe asthma and the polysymptomatic presentation of fibromyalgia. *Immun. Inflamm. Dis.* **2019**, *7*, 239–249. [CrossRef] [PubMed]

47. Mitnitski, A.B.; Mogilner, A.J.; Rockwood, K. Accumulation of deficits as a proxy measure of aging. *Sci. World J.* **2001**, *1*, 323–336. [CrossRef]
48. Rockwood, K.; Song, X.; MacKnight, C.; Bergman, H.; Hogan, D.B.; McDowell, I.; Mitnitski, A. A global clinical measure of fitness and frailty in elderly people. *CMAJ* **2005**, *173*, 489–495. [CrossRef]
49. Brummel, N.E.; Bell, S.P.; Girard, T.D.; Pandharipande, P.P.; Jackson, J.C.; Morandi, A.; Thompson, J.L.; Chandrasekhar, R.; Bernard, G.R.; Dittus, R.S.; et al. Frailty and Subsequent Disability and Mortality Among Patients With Critical Illness. *Am. J. Respir. Crit. Care Med.* **2016**, *196*, 64–72. [CrossRef]
50. Singer, J.P.; Lederer, D.J.; Baldwin, M.R. Frailty in Pulmonary and Critical Care Medicine. *Ann. Am. Thorac. Soc.* **2016**, *13*, 1394–1404. [CrossRef]

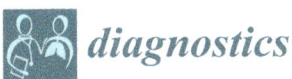

Article

Diagnostic Value of the Neutrophil-to-Lymphocyte Ratio (NLR) and Platelet-to-Lymphocyte Ratio (PLR) in Various Respiratory Diseases: A Retrospective Analysis

Milena-Adina Man [1,†], Lavinia Davidescu [2,†], Nicoleta-Stefania Motoc [1,*], Ruxandra-Mioara Rajnoveanu [1], Cosmina-Ioana Bondor [3], Carmen-Monica Pop [1] and Claudia Toma [4]

1. Department of Medical Sciences, Pulmonology, "Iuliu Hatieganu" University of Medicine and Pharmacy, 400000 Cluj Napoca, Romania; manmilena50@yahoo.com (M.-A.M.); andra_redro@yahoo.com (R.-M.R.); cpop@umfcluj.ro (C.-M.P.)
2. Faculty of Medicine and Pharmacy, University of Oradea, 410087 Oradea, Romania; lavinia.davidescu@yahoo.com
3. Department of Medical Biostatistics, "Iuliu Hatieganu" University of Medicine and Pharmacy, 400000 Cluj Napoca, Romania; cosmina_ioana@yahoo.com
4. Faculty of Medicine, Carol Davila University of Medicine and Pharmacy, 020021 Bucharest, Romania; claudia.toma@yahoo.co.uk
* Correspondence: motoc_nicoleta@yahoo.com; Tel.: +40-744-663-750
† These authors contributed equally to this work.

Abstract: The neutrophil-to-lymphocyte ratio (NLR) and platelet-to-lymphocyte (PLR) ratio are two extensively used inflammatory markers that have been proved very useful in evaluating inflammation in several diseases. The present article aimed to investigate if they have any value in distinguishing among various respiratory disorders. One hundred and forty-five patients with coronavirus disease 2019 (COVID-19), 219 patients with different chronic respiratory diseases (interstitial lung disease, obstructive sleep apnea(OSA)-chronic obstructive pulmonary disease (COPD) overlap syndrome, bronchiectasis) and 161 healthy individuals as a control group were included in the study. While neither NLR nor PLR had any power in differentiating between various diseases, PLR was found to be significant but poor as a diagnostic test when the control group was compared with the OSA-COPD group. NLR was found to be significant but poor as a diagnostic test when we compared the control group with all three groups (separately): the OSA-COPD group; interstitial lung disease group, and bronchiectasis group. NLR and PLR had poor power to discriminate between various respiratory diseases and cannot be used in making the differential diagnosis.

Keywords: respiratory diseases; inflammatory markers; neutrophil-to-lymphocyte ratio (NLR); platelet-to-lymphocyte (PLR)

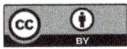

1. Introduction

The neutrophil-to-lymphocyte ratio (NLR) and platelet-to-lymphocyte ratio (PLR) are systemic inflammatory responses markers. Inflammation induces an increase in neutrophils, and platelet count accompanied by a decrease in lymphocyte count, making their ratios a valuable tool in indirectly evaluating both inflammatory status as well as cell-mediated immunity [1]. Platelets have a crucial role in the immune system due to the surface receptors that recognize pathogens and immune complexes. Activated and adherent platelets release cytokines, including chemokines that stimulate the cells' recruitment [1,2]. NLR and PLR, together or separately, have been evaluated in several conditions such as malignancies (hematological malignancies included), respiratory diseases, gastrointestinal and cardiovascular (acute coronary syndrome, intracerebral hemorrhage), systemic diseases, and lately, coronavirus disease 2019 (COVID-19) [3]. Higher values have been associated with more severe forms of the disease and worse prognosis [1–10]. Higher values have also been recorded in acute versus chronic conditions [6,8], and the most elevated values have been reported in the presence of bacteremia [7]. As far as respiratory diseases go, these markers have been studied in stable chronic obstructive pulmonary disease (COPD), acute exacerbation of COPD, sleep apnea, bronchiectasis, interstitial lung diseases, and in the last two years in COVID-19 [3–10]. Although they have been assessed in several respiratory disorders, few studies have evaluated their diagnostic value among different respiratory diseases. Additionally, a cutoff value is still to be found. Therefore, this study aimed to assess the diagnostic value of NLR and PLR in various respiratory diseases and, if possible, to find a cutoff value for each respiratory disease.

2. Materials and Methods

2.1. Study Design

The present paper was a phase II retrospective diagnostic test study of a group of several patient databases from our hospital, a clinical teaching hospital in one of the central cities of Romania, considered as cases. All patients that had neutrophil, lymphocyte, and platelet data in their files (both neutrophil-to-lymphocyte ratio and platelet-to-lymphocyte ratio could be calculated) were included in the study. Some patients were included in other studies [3,8–11]. In total, 364 patients with various respiratory diseases (145 with COVID-19-data for the entire group were published before in [3]), 36 patients with interstitial lung diseases, 98 patients with bronchiectasis, and 85 with obstructive sleep apnea (OSA)–chronic obstructive pulmonary disease (COPD) overlap syndrome) and 161 healthy individuals as the study control group were included. The control group included healthy medical staff that presented for annual evaluation. They were clinically examined and had blood tests performed. The patients were evaluated before the COVID-19 pandemic started. Data were collected between 2017–2021.

COVID-19 diagnostics were confirmed using real-time reverse-transcriptase polymerase-chain-reaction (RT-PCR) assay to test nasal and pharyngeal swab specimens according to World Health Organization (WHO) guidance. Patients' characteristics and description data were already published, and they will not be referred to in the present paper [3]. Interstitial lung disease was diagnosed according to international criteria and after a multidisciplinary meeting [9], bronchiectasis was confirmed by a chest computer scan (chest-CT) [3], and OSA–COPD overlap syndrome was defined as the presence of OSA (positive ventilatory polygraphy after the recommendations of the American Sleep Society 2007) and COPD (GOLD 2020) in the same patient [10,11]. We excluded patients with other diseases that could cause high NLR and PLR values: patients with any type of cancer, hematological diseases, severe cardiac disease (NYHA III and IV cardiac failure, recent myocardial infarction in last 3 months, unstable arrhythmia), liver disease and systemic diseases. The control group was clinically examined by a full-fledged physician and had blood tests performed. All blood tests were performed in the hospital laboratory with standard procedures. The NLR ratio was defined as the absolute count of neutrophils divided by the absolute count of lymphocytes. The PLR was defined as the absolute count of platelets divided by the absolute count of lymphocytes. CRP (C-reactive protein) and ESR (erythrocyte sedimentation rate) were also determined.

The study protocol was reviewed and approved by the Ethics Committee for Scientific Research of the Hospital 232, approved on 03 March 2020.

2.2. Statistical Method

Statistical analysis was performed using IBM SPSS STATISTICS 25.0 application. Medians (25th percentiles; 75th percentiles) were calculated for quantitative variables with a non-normal distribution. Normal distribution was tested with the Shapiro–Wilk test. The comparison of multiple means was performed using an Anova test for independent samples with equal variations depending on the Levene test result. In cases where equal variations were not found, the Kruskal–Wallis test was used. Post-hoc analysis was performed to correct type I error with Sheffe's method respective to the Bonferroni method. Frequencies were compared with the Chi-square test. For the best cutoff to discriminate between two groups in the case of a quantitative variable, the ROC (receiver operating characteristics) curve analysis was used. The area under the ROC curve (AUC) was reported. AUC was considered statistically significant when compared with 50% of the square of the area, in which case it meant that the considered parameter had the power to discriminate between the tested groups. The higher the AUC, the better the discrimination parameter. The optimal cutoff was considered when the Youden index was maximized, i.e., sensitivity (Se) plus specificity (Sp) minus 1. To evaluate the accuracy of the diagnostic test, the traditional academic point system was considered: 0.90–1 = excellent, 0.80–0.90 = good, 0.70–0.80 = fair, 0.60–0.70 = poor, 0.50–0.60 = fail [12].Other cutoffs were considered also. A p-value < 0.05 was taken to indicate statistical significance.

3. Results

We included in the study 145 patients with COVID-19, 219 patients with different chronic respiratory diseases (interstitial lung disease, OSA-COPD overlap syndrome, bronchiectasis,), and 161 healthy individuals in a control group. Their age, gender, and blood characteristics are shown in Table 1. After adjusting for type one error, NLR was significantly higher in both groups with respiratory disease compared with the control group, but with no statistically significant difference between the two groups. On the other hand, PLR was significantly different between groups. The chronic respiratory disease group was significantly lower than the control group, in which PLR was considerably lower than the COVID-19 group; statistical significance was maintained even after adjusting for type one error. White blood cells(WBC) and neutrophils were higher in the chronic respiratory disease group than in the other two groups, which were not significantly different. Lymphocytes were lower in the COVID-19 group compared with the other two groups, which were not significantly different. Platelets, CRP and ESR were statistically significantly higher in the chronic respiratory disease group compared with the control group, but we did not find a significant difference between the COVID-19 group and the controls, or between the COVID-19 group and chronic respiratory disease group. The chronic respiratory disease group was significantly older than the COVID-19 group, which was considerably older than the control group. Gender was quite different; more male patients were in the chronic respiratory disease group compared with the COVID-19 group, in which there were statistically significantly more males than in the control group.

PLR was found to be significant as a diagnostic test between the COVID-19 group and the other groups. We compared the COVID-19 group versus control group (Figure 1a), COVID-19 group versus chronic respiratory disease group (Figure 1b), and when we summed up the chronic respiratory disease group and control, also (Figure 1c). NLR was poor when discriminating between the COVID-19 and control group, but with statistic significance (Figure 1a); it failed to discriminate in the case of the COVID-19 group versus chronic respiratory disease group (AUC = 0.501, p = 0.975) (Figure 1b) and also when we summed the chronic respiratory disease group and control (AUC = 0.553, p = 0.060) (Figure 1c). PLR was poor when discriminating between the COVID-19 and control group, but with statistic significance (Figure 1a), poor also at discriminating in the case of the COVID-19 group versus chronic respiratory disease group (Figure 1b), and also when we summed the chronic respiratory disease group and control (Figure 1c).

Table 1. The characteristics of the chronic disease group compared with the control group and COVID-19 group (n = 145, data not presented, as they have already been published [3]).

	COVID-19 Group (n = 145)	Other Disease Group (n = 219)	Control Group (n = 161)	p
AGE	46 (33.5, 57) [a,b]	62 (52.5, 68) [c]	40 (29, 48)	<0.001 **
Males, number (%)	69 (47.6) [a,b]	138 (65.1) [c]	33 (20.5)	<0.001 **
NLR	2.56 (1.72, 3.79) [b]	2.48 (1.85, 3.49) [c]	2.03 (1.59, 2.59)	<0.001 **
PLR	151.85 (112.86, 211.59) [a,b]	114.1 (92.31, 150.13)	125.37 (101.78, 156.71)	<0.001 **
White blood cells	5.95 (4.89, 8.05) [a]	7.77 (6.25, 9.45) [c]	6.3 (5.54, 7.78)	<0.001 **
Lymphocytes ($10^3/\mu L$)	1.56 (1.2, 2.03) [a,b]	1.93 (1.52, 2.35)	1.96 (1.62, 2.34)	<0.001 *
Neutrophils ($10^3/\mu L$)	4.01 (2.94, 5.5) [a]	4.94 (3.94, 6.34) [c]	3.96 (3.19, 4.94)	<0.001 **
Thrombocytes (X10^3)	249 (183, 299)	231 (189, 273.5) [c]	247 (222, 279)	0.016 **
CRP	3.25 (0.99, 18.7)	4.9 (2.2, 11.8) [c]	2.55 (1.5, 4.4)	0.006 **
ESR	12 (5.5, 30)	15 (7, 28) [c]	11 (6, 15)	0.003 **

* p from Anova test between three groups: the chronic disease group, the control group, and the COVID-19 group [3] (data not shown); ** p from Kruskal–Wallis test between three groups: the chronic disease group the control group and the COVID-19 group [3] NLR—neutrophil-to-lymphocyte ratio; PLR—platelet-to-lymphocyte ratio; CRP—C-reactive protein; ESR—erythrocyte sedimentation rate; [a]—adjusted p < 0.05 for COVID-19 group compared with other disease group; [b]—adjusted p < 0.05 for COVID-19 group compared with control group; [c]—adjusted p < 0.05 for other disease group compare with control group.

The optimum cutoff for PLR was found to be 182.48 between the COVID-19 group and control group, 144.95 between the COVID-19 group and chronic respiratory disease group and 157.23 between the COVID-19 group and the other two groups (Table 2), and for NLR, was 3.02 between the COVID-19 group and control group.

PLR and NLR as Diagnostic Test for Chronic Disease: OSA-COPD Overlap, Interstitial Lung Diseases and Bronchiectasis

In our study, 85 patients had sleep apnea or COPD, 36 patients had interstitial lung diseases, and 98 patients had bronchiectasis. Their age, gender and blood characteristics are shown in Table 3. NLR was not found to be significantly different between groups with different chronic diseases after adjusting for type one error. On the other hand, PLR was significantly different between groups. The OSA-COPD group PLR was significantly lower than in the other two groups, which were not significantly different from the control group. Lymphocytes were higher in the OSA-COPD group compared with the interstitial lung disease group. Conversely, neutrophils were lower in the OSA-COPD group compared with the interstitial lung disease group. Platelets were statistically significantly higher in the bronchiectasis group compared with the OSA-COPD group. The OSA-COPD group had significantly lower ESR than the other two groups, which were not significantly different. Age and CRP were not significantly different between groups.

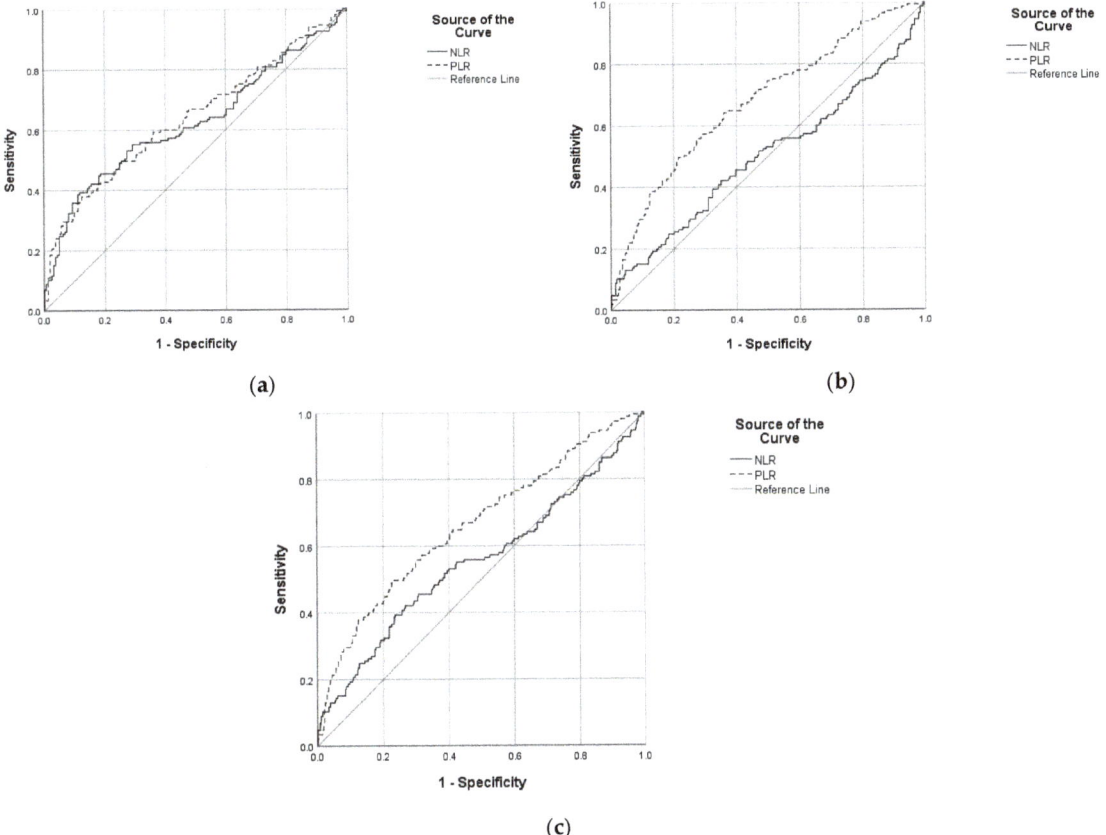

Figure 1. ROC curve with PLR and NLR (**a**) comparing COVID-19 group versus control group; (**b**) comparing COVID-19 group versus chronic respiratory disease group; (**c**) comparing COVID-19 group versus control group and chronic respiratory disease group.

PLR was found to be poor, but statistically significant as a diagnostic test when we compared the control group with the OSA-COPD group (coded with 1) (Figure 2a); but failed and was not statistically significant when we compared the control group with the interstitial lung disease group (AUC = 0.556, $p = 0.298$) (Figure 2c), or with the bronchiectasis group (AUC = 0.483, $p = 0.639$) (Figure 2e). When we compared the diseases, PLR was found to be poor also and statistically significant in the following cases: the OSA-COPD group (coded with 0) versus interstitial lung disease and bronchiectasis groups (Figure 2b); and the interstitial lung diseases group (coded with 1) versus OSA-COPD and bronchiectasis groups (Figure 2d); but failed and was not statistically significant for the bronchiectasis (coded with 1) group versus OSA-COPD and interstitial lung disease groups (AUC = 0.564, $p = 0.103$) (Figure 2e).

Table 2. Performance of PLR and NLR in the case when statistically significant difference in ROC curve was reached.

		Cutoff	Sensitivity	Specificity
PLR	COVID-19 group (codified with 1) vs. control—AUC = 0.640, $p < 0.001$	90.78	0.90	0.16
		112.52	0.75	0.35
		182.48	**0.38**	**0.88**
		190.48	0.33	0.90
	COVID-19 group (codified with 1) vs. chronic respiratory disease group—AUC = 0.677, $p < 0.001$	90.5	0.90	0.24
		112.68	0.75	0.48
		144.95	**0.56**	**0.73**
		195.84	0.30	0.90
	COVID-19 group (codified with 1) vs. control and chronic respiratory disease group—AUC = 0.662, $p < 0.001$	90.78	0.90	0.21
		112.68	0.75	0.43
		157.23	**0.49**	**0.77**
		193.55	0.30	0.90
NLR	COVID-19 group (codified with 1) vs. control—AUC = 0.624, $p < 0.001$	1.35	0.90	0.12
		1.72	0.75	0.32
		3.02	**0.39**	**0.88**
		3.15	0.36	0.90

The cutoffs with maximal sensitivity and specificity are marked in bold; NLR—neutrophil-to-lymphocyte ratio; PLR–platelet-to-lymphocyte ratio; AUC—area under the curve.

Table 3. The characteristics of the chronic disease groups.

	OSA-COPD Overlap (n = 85)	Interstitial Lung Diseases (n = 36)	Bronchiectasis (n = 98)	p
AGE	61 (51, 65)	64 (57, 69.5)	62 (54, 74)	0.177
Gender, number (%)	66 (84.6) [a,b]	20 (55.6)	52 (53.1)	<0.001
NLR	2.5 (1.87, 3.33)	2.54 (1.82, 3.76)	2.38 (1.81, 3.46)	0.808
PLR	103.93 (84.85, 129.14) [a,b]	129.8 (109.62, 165.94)	129.18 (95.18, 162.43)	0.001
Lymphocytes ($10^3/\mu L$)	2.04 (1.68, 2.38) [a]	1.71 (1.31, 2.06)	1.95 (1.47, 2.38)	0.012
Neutrophils ($10^3/\mu L$)	5.41 ± 1.77 [a]	4.61 ± 1.79	5.57 ± 2.82	0.037
Platelets (X10^3)	224 (189, 256) [b]	229.5 (175.5, 274)	241.5 (202, 295)	0.043
ESR	8 (5, 19) [a,b]	18.5 (12.5, 31)	20 (11, 34.5)	<0.001
CRP	4.8 (2.4, 11.7)	3.45 (1.85, 10.15)	6.05 (1.95, 16.65)	0.379

[a]—adjusted $p < 0.05$ for OSA-COPD group compared with interstitial lung disease group; [b]—adjusted $p < 0.05$ for OSA-COPD group compared with bronchiectasis group.

NLR was found to be poor, but statistically significant as a diagnostic test when we compared the control group with all three groups (separately): the OSA-COPD group (coded with 1) (Figure 2a); interstitial lung disease group (Figure 2c); and bronchiectasis group (Figure 2e). When we compared the diseases, NLR failed and was not statistically significant in any of the comparisons: the OSA-COPD group (coded with 0) versus interstitial lung disease and bronchiectasis groups (AUC = 0.507, $p = 0.859$) (Figure 2b); interstitial lung disease group (coded with 1) versus OSA-COPD and bronchiectasis groups (AUC = 0.534, $p = 0.516$) (Figure 2d); and bronchiectasis (coded with 1) group versus OSA-COPD and interstitial lung disease groups (AUC = 0.488, $p = 0.756$) (Figure 2e).

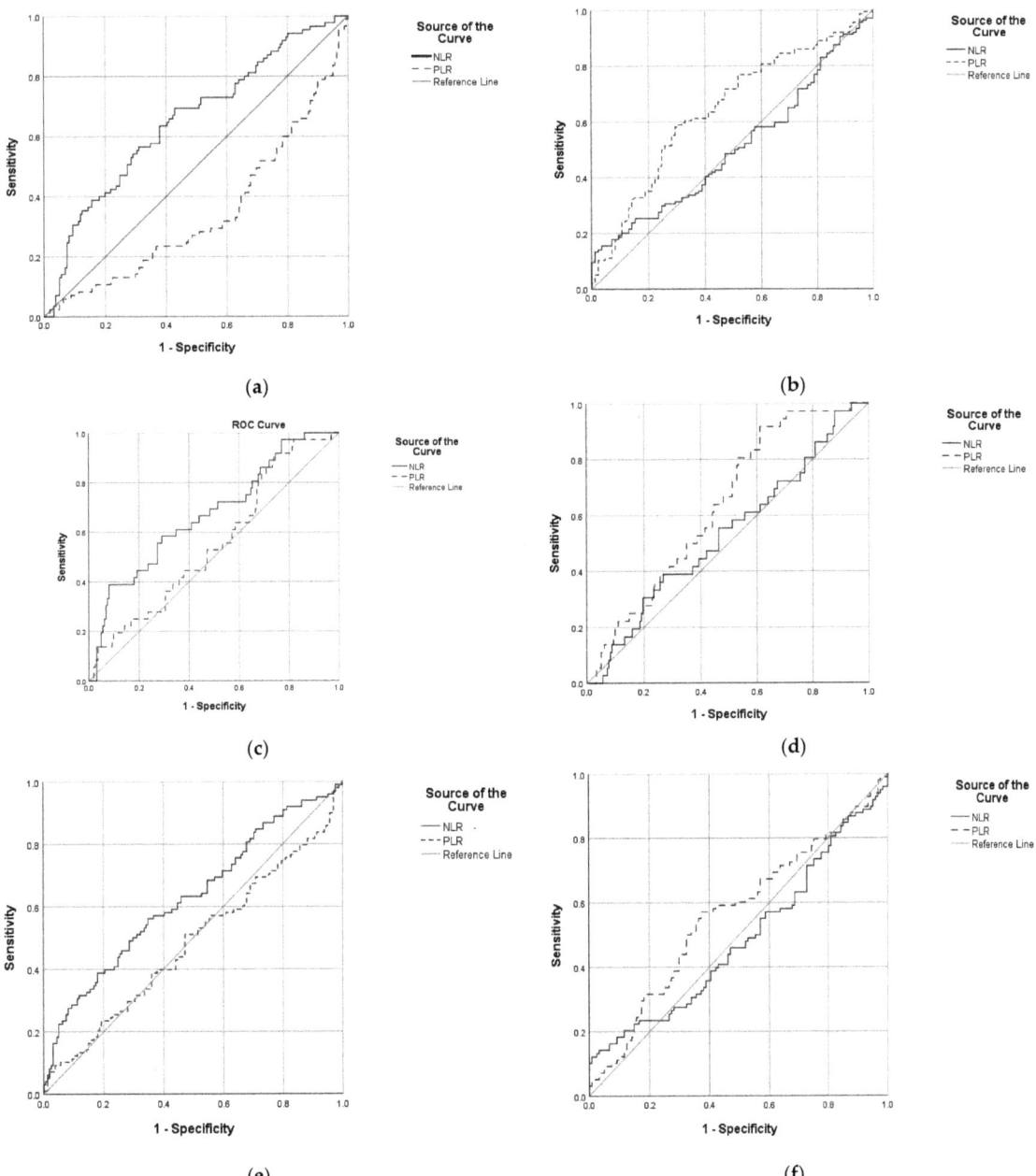

Figure 2. ROC curve with PLR and NLR (**a**) comparing OSA-COPD group (coded with 0) versus control group; (**b**) comparing OSA-COPD group (coded with 0) versus interstitial lung disease and bronchiectasis groups; (**c**) comparing interstitial lung disease group (coded with 1) versus control group; (**d**) comparing interstitial lung disease group (coded with 1) versus OSA-COPD and bronchiectasis groups; (**e**) comparing bronchiectasis (coded with 1) group versus control group; (**f**) comparing bronchiectasis (coded with 1) group versus OSA-COPD and interstitial lung disease groups.

The optimum cutoff for PLR was found to be 114.9 between the OSA-COPD group and control group, 118.38 between the OSA-COPD and interstitial lung disease and bronchiectasis groups, and 101.74 between the interstitial lung disease group (coded with 1) versus OSA-COPD and bronchiectasis groups (Table 4).

Table 4. Performance of PLR and NLR when we compare chronic respiratory disease.

		Cutoff	Sensitivity	Specificity
PLR	OSA-COPD group (codified as 0) vs. control—AUC = 0.656, $p < 0.001$	84.41	0.90	0.17
		101.82	0.75	0.48
		114.9	0.63	0.68
		172.98	0.17	0.90
	OSA-COPD group (coded with 0) versus interstitial lung disease and bronchiectasis groups—AUC = 0.645, $p < 0.001$	75.14	0.90	0.24
		102.71	0.75	0.48
		118.38	0.58	0.71
		173.78	0.19	0.90
	Interstitial lung disease group (coded with 1) versus OSA-COPD and bronchiectasis groups—AUC = 0.636, $p = 0.010$	101.74	0.92	0.39
		109.62	0.75	0.47
		148.90	0.36	0.75
		189.88	0.19	0.90
NLR	OSA-COPD group (codified with 1) vs. control—AUC = 0.652, $p < 0.001$	1.56	0.90	0.22
		2.19	0.69	0.57
		2.59	0.47	0.75
		3.15	0.31	0.90
	Interstitial lung disease group (codified with 1) vs. control—AUC = 0.672, $p = 0.001$	1.60	0.90	0.25
		1.84	0.75	0.37
		2.63	0.47	0.75
		3.31	**0.39**	**0.92**
	Bronchiectasis disease group (codified with 1) vs. control—AUC = 0.672, $p = 0.001$	1.49	0.90	0.20
		1.80	0.75	0.36
		2.31	**0.56**	**0.64**
		3.15	0.29	0.90

The cutoffs with maximal sensitivity and specificity are marked in bold; NLR—neutrophil-to-lymphocyte ratio; PLR—platelet-to-lymphocyte; AUC—area under the curve.

The optimum cutoff for NLR was found to be 2.19 between the OSA-COPD group and control group, 3.31 between interstitial lung disease group and control group, and 2.31 between bronchiectasis group and control group (Table 4).

4. Discussion

Our study aimed to analyze the diagnostic value of two widely available inflammatory markers, the neutrophil-to-lymphocyte ratio and platelet-to-lymphocyte ratio, in different respiratory diseases: COVID-19, bronchiectasis, OSA-COPD, and interstitial lung disease compared with healthy persons. NLR was found to be significantly higher in both acute (COVID-19) and chronic respiratory disease (OSA-COPD, interstitial lung disease and bronchiectasis) groups when compared with the control group, but with no statistically significant difference between the two groups. NLR was poor when discriminating between COVID-19 and the control group but statistically significant when used to discriminate between COVID-19 and the other chronic respiratory disease group (AUC = 0.501, $p = 0.975$).

The optimum cutoff for NLR was 3.02 between the COVID-19 group and the control group. NLR was found to be poor but statistically significant as a diagnostic test when we compared the control group with all three disease groups (separately): OSA-COPD group, interstitial lung disease group, and bronchiectasis group. When we compared the diseases, NLR failed and was not statistically significant in any of the comparisons. The optimum cutoff for NLR was found to be 2.19 between the OSA-COPD group and control group, 3.31 between the interstitial lung disease group and control group, and 2.31 between the bronchiectasis group and control group. There is a large amount of available data evaluating respiratory conditions such as COPD or bronchiectasis in an acute and stable phase, reporting higher values in the first category [13–16]. As NLR is a very affordable and reproducible marker, the literature is abundant with studies using NLR from sepsis to cancer to restless leg syndrome [17]. However, as it seems to be an indicator of many if not all diseases, we might conclude that it is not a reliable indicator of any disease, as it cannot be a "magical assay for every condition" [18]. We would emphasize that its use is very dependent of clinical context. For example, as mentioned before, NLR was higher in acute exacerbation of COPD and/or bronchiectasis when compared with stable conditions and, of course, when compared with the control group. Several studies that evaluated the ability of NLR to detect bacteremia showed a poor prognostic [19–23]. At a cutoff of ~10, for instance, NLR has a sensitivity of 72% and specificity of 60% for the diagnosis of bacteremia [19]. Nevertheless, its performance in this situation is superior to that of the white blood cell count [18]. Another thing that must be taken into consideration is the fact that under physiologic stress, the number of neutrophils increases, while the number of lymphocytes decreases rapidly, in under 6 h [19]. Increased levels of cortisol as well as endogenous catecholamines such as epinephrine are known to increase the neutrophil count while simultaneously decreasing the lymphocyte count [18]. Cytokines and other hormones are also likely to be involved. In conclusion, NLR is not only an indicator of infection or inflammation, but in fact may be increased by any cause of physiologic stress. The prompt response may make NLR a better reflection of acute stress than other laboratory values, making it perhaps more useful in acute rather than chronic conditions. Many patients have severe physiologic stress (with elevated NLR) without bacteremia. Alternatively, some patients with bacteremia tolerate this surprisingly well and are not very ill. In short, it is unrealistic to expect NLR to perform well in this context. This is not a failure of the test itself, but rather represents a failure to apply the test appropriately [18–20]. So, patients with inflammatory disorders may tend to present elevated NLR more than in non-inflammatory disorders and NLR in a critically ill patient may be more elevated than in a non-critical patient. As showed before, interpretation of NLR is dependent on clinical context, and there are no standard values; nevertheless, some authors [18] have suggest some values: normal NLR is roughly 1–3. An NLR of 6–9 suggests mild stress, and critically ill patients will often have an NLR of ~9 or higher. This hypothesis does not seem to be sustained by our study, where NLR values seemed to be similar in the COVID-19 group (acute condition) and chronic respiratory disease group (OSA-COPD, bronchiectasis, interstitial lung disease and pleural effusions). The explanation might be the fact that our COVID-19 population was quite heterogenousas in Romania, unlike other countries, hospitalization was compulsory for all COVID-19 patients, regardless of the severity of the disease. NLR was not able to differentiate between the chronic conditions. As NLR is influenced by steroids and acute respiratory conditions such as COPD or ILD, and in some situations COVID-19 patients might receive systemic steroids, we may ask whether this does not contribute to the elevated values.

PLR, on the other hand, was significantly different between groups.PLR was found to be significant as a diagnostic test between the COVID-19 group and the other groups. PLR was poor when used to discriminate between COVID-19 and the control group with statistical significance and also poor when used to discriminate between the COVID-19 group and chronic respiratory disease group. The optimum cutoff for PLR was found to be 182.48 between the COVID-19 group and control group, 144.95 between the COVID-19 group and chronic respiratory disease group, and 157.23 between the COVID-19 group and the other two groups. PLR was found to be poor, but statistically significant, as a diagnostic test when we used it to compare the control group with the OSA-COPD group, bur not with the interstitial lung disease group (AUC = 0.556, p = 0.298) or bronchiectasis group (AUC = 0.483, p = 0.639).

When we compared diseases, PLR was found to also be poor, but statistically significant in the following cases: the OSA-COPD group versus interstitial lung disease and bronchiectasis groups; and interstitial lung disease group versus OSA-COPD and bronchiectasis groups. However, it failed and was not statistically significant for the bronchiectasis (coded with 1) group versus OSA-COPD and interstitial lung disease groups (AUC = 0.564, p = 0.103) (Figure 2e).

The optimum cutoff for PLR was found to be 114.9 between the OSA-COPD group and control group, 118.38 between OSA-COPD and interstitial lung disease and bronchiectasis groups, and 101.74 between interstitial lung disease group (coded with 1) versus OSA-COPD and bronchiectasis groups.

PLR in the chronic respiratory disease groups was significantly lower than that of the control group, in which PLR was significantly lower than that of the COVID-19 group. The statistical significance was maintained even after adjusting for type one error. PLR was found to be significant as a diagnostic test between the COVID-19 group and the other groups. The optimum cutoff for PLR was found to be 182.48 between the COVID-19 group and control group, 144.95 between the COVID-19 group and chronic respiratory disease group, and 157.23 between the COVID-19 group and the other two groups, but the test accuracy was poorAs a discriminative marker between the COVID-19 group and control group, NLR had statistical significance but was poor as a diagnostic test. NLR was not found to be significantly different between groups of different chronic diseases after adjusting for type one error. On the other hand, PLR was significantly different between groups. The OSA-COPD group PLR was significantly lower than that of the other two groups, which were not significantly different from the control group. PLR was found to be significant in the following cases: the OSA-COPD group versus interstitial lung disease and bronchiectasis groups, and interstitial lung disease group versus OSA-COPD and bronchiectasis groups. NLR was found to be significant as a diagnostic test but poor when we compared the control group with all three groups (separately), but not when we compared among respiratory diseases groups. One can consider a cutoff with high sensitivity if they want to use NLR or PLR as screening tests. In the case of COVID-19, they can be useful as screening tests. Although both NLR and PLR can be very useful screening tools in COVID-19, it is highly unlikely that they will be used as they cannot prevent the disease, which is treated only when symptomatic. When these hematological changes appear, most likely the disease has already started. One can consider a cutoff with high specificity if they want to use NLR or PLR as a precision diagnostic test. The platelet-to-lymphocyte ratio appeared to be a more reliable diagnostic factor than NLR in the present study. PLR is used more as a diagnostic tool in cardiovascular disease (myocardial infarction and vascular diseases). Even in patients with COPD-OSA, it seems to have better discriminative value than NLR, which suggests that hypoxemia, more that inflammation, has a certain influence on the PLR value. This might explain its discriminative value among patients with conditions accompanied by hypoxemia, such as interstitial lung disease and OSA-COPD [10,11].

Our study had some limitations. It was a single-center, retrospective study. Sample size was small for the interstitial lung disease group. The groups were inhomogeneous in terms of number of participants, age, and gender. We had an acute condition as represented by a viral infection (COVID-19) and three chronic conditions (among many others). We did not have acute conditions correspondent with the above-mentioned chronic pathologies (COPD exacerbation, bronchiectasis exacerbation). Study population was quite heterogenous and not matched in age and gender, due first to differences in prevalence of the diseases among different age categories. In the COPD-OSA overlap, bronchiectasis cases were prevalent, whereas interstitial lung diseases were not. The conclusions could be influenced by the differences in age and gender between the control group and the other groups because many studies have found a positive correlation between NLR and age [23]. For comparisons with a control group, age and gender can be confounding factors and careful conclusions should be considered. As another limitation, disease severity was not evaluated in the present study. As we do know that NLR values increase with the severity of some diseases, it would be interesting to perform a subgroup analysis. We also had only one determination of both NLR and PLR. Repetitive determinations at different moments in time would be more interesting. Multiple determinations might have higher prognostic value than an isolated one.

However, ours is among the few studies that evaluated these accessible and very practical inflammatory markers for so many respiratory diseases. Although it was retrospective in nature, it was s a real-life study from a major hospital in Romania. Despite its limitations, we believe that some conclusions can be drawn:

1. NLR was found to be poor as a diagnostic test when we compared healthy persons with patients with chronic respiratory diseases, but not when we compared the diseases.
2. PLR seems to be a more reliable marker in differentiating between the evaluated chronic diseases, but as a diagnostic test, it remains poor.

5. Conclusions

The PLR has the potential to be a precision diagnostic tool for COVID-19 and a screening tool for chronic disease. However, diagnostic phase III and IV studies are needed to further evaluate its benefits and clinical relevance. Additionally, we did not manage to find any cutoff value for diagnosis.

Author Contributions: Data curation, M.-A.M., L.D., N.-S.M., C.-I.B. and C.-M.P.; Formal analysis, L.D. and C.-I.B.; Investigation, N.-S.M. and R.-M.R.; Methodology, M.-A.M., N.-S.M., R.-M.R. and C.-I.B.; Software, C.-I.B. and C.T.; Supervision, C.-I.B. and C.T.; Validation, M.-A.M., C.-M.P. and C.T.; Visualization, M.-A.M., C.-M.P. and C.T.; Writing—original draft, M.-A.M., L.D., N.-S.M., R.-M.R. and C.-I.B.; Writing—review & editing, M.-A.M., L.D., N.-S.M., R.-M.R. and C.-M.P. All authors have read and agreed to the published version of the manuscript.

Funding: This research received no external funding.

Institutional Review Board Statement: The study was conducted in accordance with the Declaration of Helsinki, and approved by the Ethics Committee for Scientific Research of the Hospital 232/03 March 2020.

Informed Consent Statement: Informed consent was obtained from all subjects involved in the study.

Conflicts of Interest: The authors declare no conflict of interest.

References

1. El-Gazzar, A.G.; Kamel, M.H.; Elbahnasy, O.K.M.; El-Naggar, M.E.-S. Prognostic value of platelet and neutrophil to lymphocyte ratio in COPD patients. *Expert Rev. Respir. Med.* **2019**, *14*, 111–116. [CrossRef] [PubMed]
2. Storey, R.; Thomas, M.R. The role of platelets in inflammation. *Thromb. Haemost.* **2015**, *114*, 449–458. [CrossRef]
3. Man, M.A.; Rajnoveanu, R.-M.; Motoc, N.S.; Bondor, C.I.; Chis, A.F.; Lesan, A.; Puiu, R.; Lucaciu, S.-R.; Dantes, E.; Gergely-Domokos, B.; et al. Neutrophil-to-lymphocyte ratio, platelets-to-lymphocyte ratio, and eosinophils correlation with high-resolution computer tomography severity score in COVID-19 patients. *PLoS ONE* **2021**, *16*, e0252599. [CrossRef] [PubMed]
4. Sun, Y.; Chen, C.; Zhang, X.; Weng, X.; Sheng, A.; Zhu, Y.; Chen, S.; Zheng, X.; Lu, C. High Neutrophil-to-Lymphocyte Ratio Is an Early Predictor of Bronchopulmonary Dysplasia. *Front. Pediatr.* **2019**, *7*, 464–481. [CrossRef]
5. Koseoglu, S.; Ozcan, K.M.; Ikinciogullari, A.; A Cetin, M.; Yildirim, E.; Dere, H. Relationship Between Neutrophil to Lymphocyte Ratio, Platelet to Lymphocyte Ratio and Obstructive Sleep Apnea Syndrome. *Adv. Clin. Exp. Med.* **2015**, *24*, 623–627. [CrossRef] [PubMed]
6. Taylan, M.; Demir, M.; Kaya, H.; Selimoglu Sen, H.; Abakay, O.; Carkanat, A.I.; Abakay, A.; Tanrikulu, A.C.; Sezgi, C. Alterations of the neutrophil-lymphocyte ratio during the period of stable and acute exacerbation of chronic obstructive pulmonary disease patients. *Clin. Respir. J.* **2017**, *11*, 311–317. [CrossRef] [PubMed]

7. Jiang, X.M.; Qian, X.S.; Gao, X.F.; Ge, Z.; Tian, N.L.; Kan, J.; Zhang, J.J. Obstructive Sleep Apnea Affecting Platelet Reactivity in Patients Undergoing Percutaneous Coronary Intervention. *Chin. Med. J.* **2018**, *9*, 1023–1030. [CrossRef] [PubMed]
8. Pascual-González, Y.; Lopez-Sanchez, M.; Dorca, J.; Santos, S. Defining the role of neutrophil-to-lymphocyte ratio in COPD: A systematic literature review. *Int. J. Chronic Obstr. Pulm. Dis.* **2018**, *13*, 3651–3662. [CrossRef]
9. Ruta, V.; Man, A.; Alexescu, T.; Motoc, N.; Tarmure, S.; Ungur, R.; Todea, D.; Coste, S.; Valean, D.; Pop, M. Neutrophil-To-Lymphocyte Ratio and Systemic Immune-Inflammation Index—Biomarkers in Interstitial Lung Disease. *Medicina* **2020**, *56*, 381. [CrossRef]
10. Motoc, N.S.; Man, M.A.; Urda, A.E.C.; Ruta, V.M.; Todea, D.A.; Pop, C.M. Neutrophil-to-Lymphocyte Ratio and Platelets-to-Lymphocytes Ratio in severe COPD exacerbation: The importance of obstructive sleep apnea. *Monit. Airw. Dis.* **2019**, *54*, PA2582. [CrossRef]
11. Motoc, N.S. The Role of Noninvasive Ventilation in Respiratory Failure: From the Acute Episode to Chronic Use. PH.D. Thesis, Iuliu Hatieganu University of Medicine and Pharmacy, Cluj Napoca, Romania, 2021.
12. Li, F.; He, H. Assessing the Accuracy of Diagnostic Tests. *Shanghai Arch. Psychiatry* **2018**, *30*, 207–212. [CrossRef] [PubMed]
13. Paliogiannis, P.; Fois, A.G.; Sotgia, S.; A Mangoni, A.; Zinellu, E.; Pirina, P.; Carru, C.; Zinellu, A. The neutrophil-to-lymphocyte ratio as a marker of chronic obstructive pulmonary disease and its exacerbations: A systematic review and meta-analysis. *Eur. J. Clin. Investig.* **2018**, *48*, e12984. [CrossRef] [PubMed]
14. Sun, W.; Luo, Z.; Jin, J.; Cao, Z.; Ma, Y. The Neutrophil/Lymphocyte Ratio Could Predict Noninvasive Mechanical Ventilation Failure in Patients with Acute Exacerbation of Chronic Obstructive Pulmonary Disease: A Retrospective Observational Study. *Int. J. Chronic Obstr. Pulm. Dis.* **2021**, *16*, 2267–2277. [CrossRef]
15. Sakurai, K.; Chubachi, S.; Irie, H.; Tsutsumi, A.; Kameyama, N.; Kamatani, T.; Koh, H.; Terashima, T.; Nakamura, H.; Asano, K.; et al. Clinical utility of blood neutrophil-lymphocyte ratio in Japanese COPD patients. *BMC Pulm. Med.* **2018**, *18*, 65. [CrossRef] [PubMed]
16. Teng, F.; Ye, H.; Xue, T. Predictive value of neutrophil to lymphocyte ratio in patients with acute exacerbation of chronic obstructive pulmonary disease. *PLoS ONE* **2018**, *13*, e0204377. [CrossRef] [PubMed]
17. Varım, C.; Acar, B.A.; Uyanık, M.S.; Acar, T.; Alagoz, N.; Nalbant, A.; Ergenc, H. Association between the neutrophil-to-lymphocyte ratio, a new marker of systemic inflammation, and restless legs syndrome. *Singap. Med. J.* **2016**, *57*, 514–516. Available online: https://www.ncbi.nlm.nih.gov/pubmed/27662970 (accessed on 30 November 2021). [CrossRef] [PubMed]
18. Farkas, J. Neutrophil-Lymphocyte Ratio (NLR): Free Upgrade to Your WBC. 2019. Available online: https://emcrit.org/pulmcrit/nlr/ (accessed on 10 October 2021).
19. Jiang, J.; Liu, R.; Yu, X.; Yang, R.; Xu, H.; Mao, Z.; Wang, Y. The neutrophil-lymphocyte count ratio as a diagnostic marker for bacteraemia: A systematic review and meta-analysis. *Am. J. Emerg. Med.* **2019**, *37*, 1482–1489. Available online: https://www.ncbi.nlm.nih.gov/pubmed/30413366 (accessed on 29 October 2021). [CrossRef]
20. Zahorec, R. Ratio of neutrophil to lymphocyte counts–rapid and simple parameter of systemic inflammation and stress in critically ill. *Bratisl. Lek. Listy* **2001**, *102*, 5–14. Available online: https://www.ncbi.nlm.nih.gov/pubmed/11723675 (accessed on 29 October 2021).
21. de Jager, C.P.C.; van Wijk, P.T.; Mathoera, R.B.; de Jongh-Leuvenink, J.; van der Poll, T. Lymphocytopenia and neutrophil-lymphocyte count ratio predict bacteremia better than conventional infection markers in an emergency care unit. *Crit. Care* **2010**, *14*, R192. Available online: https://www.ncbi.nlm.nih.gov/pubmed/21034463 (accessed on 29 October 2021). [CrossRef]
22. Lowsby, R.; Gomes, C.; Jarman, I.; Lisboa, P.; A Nee, P.; Vardhan, M.; Eckersley, T.; Saleh, R.; Mills, H. Neutrophil to lymphocyte count ratio as an early indicator of blood stream infection in the emergency department. *Emerg. Med. J.* **2015**, *32*, 531–534. Available online: https://www.ncbi.nlm.nih.gov/pubmed/25183249 (accessed on 29 October 2021). [CrossRef] [PubMed]
23. Li, J.; Chen, Q.; Luo, X.; Hong, J.; Pan, K.; Lin, X.; Liu, X.; Zhou, L.; Wang, H.; Xu, Y.; et al. Neutrophil-to-Lymphocyte Ratio Positively Correlates to Age in Healthy Population. *J. Clin. Lab. Anal.* **2015**, *29*, 437–443. [CrossRef] [PubMed]

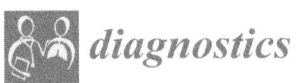

Article

Novel App-Based Portable Spirometer for the Early Detection of COPD

Ching-Hsiung Lin [1,2,3], Shih-Lung Cheng [4,5,*,†], Hao-Chien Wang [6], Wu-Huei Hsu [7], Kang-Yun Lee [8], Diahn-Warng Perng [9], Hen-I. Lin [10], Ming-Shian Lin [11], Jong-Rung Tsai [12], Chin-Chou Wang [13], Sheng-Hao Lin [1], Cheng-Yi Wang [9], Chiung-Zuei Chen [14], Tsung-Ming Yang [15], Ching-Lung Liu [16], Tsai-Yu Wang [17] and Meng-Chih Lin [13,*,†]

1. Division of Chest Medicine, Changhua Christian Hospital, Changhua 500, Taiwan; teddy@cch.org.tw (C.-H.L.); shenghao@gmail.com (S.-H.L.)
2. Institute of Genomics and Bioinformatics, National Chung Hsing University, Taichung 402, Taiwan
3. Department of Recreation and Holistic Wellness, MingDao University, Changhua 523, Taiwan
4. Department of Internal Medicine, Far Eastern Memorial Hospital, Taipei 220, Taiwan
5. Department of Chemical Engineering and Materials Science, Yuan Ze University, Zhongli, Taoyuan 320, Taiwan
6. Department of Internal Medicine, National Taiwan University Hospital, Taipei 100, Taiwan; haochienwang@gmail.com
7. Division of Pulmonary and Critical Care Medicine, Department of Internal Medicine, China Medical University Hospital, Taichung 404, Taiwan; wuhuei@gmail.com
8. Division of Pulmonary Medicine, Department of Internal Medicine, Shuang Ho Hospital, Taipei Medical University, New Taipei City 110, Taiwan; kangyenlee68@gmail.com
9. Department of Chest Medicine, Taipei Veterans General Hospital, Taipei 112, Taiwan; dwperng@vghtpe.gov.tw (D.-W.P.); chengyi@gmail.com (C.-Y.W.)
10. Department of Internal Medicine, Cardinal Tien Hospital, Fu-Jen Catholic University, Taipei 242, Taiwan; heni@gmail.com
11. Department of Internal Medicine, Ditmanson Medical Foundation Chia-Yi Christian Hospital, Chiayi 600, Taiwan; mingshian@gmail.com
12. Division of Pulmonary and Critical Care Medicine, Department of Internal Medicine, Kaohsiung Medical University Hospital, Kaohsiung 807, Taiwan; jongrung@gmail.com
13. Division of Pulmonary and Critical Care Medicine, Department of Internal Medicine, Kaohsiung Chang Gung Memorial Hospital, Chang Gung University College of Medicine, Kaohsiung 833, Taiwan; chinchou@gmail.com
14. Division of Pulmonary Medicine, Department of Internal Medicine, National Cheng Kung University, College of Medicine and Hospital, Tainan 701, Taiwan; chiungzuei@gmail.com
15. Department of Pulmonary and Critical Care Medicine, Chang Gung Memorial Hospital, Chiayi Branch 613, Taiwan; tsungming@gmail.com
16. Division of Chest Medicine, Department of Internal Medicine, MacKay Memorial Hospital, Taipei 104, Taiwan; chinglung@gmail.com
17. Department of Thoracic Medicine, Chang Gung Memorial Hospital at Linkou, Chang Gung University, College of Medicine, Taipei 333, Taiwan; tsaiyu@gmail.com
* Correspondence: shihlungcheng@gmaill.com (S.-L.C.); mengchih@cgmh.org.tw (M.-C.L.); Tel.: +886-2-89667000 (M.-C.L.); Fax: +886-2-77380708 (M.-C.L.)
† The two authors equally contributed correspondence to this work.

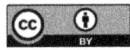

Abstract: Chronic obstructive pulmonary disease (COPD) is preventable and treatable. However, many patients remain undiagnosed and untreated due to the underutilization or unavailability of spirometers. Accordingly, we used Spirobank Smart, an app-based spirometer, for facilitating the early detection of COPD in outpatient clinics. This prospective study recruited individuals who were at risk of COPD (i.e., with age of ≥40 years, ≥10 pack-years of smoking, and at least one respiratory symptoms) but had no previous COPD diagnosis. Eligible participants were examined with Spirobank Smart and then underwent confirmatory spirometry (performed using a diagnostic spirometer), regardless of their Spirobank Smart test results. COPD was defined and confirmed using the postbronchodilator forced expiratory volume in 1 s/forced vital capacity values of <0.70 as measured by confirmatory spirometry. A total of 767 participants were enrolled and examined using Spirobank Smart; 370 participants (94.3% men, mean age of 60.9 years and mean 42.6 pack-years of smoking) underwent confirmatory spirometry. Confirmatory spirometry identified COPD in 103 participants (27.8%). At the optimal cutoff point of 0.74 that was determined using Spirobank Smart for COPD diagnosis, the area under the receiver operating characteristic was 0.903 (95% confidence interval (CI) = 0.860–0.947). Multivariate logistic regression revealed that participants who have an FEV_1/FVC ratio of <74% that was determined using Spirobank Smart (odds ratio (OR) = 58.58, 95% CI = 27.29–125.75) and old age (OR = 3.23, 95% CI = 1.04–10.07 for 60 $\leq$ age < 65; OR = 5.82, 95% CI = 2.22–15.27 for age $\geq$ 65) had a higher risk of COPD. The Spirobank Smart is a simple and adequate tool for early COPD detection in outpatient clinics. Early diagnosis and appropriate therapy based on GOLD guidelines can positively influence respiratory symptoms and quality of life.

Keywords: COPD; underdiagnosis; early detection; app-based spirometer

1. Introduction

Chronic obstructive pulmonary disease (COPD) is a leading cause of morbidity and mortality worldwide [1,2]. In Taiwan, COPD is the seventh leading cause of death, with the corresponding age-adjusted mortality rates for men and women being 19.67 and 5.70 deaths per 100,000, respectively [3]. In general, COPD is treatable and preventable when identified in the early stage; nevertheless, the underdiagnosis of COPD remains a common challenge and imposes a considerable burden on healthcare systems and patients [4,5].

Spirometry is the gold standard for diagnosing COPD and monitoring treatment response [6]; however, it is still underused or unavailable in primary care settings or non-specialized areas [4,7]. This may be attributed to various factors; for example, spirometry entails labor-intensive and time-consuming procedures and requires well-trained professionals for its execution [5,8]. Underuse of spirometry is considered a critical factor that is related to COPD underdiagnosis and results in unnecessary specialty referrals for diagnostic testing, creating barriers in COPD screening through spirometry and increasing the cost of diagnostic tests [4,9,10]. However, a report by the U.S. Preventive Services Task Force (USPSTF) revealed that the use of spirometry to screen for COPD in asymptomatic cases has no net benefit [11,12]. The early detection of COPD through a case-finding approach has been heavily advocated, and such an initiative provides opportunities for implementing interventions in the early stages, thus preventing disease progression [13,14]. Moreover, the USPSTF report suggested that COPD screening in at-risk populations has relatively high cost-effectiveness [15]. Hence, developing a feasible case-finding model that can be a suitable alternative to spirometry for identifying undiagnosed at-risk patients with COPD is urgently required.

A portable spirometer is a small and cheap device that can be a valid alternative to spirometry. Spirometers are advantageous for their ease of use, the requirement of less patient effort, and time-saving features, which render them useful for COPD screening [16–19]. Recently, the trend of integrating smart devices and portable medical devices has grown considerably and has affected the market and medical diagnosis field, including spirometry [20,21]. Systems integrating portable spirometers with smartphones can save processing power and reduce interface components, reduce medical device size and cost, and afford effective data communications [20–22]. However, only a few such systems have been validated for COPD screening, with their performance varying with the diagnostic testing procedure applied.

Spirobank Smart is an FDA-approved, app-based ultraportable device that connects to a smartphone app through Bluetooth for seamless recording of various lung function parameters, including the forced expiratory volume in one second (FEV_1), PEF, forced vital capacity (FVC), FEV_1/FVC, FEV_6, and FEF_{25-75}. Spirobank Smart can provide real-time feedback on the test quality, provide systematic and numeric visualizations of spirometer tests on the smartphone app, and afford effective data communication. A study conducted a correlation analysis between measurements obtained from Spirobank Smart and those obtained from confirmatory spirometry; the analysis indicated that this device exhibited acceptable validity and that it meets the latest ATS/ERS standards for accuracy [23]. However, the performance of Spirobank Smart in COPD screening remains unknown.

Accordingly, to fill the aforementioned knowledge gap, we conducted this study to investigate the feasibility of Spirobank Smart for the early detection of COPD. Specifically, we applied Spirobank Smart to assist in the early detection of COPD using case-finding in outpatient clinics. We determined the correlation between FEV_1/FVC values obtained by Spirobank Smart and postbronchodilator (post-BD) FEV_1/FVC ratio obtained through confirmatory spirometry (executed using a diagnostic spirometer). Furthermore, we determined the cutoff point for the FEV_1/FVC ratio and the corresponding predictive performance of Spirobank Smart in identifying COPD in high-risk populations; subsequently, we evaluated whether the FEV_1 obtained using Spirobank Smart was useful for classifying patient disease severity according to the GOLD (Global Initiative for Chronic Obstructive Lung Disease) severity stratification system.

2. Materials and Methods

2.1. Study Design

This prospective multicenter validation study was conducted for the period from April 2018 to December 2019, and the study protocol was approved by the Institutional Review Board of Changhua Christian Hospital (IRB number 190806); Institutional Review Board of Changhua Christian Hospital reviewed the project and deemed it to be exempt research because the evaluation was for a public service program and all data were de-identified. The requirement for written consent was waived. Participants were enrolled from 26 outpatient clinics in Taiwan, from which their demographic information, CAT (COPD Assessment Test) questionnaires, Spirobank Smart measurements, and diagnostic spirometer measurements were obtained.

2.2. Study Participants

The Taiwan Society of Pulmonary and Critical Care Medicine recruited participants and implemented a study, commissioned by the Taiwan Ministry of Health and Welfare, on early diagnosis of COPD. The eligibility criteria were as follows: having an age of ≥40 years, having ≥10 pack-years of smoking, exhibiting chronic respiratory symptoms (cough, phlegm, or dyspnea, or combination thereof), and not having a confirmed COPD diagnosis within the prior year. We excluded individuals who did not undergo post-BD spirometry because we could not confirm whether a given individual had a COPD diagnosis; we also excluded those who were unable to correctly operate the Spirobank Smart device. Accordingly, a total of 370 participants completed all the tests, and their data were analyzed in this study. A flowchart of the participant enrollment procedure is presented in Figure 1.

2.3. Study Procedures

All tests undertaken in the 26 outpatient settings were conducted on the same day. The participates were assessed using Spirobank Smart and required to complete a CAT questionnaire. Regarding the operation of the Spirobank Smart device, each nurse and physician who contributed to this study were adequately trained on the use of the device. The participants were also required to inhale maximally and then exhale forcibly into the mouthpiece of the device for at least 6 s until the chronometer was switched on and changed its color to green. Measurements of acceptable quality, that is those with the highest summed value (FEV_1 + FVC), were subsequently recorded; individual ratios were then calculated. Cross-contamination was minimized using disposable plastic mouthpieces. Spirometry with BD reversibility was performed independently by trained operators in accordance with the guidelines proposed by the American Thoracic Society. Lung function parameters were measured before and after 20 min of BD inhalation. At least three adequate baseline and post-BD FVC maneuvers were performed to measure the highest FEV_1 and FVC values. COPD diagnosis and COPD severity classification were conducted in accordance with GOLD definitions. The reference criterion for COPD was defined as a post-BD FEV_1/FVC value of <70%, and COPD severity was classified according to the post-BD FEV_1 percentages of the predicted values.

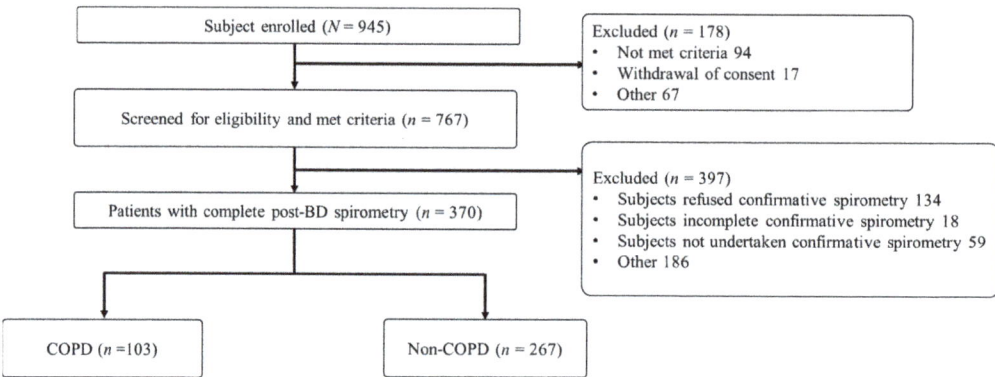

Figure 1. Flowchart of participant selection for the early detection of chronic obstructive pulmonary disease (COPD).

2.4. Devices and System

The Spirobank Smart device (MIR, Rome, Italy) used in this study can connect to smartphone apps through Bluetooth for the seamless recording of lung function parameters; it makes measurements through a bidirectional digital turbine. The turbine sensor operates based on the infrared interruption principle, which can ensure appropriate and repeatable measurement procedures. The device does not require calibration and applies a disposable turbine flow meter for its measurements. In this study, each participant's demographic information, including age, gender, height, and weight, was manually inputted into the device before the spirometry could be performed. To obtain measurements using this spirometer, each participant was required to exhale into the turbine, thus activating the motor inside the spirometer; concurrently, the speed of the rotor was recorded, and the recorded data were then adapted and transmitted to the app on the participant's smartphone. The exhalation process switched on the chronometer, and the color of the chronometer changed from orange to green after 6 s of exhalation. Accordingly, data on several parameters, including FEV_1, PEF, FVC, FEV_1/FVC, FEV_6, and FEF_{25-75}, were instantly displayed on the app. When an error occurred, the device detected and indicated the error description. Each participant was required to perform three cycles of inhalation and exhalation, and the best FEV_1 and FVC values were selected. GLI-2012-predicted values were used as the reference values (as reported in our previous study [24]) for the executed spirometry. Such predicted values can be expressed as follows: predicted value = $e^a \times H^b \times A^c \times e^{d \times group} \times e^{spline}$. In the preceding equation, "group" represents Southeast Asian.

2.5. Statistical Analysis

Data are expressed as a frequency with a percentage and as mean ± standard deviation for categorical and continuous variables, respectively. The distributions of the variables between COPD and non-COPD were compared using Student's t-test and the chi-square test. The agreement between the post-BD FEV_1/FVC values measured through confirmatory spirometry and pre-BD FEV_1/FVC values measured using Spirobank Smart was assessed using Bland–Altman plots. The optimal cutoff point for the FEV_1/FVC ratio determined by Spirobank Smart for identifying COPD in high-risk participants was determined using the Youden index derived from receiver operating characteristic (ROC) analysis. Sensitivity, specificity, positive predictive values (PPVs), negative predictive values (NPVs), and ROC curve values were then used to assess the effectiveness of the aforementioned screening tools in differentiating between COPD and non-COPD. Logistic regression analyses were performed to determine the association between potential risk factors and COPD incidence. All statistical analyses were performed using IBM SPSS 22 (IBM Corp., Armonk, NY, USA). In all analyses, two-tailed p-values < 0.05 were considered statistically significant.

3. Results

3.1. Demographic Characteristics of Study Participants

This study included data from 26 hospitals and clinics in Taiwan, including medical centers, regional hospitals, district hospitals, and clinics. The demographic characteristics of the enrolled participants are listed in Table 1. Among the participants, 103 had COPD (COPD group) and 267 did not have COPD (non-COPD group); of the participants, 94.3% were men. Participants with COPD appeared to be older, have higher pack-years of smoking, and have lower body mass index (BMI) values. The pre-BD FEV_1/FVC ratio that was determined using Spirobank Smart was significantly lower in the COPD group (63.57 ± 13.37) than it was in the non-COPD group (81.78 ± 7.44; $p < 0.001$). The COPD group had a significantly higher CAT score (12 ± 7) and lower post-BD FEV_1/FVC ratio (59.06 ± 9.04) than did the non-COPD group (CAT score: 9 ± 6; post-BD FEV_1/FVC ratio: 81.28 ± 7.19; all $p < 0.001$). These variables demonstrated statistically significant differences between the two groups.

Table 1. Demographic characteristics of eligible participants for the early detection of chronic obstructive pulmonary disease (COPD).

Characteristics	Non-COPD	COPD	Total	p-Value
Sample size	267	103	370	-
Age (mean ± SD)	59.0 ± 9.0	65.7 ± 9.8	60.9 ± 9.7	<0.001
<55 years	93 (34.8%)	17 (16.5%)	110 (29.7%)	
55–59 years	46 (17.2%)	9 (8.7%)	55 (14.9%)	<0.001
60–64 years	56 (21%)	17 (16.5%)	73 (19.7%)	
≥65 years	72 (27%)	60 (58.3%)	132 (35.7%)	
Gender				
Male	253 (94.8%)	96 (93.2%)	349 (94.3%)	0.536
Female	14 (5.2%)	7 (6.8%)	21 (5.7%)	
BMI	25.81 ± 3.86	24.38 ± 4.13	25.41 ± 3.98	0.001
Cough				
No	24 (9.0%)	4 (3.9%)	28 (7.6%)	0.096
Yes	243 (91.0%)	99 (96.1%)	342 (92.4%)	
Phlegm				
No	30 (11.2%)	9 (8.7%)	39 (10.5%)	0.483
Yes	237 (88.8%)	94 (91.3%)	331 (89.5%)	
Breathless				
No	91 (34.1%)	24 (23.3%)	115 (31.1%)	0.045
Yes	176 (65.9%)	79 (76.7%)	255 (68.9%)	

Table 1. Cont.

Characteristics	Non-COPD	COPD	Total	p-Value
CAT	9 ± 6	12 ± 7	10 ± 6	
0–9	160 (59.9%)	43 (41.7%)	203 (54.9%)	
10–19	94 (35.2%)	44 (42.7%)	138 (37.3%)	0.001
20–29	12 (4.5%)	15 (14.6%)	27 (7.3%)	
30–40	1 (0.4%)	1 (1.0%)	2 (0.5%)	
Smoking pack-years	39.4 ± 27.5	48.6 ± 29.3	42.6 ± 28.3	0.001
<50	216 (80.9%)	67 (65.0%)	283 (76.5%)	<0.001
≥50	51 (19.1%)	36 (35.0%)	87 (23.5%)	
Pre-bronchodilator FEV_1/FVC determined using Spirobank Smart	81.78 ± 7.44	63.57 ± 13.37	76.71 ± 12.49	<0.001
Post-bronchodilator FEV_1/FVC determined using a diagnostic spirometer	81.28 ± 7.19	59.06 ± 9.04	75.1 ± 12.62	<0.001

3.2. Agreement between Post-BD FEV_1/FVC Ratios Measured Using the Confirmatory Spirometry and Pre-BD FEV_1/FVC Ratios Measured Using Spirobank Smart

Bland–Altman plots (Figure 2) are useful for determining the relationship between differences and averages, which can help researchers to explore any systematic biases and identify possible outliers. In this study, we derived Bland–Altman plots to evaluate the agreement between the pre-BD FEV_1/FVC ratios measured using Spirobank Smart and the post-BD FEV_1/FVC ratios measured using the confirmatory spirometry. The plots revealed that few values (5.67%) fell outside the 95% confidence interval. The mean difference between the post-BD values derived using the confirmatory spirometry and the FEV_1/FVC values derived using Spirobank Smart was 1.6%. Additionally, the plots demonstrated that the limits of agreement were superior (narrower) for the mean of FEV_1/FVC values of <70% than they were for the mean of FEV_1/FVC values of ≥70%.

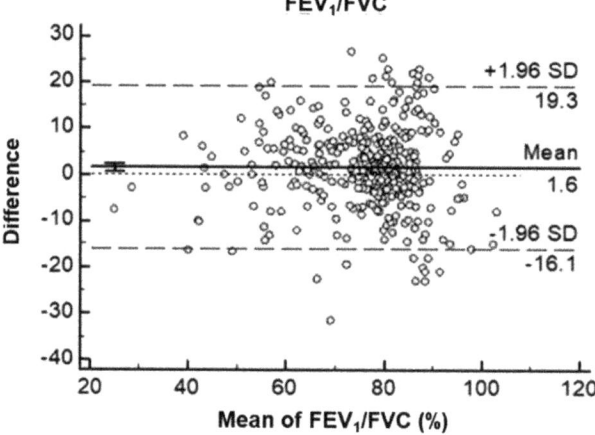

Figure 2. Bland–Altman plots illustrating the differences between the prebronchodilator (pre-BD) forced expiratory volume in 1 s (FEV_1)/forced vital capacity (FVC) values obtained using Spirobank Smart and the post-BD FEV_1/FVC values obtained using the diagnostic spirometer as a percentage of the mean difference (vertical axis) versus the mean of the two FEV_1/FVC ratios (horizontal axis).

3.3. ROC Curves and Diagnostic Accuracy for the Pre-BD FEV_1/FVC Ratios Measured Using Spirobank Smart

We constructed ROC curves (Figure 3) to assess the suitability of FEV_1/FVC measured using Spirobank Smart as a prescreening measure for COPD identification. Our results indicated that FEV_1/FVC measured by Spirobank Smart could significantly predict COPD, with the corresponding area under the ROC curve (AUROC) being 0.903 (95% CI = 0.860–0.947). According to the Youden index derived from our ROC analysis, Spirobank-Smart-measured FEV_1/FVC values of < 74% can serve as high-risk indicators of COPD, and the highest predictive ability was observed at an AUROC value of 0.873 (95% CI = 0.827–0.920).

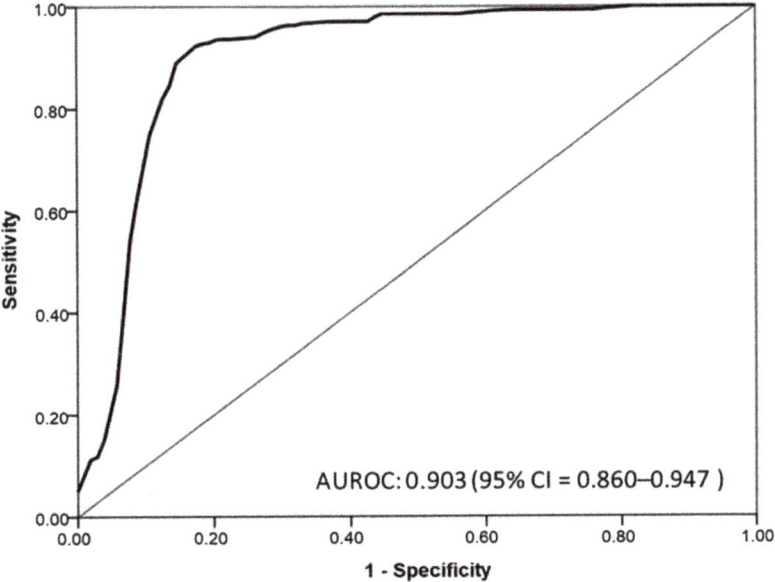

Figure 3. Receiver operating characteristic (ROC) curves for the forced expiratory volume in 1 s (FEV_1)/forced vital capacity (FVC) ratio measured using Spirobank Smart.

The cutoff values for FEV_1/FVC and the corresponding predictive performance of Spirobank Smart are presented in Table 2. As indicated in this table, at the optimal cutoff point of 0.74, the sensitivity, specificity, PPV, and NPV were 82.50%, 92.13%, 80.20%, and 93.20%, respectively. Compared with the sensitivity of Spirobank Smart with an FEV_1/FVC ratio of <70, the sensitivity of the diagnostic spirometer was as low as 70.90%; thus, most patients with COPD were underdiagnosed, despite the AUROC being 0.834 (95% CI = 0.779–0.889). The portable spirometer achieved a balance between sensitivity and specificity when the FEV_1/FVC ratio was <74%; accordingly, it exhibited the best predictive ability. Our findings revealed that Spirobank Smart could be used as a diagnostic tool in general population screening procedures for identifying patients that are at high risk of COPD.

Figure 4 illustrates the diagnostic performance, as assessed with respect to COPD severity, that was observed at the optimal cutoff point for FEV_1/FVC (<74%). Some of the participants without COPD were recorded as having COPD, resulting in false-positive results; this thus led to moderate PPV estimates (80.20%). In addition, relatively few participants with COPD were recorded as not having COPD, resulting in false-negative results; this thus led to high NPV estimates (93.20%). Of the participants for whom false-negative results were recorded, 80% had mild or only moderate COPD.

Table 2. Diagnostic accuracy of Spirobank Smart across different cutoff points.

Device Cutoff Ratio (FEV$_1$/FVC)	Sensitivity (%)	Specificity (%)	PPV (%)	NPV (%)	AUROC (95% CI)
<70%	70.90%	95.88%	86.90%	89.50%	0.834 (0.779–0.889)
<71%	73.80%	94.01%	82.60%	90.30%	0.839 (0.786–0.892)
<72%	77.70%	93.63%	82.50%	91.60%	0.857 (0.806–0.907)
<73%	80.60%	92.88%	81.40%	92.50%	0.867 (0.819–0.916)
<74%	82.50%	92.13%	80.20%	93.20%	0.873 (0.827–0.920)
<75%	86.40%	84.64%	68.50%	94.20%	0.855 (0.810–0.901)
<76%	87.40%	82.02%	65.20%	94.40%	0.847 (0.801–0.893)

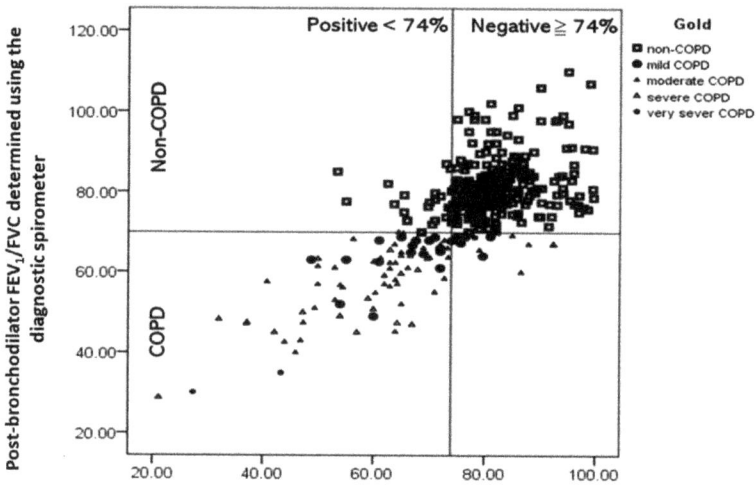

Figure 4. Scatter plots of post-bronchodilator (post-BD) forced expiratory volume in 1 s (FEV$_1$)/forced vital capacity (FVC) ratios that were determined using the diagnostic spirometer against pre-BD FEV$_1$/FVC ratios that were determined using Spirobank Smart for eligible participants. The quadrants are defined by the GOLD spirometer criteria for obstruction (post-BD FEV$_1$/FVC < 70%) and the Spirobank-Smart-measured FEV$_1$/FVC ratios that yielded optimal performance characteristics (FEV$_1$//FVC < 74%).

3.4. GOLD Classification and CAT Score of Participants Based on the FEV$_1$ Values Obtained Using Confirmatory Spirometry and Spirobank Smart

To evaluate whether the FEV$_1$ determined using Spirobank Smart could be a reliable parameter for classifying obstruction severity, we analyzed the obstruction severity by using the FEV$_1$ values obtained through confirmatory spirometry and those determined using Spirobank Smart; the analysis results are summarized in Table 3. The FEV$_1$ values obtained using the diagnostic spirometer revealed that 24.3% and 51.5% of the participants exhibited mild and moderate COPD (GOLD I and II), respectively. The classification results obtained using the FEV$_1$ values determined using Spirobank Smart were comparable to those obtained using the values determined using the diagnostic spirometer (i.e., 15.5% and 57.3% of the participants were classified as having GOLD I and II severity levels, respectively). Moreover, the CAT scores for grades III and V were higher than those for grades I and II.

Table 3. GOLD classifications and CAT scores of the patients. The scores depended on the forced expiratory volume in 1 s (FEV$_1$) values obtained using a diagnostic spirometer and Spirobank Smart. The characteristics of patients with chronic obstructive pulmonary disease (COPD) were defined according to the GOLD classification of disease severity.

GOLD Grade	Diagnostic Spirometer		Spirobank Smart	
	n (%)	CAT Score	n (%)	CAT Score
GOLD I	25 (24.3%)	10 ± 5	16 (15.5%)	10 ± 4
GOLD II	53 (51.5%)	12 ± 7	59 (57.3%)	11 ± 6
GOLD III	22 (21.3%)	11 ± 6	22 (21.4%)	13 ± 8
GOLD IV	3 (2.9%)	21 ± 19	6 (5.8%)	18 ± 12
Total	103 (100%)	12 ± 7	103 (100%)	12 ± 7

3.5. Associations of FEV$_1$/FVC Determined Using Spirobank Smart and the Participant Characteristic Variables with the COPD Incidence

Univariate logistic regression analysis revealed that factors such as an FEV$_1$/FVC ratio of <74% that was determined using Spirobank Smart, ≥50 pack-years of smoking, age, and lower BMI were positively associated with the incidence of COPD. After the multivariate adjustments, we observed that an FEV$_1$/FVC ratio of <74% that was determined using Spirobank Smart (odds ratio (OR) = 58.58, 95% CI = 27.29–125.75) and old age (OR = 3.23, 95% CI = 1.04–10.07 for 60 ≤ age < 65; OR = 5.82, 95% CI = 2.22–15.27 for age ≥ 65) remained significantly associated with the incidence of COPD (Table 4).

Table 4. Multivariate logistic regression analysis used to evaluate the associations between the forced expiratory volume in 1 s (FEV$_1$)/forced vital capacity (FVC) that was determined using Spirobank Smart, patients characteristic variables, and chronic obstructive pulmonary disease (COPD) incidence.

Variables	Crude OR (95% CI)	p-Value	Adjusted OR (95% CI)	p-Value
Portable spirometer: FEV1/FVC< 74%	55.14 (28.13–108.77)	<0.001	58.58 (27.29–125.75)	<0.001
Smoking PY ≥ 50	2.28 (1.37–3.78)	0.001	1.31 (0.57–2.98)	0.535
Age category				
Age < 55	1		1	
55 ≤ age < 60	1.07 (0.44–2.59)	0.864	1.12 (0.32–3.886)	0.864
60 ≤ age < 65	1.66 (0.79–3.51)	0.185	3.23 (1.04–10.07)	0.04
Age ≥ 65	4.56 (2.45–8.48)	<0.001	5.82 (2.22–15.27)	<0.001
CAT category				
0–9	1		1	
10–19	1.74 (1.07–2.85)	0.027	1.39 (0.65–2.98)	0.393
20–29	4.65 (2.03–10.67)	<0.001	3.43 (0.99–11.29)	0.052
30–40	3.72 (0.23–60.71)	0.356	5.89 (0.06–613.56)	0.535
BMI	0.907 (0.85–0.97)	0.002		
Gender (male)	0.759 (0.30–1.94)	0.759		

4. Discussion

Earlier detection of COPD in patients can improve the short- and long-term patient outcomes when treated using current therapies. Although spirometry is the gold standard for COPD diagnosis, it is often perceived as an expensive and time-consuming process, leading to the underdiagnosis or misdiagnosis of COPD. Furthermore, spirometry is not cost-effective for screening for COPD in a population of truly asymptomatic smokers. To the best of our knowledge, few efficacious strategies have been designed for identifying patients with undiagnosed COPD who are most likely to benefit from current therapies, especially in Taiwan [19]. Accordingly, to bridge this gap, we used an app-based portable spirometer, namely, Spirobank Smart, to identify undiagnosed COPD in at-risk populations as the first step in determining which patients should be referred for further COPD diagnostic evaluation.

We validated the feasibility and suitability of Spirobank Smart for deriving FEV_1/FVC values for screening undiagnosed patients who were at risk of COPD. Based on our knowledge, this is the first study in Taiwan to evaluate the accuracy and feasibility of an app-based spirometer for early COPD detection. The principal findings of this study regarding at-risk population outcomes are outlined as follows. First, we found that 27.8% of the participants were newly diagnosed with COPD using confirmatory spirometry at tertiary hospitals, and nearly 70% of the newly diagnosed patients had mild or moderate COPD. Second, the AUROC value for COPD identification using Spirobank-Smart-derived was 0.903. Third, patients who have an FEV_1/FVC ratio of <74% that was determined using Spirobank Smart (odds ratio (OR) = 60.70, 95% CI = 27.95–131.83) and old age (OR = 3.23, 95% CI = 1.04–10.07 for $60 \leq$ age < 65; OR = 5.82, 95% CI = 2.22–15.27 for age $\geq$ 65) exhibited a higher risk of COPD; this indicates that COPD incidence was associated with increased age and FEV_1/FVC ratio < 74% determined by Spirobank-Smart. These findings support the claim that Spirobank Smart is an acceptable and feasible screening tool for the early detection of COPD.

A previous study reported a COPD prevalence of 18.9% when respiratory symptoms were not considered in the inclusion criteria [25]. When respiratory symptoms were considered in the inclusion criteria, the prevalence of COPD increased to 25–52.9% [16,18]. In Taiwan, a nationwide survey of the general population revealed an estimated COPD prevalence of 6% [26]; however, a case-finding study reported that the COPD prevalence in an at-risk population was 48.8% [27]. The present study indicated a COPD prevalence of 27.85% in smokers who were aged >40 years and had $\geq$10 pack-years of smoking and at least one symptom. Kjeldgaard et al. used a similar study design and similar inclusion criteria to those of the present study; they determined the COPD prevalence to be 32% in an at-risk population (aged $\geq$40 years with smoking history and at least one respiratory symptom) [18]. Kim et al. measured the COPD prevalence in smokers who had 10 pack-years of smoking and were aged >40 years in a primary care setting; they reported that the prevalence of COPD was 23.7% [28]. These findings suggest that the prevalence would be significantly influenced by the inclusion criteria that are used to define COPD and that screening for high-risk individuals can detect high proportions of patients that are undiagnosed as having COPD. Furthermore, our findings demonstrate that Spirobank Smart could be used for early detection of COPD in an outpatient clinical setting, as evidenced by a follow-up diagnostic spirometer test used for confirmation; the concomitant presence of respiratory symptoms increased the likelihood of identifying COPD.

In the present study, the level of agreement between the pre-BD FEV_1/FVC values that were determined using Spirobank Smart and the post-BD FEV_1/FVC values that were determined using the diagnostic spirometer was satisfactory; this thus demonstrates that Spirobank Smart is an acceptable alternative screening tool for early detection of COPD. Notably, the limits of agreement for the FEV_1/FVC values of <70% were narrower than those for FEV_1/FVC values of $\geq$70%, implying that FEV_1/FVC values of $\geq$70% may lead to slight underestimations. In other words, the underdiagnosis of obstruction may occur in younger adults or those with mild COPD. Therefore, we suggest that FEV_1/FVC values of <0.74, instead of FEV_1/FVC values of <0.70 (the conventional GOLD definition), be used along with Spirobank Smart for optimal screening; additionally, this cutoff resulted in the achievement of a balance between false-positive and false-negative results in our study population, thereby reducing the possibility of underdiagnosis or misdiagnosis.

Few reports are available on the feasibility and reliability of portable devices for COPD screening in clinical settings. Frith et al. evaluated the feasibility of piko-6 in the early detection of COPD without including a BD test [29]. Two other studies have also used COPD-6 and piko-6 screening devices. These three studies have indicated that COPD-6 and piko-6 implemented with FEV_1/FEV_6 for COPD screening in at-risk populations had AUROC values of 0.75 and 0.86, respectively, validating these screening devices as acceptable tools for COPD screening in at-risk populations [16–19,29]. These findings are similar to those of the present study. Although FEV_6 is an acceptable surrogate for FVC in spirometry, FEV_6 has some drawbacks, such as the underestimation of mild airway obstruction [30–32]. Hernández et al. reported that FEV_1/FVC values of <0.7 determined using a smartphone-based spirometer, namely Air-Smart, for detecting obstructive airway diseases had a sensitivity of 94.0% and a specificity of 97.2% [20]. Although the use of portable devices to diagnose COPD or obstructive airway diseases has been validated, the results cannot be compared with those of the current study due to the differences in experimental design and spirometry procedures between the studies.

ROC analysis for the FEV_1/FVC values that were determined using Spirobank Smart demonstrated that this parameter could differentiate between the COPD and non-COPD groups with moderate to good AUROC values (0.903 (95% CI = 0.860–0.947)). The optimal cutoff point (FEV_1/FVC value of <74.0%) with a score of 0.757 was determined according to the Youden index. A screening method with perfect sensitivity, specificity, PPV, and NPV is not usually available. In COPD screening, high sensitivity, rather than high specificity, is prioritized because identifying more potential patients with COPD-like conditions is crucial. The PPVs derived in this study revealed that approximately 20% of patients had post-BD FEV_1/FEV values below the optimal cutoff point of <0.7; therefore, the PPV is useful for avoiding unnecessary, excessive examination of participants due to false positives. Additionally, high NPVs were observed in this study, indicating that 90% of patients had FEV_1/FVC values of $\geq$74.0%, as determined using Spirobank Smart; therefore, we could feasibly determine whether a participant could have COPD and require further testing. Our results are similar to those of a previous study that examined the COPD screening accuracy of a handheld spirometer according to the AUROC, sensitivity, specificity, PPV, and NPV at a specified cutoff point. Additional studies are warranted to determine the clinically sensible cutoff point of the parameter in Spirobank Smart in other cohorts and thereby confirm its clinical usefulness for COPD screening. The use of a spirometer alongside a BD is the gold standard for COPD diagnosis. However, a BD is not sufficiently safe for implementation in primary clinics or nonspecialist areas due to insufficient monitoring and emergency procedures [28]. Therefore, we suggest that for individuals who are at risk of COPD and have abnormal testing results from Spirobank Smart, another diagnostic procedure executed using a spirometer alongside a BD should be used. Accordingly, Spirobank Smart may reduce inappropriate BD use in COPD diagnoses and provide a feasible screening process.

The conventional GOLD definition may lead to the underdiagnosis of obstruction in younger adults and overdiagnosis of obstruction in older adults [33,34]. Therefore, scholars have suggested the use of a lower limit of normal (LLN)-based diagnosis of COPD [33–35]. However, a previous study reported that LLN-based definitions tend to underdiagnose COPD in symptomatic patients [4]. In our study design, we used a case-finding strategy based on symptom screening. The conventional GOLD definition may, therefore, be the appropriate choice for reducing the underdiagnosis of COPD in our screening strategy. In addition, previous studies have indicated that the LLN-based diagnosis of COPD generated fewer false positives and more false negatives compared with the conventional GOLD definition. False negatives lead to the undertreatment of patients with COPD during disease stages (e.g., GOLD I and II) when they are likely to benefit most. Moreover, LLN tends to categorize elderly adults with mild obstruction into a non-COPD category (due to its high specificity and low sensitivity) [36]. In our study population, the mean age was 60.9 years, and a large proportion of the participants had COPD in GOLD I and II; thus, the use of the conventional GOLD definition may help to avoid potential false-negative results. A previous study revealed that compared with diagnoses executed using fixed cutoff values, diagnoses based on the LLN involved slightly higher NPVs [37]. Considering the potential false positives that can result from using the conventional GOLD definition and considering the evolving understanding of strategies for airflow obstruction detection, the use of the LLN-based definitions as a gold standard in spirometry to validate the FEV_1/FVC values that were determined using Spirobank Smart could be valuable and warrants further study.

A CAT score of ≥ 10 points is used to classify patients with COPD as highly symptomatic. In the present study, 41.7% of patients that were newly diagnosed as having COPD had CAT scores of <10, which indicated that the presence of fewer symptoms may contribute to diagnostic confusion and clinical neglect. Moreover, studies have reported that handheld spirometers are useful for determining obstruction severity. In our study, we assessed the feasibility of evaluating COPD severity in an at-risk population by using FEV_1. We determined that nearly 70% of the newly diagnosed COPD cases were classified as GOLD I or II based on the FEV_1 values that were measured using Spirobank Smart. The frequency of GOLD classifications was similar to that of the diagnostic spirometer. Our findings also demonstrate that the prevalence of COPD in GOLD I was 24.3%, which is similar to that (27.2%) observed in a previous study conducted at a single medical center in Taiwan [23]; this suggests that Spirobank Smart is useful for identifying undiagnosed COPD with mild or moderate airway limitations in at-risk populations and can help to raise awareness of current perceptions of COPD. Based on our study findings, to provide the appropriate intervention, we propose the following clinical procedure for the triage of participants who are at risk of COPD: (1) if the FEV_1/FVC ratio is <0.74, the patient should be referred to a pulmonologist for further diagnosis; (2) if the FEV_1/FVC ratio is ≥ 0.74, a diagnosis alternative to COPD should be considered, and smoking cessation should be recommended to the patient; (3) if a patient is newly diagnosed as having COPD, they should be invited to join the COPD pay-for-performance program that is implemented by the National Health Insurance Administration to encourage physicians to provide patient-centered care plans; (4) if an individual is diagnosed as not having COPD, they should be advised to cease smoking (Figure 5). Furthermore, our findings indicated that patients with known smoking history who are old age had a higher risk of COPD. The English Longitudinal Study of Ageing (ELSA) demonstrated that nearly all smoking-related deaths (99%) were due to the occurrence of COPD in people aged >50 years, and the mean duration of smoking for current smokers was 42 years [38]. These findings suggest that an age of >40 years and a smoking history of ≥ 10 pack-years are adequate criteria for early COPD detection. In our study, we believe that symptomatic individuals who are aged >60 years with smoking history have greater risk of COPD and deserve closely routine COPD screening.

Limitations regarding the implementation of Spirobank Smart should be acknowledged. The data were collected from only a limited number of participants enrolled in hospital-based facilities, including medical centers and regional hospitals, which may not reflect the entire COPD population, especially those who have never visited hospitals for COPD testing. Additional studies including more types of medical facilities, such as primary care facilities, are warranted to assess the validity of Spirobank Smart. Moreover, the FEV_1 measurements that were obtained using Spirobank Smart were underestimated by up to 5%, and the FEV_1/FVC ratios were underestimated by 3–4%. These underestimations may cause by the inaccuracy of the portable device. However, Spirobank Smart complies with the latest documented ATS/ERS standards for accuracy, and our ROC analysis indicated that Spirobank Smart was sufficiently accurate for COPD identification through the case-finding strategy. Finally, the interday repeatability of the lung function test, even in the clinical trial population, was determined to be considerable, which may be a limitation of our study. A previous study highlighted the obscurity of lung function values from a single spirometry procedure. The results indicated that approximately 1% of the participants' values changed from the lowest to highest quintiles (and vice versa), and only approximately half of the participants allocated to different lung function quintiles at screening were grouped into the same quintile at baseline. A possible explanation for this is the methodological variability of lung function measurements and the physiological variability of the airway caliber [39].

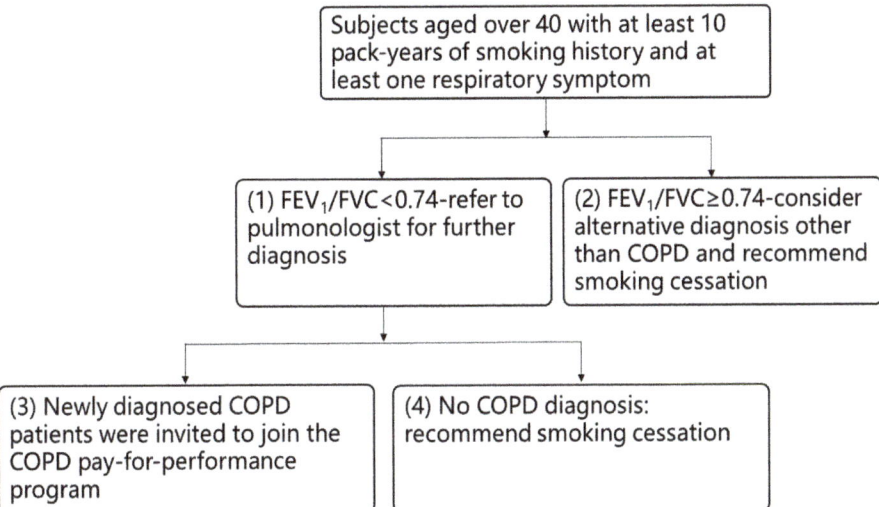

Figure 5. Clinical procedure for the triage of participants who are at risk of chronic obstructive pulmonary disease (COPD) based on the results obtained in this study using a lung function test and Spirobank Smart.

In conclusion, Spirobank Smart was determined to be a simple and feasible device for screening undiagnosed COPD in at-risk populations in outpatient clinical settings. We observed that measurements obtained from the device had a moderate correlation with those obtained from a diagnostic spirometer and that the device had acceptable accuracy in identifying undiagnosed COPD in our at-risk population. The use of an app-based spirometer is a potential strategy for improving the early detection of COPD. We suggest that individuals who are aged >40 years and have >10 pack-years of smoking and at least one respiratory symptom should receive a lung function evaluation using an app-based spirometer. Furthermore, we suggest that participants who have abnormal test results, as determined using Spirobank Smart with FEV_1/FVC values of <0.74, should undergo diagnostic spirometrer to confirm the COPD diagnosis and initiate an appropriate intervention in the early stages of the disease.

Author Contributions: Task, C.-H.L., S.-L.C., and H.-C.W.; formal analysis, C.-H.L., S.-L.C., and C.-Z.C.; investigation, D.-W.P., H.-I.L., M.-S.L., J.-R.T., C.-C.W., S.-H.L., H.-C.W., C.-Z.C., T.-M.Y., C.-L.L., and T.-Y.W.; resources, D.-W.P., H.-I.L., M.-S.L., J.-R.T., C.-C.W., S.-H.L., H.-C.W., C.-Z.C., T.-M.Y., C.-L.L., and T.-Y.W.; data curation, C.-H.L., S.-L.C., K.-Y.L., C.-Y.W.; writing—original draft preparation, C.-H.L. and S.-L.C.; writing—review and editing, H.-C.W.; visualization, C.-H.L.; supervision, H.-C.W. and M.-C.L.; project administration, W.-H.H. and M.-C.L. All authors have read and agreed to the published version of the manuscript.

Funding: This research was funded by Health Promotion Administration of Taiwan, grant number D1070206-108; The APC was funded by 109-CCH-MST-175.

Institutional Review Board Statement: The study was conducted according to the guidelines of the Declaration of Helsinki and approved by the Institutional Review Board (or Ethics Committee) of Changhua Christian Hospital (protocol code 190806 and date 10-08-2019).

Informed Consent Statement: Institutional Review Board of Changhua Christian Hospital reviewed the project and deemed it to be exempt research because the evaluation was for a public service program and all data were de-identified. The requirement for written consent was waived.

Data Availability Statement: The data presented in this study are available on request from the corresponding author. The data are not publicly available due to ethical reasons.

Conflicts of Interest: All authors declare no conflict of interest related to the data collected and procedures in this study.

Abbreviations

Abbreviations
COPD chronic obstructive pulmonary disease
FVC forced vital capacity
FEV_1 forced expiratory volume in 1 s
FEV_6 forced expiratory volume in 6 s
ROC receiver operating characteristic
AUROC area under the ROC curve

References

1. Lozano, R.; Naghavi, M.; Foreman, K.; Lim, S.; Shibuya, K.; Aboyans, V.; Abraham, J.; Adair, T.; Aggarwal, R.; Ahn, S.Y.; et al. Global and regional mortality from 235 causes of death for 20 age groups in 1990 and 2010: A systematic analysis for the Global Burden of Disease Study 2010. *Lancet* **2012**, *380*, 2095–2128. [CrossRef]
2. Contreras-Garza, B.M.; Xiong, W.; Guo, X.; Orozco-Hernández, J.P.; Pacheco-Gallego, M.; Montoya-Martínez, J.J.; Celli, B.R.; A Wedzicha, J. Update on Clinical Aspects of COPD. *N. Engl. J. Med.* **2019**, *381*, 2484–2486. [CrossRef]
3. Hwang, S.L.; Lin, Y.C.; Guo, S.E.; Chi, M.C.; Chou, C.T.; Lin, C.M. Prevalence of chronic obstructive pulmonary disease in Southwest-ern Taiwan: A population-based study. *J. Respir. Pulm. Med.* **2016**, *3*, 1–4.
4. Diab, N.; Gershon, A.S.; Sin, D.D.; Tan, W.C.; Bourbeau, J.; Boulet, L.P.; Aaron, S.D. Underdiagnosis and Overdiagnosis of Chronic Ob-structive Pulmonary Disease. *Am. J. Respir. Crit. Care Med.* **2018**, *198*, 1130–1139. [CrossRef] [PubMed]
5. Kaplan, A.; Thomas, M. Screening for COPD: The gap between logic and evidence. *Eur. Respir. Rev.* **2017**, *26*, 160113. [CrossRef] [PubMed]
6. Rodriguez-Roisin, R.; Rabe, K.F.; Vestbo, J.; Vogelmeier, C.; Agustí, A.; all previous and current members of the Science Committee and the Board of Directors of GOLD (goldcopd.org/committees/). Global Initiative for Chronic Obstructive Lung Disease (GOLD) 20th Anniversary: A brief history of time. *Eur. Respir. J.* **2017**, *50*, 1700671. [CrossRef]
7. Heffler, E.; Crimi, C.; Mancuso, S.; Campisi, R.; Puggioni, F.; Brussino, L.; Crimi, N. Misdiagnosis of asthma and COPD and underuse of spirometry in primary care unse-lected patients. *Respir. Med.* **2018**, *142*, 48–52. [CrossRef]
8. Fujita, M.; Nagashima, K.; Takahashi, S.; Suzuki, K.; Fujisawa, T.; Hata, A. Handheld flow meter improves COPD detectability regardless of using a conventional questionnaire: A split-sample validation study. *Respirology* **2019**, *25*, 191–197. [CrossRef]
9. Blain, E.; Craig, T. The Use of Spirometry in a Primary Care Setting. *J. Allergy Clin. Immunol.* **2008**, *121*, S81. [CrossRef]
10. Schermer, T.R.; Vatsolaki, M.; Behr, R.; Grootens, J.; Cretier, R.; Akkermans, R.; Denis, J.; Poels, P.; Bemt, L.V.D. Point of care microspirometry to facilitate the COPD diagnostic process in primary care: A clustered randomised trial. *NPJ Prim. Care Respir. Med.* **2018**, *28*, 17. [CrossRef]
11. US Preventive Services Task Force (USPSTF); Siu, A.L.; Bibbins-Domingo, K.; Grossman, D.C.; Davidson, K.W.; Epling, J.W., Jr.; García, F.A.; Gillman, M.; Kemper, A.R.; Krist, A.H.; et al. Screening for Chronic Obstructive Pulmo-nary Disease: US Preventive Services Task Force Recommendation Statement. *JAMA* **2016**, *315*, 1372–1377. [PubMed]
12. Guirguis-Blake, J.M.; Senger, C.A.; Webber, E.M.; Mularski, R.A.; Whitlock, E.P. Screening for Chronic Obstructive Pulmonary Dis-ease: Evidence Report and Systematic Review for the US Preventive Services Task Force. *JAMA* **2016**, *315*, 1378–1393. [CrossRef]
13. Yawn, B.P.; Martinez, F.J. POINT: Can Screening for COPD Improve Outcomes? Yes. *Chest* **2020**, *157*, 7–9. [CrossRef]
14. Hemmingsen, U.B.; Stycke, M.; Dollerup, J.; Poulsen, P.B. Guideline-Based Early Detection of Chronic Obstructive Pulmonary Disease in Eight Danish Municipalities: The TOP-KOM Study. *Pulm. Med.* **2017**, *2017*, 7620397. [CrossRef]
15. Martinez, F.J.; O'Connor, G.T. Screening, Case-Finding, and Outcomes for Adults with Unrecognized COPD. *JAMA* **2016**, *315*, 1343–1344. [CrossRef] [PubMed]
16. Sierra, V.H.; Mezquita, M.Á.H.; Cobos, L.P.; Sánchez, M.G.; Castellanos, R.D.; Sánchez, S.J.; Pérez, R.C.; Ferrero, M. Usefulness of The Piko-6 Portable Device for Early COPD Detection in Primary Care. Utilidad del dispositivo portátil Piko-6 para la detección precoz de la enfermedad pul-monar obstructiva crónica en atención primaria. *Arch Bronconeumol.* **2018**, *54*, 460–466. [CrossRef]
17. Sichletidis, L.; Spyratos, D.; Papaioannou, M.; Chloros, D.; Tsiotsios, A.; Tsagaraki, V.; Haidich, A.B. A combination of the IPAG questionnaire and PiKo-6®flow meter is a val-uable screening tool for COPD in the primary care setting. *Prim. Care Respir. J.* **2011**, *20*, 184–189. [CrossRef] [PubMed]

18. Kjeldgaard, P.; Lykkegaard, J.; Spillemose, H.; Ulrik, C.S. Multicenter study of the COPD-6 screening device: Feasible for early detection of chronic obstructive pulmonary disease in primary care? *Int. J. Chronic Obstr. Pulm. Dis.* **2017**, *12*, 2323–2331. [CrossRef]
19. Dickens, A.P.; Fitzmaurice, D.A.; Adab, P.; Sitch, A.; Riley, R.D.; Enocson, A.; Jordan, R.E. Accuracy of Vitalograph lung monitor as a screening test for COPD in primary care. *NPJ Prim. Care Respir. Med.* **2020**, *30*, 1–8. [CrossRef]
20. Ramos Hernández, C.; Núñez Fernández, M.; Pallares Sanmartín, A.; Mouronte Roibas, C.; Cerdeira Domínguez, L.; Botana Rial, M.I.; Cid, N.B.; Villar, A.F. Validation of the portable Air-Smart Spirometer. *PLoS ONE* **2018**, *13*, e0192789. [CrossRef]
21. Exarchos, K.P.; Gogali, A.; Sioutkou, A.; Chronis, C.; Peristeri, S.; Kostikas, K. Validation of the portable Bluetooth®Air Next spirometer in patients with different respiratory diseases. *Respir. Res.* **2020**, *21*, 79. [CrossRef] [PubMed]
22. Ring, B.; Burbank, A.J.; Mills, K.; Ivins, S.; Dieffenderfer, J.; Hernandez, M.L. Validation of an app-based portable spirometer in ad-olescents with asthma. *J. Asthma* **2019**, *58*, 497–504. [CrossRef] [PubMed]
23. Degryse, J.; Buffels, J.; Van Dijck, Y.; Decramer, M.; Nemery, B. Accuracy of office spirometry performed by trained primary-care physicians using the MIR Spirobank Smart hand-held spirometer. *Respiration* **2012**, *83*, 543–552. [CrossRef] [PubMed]
24. Quanjer, P.; Stanojevic, S.; Cole, T.; Baur, X.; Hall, G.; Culver, B.; Enright, P.; Hankinson, J.L.; Ip, M.S.; Zheng, J.; et al. Multi-ethnic reference values for spirometry for the 3–95-yr age range: The global lung function 2012 equations. *Eur. Respir. J.* **2012**, *40*, 1324–1343. [CrossRef]
25. Tinkelman, D.G.; Price, D.B.; Nordyke, R.J.; Halbert, R.J. COPD screening efforts in primary care: What is the yield? *Prim. Care Respir. J.* **2007**, *16*, 41–48. [CrossRef]
26. Hang, L.W.; Hsu, J.Y.; Chang, C.J.; Wang, H.C.; Cheng, S.L.; Lin, C.H.; Chan, M.C.; Wang, C.C.; Perng, D.W.; Yu, C.J. Predictive factors warrant screening for obstructive sleep apnea in COPD: A Taiwan National Survey. *Int. J. Chronic Obstr. Pulm. Dis.* **2016**, *30*, 665–673.
27. Su, K.-C.; Ko, H.-K.; Chou, K.-T.; Hsiao, Y.-H.; Su, V.Y.-F.; Perng, D.-W.; Kou, Y.R. An accurate prediction model to identify undiagnosed at-risk patients with COPD: A cross-sectional case-finding study. *NPJ Prim. Care Respir. Med.* **2019**, *29*, 22. [CrossRef]
28. Kim, J.K.; Lee, C.M.; Park, J.Y.; Kim, J.H.; Park, S.H.; Jang, S.H.; Jung, K.; Yoo, K.H.; Park, Y.B.; Rhee, C.K.; et al. Active case finding strategy for chronic obstructive pulmonary disease with handheld spirometry. *Medicine* **2016**, *95*, e5683. [CrossRef]
29. Frith, P.; Crockett, A.; Beilby, J.; Marshall, R.; Attewell, R.; Ratnanesan, A.; Gavagna, G. Simplified COPD screening: Validation of the PiKo-6®in primary care. *Prim. Care Respir. J.* **2011**, *20*, 190–198. [CrossRef]
30. Melbye, H.; Medbø, A.; Crockett, A. The FEV1/FEV6 ratio is a good substitute for the FEV1/FVC ratio in the elderly. *Prim. Care Respir. J.* **2006**, *15*, 294–298. [CrossRef]
31. Wang, S.; Gong, W.; Tian, Y.; Zhou, J. FEV1/FEV6 in Primary Care Is a Reliable and Easy Method for the Diagnosis of COPD. *Respir. Care* **2015**, *61*, 349–353. [CrossRef] [PubMed]
32. Demir, T.; Ikitimur, H.D.; Koc, N.; Yildirim, N. The role of FEV6 in the detection of airway obstruction. *Respir. Med.* **2005**, *99*, 103–106. [CrossRef] [PubMed]
33. Smith, L.J. The lower limit of normal versus a fixed ratio to assess airflow limitation: Will the debate ever end? *Eur. Respir. J.* **2018**, *51*, 1800403. [CrossRef] [PubMed]
34. Enright, P.; Brusasco, V. Counterpoint: Should we abandon $FEV_1/FVC < 0.70$ to detect airway obstruction? Yes. *Chest* **2010**, *138*, 1040–1042.
35. Swanney, M.P.; Ruppel, G.; Enright, P.L.; Pedersen, O.F.; Crapo, R.O.; Miller, M.R.; Jensen, R.L.; Falaschetti, E.; Schouten, J.P.; Hankinson, J.L.; et al. Using the lower limit of normal for the FEV1/FVC ratio reduces the misclassification of airway obstruction. *Thorax* **2008**, *63*, 1046–1051. [CrossRef]
36. Güder, G.; Brenner, S.; Angermann, C.E.; Ertl, G.; Held, M.; Sachs, A.P.; Lammers, J.-W.; Zanen, P.; Hoes, A.W.; Störk, S.; et al. GOLD or lower limit of normal definition? a comparison with expert-based diagnosis of chronic obstructive pulmonary disease in a prospective cohort-study. *Respir. Res.* **2012**, *13*, 13. [CrossRef]
37. van den Bemt, L.; Wouters, B.C.; Grootens, J.; Denis, J.; Poels, P.J.; Schermer, T.R. Diagnostic accuracy of pre-bronchodilator FEV1/FEV6 from microspirometry to detect airflow obstruction in primary care: A randomised cross-sectional study. *NPJ Prim. Care Respir. Med.* **2014**, *14*, 14033. [CrossRef]
38. Lewer, D.; McKee, M.; Gasparrini, A.; Reeves, A.; De Oliveira, C. Socioeconomic position and mortality risk of smoking: Evidence from the English Longitudinal Study of Ageing (ELSA). *Eur. J. Public Health* **2017**, *27*, 1068–1073. [CrossRef]
39. Bikov, A.; Lange, P.; Anderson, J.A.; Brook, R.D.; Calverley, P.M.A.; Celli, B.R.; Cowans, N.J.; Crim, C.; Dixon, I.J.; Martinez, F.J.; et al. FEV1 is a stronger mortality predictor than FVC in patients with moderate COPD and with an increased risk for cardiovascular disease. *Int. J. Chronic Obstr. Pulm. Dis.* **2020**, *15*, 1135–1142. [CrossRef]

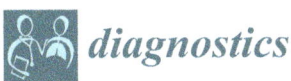

Article

Is the 1-Minute Sit-to-Stand Test a Good Tool to Evaluate Exertional Oxygen Desaturation in Chronic Obstructive Pulmonary Disease?

Ana L. Fernandes *, Inês Neves, Graciete Luís, Zita Camilo, Bruno Cabrita, Sara Dias, Jorge Ferreira and Paula Simão

Pulmonology Department, Pedro Hispano Hospital, 4464-513 Matosinhos, Portugal; inesmaria.neves@ulsm.min-saude.pt (I.N.); graciete.teixeira@ulsm.min-saude.pt (G.L.); zita.camilo@ulsm.min-saude.pt (Z.C.); bruno.cabrita@ulsm.min-saude.pt (B.C.); sara.pimentadias@ulsm.min-saude.pt (S.D.); jorge.ferreira@ulsm.min-saude.pt (J.F.); paula.simao@ulsm.min-saude.pt (P.S.)
* Correspondence: analuisafernandes22@gmail.com; Tel.: +351-916-701-756

Abstract: Background: Chronic obstructive pulmonary disease (COPD) is frequently associated with exertional oxygen desaturation, which may be evaluated using the 6-minute walking test (6MWT). However, it is a time-consuming test. The 1-minute sit-to-stand test (1STST) is a simpler test, already used to evaluate the functional status. The aim of this study was to compare the 1STST to the 6MWT in the evaluation of exertional desaturation. Methods: This was a cross-sectional study including 30 stable COPD patients who performed the 6MWT and 1STST on the same day. Six-minute walking distance (6MWD), number of 1STST repetitions (1STSTr), and cardiorespiratory parameters were recorded. Results: A significant correlation was found between the 6MWD and the number of 1STSTr (r = 0.54; p = 0.002). The minimum oxygen saturation (SpO_2) in both tests showed a good agreement (intraclass correlation coefficient (ICC) 0.81) and correlated strongly (r = 0.84; p < 0.001). Regarding oxygen desaturation, the total agreement between the tests was 73.3% with a fair Cohen's kappa (κ = 0.38; p = 0.018), and 93.33% of observations were within the limits of agreement for both tests in the Bland–Altman analysis. Conclusion: The 1STST seems to be a capable tool of detecting exercise-induced oxygen desaturation in COPD. Because it is a less time- and resources-consuming test, it may be applied during the outpatient clinic consultation to regularly evaluate the exercise capacity and exertional desaturation in COPD.

Keywords: COPD; 6MWT; STST; exercise capacity; oxygen desaturation; prognosis

Citation: Fernandes, A.L.; Neves, I.; Luís, G.; Camilo, Z.; Cabrita, B.; Dias, S.; Ferreira, J.; Simão, P. Is the 1-Minute Sit-to-Stand Test a Good Tool to Evaluate Exertional Oxygen Desaturation in Chronic Obstructive Pulmonary Disease?. *Diagnostics* **2021**, *11*, 159. https://doi.org/10.3390/diagnostics11020159

Academic Editor: Koichi Nishimura

Received: 27 December 2020
Accepted: 19 January 2021
Published: 22 January 2021

Publisher's Note: MDPI stays neutral with regard to jurisdictional claims in published maps and institutional affiliations.

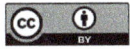

Copyright: © 2021 by the authors. Licensee MDPI, Basel, Switzerland. This article is an open access article distributed under the terms and conditions of the Creative Commons Attribution (CC BY) license (https://creativecommons.org/licenses/by/4.0/).

1. Introduction

Chronic obstructive pulmonary disease (COPD) is a leading cause of morbidity and mortality worldwide, with an economic and social burden that is both substantial and increasing [1]. Sedentarism in COPD is a consequence of constitutional and respiratory symptoms, which progressively affect functional status, exercise capacity, and health-related quality of life. Physical activity limitations and desaturation with exertion are important clinical markers in COPD patients and are associated with a poorer prognosis and higher number of exacerbations [2,3].

The 6-minute walking test (6MWT) is considered a validated and reliable test to evaluate the cardiopulmonary and musculoskeletal function in COPD [4]. However, it is not often assessed in investigational, inpatient, outpatient, or primary care settings due to the time, resources, and space needed to conduct it.

In recent years, new tests have been developed to facilitate exercise capacity in COPD. In this context, the sit-to-stand test (STST) has been proposed. The STST, first described in 1985 by Csuka and McCarty [5], measures a movement commonly performed in everyday life. Two main types of STST have been developed; one measures the number of repetitions in a set time (the 1-minute STST (1STST)) and the other the time taken to perform a set number of repetitions (the 5-repetition STST) [6]. The best protocol, however, was determined to be the 1STST in subjects with COPD [7,8].

The 1STST is accepted as an evaluation tool for the functional status and fall risk prediction of the elderly [9]. In particular, in recent studies, 1STST has shown predictive validity as a strong and independent predictor of mortality and health-related quality of life in COPD patients [10]. Some studies have demonstrated a significant correlation between the number of repetitions (1STSTr) and the 6-min walked distance (6MWD), the quadriceps muscle strength, and the level of physical activity in COPD patients, indicating that the 1STST may be valid for measuring exercise capability after respiratory rehabilitation [11–16]. Recently, Crook et al. reported that the 1STST is a reliable test for exercise capacity measurement in COPD with a minimal important difference of three repetitions [13]. Moreover, the 1STST has also been studied to evaluate exercise capacity and oxygen desaturation in interstitial lung disease and cystic fibrosis [17,18].

To our knowledge, a few studies have focused on evaluating the oxygen desaturation during the 1STST in COPD. Therefore, we aimed to compare the 1STST to the 6MWT for the ability to assess exercise-induced oxygen desaturation in COPD.

2. Materials and Methods

2.1. Subjects

Consecutive patients with COPD, according to the Global Initiative for Chronic Obstructive Lung Disease (GOLD) [1], followed in a pulmonology outpatient department were referred for consideration to our pulmonary function laboratory between August 2017 and February 2019. The exclusion criteria were chronic respiratory failure with long-term oxygen therapy, recent exacerbation (less than one month), patients without a recent lung function test (less than six months), and cardiovascular or orthopedic conditions that limit the ability to perform the tests.

2.2. Study Design

The study design was a cross-sectional study including stable COPD patients who performed the 6MWT and 1STST on the same day, with a 30-min resting period and accompanied by a cardiopulmonary technician. The sequence of the tests was random.

A 6-minute walking distance (6MWD) and the number of repetitions (1STSTr) were assessed. Regarding cardiorespiratory parameters, systolic blood pressure (sBP), diastolic blood pressure (dBP), dyspnea, and lower limb fatigue (modified Borg scale [19]) were recorded before and after both tests. Heart rate (HR) and peripheral arterial saturation (SpO_2) were continuously measured during the tests and for three minutes after the end of each test using Spirodoc® (Medical International Research, New Berlin, WI, USA). Oxygen desaturation (ΔSpO_2) for each test was defined as the difference between baseline SpO_2 and the minimum SpO_2. After a literature review, a $\Delta SpO_2 \geq 4\%$ was considered clinically significant for this study [17].

Demographic, clinical, and lung function data were collected by chart review. Forced vital capacity (FVC), expiratory volume in the first second (FEV_1), residual volume (RV) and total lung capacity (TLC) were performed by spirometry and plethysmography using Jaeger cabin®. Diffusing capacity for carbon monoxide (DLCO) was measured using the single breath method, and arterial partial pressure of oxygen (PaO_2) and arterial partial pressure of carbon dioxide ($PaCO_2$) from arterial blood gas were obtained.

The protocol of this study was approved by the local ethics committee. The aim of the study was explained to all participants and all signed an informed consent.

2.3. Outcome Measurements

2.3.1. Six-Minute Walking Test (6MWT)

Patients performed the 6MWT, according to the guidelines of the European Respiratory Society (ERS)/American Thoracic Society (ATS) [4]. The 6MWT was performed in a 30-

meter indoor corridor. A cardiopulmonary technician timed the walk and recorded the distance, using standardized encouragement strategy. None of the patients used a walking aid in daily life.

2.3.2. One-Minute Sit-to-Stand Test (1STST)

The 1STST was performed in a standard height chair (46 cm) without arm rests, according to the previously described protocols [13]. The test was first demonstrated by the staff and then performed by the participant. The patient was seated upright in the chair with knees and hips flexed at 90°, feet placed flat on the floor at hip width apart, and arms held stationary by placing their hands on their hips. Patients were asked to perform repetitions of standing upright and then sitting down in the same position at a self-paced speed (safe and comfortable) as many times as possible for 1 min. They were instructed not to use their arms for support while rising or sitting. The number of completed repetitions was manually recorded.

2.4. Statistical Analysis

All analyses were conducted using SPSS (version 22.0, software IBM, Armonk, NY, USA) for Windows. Descriptive data on continuous variables were reported as mean (M) and standard deviation (SD), depending on the normality of the variable distribution. Normality was verified by asymmetry coefficient and graphic analysis. For categorical variables, absolute (n) and relative (%) frequencies were used. The relationship between the 6MWD and the 1STSTr and the minimum SpO_2 of both tests was calculated by Pearson's correlation coefficient. This coefficient was also used to evaluate a relationship between 6MWD, 1STSTr, or minimum SpO_2 of both tests and clinical or lung function variables. The correlation value (r) was evaluated as: 0–0.25 = very weak, 0.26–0.50 = weak, 0.51–0.75 = moderate, 0.76–0.90 = strong, and 0.91–1.0 = very strong. The ANOVA test was used to measure the differences and evolution in the cardiorespiratory parameters, dyspnea, and lower limb fatigue (modified Borg scale) during the 6MWT and the 1STST. Agreement between the values obtained in the 6MWT and the 1STST were evaluated with the intraclass correlation coefficient (ICC). Agreement between the ability of the two exercise tests to detect desaturation ≥4% was assessed using Cohen's kappa coefficient (κ). The κ values of < 0, 0–0.20, 0.21–0.40, 0.41–0.60, 0.61–0.80, and 0.81–1 were considered to indicate no, slight, fair, moderate, substantial, and almost perfect agreement, respectively. A Bland–Altman analysis was conducted to graphically represent the limits of agreement between the minimum SpO_2 in the 6MWT and 1STST. A p value of less than 0.05 was considered significant.

3. Results

3.1. Participants

Thirty patients were included in the analysis, mainly males (26–86.7%) with a mean age of 67.57 ± 9.10 years and former smokers (15–50.0%). The mean body mass index (BMI) was 25.17 ± 4.98 kg/m². Most patients were included in the moderate-to-severe GOLD category [1] (GOLD 1: 1 (3.3%), GOLD 2: 16 (53.3%), GOLD 3: 12 (40%), GOLD 4: 1 (3.3%)). Demographic, clinical, and lung function characteristics are represented in Table 1.

Table 1. Patients' baseline characteristics, lung function tests, and results of the 1STST and the 6MWT. (M = mean; SD = standard deviation; 1STST = 1-min sit-to-stand test; 6MWT = 6-min walking test; mMRC = modified Medical Research Council; BODE = index with BMI, FEV_1, 6MWD, and mMRC; L= liters).

Variable	M/n	SD/%	Minimum	Maximum
Male gender	26	86.7	–	–
Smoking status				
Former smoker ǀ smoker ǀ non-smoker	15ǀ13ǀ2	50.0ǀ43.3ǀ6.7	–	–
Age (years)	67.57	9.10	48	83
Body mass index (BMI) (kg/m^2)	25.17	4.98	15.05	36.05
mMRC dyspnea scale	1.60	0.81	0	3
BODE index	2.70	1.75	0	6
Forced vital capacity (FVC) (liters (L))	2.51	0.76	1.42	4.56
Forced vital capacity (% predicted)	73.05	15.31	48.00	107.00
Forced expiratory volume in 1st second (FEV_1) (L)	1.41	0.52	0.60	2.78
Forced expiratory volume in 1st second (% predicted)	50.83	14.49	24.70	78.00
Residual volume (RV) (L)	4.47	1.43	2.66	9.31
Residual volume (% predicted)	191.87	58.32	106.00	354.00
Total lung capacity (TLC) (L)	7.09	1.77	4.87	12.59
Total lung capacity (% predicted)	116.37	19.97	78.90	172.00
Diffusing capacity for carbon monoxide (DLCO) (% predicted)	45.14	20.47	15.00	100.00
Arterial partial pressure of oxygen (PaO2) (mmHg)	69.80	13.80	34.00	91.00
Arterial partial pressure of carbon dioxide (PaCO2) (mmHg)	44.36	7.47	33.00	64.00
6-minute walking distance (6MWD) (meters)	409.37	103.23	240.00	630.00
Percentage of 6MWD (%)	84.23	20.65	52.00	134.00
Baseline SpO$_2$ 6MWT (%)	94.47	2.60	88.00	99.00
Minimum SpO$_2$ 6MWT (%)	86.47	6.55	68.00	96.00
Number of repetitions during 1STST (1STSTr)	18.13	5.46	9.00	34.00
Baseline SpO$_2$ 1STST (%)	94.67	2.58	89.00	99.00
SpO$_2$ minimum 1STST (%)	89.73	5.01	77.00	98.00

3.2. Comparison of Exercise Capacity and Cardiorespiratory Parameters between the 1STST and the 6MWT

The average number for the 1STSTr was 18.13 ± 5.46 in our population (Table 1). Regarding the 1STST, the number of repetitions presented a negative and statistical correlation with age (r = −0.53; p = 0.002), but it did not correlate with BMI or lung function parameters (FVC, FEV1, RV, TLC, or DLCO).

The mean 6MWD was 409.37 ± 103.23 m (Table 1). There was a statically negative correlation between 6MWD with age (r = −0.36; p = 0.049) and a positive correlation with FVC (r = 0.37; p = 0.044) and DLCO (r = 0.40; p = 0.036). No correlation was found with BMI or other lung function parameters.

Furthermore, there was a statistically significant positive correlation between the 6MWD and the 1STSTr (r = 0.54; p = 0.002) (Figure 1).

The results of the cardiorespiratory parameters, Borg dyspnea, and lower limb fatigue obtained during the 1STST and 6MWT are presented in Table 2. The evolution of the parameters resembles a polynomial function of the quadratic type (Figure 2). A significant increase in systolic blood pressure (sBP) (p < 0.001), diastolic blood pressure (dBP) (p < 0.001), heart rate (HR) (p < 0.001), Borg dyspnea (p < 0.001), and Borg lower limb fatigue (p < 0.001) were noted during the 6MWT and the 1STST. A significant decrease in SpO$_2$ was observed with both tests, as well as an increase in HR. After three minutes, the previously stated variables were similar to the baseline values. An interaction effect was observed in the evolution of sBP that registered a higher value at the end of the 6MWT (M = 160.17; SD = 21.93) compared to the 1STST (M = 154.17; SD = 23.77). The evolution of dBP (p = 0.182), HR (p = 0.126), SpO$_2$ (p = 0.148), Borg dyspnea (p = 0.103), and Borg lower limbs' fatigue (p = 0.238) was similar in both groups.

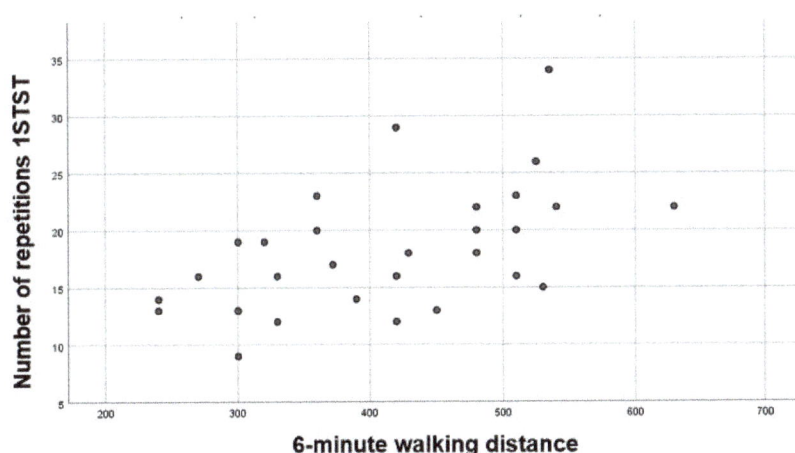

Figure 1. Correlation between 6MWD and 1STSTr (1STSTr = number of repetitions during 1-min sit-to-stand test; 6MWD = 6-min walking distance).

Table 2. ANOVA of repetitive measurements for the evolution of systolic blood pressure, diastolic blood pressure, heart rate, oxygen saturation, Borg dyspnea, and lower limbs' fatigue in the 6MWT and the 1STST. (1STST = 1-min sit-to-stand test; 6MWT = 6-min walking test; sBP = systolic blood pressure; dBP = diastolic blood pressure; HR = heart rate; SpO_2 = oxygen saturation).

Variable	Test	Baseline	Maximum Minimum	End	After 3 min	Variance Analysis		
						Evolution	Test	Interaction
sBP [&]	6MWT	129.93 (13.38)	–	160.17 (21.93)	136.20 (17.72)	$p < 0.001$ *	$p = 0.179$	$p = 0.005$ *
	STST	130.17 (17.38)	–	154.17 (23.77)	136.33 (20.16)			
dBP [&]	6MWT	71.87 (9.70)	–	79.67 (10.68)	76.27 (10.64)	$p < 0.001$ *	$p = 0.941$	$p = 0.182$
	STST	74.87 (11.80)	–	78.37 (10.68)	74.83 (10.54)			
HR [&]	6MWT	81.03 (14.24)	109.80 (14.24)	104.03 (16.04)	87.00 (12.66)	$p < 0.001$ *	$p = 0.007$ *	$p = 0.126$
	STST	80.87 (13.69)	105.60 (15.09)	96.13 (14.36)	82.60 (12.60)			
SpO_2 [&]	6MWT	94.47 (2.60)	86.47 (6.55)	90.00 (6.80)	94.03 (2.91)	$p < 0.001$ *	$p = 0.020$ *	$p = 0.148$
	STST	94.67 (2.58)	89.73 (5.01)	90.10 (5.42)	95.03 (2.81)			
Borg Dyspnea [#]	6MWT	1.27 (0.91)	–	3.33 (2.06)	–	$p < 0.001$ *	$p = 0.095$	$p = 0.103$
	STST	1.23 (0.97)	–	2.90 (1.77)	–			
Borg Limbs [#]	6MWT	1.27 (0.87)	–	3.23 (1.89)	–	$p < 0.001$ *	$p = 0.668$	$p = 0.238$
	STST	1.00 (0.83)	–	3.30 (1.64)	–			

Values represented as mean and standard deviation; [&] quadratic adjustment; [#] linear adjustment; * statistically significant.

When analyzing the differences between the 6MWT and the 1STST, we verified that the HR obtained a slightly higher but statistically significant value in the 6MWT ($p = 0.007$). Regarding SpO_2, the 6MWT obtained a significantly lower value comparing to the 1STST ($p = 0.02$).

The agreement values for cardiorespiratory parameters between the 6MWT and the 1STST are presented in Table 3. Moderate or strong agreement values were obtained for most variables. The minimum SpO_2 showed a substantial agreement between tests (ICC = 0.810) as did the end-test Borg dyspnea (ICC 0.750).

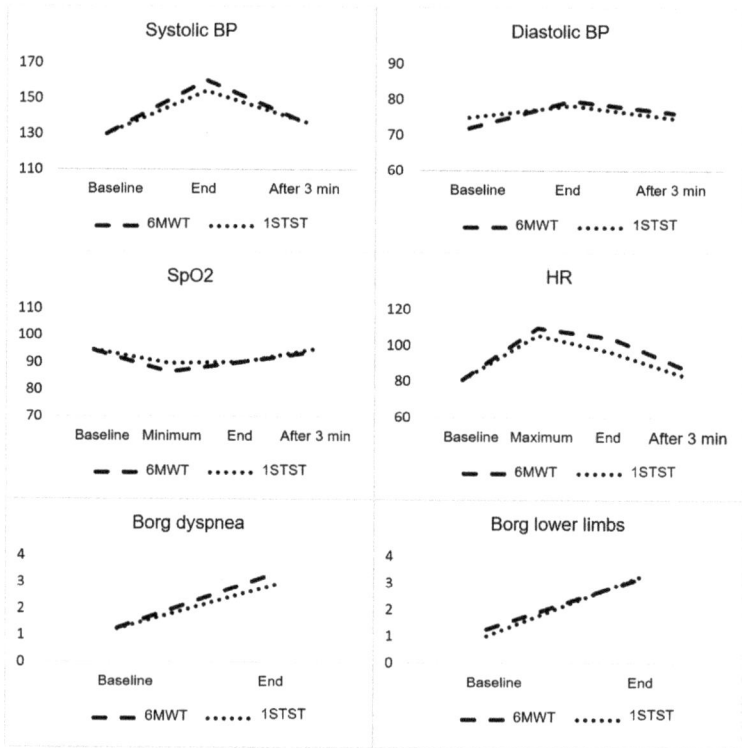

Figure 2. Evolution of cardiorespiratory parameters, Borg dyspnea, and lower limb fatigue during the 6MWT and the 1STST. (1STST = 1-min sit-to-stand test; 6MWT = 6-min walking test; sBP = systolic blood pressure; dBP = diastolic blood pressure; HR = heart rate; SpO_2 = oxygen saturation).

Table 3. Agreement on cardiorespiratory parameters between 1STST and 6MWT evaluated by intraclass correlation coefficient (ICC). (1STST = 1-min sit-to-stand test; 6MWT = 6-min walking test; sBP = systolic blood pressure; dBP = diastolic blood pressure; HR = heart rate; SpO_2 = oxygen saturation).

Variable	Baseline	Minimum	Maximum	End	After 3 min
sBP	0.780	-	-	0.870	0.866
dBP	0.739	-	-	0.754	0.340
HR	0.891	-	0.665	0.484	0.789
SpO_2	0.833	0.810	-	0.506	0.764
Borg dyspnea	0.942	-	-	0.750	-
Borg limbs	0.669	-	-	0.555	-

3.3. Comparison of Oxygen Desaturation between the 1STST and 6MWT

The minimum SpO_2 on STST was 89.73 ± 5.01 and 18 patients (60.0%) presented an oxygen desaturation (ΔSpO_2) ≥ 4%. Four patients (13.3%) registered their minimum SpO_2 during the three minutes after the end of the test, mostly during the first minute. There were statistical correlations between minimum SpO_2 in 1STST with TLC (r = 0.41; p = 0.025) and paO2 (r = 0.52; p = 0.007). No correlation was found with age, BMI, or other lung function parameters.

The minimum SpO_2 on 6MWT was 86.47 ± 6.55 and 26 patients (86.7%) presented a desaturation (ΔSpO_2) ≥ 4%. In one participant (3.0%), the minimum SpO_2 was obtained after the end of the test. A statistically significant correlation was verified between minimum SpO_2 in the 6MWT with paO2 (r = 0.67; $p < 0.001$), FVC (r = 0.38; $p = 0.036$), FEV1 (r = 0.38; $p = 0.037$), and DLCO (r = 0.38; $p = 0.043$). No correlation was found with age, BMI, and other lung function parameters. Individual SpO_2 measurements during the 6MWT and the 1STST are presented in Table S1.

A significant, strong, and positive correlation was found between the minimum SpO_2 registered in the 1STST and the 6MWT (r = 0.84; $p < 0.001$) (Figure 3).

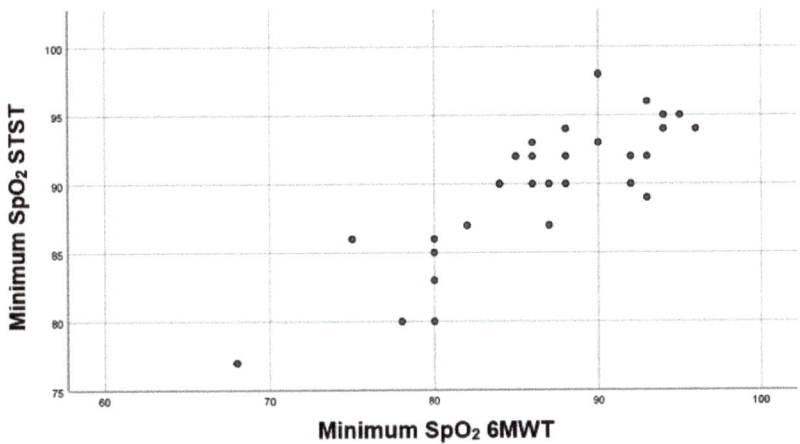

Figure 3. Correlation between minimum SpO_2 registered during the 1STST and the 6MWT. (SpO_2 = oxygen saturation; 1STST = 1-min sit-to-stand test; 6MWT = 6-min walking test).

Regarding oxygen desaturation (ΔSpO_2), the total agreement between the 1STST and the 6MWT was 73.3% with a fair Cohen's kappa, as shown in Table 4.

Table 4. Agreement between $\Delta SpO_2 \geq 4\%$ in the 1STST and the 6MWT, evaluated by Cohen's kappa (k). (1STST = 1-min sit-to-stand test; 6MWT = 6-min walking test; SpO_2 = oxygen saturation).

Variables	$\Delta SpO_2 \geq 4\%$ (1STST)		Agreement Analysis
$\Delta SpO_2 \geq 4\%$ (6MWT)	No	Yes	% total agreement = 73.3% ($p = 0.018$)
No	4 (13.3%)	0 (0%)	Cohen's kappa = 0.38
Yes	8 (26.7%)	18 (60.0%)	

Moreover, the agreement between the minimum SpO_2 values of the two tests was evaluated by the Bland–Altman plot (Figure 4). The limit of agreement was calculated as $M \pm 1.96 \times SD$, which created the interval] $-3.27 - 1.96 \times 3.60$; $-3.27 + 1.96 \times 3.60$ [=] -10.33; $3.79 \times$ [. A total of 93.33% of observations were within the limits of agreement, as demonstrated in Figure 4.

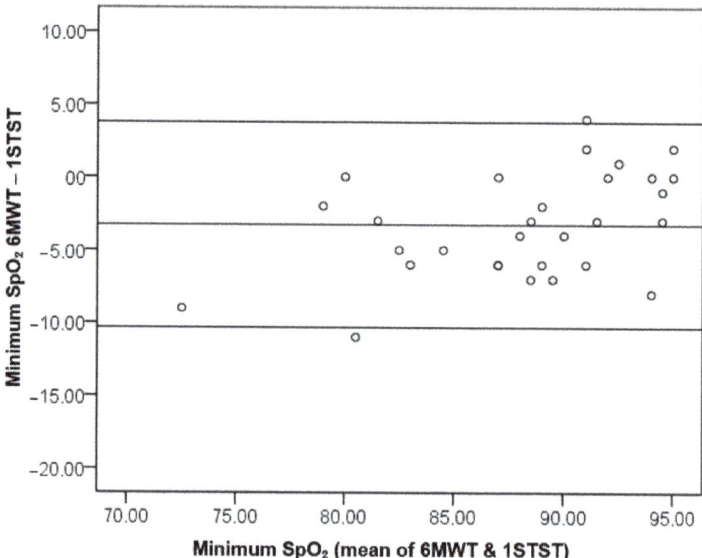

Figure 4. Bland–Altman plot of the difference in the minimum SpO$_2$ between the 6MWT and 1STST as a function of the mean minimum SpO$_2$ in both tests. (SpO$_2$ = oxygen saturation; 6MWT = 6-min walking test; 1STST = 1-min sit-to-stand test).

4. Discussion

The purpose of this study was to compare the utility of the 1STST with the 6MWT in the evaluation of exertional oxygen desaturation in patients with COPD. Our study established that the 1STST seems to be a reliable test to estimate exercise-induced oxygen desaturation in COPD, as demonstrated by the existence of a strong correlation and agreement between minimum SpO$_2$ in the 1STST and in the 6MWT and a good total concordance between oxygen desaturation recorded during both tests.

In various chronic respiratory disorders, mortality and morbidity have been associated with measurements during the 6MWT or the cardiopulmonary exercise testing (CPET), including oxygen desaturation and minimum SpO$_2$. This suggests that exercise-induced oxygen desaturation may be a key element in the prognostic evaluation and follow-up in COPD [20–22]. Moreover, some studies have demonstrated that regular monitoring of physiological variables during effort, such as oxygen desaturation and heart rate, may help to detect an exacerbation earlier [3,23].

The 6MWT is acknowledged as a simple test to evaluate exercise capacity and desaturation on exertion. As COPD is a highly prevalent disease [1], the follow-up of many patients is widely performed by the general practitioner or in office-based practices. In these settings, it may be difficult to guarantee the necessary conditions to complete a 6MWT, which may contribute to the undervaluation of exercise capacity.

The 1STST is less time consuming and does not need specific equipment, as it may be performed at the outpatient setting using a portable oximeter. Our results demonstrate that moderate-to-severe COPD patients (GOLD 2 and 3) performed a mean of 18.13 ± 5.46 repetitions. Moreover, a moderate, positive, and significant correlation was found between 6MWD and the 1STSTr. This is in line with previous publications and corroborates the utility of the 1STST for evaluating exercise capacity [11–13].

To our knowledge, few studies have focused on evaluating oxygen desaturation with the 1STST in COPD. Contradicting results regarding the SpO$_2$ decline in 1STST have been described in the literature. On the one hand, studies by Meriem and Ozalevli did not report a significant change of SpO$_2$ during the STST in their publications [11,12]. On the other hand, Crook et al. observed that the SpO_2 during the 1STST may continue to decline after the end of the test. When using the minimum SpO_2 instead of the end-test SpO_2, they detected desaturation during the 1STST in all patients who had desaturation in the 6MWT [13]. In our study, we verified a significant decrease in SpO_2 during the 6MWT and the 1STST; however, the oxygen desaturation was higher during the 6MWT, which is similar to previous articles [13,17,18]. This could be due to the shorter duration of the 1STST or the higher muscle demand during the 6MWT. We also demonstrated that the minimum SpO_2 was concordant in both tests and strongly correlated. Furthermore, we observed that the 1STST and the 6MWT could detect a desaturation ≥4%, which was considered a significant threshold for SpO_2 variability in both tests.

In some studies, the cardiovascular demand seemed to be greater during the 6MWT than in the 1STST [11,12]. Other publications have demonstrated a comparable end-exercise HR response in both tests, but blood pressure parameters were not evaluated [13,17]. We reported a higher increase in sBP, dBP, and HR in 6MWT than in the 1STST; however, the results only reached a statistically significant difference for HR. Duration and demand of peripheral muscles is different between these tests, which may partially explain the distinct cardiovascular response [11,12]. Lower limb fatigue was not statistically different in our study, but the mean result obtained was slightly higher at the end of the 1STST.

We tried to explore the results obtained in both tests and the clinical and functional measurements. Age was correlated with impaired exercise capacity in 1STST and 6MWT in concordance with previous studies. No correlation was found between 1STST outcomes and lung function parameters. Despite the fact that FEV1 has been considered a poor predictor of disease status, lung function is routinely used to assess COPD severity. A correlation between lung function and the 1STST would mean that the 1STSTr or the minimum SpO_2 could be useful severity surrogates as the 1STST is an easier test to perform.

Several STST protocols have been published in the literature [7]. The availability of multiple protocols has probably slowed the acceptance by the scientific community and the development of standardized criteria for this test. The 1STST is the most used test and seems to be practical enough for regular usage in the daily outpatient routine. Furthermore, it is sufficiently long to detect oxygen desaturation [13,17]. In some patients, the SpO_2 continues to decline after the end of the test, although it is fundamental to maintain a continuous SpO_2 monitoring during and for some minutes after the end of the test [13].

The main limitation of our study was the sample size and the absence of a control group of healthy subjects for comparison with the 1STST results. Recently, the 1STST was validated in a COPD cohort for measuring functional capacity, and reference values for the 1STST were published. However, no validity for oxygen desaturation or SpO_2 values were studied [13,24]. Another limitation was the possibility of an impact on results according to the order of the tests. A learning effect of 27 meters has been reported for the 6MWT and of 0.8 repetitions for the 1STST in COPD [13,25]. However, we found no studies evaluating this subject and in our study the order of the tests was completely random to minimize this possible effect on SpO_2.

In the future, it would be interesting to assess the impact of using 1STST as a triage tool to prioritize a formal evaluation of oxygen desaturation with a 6MWT or CPET in COPD patients. Another attractive possibility may be to perform 1STST sequentially to assess its effect on exacerbations and survival in COPD. Additionally, the role of the 1STST may also be studied in other chronic respiratory and cardiovascular disorders.

5. Conclusions

Our study highlights the ability of the 1STST to detect exercise-induced oxygen desaturation. The 1STST is an easy-to-perform and well-tolerated test and does not need specialized equipment (only a portable oximeter). Hence, it is ideal for implementation by general practitioners and outpatient routine consultations to evaluate exercise capacity oxygen desaturation, which is a negative marker for COPD prognosis. Larger studies will be needed to confirm our described results in COPD.

Supplementary Materials: The following are available online at https://www.mdpi.com/2075-4418/11/2/159/s1, Table S1: Individual SpO$_2$ measurements during the 6MWT and the 1STST. (SpO$_2$: oxygen saturation; 6MWT: 6-minute walking test; 1STST: 1-minute sit-to-stand test).

Author Contributions: Conceptualization, J.F. and P.S.; Methodology, Z.C. and G.L.; formal analysis, Z.C., G.L., and B.C.; investigation, A.L.F., B.C., and S.D.; data curation, A.L.F. and P.S.; writing—original draft preparation, A.L.F. and I.N.; writing—review and editing, Z.C., G.L., I.N., B.C., S.D., J.F., and P.S.; visualization, Z.C., G.L., I.N., B.C., S.D., J.F., and P.S.; supervision, I.N. and P.S.; project administration, P.S. All authors have read and agreed to the published version of the manuscript.

Funding: This research received no external funding.

Institutional Review Board Statement: The study was conducted according to the guidelines of the Declaration of Helsinki and approved by the Institutional Ethics Committee of Hospital Pedro Hispano (protocol code 57/CE/JAS, 9 July 2017).

Informed Consent Statement: Written, informed consent was obtained from the patients to publish this paper.

Acknowledgments: We would like to thank Joana Amado for the help during this work.

Conflicts of Interest: The authors declare no conflict of interest.

References

1. Global Initiative for Chronic Obstructive Lung Disease—Global Initiative for Chronic Obstructive Lung Disease—GOLD. Available online: https://goldcopd.org/ (accessed on 25 December 2020).
2. Waatevik, M.; Johannessen, A.; Real, F.G.; Aanerud, M.; Hardie, J.A.; Bakke, P.S.; Eagan, T.M.L. Oxygen Desaturation in 6-Min Walk Test is a Risk Factor for Adverse Outcomes in COPD. *Eur. Respir. J.* **2016**, *48*, 82–91. [CrossRef] [PubMed]
3. Gonçalves, I.; Guimarães, M.J.; van Zeller, M.; Menezes, F.; Moita, J.; Simão, P. Clinical and Molecular Markers in COPD. *Pulmonology* **2018**, *24*, 250–259. [CrossRef] [PubMed]
4. Holland, A.E.; Spruit, M.A.; Troosters, T.; Puhan, M.A.; Pepin, V.; Saey, D.; McCormack, M.C.; Carlin, B.W.; Sciurba, F.C.; Pitta, F.; et al. An Official European Respiratory Society/American Thoracic Society Technical Standard: Field Walking Tests in Chronic Respiratory Disease. *Eur. Respir. J.* **2014**, *44*, 1428–1446. [CrossRef] [PubMed]
5. Csuka, M.; McCarty, D.J. Simple Method for Measurement of Lower Extremity Muscle Strength. *Am. J. Med.* **1985**, *78*, 77–81. [CrossRef]
6. Jones, S.E.; Kon, S.S.C.; Canavan, J.L.; Patel, M.S.; Clark, A.L.; Nolan, C.M.; Polkey, M.I.; Man, W.D.C. The Five-Repetition Sit-to-Stand Test as a Functional Outcome Measure in COPD. *Thorax* **2013**, *68*, 1015–1020. [CrossRef]
7. Vaidya, T.; Chambellan, A.; de Bisschop, C. Sit-to-Stand Tests for COPD: A Literature Review. *Respir. Med.* **2017**, *128*, 70–77. [CrossRef]
8. Morita, A.A.; Bisca, G.W.; Machado, F.V.C.; Hernandes, N.A.; Pitta, F.; Probst, V.S. Best Protocol for the Sit-to-Stand Test in Subjects with Copd. *Respir. Care* **2018**, *63*, 1040–1049. [CrossRef]
9. Chorin, F.; Cornu, C.; Beaune, B.; Frère, J.; Rahmani, A. Sit to Stand in Elderly Fallers vs Non-Fallers: New Insights from Force Platform and Electromyography Data. *Aging Clin. Exp. Res.* **2016**, *28*, 871–879. [CrossRef]
10. Puhan, M.A.; Siebeling, L.; Zoller, M.; Muggensturm, P.; ter Riet, G. Simple Functional Performance Tests and Mortality in COPD. *Eur. Respir. J.* **2013**, *42*, 956–963. [CrossRef]
11. Ozalevli, S.; Ozden, A.; Itil, O.; Akkoclu, A. Comparison of the Sit-to-Stand Test with 6 Min Walk Test in Patients with Chronic Obstructive Pulmonary Disease. *Respir. Med.* **2007**, *101*, 286–293. [CrossRef]
12. Meriem, M.; Cherif, J.; Toujani, S.; Ouahchi, Y.; Hmida, A.B.; Beji, M. Sit-to-Stand Test and 6-Min Walking Test Correlation in Patients with Chronic Obstructive Pulmonary Disease. *Ann. Thorac. Med.* **2015**, *10*, 269–273. [CrossRef] [PubMed]
13. Crook, S.; Büsching, G.; Schultz, K.; Lehbert, N.; Jelusic, D.; Keusch, S.; Wittmann, M.; Schuler, M.; Radtke, T.; Frey, M.; et al. A Multicentre Validation of the 1-Min Sit-to-Stand Test in Patients with COPD. *Eur. Respir. J.* **2017**, *49*. [CrossRef] [PubMed]
14. Reychler, G.; Boucard, E.; Peran, L.; Pichon, R.; le Ber-Moy, C.; Ouksel, H.; Liistro, G.; Chambellan, A.; Beaumont, M. One Minute Sit-to-Stand Test Is an Alternative to 6MWT to Measure Functional Exercise Performance in COPD Patients. *Clin. Respir. J.* **2018**, *12*, 1247–1256. [CrossRef] [PubMed]
15. Vaidya, T.; de Bisschop, C.; Beaumont, M.; Ouksel, H.; Jean, V.; Dessables, F.; Chambellan, A. Is the 1-Minute Sit-to-Stand Test a Good Tool for the Evaluation of the Impact of Pulmonary Rehabilitation? Determination of the Minimal Important Difference in COPD. *Int. J. COPD* **2016**, *11*, 2609–2616. [CrossRef] [PubMed]
16. Zanini, A.; Aiello, M.; Cherubino, F.; Zampogna, E.; Azzola, A.; Chetta, A.; Spanevello, A. The One Repetition Maximum Test and the Sit-to-Stand Test in the Assessment of a Specific Pulmonary Rehabilitation Program on Peripheral Muscle Strength in COPD Patients. *Int. J. COPD* **2015**, *10*, 2423–2430. [CrossRef]
17. Briand, J.; Behal, H.; Chenivesse, C.; Wémeau-Stervinou, L.; Wallaert, B. The 1-Minute Sit-to-Stand Test to Detect Exercise-Induced Oxygen Desaturation in Patients with Interstitial Lung Disease. *Ther. Adv. Respir. Dis.* **2018**, *12*. [CrossRef]

18. Gruet, M.; Peyré-Tartaruga, L.A.; Mely, L.; Vallier, J.M. The 1-Minute Sit-to-Stand Test in Adults with Cystic Fibrosis: Correlations with Cardiopulmonary Exercise Test, 6-Minute Walk Test, and Quadriceps Strength. *Respir. Care* **2016**, *61*, 1620–1628. [CrossRef]
19. Muza, S.R.; Silverman, M.T.; Gilmore, G.C.; Hellerstein, H.K.; Kelsen, S.G. Comparison of Scales Used to Quantitate the Sense of Effort to Breathe in Patients with Chronic Obstructive Pulmonary Disease. *Am. Rev. Respir. Dis.* **1990**, *141*, 909–913. [CrossRef]
20. Waatevik, M.; Johannessen, A.; Hardie, J.A.; Bjordal, J.M.; Aukrust, P.; Bakke, P.S.; Eagan, T.M.L. Different COPD Disease Characteristics Are Related to Different Outcomes in the 6-Minute Walk Test. *COPD J. Chronic Obstr. Pulm. Dis.* **2012**, *9*, 227–234. [CrossRef]
21. Golpe, R.; Pérez-de-Llano, L.A.; Méndez-Marote, L.; Veres-Racamonde, A. Prognostic Value of Walk Distance, Work, Oxygen Saturation, and Dyspnea during 6-Minute Walk Test in COPD Patients. *Respir. Care* **2013**, *58*, 1329–1334. [CrossRef]
22. Casanova, C.; Cote, C.; Marin, J.M.; Pinto-Plata, V.; de Torres, J.P.; Aguirre-Jaíme, A.; Vassaux, C.; Celli, B.R. Distance and Oxygen Desaturation during the 6-Min Walk Test as Predictors of Long-Term Mortality in Patients with COPD. *Chest* **2008**, *134*, 746–752. [CrossRef] [PubMed]
23. Gálvez-Barrón, C.; Villar-Álvarez, F.; Ribas, J.; Formiga, F.; Chivite, D.; Boixeda, R.; Iborra, C.; Rodríguez-Molinero, A. Effort Oxygen Saturation and Effort Heart Rate to Detect Exacerbations of Chronic Obstructive Pulmonary Disease or Congestive Heart Failure. *J. Clin. Med.* **2019**, *8*, 42. [CrossRef] [PubMed]
24. Strassmann, A.; Steurer-Stey, C.; Lana, K.D.; Zoller, M.; Turk, A.J.; Suter, P.; Puhan, M.A. Population-Based Reference Values for the 1-Min Sit-to-Stand Test. *Int. J. Public Health* **2013**, *58*, 949–953. [CrossRef] [PubMed]
25. Hernandes, N.A.; Wouters, E.F.M.; Meijer, K.; Annegarn, J.; Pitta, F.; Spruit, M.A. Reproducibility of 6-minute walking test in patients with COPD. *Eur. Respir. J.* **2011**, *38*, 261–267. [CrossRef]

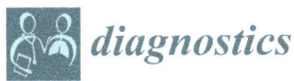

Article

Characterization of the COPD Salivary Fingerprint through Surface Enhanced Raman Spectroscopy: A Pilot Study

Cristiano Carlomagno, Alice Gualerzi, Silvia Picciolini, Francesca Rodà, Paolo Innocente Banfi, Agata Lax and Marzia Bedoni *

IRCCS Fondazione Don Carlo Gnocchi ONLUS, Via Capecelatro 66, 20148 Milan, Italy; ccarlomagno@dongnocchi.it (C.C.); agualerzi@dongnocchi.it (A.G.); spicciolini@dongnocchi.it (S.P.); froda@dongnocchi.it (F.R.); pabanfi@dongnocchi.it (P.I.B.); alax@dongnocchi.it (A.L.)
* Correspondence: mbedoni@dongnocchi.it; Tel.: +39-0240308874

Citation: Carlomagno, C.; Gualerzi, A.; Picciolini, S.; Rodà, F.; Banfi, P.I.; Lax, A.; Bedoni, M. Characterization of the COPD Salivary Fingerprint through Surface Enhanced Raman Spectroscopy: A Pilot Study. Diagnostics 2021, 11, 508. https://doi.org/10.3390/diagnostics11030508

Academic Editor: Koichi Nishimura

Received: 24 February 2021
Accepted: 11 March 2021
Published: 12 March 2021

Publisher's Note: MDPI stays neutral with regard to jurisdictional claims in published maps and institutional affiliations.

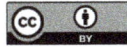

Copyright: © 2021 by the authors. Licensee MDPI, Basel, Switzerland. This article is an open access article distributed under the terms and conditions of the Creative Commons Attribution (CC BY) license (https://creativecommons.org/licenses/by/4.0/).

Abstract: Chronic Obstructive Pulmonary Disease (COPD) is a debilitating pathology characterized by reduced lung function, breathlessness and rapid and unrelenting decrease in quality of life. The severity rate and the therapy selection are strictly dependent on various parameters verifiable after years of clinical observations, missing a direct biomarker associated with COPD. In this work, we report the methodological application of Surface Enhanced Raman Spectroscopy combined with Multivariate statistics for the analysis of saliva samples collected from 15 patients affected by COPD and 15 related healthy subjects in a pilot study. The comparative Raman analysis allowed to determine a specific signature of the pathological saliva, highlighting differences in determined biological species, already studied and characterized in COPD onset, compared to the Raman signature of healthy samples. The unsupervised principal component analysis and hierarchical clustering revealed a sharp data dispersion between the two experimental groups. Using the linear discriminant analysis, we created a classification model able to discriminate the collected signals with accuracies, specificities, and sensitivities of more than 98%. The results of this preliminary study are promising for further applications of Raman spectroscopy in the COPD clinical field.

Keywords: SERS; COPD; multivariate analysis; saliva

1. Introduction

Chronic Obstructive Pulmonary Disease (COPD) is a chronic and unrelenting lung syndrome that causes limitations in physiological air flows, leading to airway remodeling, pulmonary emphysema, and to death in the 20% of the cases, with an incidence between 4% and 10% and smoking habits recognized as one of the principal risk factors [1]. Despite the fast diagnostic procedure that involves the Forced Expiratory Volume in 1 s/Forced Vital Capacity (FEV1/FEV), there are still substantial issues regarding the management of COPD. Some examples are provided by the definition of the COPD phenotypes, which nowadays is performed following a combination of parameters with clinical significance including symptoms, exacerbations, responses to rehabilitation treatments, progression rates or death, in a time-consuming procedure [2]. The exacerbation and hospitalization risks associated with a single patient or to a specific COPD phenotype have not yet been assessed, whereas the therapy effectiveness also relies mainly on the continuous monitoring of patients clinical symptoms during the hospitalizations [1,3]. A correlated critical issue regarding the management of COPD includes the therapy adherence and the personalized respiratory rehabilitation; in fact, treatments effectiveness relies mainly on the characterization of the COPD phenotype and on the adherence to the prescribed therapies [4]. The non-adherence of patients to the continuous therapy regards not only the disadvantages for the affected subjects, but also the important costs for the national health system [5]. Trying to overcome all the listed problems related to COPD, researchers are focused on the identification of a new, fast, and highly informative approach able to identify a biomarker that could allow to evaluate and monitor the therapy and respiratory rehabilitation effectiveness or adherence, and to fully characterize the patients' biochemical equilibrium in the physiological and pathological state. In recent years, the vibrational Raman Spectroscopy (RS) has been gradually adapted to the characterization of proteins, lipids, nucleic acids, metabolites, and hormones inside specific biofluids with the aim to individuate a specific fingerprint for a pathological onset [6]. RS represents in this frame an ideal methodology due to the rapidity of the analysis, the elevated sensitivity, and the minimal or no sample preparation required. The output signal represents a complex combination of all the concentrations, interactions, modifications, presences, and environments of physiological or pathological biomolecules present in the sample of interest, thus giving a biochemical profile of the sample [7]. The deep analysis of the Raman spectra can not only provide information about the vibrational modes of the molecules, but also about the macro-organization and assembly of the most represented biological species investigated. In many cases, the application of metal nanostructures for the Raman analysis al-lowed to obtain more biochemical information thanks to the enhancement of the signals intensity, due to the Surface Enhanced Raman Scattering (SERS) effect. The SERS effect can be induced by metallic nanostructures such as nanoparticles or by metallic nanostructured materials. Besides gold and silver nanoparticles, aluminum foils demonstrated their potential application in this field due to the detailed SERS signal provided from biological fluids and due to the cheapness of the material [8]. Consequently, the comparative Raman and SERS investigation is able to characterize the different families (or in specific cases also the single molecules) responsible for the main differences between biofluids collected from healthy or pathological subjects [8]. Due to the signal complexity, analytical procedures have been associated to RS for the reduction of the collected data amount and for the decryption of common trends and differential spectral regions [9]. Multivariate Analysis (MVA), in particular Principal Component Analysis (PCA) and Linear Discriminant Analysis (LDA), allows to reduce the Raman data dimensionality extrapolating informative variables uniquely associated to the relative spectrum, that can be used to evaluate the differences in the signals and to create a classification model [10]. Both Raman and SERS regimen combined with MVA have been already proposed and used for the identification of significant differences in Raman spectra of various pathologies including neurodegenerative diseases, cancers, viral, and bacterial infections analyzing various biofluids among which are blood, serum, plasma, extracellular vesicles, cerebrospinal fluid, saliva, and urine [8,11–17]. One of the most promising results has been reached using saliva as ideal biofluid, due to the variety of significant molecules contained and to the easiness and repeatability of the collection procedure. Saliva is a complex biofluid with a large pattern of biological molecules shared with the blood stream, some of which have been identified as potential COPD biomarkers, such as C-reactive protein, neutrophil elastases, molecules related to the Radical Oxygen Species (ROS) stress, and procalcitonin [18–22]. In this work, RS in SERS regimen has been used for the analysis of saliva collected from 15 patients affected by COPD and from 15 age- and sex- matched healthy subjects (CTRL). The analytical procedure was optimized taking into consideration two Raman substrates and evaluating the effects of saliva deposition and acquisition procedure. Once optimized, the protocol was adopted for the creation of a Raman database used for the MVA. The final classification model was able to determine the single spectrum membership with accuracy, sensitivity, specificity, and precision of more than 98%. The obtained results represent a proof-of-concept for the potential application of Raman analysis used as diagnostic and monitoring tool in the clinical field.

2. Materials and Methods

2.1. Materials

All the materials were purchased from Merck KGaA (Merck KGaA, Darmstadt, Germany) and used as received, if not specified. Raman-grade calcium fluoride disks (CaF2) were purchased from Crystran LTD (Crystran LTD, Poole, United Kingdom) and used without further purification steps. For the collection of saliva, Salivette® swabs were purchased from Sarstedt (Sarstedt AG & CO, Numbrecht, Germany). Aluminum foil was purchased from Merck KGaA (Merck KGaA, Darmstad, Germany) and used as received to cover the glass substrate for the SERS analysis. All the materials were used following the manufacturer's instructions.

2.2. Patients Selection and Saliva Collection

All the participants provided written informed consent after the approval of the study from the institutional review board at IRCCS Fondazione Don Carlo Gnocchi ONLUS on 11th December 2019. For the proposed pilot study, a total number of 15 COPD patients (n = 15) and 15 CTRL (n = 15) were recruited for this study at IRCCS Fondazione Don Carlo Gnocchi ONLUS, Milan (Italy). COPD patients were recruited with a postbronchodilator ratio of FEV1/FEV < 0.7. The severity of airflow limitation and phenotypes were defined as described by the GOLD grading system [5], including Grade 2, 3, or 4 and subgrades. Exclusion criteria were the combination with obstructive sleep apnea, cancer, minimum state examination < 24, at least 4 weeks from the last acute exacerbation, gingivitis, periodontal diseases, general bleeding of the gum, oral bacterial or/and fungal infections, recent dental operations, and other important comorbidities including cardiovascular, neurologic, and kidney diseases, age < 18. Frequent exacerbators were defined by at least two treated exacerbations per year. Smoking habits were collected and defined as actual smoker or ex-smoker (at least one year without smoking). Sex and age-matched CTRL were recruited. A detailed description of inclusion and exclusion criteria, as well as of the analytical procedure, is reported on ClinicalTrials.gov (ClinicalTrials.gov Identifier: NCT04628962; Title: Raman Analysis of Saliva as Biomarker of COPD). The saliva collection procedure was performed following the instructions provided by Sarstedt. Briefly, a swab was placed in the mouth and chewed for one minute, in order to stimulate salivation. To maintain data comparability, avoiding fluctuations of specific molecules during the day (e.g., cortisol), the collection procedure was performed at fixed time point at least two hours after the last meal and teeth brushing. The collection time was fixed between 3 and 5 pm on Tuesday during the clinical controls at Santa Maria Nascente Hospital (IRCCS Fondazione Don Carlo Gnocchi). Storage time and temperature, participants smoking and particular dietary habits, and time between the collection and the Raman analysis were recorded. Collected samples were stored at $-20\ °C$ before the Raman analysis.

2.3. Raman Analysis

Before the analysis, saliva samples were towed and centrifuged at $1000 \times g$ for 5 min in order to recover the biofluid. A drop of saliva (3 µL) was deposited on a CaF2 disk or on a commercially available aluminum foil to provide the Raman signal enhancement (SERS) thanks to its metallic nature and to the micro- nano-structure, slightly modifying our previous protocol [8]. In this work, the filtration step using filters with different cut-offs was avoided, in order to keep the physiological and pathological amount of biological molecules inside saliva. After the deposition step, saliva was dried at room temperature. The Raman analysis was performed using a Raman microscope Aramis (Horiba Jobin-Yvon, France), equipped with a 785 nm laser source emitting at 512 mW. The silicon reference band at 520.7 cm^{-1} was used as reference for the calibration procedure. For all the analysis, a 50× objective (Olympus, Japan) was used, with acquisition time of 30 s, grating at 600 and hole at 400. The spectral range was set between 400 and 1600 cm^{-1} while the range was restricted to 400–1500 cm^{-1} for the analysis on calcium fluoride. The final spectral resolution was 0.8 cm^{-1}/step. For each subject involved in the study, the Raman acquisition was performed following a square-map with at least 25 points (60 µm × 80 µm) or, in the CaF2 cases, focalizing all the points on the interest area. All the methods and procedures described in this work were performed in accordance with the relevant guidelines and regulations.

2.4. Data Processing and Statistical Analysis

Before the MVA process, all the spectra were pre-processed in order to uniform and homogenize the Raman dataset. In particular, the raw acquired data were fitted with a fifth-degree polynomial baseline, using 79 points to interpolate the baseline and 21 points to determine the noise. All the spectra were resized on the reference band at 1001.5 cm^{-1} and smoothed using a second-degree Savitzky–Golay method in order to remove non-informative spikes. Data were extracted with a final resolution of 0.98 cm^{-1}/step, acquiring 985 points for single spectrum. The contribution of the aluminum substrate was removed from all the spectra acquired on the same substrate. Artifact spectra due to fluorescence or Raman z-axis de-focus, were removed resulting in a 468 spectral set. Once pre-processed, the spectra collected from the two experimental groups were used as means to show the average signal obtained from COPD and CTRL. LDA was performed in order to assess a preliminary difference between the groups, reducing data dimensionality extracting and characterizing the Principal Components (PCs) with the highest loading. The first 15 PCs (cumulative loading 86.28%) were used to create the LDA-based classification model avoiding the classification overfitting and extracting the informative Canonical Variables (CVs) used for the Leave-One Out Cross-Validation (LOOCV), hierarchical clustering, and related confusion matrix. LOOCV was applied on the single spectrum collected, not considering the spectral pattern associated to the subject, in order to verify the effective differences between the Raman datasets. The Receiver Operating Characteristic (ROC) curve was calculated using the sensitivities and specificities associated to the confusion matrix, as described in literature [23], reporting the obtained Area Under the Curve (AUC). Matthews Correlation Coefficient (MCC) was calculated in order to assess the quality of the binary classification model. ANOVA test was used to assess the statistical relevant differences between the analyzed groups. All the statistical tests were performed using OriginPro 2018 (OriginLab, Northampton, version 2021, USA) and MedCalc (MedCalc Software, Ostend, version14.8.1., Belgium).

3. Results

3.1. SERS Methodology

The Raman analysis of saliva was performed optimizing the analytical protocol developed by our group, reporting the effects of the different acquisition parameters [8]. The previous selective filtering procedure (cut-off 3kDa) was avoided in order to (i) decrease the time for sample preparation, (ii) make the analysis cheaper, and, more importantly, (iii) to preserve the original biochemical pattern of molecules inside the biofluid. The first analysis was performed on a drop of saliva (3 µL), dried at room temperature, and deposited on a CaF2 disk. CaF2 is a Raman standard substrate, chosen for its negligible Raman signal. After the drying procedure, all the biomaterials present in saliva create regular aggregates as a result of the evaporating concentration gradient affected by the presence of organic mucin matrices (Figure 1A) [24,25]. The Raman spectra were collected on the volumetric deposition, obtaining a detailed and intense Raman signal respect to the spot on the drop plane. Figure 1B shows the Raman spectrum collected from the volume deposition in dried saliva samples. The spectrum shows all the characteristic salivary peaks: 441, 517, 599, 715, 750, 866, 920, 978, 1001, 1047, 1157, 1203, 1244, 1268, 1346, and 1444 cm^{-1}. The most important signal attribution regards the peak at 750 cm^{-1} related to the O-O stretching vibration in oxygenated proteins. The peaks at 866 and 1157 cm^{-1} can be attributed to the C-N stretching and to the CH3 rocking in protein backbone, respectively, while the peak at 1001 cm^{-1} is related to the ring breathing of aromatic amino acids and the signal at 1444 cm^{-1} can be assigned to the C-H stretching of glycoproteins, mostly obtained from mucines [24].

Despite the intense and detailed Raman signal, analysis on CaF2 presents some limitations including the cost of the material and the formation of the double structure after the drying procedure (spot on the drop plane and volume deposition). This last phenomenon highly influences the collection of a repeatable spectrum, generating high variability (Figure 1B, standard deviation), favoring the presence of artefact spectra and providing a low-intensity signal. In order to overcome these limitations, commercially available aluminum was used as Raman substrate for the saliva analysis, modifying the procedure reported by Muro et al. [26]. After the drying step on aluminum, the saliva drop presents a remarked edge, which separates the substrate from the sample. The saliva drop observed with the optical microscope presents a homogeneous surface without volume deposits and spots on the drop plane (Figure 2A, in box), with the Raman signal of a comparable intensity all over the sample and with a lower number of artefact spectra. The signals collected from each region are highly homogenous, as indicated by the low standard deviation associated to the spectrum (Figure 2A). The identified peaks normally correspond to the signals collected using calcium fluoride as substrates, with the most intense bands at 441, 524, 543, 587, 621, 715, 746, 778, 812, 924, 1001, 1051, 1126, 1161, 1267, 1284, 1301, 1382, 1409, and 1454 cm^{-1} (Figure 2A, black arrows). The slight changes in peaks shift and intensities are due to the SERS induced by the metallic substrate provided by the used SERS inducer, with results comparable with the other present in literature about the SERS enhancing [26]. The comparison between the spectra obtained using the two different substrates is shown in Figure 2B. The attribution of the peaks, based on previous studies on saliva and on biological tissues, is reported in Table 1 [7,24,26].

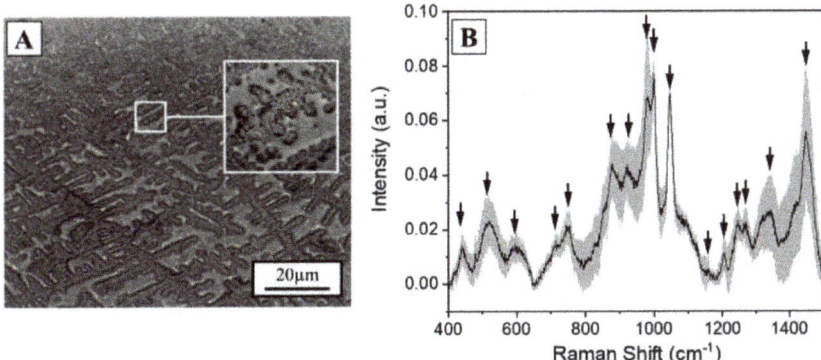

Figure 1. (A) Optical microscopy image (10×) of a saliva drop (3µL) dried at room temperature on a Calcium Fluoride disk. Scale bar 20 µm. In box, magnification (50×) of the volumetric mass after the drying procedure. (B) Average Raman spectrum of the saliva sample collected on the volumetric mass. The grey band represents the standard deviation. The black arrows indicate the most prominent peaks of interest.

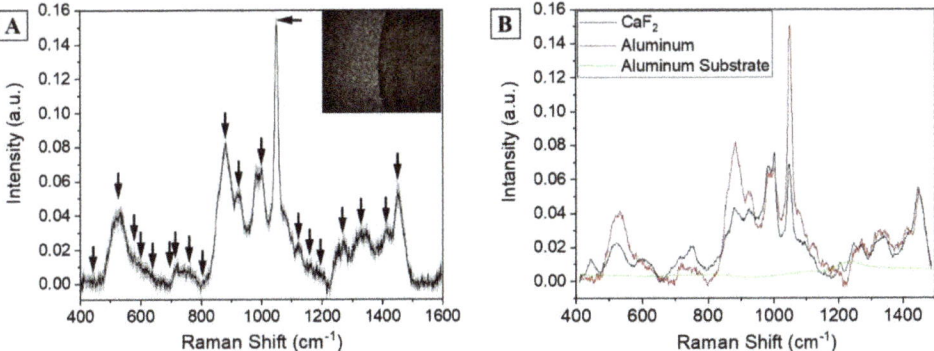

Figure 2. (A) Raman average spectra of a drop of saliva dried on aluminum substrate. The grey band represents the standard deviation. The box shows the optical microscopic image of the sample (objective 50×). The black arrows indicate the attributed peaks. (B) Comparison between the salivary spectra obtained using CaF2 and aluminum as Raman substrates and the signal of the aluminum substrate without saliva (green line).

Table 1. Attribution of the most prominent peaks obtained from Raman salivary analysis (± 4 cm-1), based on reported literature [7,24,26].

Raman Shift	Attribution			
	Protein	Lipids	Nucleotides	Carbohydrates
441 cm^{-1}		Sterols stretching		
524 cm^{-1}		Phosphatidylserine		
543 cm^{-1}				Glucose/Saccharides
587 cm^{-1}		Phosphatidylinositol		
621 cm^{-1}	Phenylalanine			
715 cm^{-1}		C-N phospholipids		
746 cm^{-1}			Ring breathing DNA/RNA	
778 cm^{-1}			Ring breathing C, U, T	
812 cm^{-1}			Phosphodiester bonds	
924 cm^{-1}				Glucose/Glycogen
1001 cm^{-1}	Phenylalanine, Tryptophan			
1051 cm^{-1}				Glycogen
1126 cm^{-1}		Stretching of acyl backbone		
1161 cm^{-1}	Tyrosine			
1267 cm^{-1}	Amide III			
1284 cm^{-1}	C-H bending			
1301 cm^{-1}			C-H vibration	
1382 cm^{-1}	C-H rocking			
1409 cm^{-1}	Bending of methyl groups			
1454 cm^{-1}		Phospholipids		

Most of the identified peaks are related to the protein content of saliva (specific amino acids, protein backbone, and secondary structure), lipids carbon signals, nucleotide modes, and glucose or glycogen (Table 1). The abundance of information is related to the high concentration of biomolecules inside the biofluid, and to the strength of the Raman signal provided. Proteins and lipids possess strong Raman effects, deeply described in literature, allowing the precise attribution of the peaks. Examples are provided by the Amide III band that represents the amount and percentage of C-N stretch and N-H bend at 1267 cm^{-1}, and by the strong signal of aromatic amino acids such as tryptophan and phenylalanine (Table 1). Depending on the position of the Amide III identified band, the Raman spectra can provide information regarding the secondary structure of the most abundant protein. In this case, the position at 1267 cm^{-1} indicates a most prominent α-helix conformation [27]. Combined with the information collected about the aromatic amino acids, the partial identification of the most abundant group of proteins can be done on the base of the secondary structure and the percentage of specific peptides. Similarly, peaks at specific positions attributed to different molecules can provide information regarding the species involved (Table 1). Several biological molecules have been already attributed to specific Raman signals, which can be altered in specific physiological or pathological conditions, contributing to the identification of alterations in metabolic pathways, damaged products, and metabolic pathways. Phosphatidylserine and phosphatidylinositol are membrane lipids involved in several communication and metabolic pathways, usually interconnected in the protein transportation. The concentration and modifications of these molecules have been connected to the onset of different pathologies including diabetes, cancer, cognitive impairment, and lung disorders such as COPD [28–31]. Other important information can be deduced from the position of specific peaks attributed to lipids and nucleic acids damaged of differentially expressed because of the damages produced by ROS in stress conditions, specifically [24,32,33]. The Raman signals provided by saccharides, mostly by glucose and glycogen, are indicators of the different accumulation and metabolism inside the body. These markers have been associated to different pathologies related to the altered glucose metabolism, release, and accumulation. Besides diabetes, in COPD onset, the levels and fluctuations of glucose and glycogen have also been associated to different pathological events [34,35]. Considering the increased homogeneity and quality of the Raman spectra of the saliva samples analyzed on the aluminum compared to the difficulty on calcium fluoride, aluminum was selected as substrate for further analysis of clinical samples.

3.2. Clinical Analysis

Subjects included in the study were 15 COPD patients (n = 15) and 15 CTRL (n = 15) with the clinical and demographic characteristics reported in Table 2. Number and demographic data of the two experimental groups were comparable, with a good distribution of the GOLD classification among the COPD patients. The individuated COPD phenotypes were classified as COPD with emphysema (n = 7) and COPD with bronchitis (n = 8), without any patient affected by overlapped COPD/Asthma and avoiding the potential signal contamination by other comorbidities.

Table 2. Demographic characteristics of the subjects involved in the study. Data are presented as average with the standard deviation (± SD) or percentages (n %) and with the two-sided p—Values (p). Smoking habits are defined as actual smokers (Yes), never smoked (No) or previous smoking habits before the last year (Ex). COPD phenotypes and GOLD classification were attributed following [5]. Frequent exacerbators presented at least two treated exacerbations per year. Differences between the groups were analyzed using Chi-square test and Fisher Exact test.

	COPD	CTRL	p-Value
Number	15	15	–
Sex (male)	53.3% (8)	53.3% (8)	1.23
Age (years)	66 ± 10	60 ± 6	0.06
Smoker	Yes = 46.6% (7) Ex = 54.4% (8)	Yes = 33.3% (5) No = 66.7% (10)	0.27
COPD Phenotype	With Emphysema = 46.6% (7) With Bronchitis = 54.4% (8)	–	0.59
Frequent exacerbator	Yes = 60% (9) No = 40% (6)	–	0.12
GOLD Classification	2 A = 6.6% (1) 2 B = 20% (3) 2 C = 6.6% (1) 2 D = 6.6% (1) 3 C = 6.6% (1) 3 D = 26.6% (4) 4 B = 13.3% (2) 4 D = 13.3% (2)	–	–

Taking advantage of the fast analytical Raman procedure and of the large amount of information provided by the salivary spectral analysis, the optimized protocol was adopted for the analysis of saliva collected from 15 patients affected by COPD and 15 CTRL. The aim of the procedure was to ascertain and determine the main differences be-tween the two experimental groups, laying the foundations for the identification of a specific COPD salivary fingerprint. In Figure 3, the average Raman spectra collected from the two groups are presented. The COPD average spectrum presents a uniform shape, with the lower values of calculated standard deviations respect to the CTRL (Figure 3). The peaks attribution reflect the values presented in Table 1, with slight shifts always included between ±4 cm^{-1}. The tapered curve collected from COPD indicates a homogeneous spectral trend between the analyzed subjects, promoting the conception of a salivary Raman COPD signature, able to identify the pathological onset.

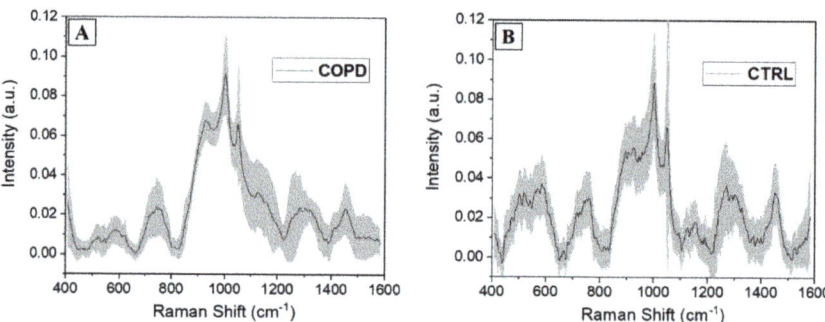

Figure 3. Average salivary Raman spectra collected from the experimental (**A**) COPD and (**B**) CTRL groups. The grey bands represent the standard deviations.

On the other hand, the signals collected from the CTRL group present a more jagged shape indicating, together with the higher standard deviation values, the disparate distribution of the collected spectra. The main differences comparing the two groups are presented in Figure 4. The overlap of the two average spectra revealed regions of particular interest, in which the signal was different in terms of intensities, peak positions, and presence (Figure 4A, grey boxes). Regions between 500 and 600 cm^{-1}, normally due to the signals of lipids and carbohydrates, were more intense and structured in CTRL group with respect to the COPD counterpart. Similarly, the region between 1250 and 1350 cm^{-1} was more prominent in CTRL. As a result of the uniform shape in COPD spectra, only regions between 900 and 950 cm^{-1} and 1100 and 1200 cm^{-1} were more prominent in the COPD group with respect to the CTRL. These two regions were attributed principally to proteins, carbohydrates, and nucleotides vibrational modes. A deeper analysis was performed subtracting the two averages spectra and calculating the associated error propagation, identifying in this way the peaks and bands responsible for the differences between the two experimental groups (Figure 4B). The individuated peaks, belonging to the class in which they were more abundant, are presented in Table 3.

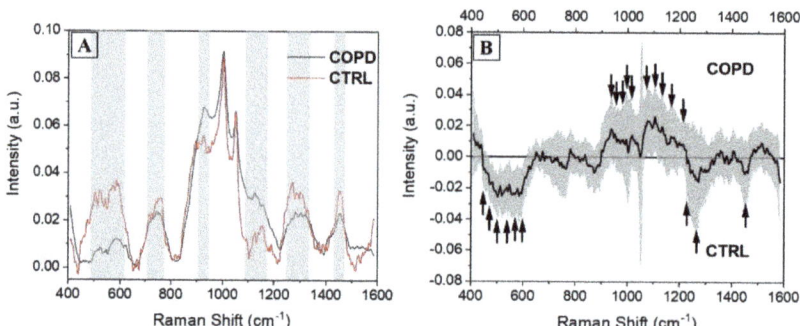

Figure 4. (**A**) Overlapped average Raman spectra collected from COPD (black) and CTRL (red) subjects, with the indications of the regions with the main differences (grey boxes). (**B**) Subtraction spectrum between COPD and CTRL groups. The grey band represents the error propagation calculated from the spectral standard deviations. The black arrows indicate the most important peaks.

Table 3. Attribution of the principal Raman peaks due to the differences in the subtraction spectrum, following the attribution of [7,24,26]. The Raman shifts are presented under CTRL or COPD depending on the abundance (±0.005 ΔI) in the considered group.

Raman Shift CTRL	Attribution	Raman Shift COPD
441 cm^{-1}	Sterols stretching	—
471 cm^{-1}	Polysaccharides	—
499 cm^{-1}	Glycogen	—
524 cm^{-1}	Phosphatidylserine	—
543 cm^{-1}	Glucose/Saccharides	—
560 cm^{-1}	Tryptophan	—
587 cm^{-1}	Phosphatidylinositol	—
—	Glucose/Glycogen	924 cm^{-1}
—	Proline	937 cm^{-1}
—	Proline and Valine	948 cm^{-1}
—	Phosphate monoester groups	962 cm^{-1}
—	C-H bending in lipids	979 cm^{-1}
—	Phenylalanine, Tryptophan	1001 cm^{-1}
—	Glycogen	1051 cm^{-1}
—	C-C of lipids	1077 cm^{-1}
—	Phenylalanine	1104 cm^{-1}
—	Stretching of acyl backbone	1126 cm^{-1}
—	Tyrosine	1161 cm^{-1}
—	Nucleotides breathing	1195 cm^{-1}
1242 cm^{-1}	Amide III	—
1267 cm^{-1}	Amide III/Lipids	—
1450 cm^{-1}	C-H deformations in lipids	—
—	Cytosine	1515 cm^{-1}

After a general overview, signals related to lipids and protein were more abundant in COPD with respect to the CTRL group, where the saccharides part was more concentrated (Figure 4B and Table 3). In particular, the signals collected from phosphatidylserine and phosphatidylinositol were more intense in CTRL respect to the COPD. The general alteration and loss of lipids, in particular phospholipids, has been widely demonstrated after COPD onset [36]. Availability of phospholipids, in particular phosphatidylserine and phosphatidylinositol, strongly correlates with pulmonary function, consecutively inducing a loss of phosphorylated lipids during the pathological onset [37]. Peaks related to saccharides, including glucose and glycogen, are more represented in the COPD average spectrum (Figure 4B, Table 3) with respect to the CTRL group, probably indicating an accumulation of the molecules. The described scenario reflects the metabolic alterations occurring in COPD onset. Acute hyperglycemia is associated with poor outcomes for different acute and chronic diseases including COPD, where progressive insulin-resistance, altered glucose metabolism, and glucose-mediated hormones responses have been deeply characterized [38,39]. Moreover, plasmatic glucose levels have been proposed as potential biomarkers for the definition and prediction of the exacerbation events in COPD [34]. The hallmarks of protein in the subtraction spectra present in COPD reveal a similar situation, in which the signals related to the single aromatic amino acids and to the vibrational mode of the secondary structure are more significant in the pathological state (Figure 4B, Table 3). The chronic inflammatory and oxidative stressful state induced by COPD generates an overexpression and consecutively a higher presence of specific molecules circulating in different biofluids (e.g., blood, saliva). These molecules are related to the inflammatory system and to the product of the inflammatory response. Different proteins have been characterized in saliva, allowing to discriminate the saliva collected from COPD from the one collected from healthy controls with their higher expression patterns. An example is provided by the work of Patel et al. [40] where higher levels of C-reactive protein, procalcitonin, and neutrophil elastase in saliva were able to highly discriminate the biofluid collected from COPD patients respect to the CTRL group. The same scenario has been characterized in our results, with the contributions of a higher methodological sensitivity provided by RS (up to 10–15 M in SERS regimen) and of the concomitant detection of multiple molecules respect to the ELISA method that can determine the differences between the two groups. Several peaks related to the signal provided by lipids and nucleic acids can be attributed to the damages in the biological structures caused by ROS, highlighted in the COPD spectrum respect to the CTRL (Figure 4B, Table 3). Especially during the continuous stress situations, such as chronic pathologies, the damages due to the ROS increase the products related to this pathway [19]. During the COPD onset and progression, the ROS-related molecules, including lipids and nucleic acids, assume a defined expression pattern allowing the identification of the pathological state [41]. The global overview provided by the grouped analysis of saliva could be able to generate specific information about the biological species involved at the onset of the pathology and during the progression and, once completely interpreted, also revealing useful information regarding the pathological mechanisms and the targets of new therapies. These results can be used to identify a Raman salivary fingerprint that could be used to assess the pathological onset, the identification of different phenotypes, the effects of the prescribed therapies, and to monitor the respiratory rehabilitation efficacy.

3.3. Multivariate Analysis and Classification Model

The differences and the particular spectral patterns detected by means of the RS in the COPD and CTRL groups were computed using MVA in order to reduce the volume of data and to extract coefficients that are able to maximize the variance between each spectrum. The PCA is an unsupervised data transformation procedure of complex data that reduces the input variables in a set of independent and orthogonal PCs maximizing the variance [9]. The application of the LDA model on the PCA leads to the identification of the discriminant axes that optimally classify the extracted data on the base of their relationships. As result, the CVs are the coefficients that best describe the optimal data dispersion for potential differences. Consecutively, once the effective different dispersions of PCs and CVs was tested, a LOOCV-based classification model was performed assessing the capability of the Raman signature to be exploited as discriminant marker for the COPD.

Figure 5 shows the results obtained from the PCA procedure. The cumulative loading obtained from the first three extracted PCs was 60.3%, identifying a great part of the detected differences in these data. The areas concerning the different PCs interest all the spectra, with particular regions of dispersion, which highlight the relationship between the variables in the areas of the three considered PCs (Figure 5A). The 3-D distribution of PC1, PC2 and PC3 demonstrated two defined spatial groups clearly indicating the difference between the data (Figure 5B). The uniform shape of the average COPD Raman spectra (Figure 3A) is translated in the more centered dispersion of the PCs collected from the COPD group (Figure 3B). The statistical test performed regarding the influence of the smoking habits on the collected data, revealed a statistical difference (Mann–Whitney test, $p < 0.05$, Data not shown) between the subjects without smoking habits and with past smoking habits. Despite the weak evidence individuated, an increase in subjects' numerosity will probably decrease the difference encountered due also to the missing statistical differences between subjects with smoking habits and without smoking habits. Similarly, considering the Raman data processed through PCA, the analysis based on the patients severity stages (Table 2) was not performed due to the explorative character of the study and due to the almost single presence of patient in each clinical stage. After the PCA, LDA was performed in order to extract the coefficients for the creation of the classification model. Considering that the LDA is a supervised method, CVs were firstly processed through unsupervised hierarchical clustering, assessing the effective grouping of the collected variable without the labelling procedure (Figure 6A). The resulting dendogram shows the automatic aggregation of the CVs into two groups (COPD and CTRL) at a relatively short distance, confirming the effective belonging to two different classes. The statistical analysis performed on the same data revealed a significant difference between the CVs dispersions of COPD and CTRL (Figure 6B, $p < 0.001$). The further analysis of the CVs dispersion revealed no overlapping between the two groups, with no points indicated as outliers (Figure 6A). After the validation of the data used to create the classification model, LOOCV was applied with the purpose to train the algorithm with the detected differences leading to the independent identification and attribution of each single spectrum collected during the Raman analysis. Each single spectrum was used for the LOOCV at the spectral level, in order to verify the existing differences between the collected datasets, avoiding the single patient labelling. The application of the LOOCV model to the spectral dataset is aimed at the identification of repetitive and constant spectral variations for the creation of a single-spectrum classification model. Despite the identified significant differences, a LOOCV model based on the total spectral pattern of each subject involved in this study (patient-level classification model) cannot be adopted due to the experimental groups' numerosity. Our scope was to set up a proof-of-concept with the proposed preliminary study, investigating if the analyzed spectral differences can be applied for the creation of a classification model, confirming the spectral difference constancy. Further patients' enrolment are needed for the definitive validation of the technique at the patient level. The performances of the classification model are reported in Table 4.

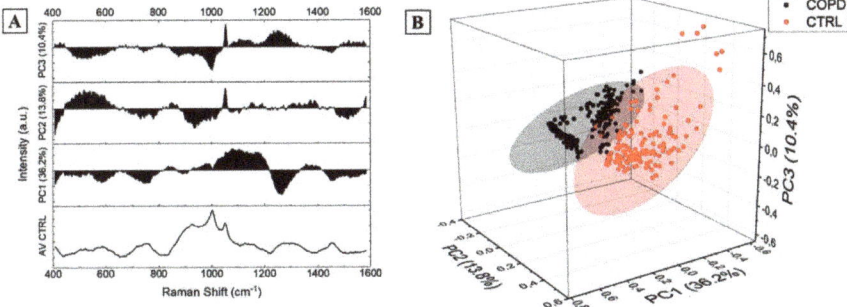

Figure 5. Results of the Principal Component Analysis showing (**A**) the loadings and (**B**) the 3-D distribution with the 95% confidence ellipse of the Principal Component 1 (36.2%), Principal Component 2 (13.8%), and Principal Component 3 (10.4%) cumulatively representing the 60.3% of the components.

Table 4. Results of the model based on Leave-One out Cross-Validation for the assignment of the single spectra to the experimental group. Error-Rate for cross-validation of training data (ER); Matthews Correlation Coefficient (MCC); Receiver Operating Characteristic Area Under the Curve (ROC-AUC).

	Accuracy	Sensitivity	Specificity	Precision	ER	MCC	ROC-AUC
LOOCV Model	98%	98%	99%	98%	0.85%	0.97	0.975

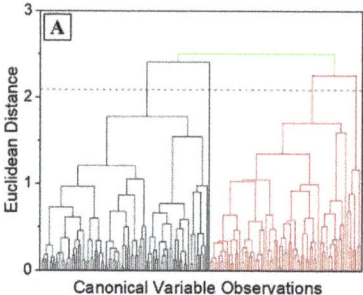
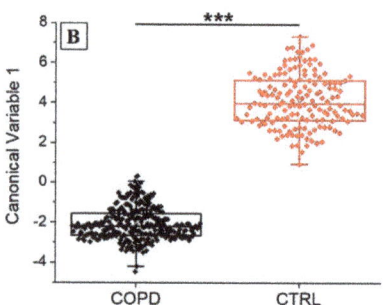

Figure 6. (**A**) Hierarchical clustering dendogram representing the unsupervised grouping of the Canonical Variables on the base of the Euclidean distance. The dashed line represents the convergence distance. (**B**) Dispersion of the Canonical Variable 1 for COPD and CTRL. *** $p < 0.001$ One-Way ANOVA test.

Accuracy, sensitivity, specificity, and precision were all equal or more than 98% due to the Error-Rate for cross validation of training data (ER) of 0.85% indicating a minimal error in the spectral attribution process (Table 4). MCC is an indicator used to assess the reliability and the quality of a binary classification calculated on the values of true and false positives and negatives. The obtained value of 0.97 confirmed the ability of the system. As further confirmation, we analyzed the ROC curve, estimating the AUC to 0.975 with a confidence interval of the 95% (Table 4). All the data regarding the performances of the classification model, based on the single Raman spectrum, confirm the ability of the RS to accurately discriminate the signal collected from COPD respect to the CTRL. This finding was firstly highlighted by the different shape of the average Raman spectra collected from the experimental group and definitively confirmed by the deeper MVA. Despite different studies reported in literature about the characterization of several potential circulating biomarkers for the COPD, the main limitations regarding these studies concern the individuation of one, or few, molecules each time using single molecule detection techniques such as ELISA, mass spectroscopy, or nucleic acids amplification [18,29,42,43].

The main advantage of RS regards the detection of the entire biomolecular pattern present in a specific biofluid, treating the entire informative spectrum as whole biomarker. In this way, it is possible to collect information regarding the content and quality of circulating proteins, molecules of the inflammatory system, products of the ROS pathways, structural and signaling lipids, carbohydrates, and alterations in the nucleic acids content. The complexity of the obtained signal combined with the high data volume require a computational technique to deeply investigate the extractable information. The application of MVA to the Raman database has been already proposed and used for almost all the techniques involving RS as diagnostic or body fluids investigative tool [9]. Besides the accuracy and sensitivity, RS is taken into high consideration also for the velocity of the test and for the minimal sample preparation required before the analysis. In the proposed study, the entire analytical process, starting from the collection of saliva to the obtaining of the final result after the MVA, lasts approximately 30 min, with different steps that can be easily reduced (e.g., drying procedure, acquisition time, number of acquired spectra for each patient). Despite the limited number of participants involved in the study, the results in terms of Raman profiles and discriminant power of the final classification model were extremely encouraging, confirming the potential of the proposed methodology. A larger cohort of patients will be fundamental for the standardization of the procedure, introducing more experimental groups in order to characterize the slight changes in Raman spectral structures that define, for example, the patients that completely adhere to the therapy, the risk of exacerbation associated to the single patient, or the different COPD phenotypes for a fast phenotypic identification. This last point is a critical issue in COPD management, nowadays being the identification of phenotypes time-consuming, expensive, and not accurate [2]. The identification of the COPD phenotype involves the clinical observation of the patients, reporting the combination of exacerbation events, respiratory afflictions, other related symptoms, responses to the pharmacological and rehabilitative therapies, and to the survival rate of the patient in a time-consuming (2/3 years) process [2]. Moreover, similar to other pathologies, each phenotype responds in a different way to the prescribed pharmacological and rehabilitative therapies, without a quantifiable biomarker that is able to indicate the optimal route. Once well characterized and validated with more patients and more experimental groups treated with different therapies and analyzed in a transversal and longitudinal study, the RS-based approach could provide a fast and sensitive investigative tool for the clinicians, helping the management of a complex and chronic respiratory pathology. The creation of a Leave-One Patient Out Cross-Validation-based classification model will be of crucial importance to assess the feasibility of the diagnostic and monitoring Raman platform.

4. Conclusions

In conclusion, in this pilot study, we proposed the characterization of the COPD salivary Raman fingerprint. Saliva was selected as investigative biofluid due to the highly informative biochemical composition and due to the minimally invasive and easy collection procedure. We evaluated different acquisition parameters taking into consideration both the details and information of the final spectrum and the optimization of an easy-to-acquire and not expensive sample preparation. The analysis on the average spectrum led to the potential attribution of the main biochemical species responsible for the differences between the COPD and CTRL groups, identifying specific protein families, lipids, and saccharides in common with previous studies reporting modifications in the biochemical equilibrium after COPD onset. The consecutive MVA allowed the creation of a classification model able to discriminate the single Raman signal collected from the two experimental groups with accuracy, sensitivity, specificity, and precision of more than 98%. Due to the low number of subjects involved in this preliminary and pilot study, more patients, as well as more healthy subjects and the recruitment of a comparable pathological control group, must be included to definitively assess the application of the RS as diagnostic and monitoring tool in COPD at the patient level. Our preliminary results demonstrated the potentiality of a Raman-based approach that could be use in future not only to assess the COPD pathological onset, but also to identify different phenotypes, evaluate the effects of the prescribed therapies, and to monitor the respiratory rehabilitation efficacy starting from an easily collectable biological fluid.

Author Contributions: Conceptualization, C.C., P.I.B., and M.B.; methodology, C.C. and A.G.; validation, C.C., S.P., and F.R.; investigation, C.C., S.P., and F.R.; resources, P.I.B. and M.B.; clinical data curation, P.I.B. and A.L.; statistical analysis, C.C., A.G., S.P., and F.R. writing—original draft preparation, C.C.; writing—review and editing, All the authors; supervision, M.B. and P.I.B. All authors have read and agreed to the published version of the manuscript.

Funding: This research was supported by the Italian Ministry of Health, Ricerca Corrente 2020.

Institutional Review Board Statement: The study was conducted according to the guidelines of the Declaration of Helsinki, and approved by the Ethics Committee of Fondazione Don Carlo Gnocchi on 11 December 2019, CE_FDG_11.12.2019.

Informed Consent Statement: Informed consent was obtained from all subjects involved in the study.

Data Availability Statement: All the data can be obtain after reasonable requests, contacting C.C. or M.B. Information regarding the study can be also found at ClinicalTrials.gov; Identifier: NCT04628962; Title: Raman Analysis of Saliva as Biomarker of COPD.

Acknowledgments: Authors acknowledge Chiesi Farmaceutici S.p.A. for the support.

Conflicts of Interest: The authors declare no conflict of interest.

References

1. Golpe, R.; Suárez-Valor, M.; Martín-Robles, I.; Sanjuán-López, P.; Cano-Jiménez, E.; Castro-Añón, O.; Llano, L.A.P.D. Mortality in COPD patients according to clinical phenotypes. *Int. J. Chronic Obstr. Pulm. Dis.* **2018**, *13*, 1433–1439. [CrossRef]
2. Miravitlles, M.; Calle, M.; Soler-Cataluña, J.J. Clinical Phenotypes of COPD: Identification, Definition and Implications for Guidelines. *Arch. Bronconeumol.* **2012**, *48*, 86–98. [CrossRef] [PubMed]
3. Caramori, G.; Casolari, P.; Carone, M.; Bertorelli, G.; Banfi, P.; Andò, F. Personalised treatment of stable COPD patients. *Rass. Patol. Appar. Respir.* **2016**, *31*, 83–90.
4. Calzetta, L.; Rogliani, P.; Matera, M.G.; Cazzola, M. A Systematic Review With Meta-Analysis of Dual Bronchodilation With LAMA/LABA for the Treatment of Stable COPD. *Chest* **2016**, *149*, 1181–1196. [CrossRef]
5. WHO. *Global Initiative for Chronic Obstructive Lung Disease*; WHO: Geneva, Switzerland, 2019.
6. Chisanga, M.; Muhamadali, H.; Ellis, D.I.; Goodacre, R. Enhancing Disease Diagnosis: Biomedical Applications of Surface-Enhanced Raman Scattering. *Appl. Sci.* **2019**, *9*, 1163. [CrossRef]
7. Movasaghi, Z.; Rehman, S.; Rehman, I.U. Raman Spectroscopy of Biological Tissues. *Appl. Spectrosc. Rev.* **2007**, *42*, 493–541. [CrossRef]
8. Carlomagno, C.; Banfi, P.I.; Gualerzi, A.; Picciolini, S.; Volpato, E.; Meloni, M.; Lax, A.; Colombo, E.; Ticozzi, N.; Verde, F.; et al. Human salivary Raman fingerprint as biomarker for the diagnosis of Amyotrophic Lateral Sclerosis. *Sci. Rep.* **2020**, *10*, 1–13. [CrossRef] [PubMed]
9. Gautam, R.; Vanga, S.; Ariese, F.; Umapathy, S. Review of multidimensional data processing approaches for Raman and infrared spectroscopy. *EPJ Tech. Instrum.* **2015**, *2*, 8. [CrossRef]
10. Ryzhikova, E.; Ralbovsky, N.M.; Halámková, L.; Celmins, D.; Malone, P.; Molho, E.; Quinn, J.; Zimmerman, E.A.; Lednev, I.K. Multivariate Statistical Analysis of Surface Enhanced Raman Spectra of Human Serum for Alzheimer's Disease Diagnosis. *Appl. Sci.* **2019**, *9*, 3256. [CrossRef]
11. Devitt, G.; Howard, K.; Mudher, A.; Mahajan, S. Raman Spectroscopy: An Emerging Tool in Neurodegenerative Disease Research and Diagnosis. *ACS Chem. Neurosci.* **2018**, *9*, 404–420. [CrossRef] [PubMed]
12. Gniadecka, M.; Philipsen, P.A.; Wessel, S.; Gniadecki, R.; Wulf, H.C.; Sigurdsson, S.; Nielsen, O.F.; Christensen, D.H.; Hercogova, J.; Rossen, K.; et al. Melanoma Diagnosis by Raman Spectroscopy and Neural Networks: Structure Alterations in Proteins and Lipids in Intact Cancer Tissue. *J. Investig. Dermatol.* **2004**, *122*, 443–449. [CrossRef] [PubMed]
13. Choi, S.; Moon, S.W.; Shin, J.-H.; Park, H.-K.; Jin, K.-H. Label-Free Biochemical Analytic Method for the Early Detection of Adenoviral Conjunctivitis Using Human Tear Biofluids. *Anal. Chem.* **2014**, *86*, 11093–11099. [CrossRef] [PubMed]
14. Connolly, J.M.; Davies, K.; Kazakeviciute, A.; Wheatley, A.M.; Dockery, P.; Keogh, I.; Olivo, M. Non-invasive and label-free detection of oral squamous cell carcinoma using saliva surface-enhanced Raman spectroscopy and multivariate analysis. *Nanomed. Nanotechnol. Biol. Med.* **2016**, *12*, 1593–1601. [CrossRef] [PubMed]
15. Derruau, S.; Robinet, J.; Untereiner, V.; Piot, O.; Sockalingum, G.D.; Lorimier, S. Vibrational Spectroscopy Saliva Profiling as Biometric Tool for Disease Diagnostics: A Systematic Literature Review. *Molecules* **2020**, *25*, 4142. [CrossRef]
16. Gualerzi, A.; Picciolini, S.; Carlomagno, C.; Terenzi, F.; Ramat, S.; Sorbi, S.; Bedoni, M. Raman profiling of circulating extracellular vesicles for the stratification of Parkinson's patients. *Nanomed. Nanotechnol. Biol. Med.* **2019**, *22*, 102097. [CrossRef]
17. Carlomagno, C.; Cabinio, M.; Picciolini, S.; Gualerzi, A.; Baglio, F.; Bedoni, M. SERS-based biosensor for Alzheimer disease evaluation through the fast analysis of human serum. *J. Biophotonics* **2020**, *13*, e201960033. [CrossRef]
18. Dong, T.; Santos, S.; Yang, Z.; Yang, S.; Kirkhus, N.E. Sputum and salivary protein biomarkers and point-of-care biosensors for the management of COPD. *Analyst* **2020**, *145*, 1583–1604. [CrossRef] [PubMed]
19. Yigla, M.; Berkovich, Y.; Nagler, R.M. Oxidative stress indices in COPD—Broncho-alveolar lavage and salivary analysis. *Arch. Oral Biol.* **2007**, *52*, 36–43. [CrossRef] [PubMed]
20. Carmicheal, J.; Hayashi, C.; Huang, X.; Liu, L.; Lu, Y.; Krasnoslobodtsev, A.; Lushnikov, A.; Kshirsagar, P.G.; Patel, A.; Jain, M.; et al. Label-free characterization of exosome via surface enhanced Raman spectroscopy for the early detection of pancreatic cancer. *Nanomed. Nanotechnol. Biol. Med.* **2019**, *16*, 88–96. [CrossRef] [PubMed]
21. Inonu, H.; Doruk, S.; Sahin, S.; Ünal, E.; Celik, D.; Celikel, S.; Seyfikli, Z. Oxidative Stress Levels in Exhaled Breath Condensate Associated With COPD and Smoking. *Respir. Care* **2012**, *57*, 413–419. [CrossRef]
22. Salamzadeh, J.; Dadashzadeh, S.; Habibi, M.; Estifaie, S. Serum and Saliva Theophylline Levels in Adult Outpatients with Asthma and Chronic Obstructive Pulmonary Disease (COPD): A Cross-Sectional Study. *Iran. J. Pharm. Res.* **2010**, *7*, 83–87.
23. DeLong, E.R.; DeLong, D.M.; Clarke-Pearson, D.L. Comparing the areas under two or more correlated receiver operating characteristic curves: A nonparametric approach. *Biometrics* **1988**, *44*, 837–845. [CrossRef]
24. Gonchukov, S.; Sukhinina, A.; Bakhmutov, D.; Minaeva, S. Raman spectroscopy of saliva as a perspective method for periodontitis diagnostics. *Laser Phys. Lett.* **2012**, *9*, 73–77. [CrossRef]
25. Carlomagno, C.; Speranza, G.; Aswath, P.; Sorarù, G.D.; Migliaresi, C.; Maniglio, D. Breath figures decorated silica-based ceramic surfaces with tunable geometry from UV cross-linkable polysiloxane precursor. *J. Eur. Ceram. Soc.* **2018**, *38*, 1320–1326. [CrossRef]
26. Muro, C.K.; Fernandes, L.D.S.; Lednev, I.K. Sex Determination Based on Raman Spectroscopy of Saliva Traces for Forensic Purposes. *Anal. Chem.* **2016**, *88*, 12489–12493. [CrossRef] [PubMed]
27. Rygula, A.; Majzner, K.; Marzec, K.M.; Kaczor, A.; Pilarczyk, M.; Baranska, M. Raman spectroscopy of proteins: A review. *J. Raman Spectrosc.* **2013**, *44*, 1061–1076. [CrossRef]

28. Sharma, B.; Kanwar, S.S. Phosphatidylserine: A cancer cell targeting biomarker. *Semin. Cancer Biol.* **2018**, *52*, 17–25. [CrossRef] [PubMed]
29. Liu, D.; Meister, M.; Zhang, S.; Vong, C.I.; Wang, S.; Fang, R.; Li, L.; Wang, P.G.; Massion, P.; Ji, X. Identification of lipid biomarker from serum in patients with chronic obstructive pulmonary disease. *Respir. Res.* **2020**, *21*, 242. [CrossRef]
30. Knowles, E.E.; Meikle, P.J.; Huynh, K.; Göring, H.H.; Olvera, R.L.; Mathias, S.R.; Duggirala, R.; Almasy, L.; Blangero, J.; Curran, J.E.; et al. Serum phosphatidylinositol as a biomarker for bipolar disorder liability. *Bipolar Disord.* **2017**, *19*, 107–115. [CrossRef]
31. Zhu, C.; Liang, Q.-L.; Hu, P.; Wang, Y.-M.; Luo, G.-A. Phospholipidomic identification of potential plasma biomarkers associated with type 2 diabetes mellitus and diabetic nephropathy. *Talanta* **2011**, *85*, 1711–1720. [CrossRef] [PubMed]
32. Kirkham, P.A.; Barnes, P.J. Oxidative Stress in COPD. *Chest* **2013**, *144*, 266–273. [CrossRef] [PubMed]
33. Taniguchi, M.; Iizuka, J.; Murata, Y.; Ito, Y.; Iwamiya, M.; Mori, H.; Hirata, Y.; Mukai, Y.; Mikuni-Takagaki, Y. Multimolecular Salivary Mucin Complex Is Altered in Saliva of Cigarette Smokers: Detection of Disulfide Bridges by Raman Spectroscopy. *BioMed Res. Int.* **2013**, *2013*, 1–7. [CrossRef]
34. Baker, E.H.; Bell, D. Blood glucose: Of emerging importance in COPD exacerbations. *Thorax* **2009**, *64*, 830–832. [CrossRef]
35. Ngkelo, A.; Hoffmann, R.F.; Durham, A.L.; Marwick, J.A.; Brandenburg, S.M.; De Bruin, H.G.; Jonker, M.R.; Rossios, C.; Tsitsiou, E.; Caramori, G.; et al. Glycogen synthase kinase-3β modulation of glucocorticoid responsiveness in COPD. *Am. J. Physiol. Cell. Mol. Physiol.* **2015**, *309*, L1112–L1123. [CrossRef]
36. Dai, W.-C.; Zhang, H.-W.; Yu, J.; Xu, H.-J.; Chen, H.; Luo, S.-P.; Zhang, H.; Liang, L.-H.; Wu, X.-L.; Lei, Y.; et al. CT Imaging and Differential Diagnosis of COVID-19. *Can. Assoc. Radiol. J.* **2020**, *71*, 195–200. [CrossRef] [PubMed]
37. Agudelo, C.W.; Kumley, B.K.; Area-Gomez, E.; Xu, Y.; Dabo, A.J.; Geraghty, P.; Campos, M.; Foronjy, R.; Garcia-Arcos, I. Decreased surfactant lipids correlate with lung function in chronic obstructive pulmonary disease (COPD). *PLoS ONE* **2020**, *15*, e0228279. [CrossRef] [PubMed]
38. Bolton, C.E.; Evans, M.; Ionescu, A.A.; Edwards, S.M.; Morris, R.H.K.; Dunseath, G.; Luzio, S.; Owens, D.R.; Shale, D.J. Insulin Resistance and inflammation—A Further Systemic Complication of COPD. *COPD J. Chronic Obstr. Pulm. Dis.* **2007**, *4*, 121–126. [CrossRef]
39. Hjalmarsen, A.; Aasebø, U.; Birkeland, K.; Sager, G.; Jorde, R. Impaired glucose tolerance in patients with chronic hypoxic pulmonary disease. *Diabetes Metab.* **1996**, *22*, 37–42.
40. Patel, N.; Belcher, J.; Thorpe, G.; Forsyth, N.R.; Spiteri, M.A. Measurement of C-reactive protein, procalcitonin and neutrophil elastase in saliva of COPD patients and healthy controls: Correlation to self-reported wellbeing parameters. *Respir. Res.* **2015**, *16*, 62. [CrossRef]
41. Langen, R.; Korn, S.; Wouters, E. ROS in the local and systemic pathogenesis of COPD. *Free. Radic. Biol. Med.* **2003**, *35*, 226–235. [CrossRef]
42. Man, S.F.P.; Xing, L.; Connett, J.E.; Anthonisen, N.R.; Wise, R.A.; Tashkin, D.P.; Zhang, X.; Vessey, R.; Walker, T.G.; Celli, B.R.; et al. Circulating fibronectin to C-reactive protein ratio and mortality: A biomarker in COPD? *Eur. Respir. J.* **2008**, *32*, 1451–1457. [CrossRef]
43. Stolz, D.; Christ-Crain, M.; Morgenthaler, N.G.; Leuppi, J.; Miedinger, D.; Bingisser, R.; Müller, C.; Struck, J.; Müller, B.; Tamm, M. Copeptin, C-Reactive Protein, and Procalcitonin as Prognostic Biomarkers in Acute Exacerbation of COPD. *Chest* **2007**, *131*, 1058–1067. [CrossRef] [PubMed]

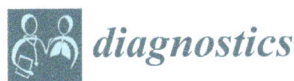

Article

Combination of Systemic Inflammatory Biomarkers in Assessment of Chronic Obstructive Pulmonary Disease: Diagnostic Performance and Identification of Networks and Clusters

Iva Hlapčić [1], Daniela Belamarić [2], Martina Bosnar [2], Domagoj Kifer [3], Andrea Vukić Dugac [4,5] and Lada Rumora [1,*]

1. Department of Medical Biochemistry and Haematology, Faculty of Pharmacy and Biochemistry, University of Zagreb, 10000 Zagreb, Croatia; iva.hlapcic@pharma.unizg.hr
2. Fidelta Ltd., 10000 Zagreb, Croatia; daniela.belamaric@glpg.com (D.B.); Martina.Bosnar@glpg.com (M.B.)
3. Department of Biophysics, Faculty of Pharmacy and Biochemistry, University of Zagreb, 10000 Zagreb, Croatia; domagoj.kifer@pharma.unizg.hr
4. Clinical Department for Lung Diseases Jordanovac, University Hospital Centre Zagreb, 10000 Zagreb, Croatia; avukic@kbc-zagreb.hr
5. School of Medicine, University of Zagreb, 10000 Zagreb, Croatia
* Correspondence: lada.rumora@pharma.unizg.hr; Tel.: +385-16394782; Fax: +385-14612716

Received: 30 October 2020; Accepted: 28 November 2020; Published: 30 November 2020

Abstract: Interleukin (IL)-1α, IL-1β, IL-6, IL-8 and tumor necrosis factor (TNF)α contribute to inflammation in chronic obstructive pulmonary disease (COPD). We wanted to investigate their interrelations and association with disease severity, as well as to combine them with other inflammation-associated biomarkers and evaluate their predictive value and potential in identifying various patterns of systemic inflammation. One hundred and nine patients with stable COPD and 95 age- and sex-matched controls were enrolled in the study. Cytokines' concentrations were determined in plasma samples by antibody-based multiplex immunosorbent assay kits. Investigated cytokines were increased in COPD patients but were not associated with disease or symptoms severity. IL-1β, IL-6 and TNFα showed the best discriminative values regarding ongoing inflammation in COPD. Inflammatory patterns were observed in COPD patients when cytokines, C-reactive protein (CRP), fibrinogen (Fbg), extracellular adenosine triphosphate (eATP), extracellular heat shock protein 70 (eHsp70) and clinical data were included in cluster analysis. IL-1β, eATP and eHsp70 combined correctly classified 91% of cases. Therefore, due to the heterogeneity of COPD, its assessment could be improved by combination of biomarkers. Models including IL-1β, eATP and eHsp70 might identify COPD patients, while IL-1β, IL-6 and TNFα combined with CRP, Fbg, eATP and eHsp70 might be informative regarding various COPD clinical subgroups.

Keywords: chronic obstructive pulmonary disease; cytokines; systemic inflammation; clusters; adenosine triphosphate; heat shock protein 70

1. Introduction

Cytokines are small proteins (5–30 kDa) with a short half-life and they are usually circulating in body fluids in picomolar concentrations. While being produced by a variety of cells, their main role is regulation of the immune system, so they or their receptors are often being recognized as targets for potential therapeutic interventions in many different diseases [1]. Cytokines are not disease-specific biomarkers, yet they are considered to be surrogate biomarkers for inflammation in chronic obstructive pulmonary disease (COPD), as it seems they have an important role in

COPD-associated inflammatory responses [2]. COPD is a complex, heterogeneous disease at the genetic (e.g., alpha-1 antitrypsin deficiency), cellular and molecular levels, and its manifestations are both pulmonary and extrapulmonary [3]. Currently, it is the fourth leading cause of death in the world, and it represents an important public health challenge as its global prevalence of 11.7% is expected to rise for many years to come [4]. Although COPD is characterized by respiratory symptoms and airflow limitation, systemic inflammation may be developed in some patients and it contributes to the progression of the disease and development of comorbidities that might have an impact on morbidity and mortality [5–9]. Various clinical studies reported elevated levels of inflammatory cytokines in respiratory tract and/or peripheral blood of COPD patients in comparison to healthy controls [2,7,10–12]. Our study focused on several cytokines as it follows: interleukin (IL)-1α, IL-1β, IL-6, IL-8 and tumor necrosis factor (TNF)α.

IL-1 is mainly produced by the airway epithelium and macrophages, and it is released along with IL-6, IL-8 and TNFα. It causes neutrophilia, macrophage activation and responses by T cells [13]. Both pro-IL-1α and its mature IL-1α form are biologically active [14]. Contrary to this, pro-IL-1β has to be cleaved to be biologically active, mostly by caspase-1 through nucleotide-binding domain (NOD)-like receptor protein (NLRP)3 inflammasome activation [15]. IL-6 is a pro-inflammatory cytokine synthesized by the airway epithelium, macrophages, and other cells at the site of inflammation in response to environmental stressful stimuli such as smoking, and it is participating in the activation, proliferation and differentiation of T cells [6,16,17]. IL-8 is a multifunctional chemokine involved in inflammatory processes including neutrophil infiltration and chemotaxis [16,18]. It is secreted from macrophages, T cells, airway epithelium and neutrophils [19]. TNFα is produced by T cells, mast cells, and cells of airway epithelium. Its main functions are control of cellular migration and stimulation of secretion of other cytokines [20].

There are inconsistent observations regarding the association of cytokines with COPD severity, prognostic value and cytokine-targeted therapeutic approach. In addition, due to the disease complexity and different underlying mechanisms, clinical manifestations of COPD are presented differently. Therefore, instead of one, a group of biomarkers might better represent a specific COPD phenotype. In line with this, it was shown that persistent systemic inflammation is present in some of COPD patients and accompanied with an increase in CRP, fibrinogen (Fbg), white blood cells (WBC) and inflammatory cytokines [9]. Agusti et al. investigated six inflammatory parameters (CRP, Fbg, WBC, IL-6, IL-8 and TNFα) which form "inflammome" and showed that 70% of COPD patients had some of the components of systemic inflammation. Among them, in 16% of COPD patients inflammation was persistent, and associated with mortality and exacerbations [21]. From our previous studies, we observed that our COPD cohort might also show characteristics of systemic inflammation because of increased concentrations of CRP and Fbg [22] that are being common inflammatory parameters as well as extracellular adenosine triphosphate (eATP) [23] and extracellular heat shock protein 70 (eHsp70) [24] which act like damage-associated molecular patterns (DAMPs). In addition, a previous investigation showed that there were significant associations between the aforementioned parameters with lung function and disease severity, as well as symptoms severity and history of exacerbations, and different multicomponent clinical parameters used for the assessment of dyspnoea, exacerbations and lung impairment. These parameters have not been studied together before, and we wanted to evaluate their combined performances. First, our aim was to determine concentrations of cytokines IL-1α, IL-1β, IL-6, IL-8 and TNFα in COPD patients in comparison to healthy subjects and to investigate their association with disease and symptoms severity. As cytokines exhibit pleiotropy and redundancy, we also wanted to assess relations between them in healthy non-smokers, healthy smokers and COPD patients. We hypothesized that the combination of common inflammatory biomarkers (CRP and Fbg), DAMPs (eATP and eHsp70) and cytokines might ameliorate the understanding of relations between different inflammatory parameters and help to identify some potential COPD subgroups regarding systemic inflammation. Finally, we wanted to suggest a model of combined parameters for recognizing COPD patients based on predictive value.

2. Materials and Methods

2.1. Participants

The current cross-sectional case-control study included 109 patients with stable COPD and 95 healthy individuals. For the additional analyses that involved eATP, one COPD patient was excluded because the plasma sample for the determination of eATP could not be obtained. For the determination of eATP and eHsp70, all individuals from the study (137 COPD patients and 95 controls) were recruited during 2017 and 2018 at the Clinical Department for Lung Diseases Jordanovac, University Hospital Centre Zagreb (Zagreb, Croatia) according to the predefined inclusion and exclusion criteria, while additional recruitment for the investigation of common inflammatory biomarkers and cytokines was performed during 2019 (109 COPD patients and 95 controls). During the second recruitment, not all participants were suitable to be included in the study because some of them died ($n = 10$), while others did not match inclusion criteria (lung transplantation, $n = 5$; acute exacerbations, $n = 4$) or could not be reached ($n = 9$). All participants agreed to take a part in the study as volunteers and confirmed it by signing an informed consent. The study was approved by the Ethics Committee of University of Hospital Centre Zagreb and Ethics Committee for Experimentation of Faculty of Pharmacy and Biochemistry, University of Zagreb (Zagreb, Croatia) (Approval Protocol Numbers: 02/21/JG on 29 August 2014 and 251-62-03-14-78 on 10 September 2014, respectively). Pulmonology specialists confirmed diagnosis of COPD after symptoms evaluation and spirometry measurements according to the guidelines by the Global Initiative for Chronic Obstructive Pulmonary Disease (GOLD) [4]. All patients were in the stable phase of the disease with no exacerbations in the last three months since the recruitment, no changes in therapy and no symptoms of infection in lower respiratory tract. On the other hand, healthy individuals were included in the study based on anamnestic data and spirometry results that were among normal values. They were age- and gender-matched to the COPD patients. Exclusion criteria were same for all participants and they included as follows: age under 40, lung diseases other than COPD (except COPD for COPD patients), systemic inflammatory diseases, acute infections, diabetes with severe complications, severe liver diseases, severe kidney insufficiency, malignant diseases, transplantations, and other specific or non-specific acute inflammations. In addition, smoking data was obtained from all participants. COPD patients were divided in GOLD 2-4 stages according to the level of airflow limitation, as suggested by GOLD guidelines [4]. Besides forced expiratory volume in one second (FEV_1)-based disease severity, COPD patients were divided in GOLD A-D groups based on the assessment of symptoms severity and history of exacerbations. Evaluation of the symptoms and health-related quality of life was assessed by COPD Assessment Test (CAT), modified Medical Research Council (mMRC) Dyspnoea Scale as well as St George Respiratory Questionnaire for COPD patients (SGRQ-C). Additionally, data about previous exacerbations were obtained from the COPD patients. Finally, the Charlson comorbidity index was matched to every COPD patient, so that the multicomponent parameter CODEx could be established. CODEx stands for comorbidities (Charlson index), airflow obstruction, dyspnoea, and previous exacerbations [25].

2.2. Evaluation of Lung Function

Diagnosis of airflow limitation was established by spirometry when FEV_1 and forced vital capacity (FVC) ratio was <0.70. Measurements were performed by trained technicians at the Clinical Department for Lung Diseases Jordanovac, University Hospital Centre Zagreb. Moreover, the pulmonary diffusion capacity for carbon monoxide (DLCO) was measured for the assessment of lung function in COPD patients. Both procedures were performed as already described in detail in [23].

2.3. Blood Sampling and Cytokine Determination

Peripheral venous blood was collected from 7 a.m. to 9 a.m. by venepuncture of a large antecubital vein after overnight fasting. Tubes with K_3-ethylenediaminetetraacetic acid (K_3 EDTA) anticoagulant (Greiner Bio-One, Kremsmünster, Austria) were used for the blood collection. Afterwards, tubes were mixed by an inversion 8×, and centrifuged immediately, as recommended by the Clinical and Laboratory Standards Institute (CLSI) guidelines [26]. Obtained EDTA plasma samples were stored at −80 °C until the analysis. Concentration of IL-1α in plasma was determined by Platinum Procarta Plex Kit (Thermo Fischer Scientific, Waltham, MA, USA), while levels of IL-1β, IL-6, IL-8 and TNFα were determined by Procarta Plex High Sensitivity Luminex kit (Thermo Fischer Scientific), according to manufacturer's recommendations. Antibody-coated magnetic beads were transferred to wells of a 96-well plate and washed. Afterwards, 25 μL of assay buffer was added to wells followed by addition of 25 μL of samples or standards. For IL-1α, determination plate was incubated for 120 min at room temperature (RT) with shaking, while for determination of the other cytokines, plates were incubated for 30 min at RT followed by an overnight incubation at 4 °C. At the end of incubation, plates were washed and 25 μL of detection antibodies were added to wells. Plates were then incubated for 30 min at RT, with shaking. After the washing step, 50 μL of streptavidin-phycoerythrin conjugate was added to wells and plates were incubated for 30 min at RT with shaking. At the end of incubation, plates for IL-1α determination were washed, 120 μL of reading buffer was added to wells and samples were analyzed by use of Luminex 200 instrument (Luminex Corporation, Austin, TX, USA). On the other hand, for IL-1β, IL-6, IL-8 and TNFα determination, 50 μL of amplification reagent 1 was added to wells. After 30 min incubation, 50 μL of amplification reagent 2 was added to wells and incubation continued for additional 30 min. Finally, plates were washed, beads were resuspended in 120 μL of reading buffer, and samples were analyzed by a Luminex 200 instrument. Cytokines concentrations were determined by interpolation from a standard curve using the xPONENT software package (Luminex Corporation).

2.4. Statistics

Normality of all data was tested by Kolmogorov–Smirnov test, and since all data failed a normality test, results were shown as median with interquartile range (IQR). Only age was shown as median with minimum and maximum, while gender was shown in absolute numbers. Non-parametric Mann–Whitney test and Kruskal–Wallis test were used for the analyses of differences between the groups of interest. Gender was tested by Chi-squared test. Univariate and multivariate logistic regression analyses were used to investigate COPD-inflammation contributing factors, and odds ratio (OR) with 95% confidence interval (CI) were obtained. Variables were added in the binary logistic regression analysis as continuous variables. Described analysis were performed in MedCalc statistical software version 17.9.2. (MedCalc Software, Ostend, Belgium).

Network analysis was used for the assessment of relations between investigated parameters. Values of the 95th percentile of each parameter in healthy non-smokers were considered as the criteria for the evaluation of the patterns between the parameters in healthy non-smokers, healthy smokers and COPD patients. Differences in the number of patients with abnormal levels between the groups were analyzed using Fisher's exact tests. Prior hierarchical clustering, variables were transformed to standard normal distribution by inverse transformation of ranks to normality (R package "Gen ABEL") [27]. Distance between the subjects was calculated using Euclidian method, and group of subjects were merged by complete linkage method. Optimal number of clusters was determined combining 30 indices apply NbClust function (R package "NbClust") [28]. Variables used for clustering and reference variables presented next to cluster were compared using a Kruskal–Wallis test or Fisher's exact test, depending on the data type. Network and clustering analyses were performed in R programming software (R Core Team) [29]. For all analyses, the false discovery rate was controlled using the Benjamini–Hohcberg method at significance level of 0.05.

3. Results

3.1. Basic Characteristics and Cytokines' Concentrations of All Participants

One hundred and nine patients with stable COPD were compared to age- and gender-matched healthy subjects (total healthy participants and only healthy non-smokers). COPD patients showed to have declined lung function in comparison to controls assessed by spirometry parameters. All investigated cytokines were elevated in peripheral circulation of COPD patients when compared to healthy individuals (Table 1). As smoking data were obtained from all participants, it was shown that only TNFα was increased in healthy smokers in comparison to healthy non-smokers. In addition, concentrations of TNFα and IL-6 were increased in both COPD former smokers and COPD smokers when they were compared to healthy controls regarding their smoking status as well as to COPD non-smokers. On the other hand, IL-1α was increased only in COPD smokers in comparison to both non-smoking controls and smoking controls, while IL-1β showed to be increased in each of COPD groups regarding smoking status when compared to healthy non-smokers and healthy smokers (see Supplementary Table S1).

Table 1. Demographic characteristics, spirometry parameters and cytokines' concentrations in participants from the study.

	Total Healthy Subjects $n = 95$	Healthy Non-Smokers $n = 48$	COPD Patients $n = 109$	p_1	p_2
age	64 (46–83)	65 (52–83)	65 (45–87)	0.069	0.600
gender male female	49 46	23 25	69 40	0.121	0.104
FEV$_1$ (L)	2.60 (2.12–3.19)	2.82 (2.28–3.19)	1.08 (0.69–1.60)	<0.001	<0.001
FEV$_1$ (% pred.)	93.3 (86.4–104.2)	101.1 (90.6–110.4)	40.8 (27.9–61.7)	<0.001	<0.001
FVC (L)	3.35 (2.77–4.16)	3.58 (2.76–4.18)	2.28 (1.74–2.77)	<0.001	<0.001
FEV$_1$/FVC (%)	80.6 (76.8–87.6)	83.0 (78.1–91.8)	51.3 (40.7–58.7)	<0.001	<0.001
IL-1α (pg/mL)	0.30 (0.30–0.97)	0.31 (0.31–0.71)	0.43 (0.30–2.13)	0.003	0.007
IL-1β (pg/mL)	0.10 (0.10–0.61)	0.10 (0.10–0.17)	6.90 (0.61–23.91)	<0.001	<0.001
IL-6 (pg/mL)	4.85 (3.45–7.09)	4.41 (3.29–6.17)	32.17 (10.64–64.30)	<0.001	<0.001
IL-8 (pg/mL)	6.36 (4.07–11.17)	6.22 (4.34–11.33)	8.73 (3.56–17.76)	0.040	0.049
TNFα (pg/mL)	0.40 (0.35–1.36)	0.35 (0.35–0.53)	8.24 (0.35–19.23)	<0.001	<0.001

Age was shown as median with minimum and maximum, while gender was presented as an absolute number. Results of spirometry and cytokines' measurements were shown as median with interquartile range (IQR). Comparison of males and females was performed by Chi-squared test, while all other parameters were tested by Mann–Whitney Rank Sum test. Data were considered significant if $p < 0.05$. FEV$_1$–forced expiratory volume in one second; FVC–forced vital capacity; IL-1α–interleukin-1alpha; IL-1β–interleukin-1beta; IL-6–interleukin-6; IL-8–interleukin-8; TNFα–tumor necrosis factor alpha. alpha; p_1–statistical significance of differences between total healthy subjects and chronic obstructive pulmonary disease (COPD) patients; p_2–statistical significance of differences between healthy non-smokers and COPD patients. All p-values that are <0.05 are in bold.

3.2. Association of Cytokines' Concentrations with the Severity of Airflow Limitation and Symptoms Severity

All the cytokines were investigated regarding the severity of COPD based on GOLD guidelines (Table 2). None of the cytokines was associated with the severity of airflow obstruction or the symptoms severity and history of exacerbations, since the concentrations were only elevated in each of GOLD 2-4 stages and GOLD A-D groups when being compared to healthy subjects but did not differ between GOLD 2-4 or GOLD A-D. IL-8 was the only cytokine whose level did not show significant difference between healthy subjects and COPD patients with moderate COPD in GOLD 2 stage, and there was no change of IL-8 concentration in either of GOLD A-D groups. As well as in combined ABCD assessment, we have compared cytokines' concentrations in COPD frequent exacerbators and non-frequent exacerbators, but no statistically significant difference was found (data not shown). In addition, cytokines' concentrations were similar in men and women (in both healthy and COPD groups). Regarding comorbidities (cardiovascular diseases or metabolic diseases), we also found no statistically significant difference in circulating cytokines' levels.

Table 2. Concentration of cytokines in healthy participants and COPD patients regarding the severity of airflow obstruction assessed by FEV_1 (GOLD 2-4 stages) and the severity of symptoms and exacerbation history (GOLD A-D groups).

	IL-1α (pg/mL)	IL-1β (pg/mL)	IL-6 (pg/mL)	IL-8 (pg/mL)	TNFα (pg/mL)
controls $n = 95$	0.30 (0.30–0.97)	0.10 (0.10–0.61)	4.85 (3.45–7.09)	6.36 (4.07–11.17)	0.40 (0.35–1.36)
GOLD 2 $n = 39$	0.40 (0.30–2.37)[1]	8.77 (0.70–20.40)[1]	30.14 (10.54–58.01)[1]	6.98 (3.27–15.25)	11.04 (0.39–19.37)[1]
GOLD 3 $n = 36$	0.63 (0.30–2.04)[1]	7.57 (0.75–22.63)[1]	34.75 (8.25–56.75)[1]	8.77 (3.50–23.59)[1]	7.40 (0.77–14.08)[1]
GOLD 4 $n = 34$	0.48 (0.30–1.60)[1]	5.54 (0.56–42.23)[1]	27.23 (12.51–106.87)[1]	9.74 (4.56–22.89)[1]	6.63 (0.35–31.37)[1]
p_1	**0.031**	**<0.001**	**<0.001**	**0.041**	**<0.001**
GOLD A $n = 14$	2.04 (0.30–3.09)[1]	8.72 (3.55–20.63)[1]	33.33 (11.95–56.65)[1]	6.07 (3.55–14.00)	12.31 (3.34–18.65)[1]
GOLD B $n = 63$	0.40 (0.30–1.84)[1]	8.27 (0.56–25.78)[1]	33.36 (10.85–71.16)[1]	9.40 (3.64–19.89)	8.60 (0.35–19.46)[1]
GOLD D $n = 32$	0.48 (0.30–2.56)[1]	4.25 (0.53–21.72)[1]	24.07 (8.25–52.93)[1]	8.20 (3.37–18.60)	4.29 (0.35–17.28)[1]
p_2	**0.018**	**<0.001**	**<0.001**	0.398	**<0.001**

Data were presented as median with IQR after performing Kruskal–Wallis one-way analysis of variance test. Data were considered significant if $p < 0.05$. Afterwards, post-hoc analysis was performed. GOLD–Global Initiative for chronic obstructive pulmonary disease; IL-1α—interleukin-1alpha; IL-1β—interleukin-1beta; IL-6–interleukin-6; IL-8—interleukin-8; TNFα—tumor necrosis factor alpha; p_1—statistical significance of differences between controls, GOLD 2, GOLD 3 and GOLD 4; p_2—statistical significance of differences between controls, GOLD A, GOLD B and GOLD D. [1] statistically significant in comparison to controls. All p-values that are <0.05 are in bold.

3.3. Cytokines' Interrelations

Network analysis was performed for the assessment of relations between investigated cytokines. Every cytokine was presented by an individual node, and its size was proportional to the percentage of defined abnormal values, as described (see Supplementary Table S2). Links between the nodes were present when at least 1% of the participants shared abnormal values for linked parameters. Moreover, the width of the link presented the percentage of the participants sharing abnormal values (Figure 1). There were no significant cytokine-based interrelations in healthy non-smokers as the nodes were small and the links between them were rare. Interestingly, healthy smokers showed to have larger nodes of IL-1β ($p < 0.05$) and TNFα ($p < 0.01$), and there were more linking nodes in comparison to healthy non-smokers. The cytokine network is even more developed in COPD patients with increased nodes of IL-1β, IL-6 and TNFα ($p < 0.001$ in comparison to both healthy non-smokers and healthy smokers for all three parameters) as well as IL-8 ($p < 0.05$ in comparison to healthy non-smokers).

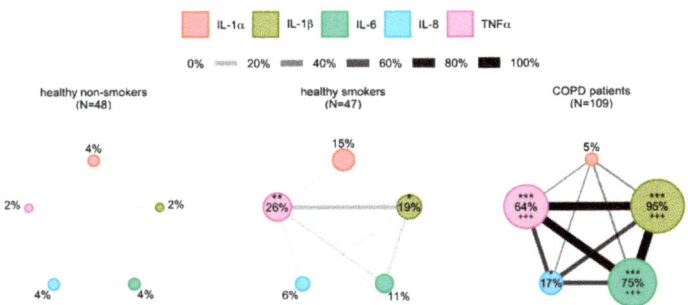

Figure 1. Network layout of cytokines determined in healthy non-smokers, healthy smokers and COPD patients. Cytokines are shown as different nodes of the network whose size is in proportion with the prevalence of their abnormal values defined by 95th percentile of healthy non-smokers. Two nodes are linked when more than 1% of participants in the network share abnormal values of these two parameters, and width of a line is proportional to that proportion. IL-1α–interleukin-1alpha; IL-1β–interleukin-1beta; IL-6–interleukin-6; IL-8–interleukin-8; TNFα–tumor necrosis factor alpha. * $p < 0.05$, ** $p < 0.01$, *** $p < 0.001$ in comparison to healthy non-smokers, +++ $p < 0.001$ in comparison to healthy smokers.

3.4. The Potential of Cytokines in Identifying COPD Patients

To determine the potential of cytokines regarding identifying COPD patients, univariate logistic regression analysis was performed for cytokines whose concentrations were determined in plasma of all participants from the study. IL-1α had no statistically significant predictive performances, while IL-8 showed to have the lowest OR as well as number of correctly classified cases. ORs of IL-1β, IL-6 and TNFα were 5.53, 1.14 and 1.27 ($p < 0.001$ for all) (Table 3).

Table 3. Univariate logistic regression analysis of all cytokines investigated.

	OR	p	95% CI	Cases Correctly Classified (%)
IL-1α	1.00	0.536	0.99–1.01	53
IL-1β	5.53	**<0.001**	2.05–14.90	84
IL-6	1.14	**<0.001**	1.08–1.19	80
IL-8	1.03	**0.010**	1.01–1.05	56
TNFα	1.27	**<0.001**	1.16–1.40	74

OR—odds ratio; CI—confidence interval; IL-1α—interleukin-1alpha; IL-1β—interleukin-1beta; IL-6—interleukin-6; IL-8—interleukin-8; TNFα—tumor necrosis factor alpha. All p-values that are <0.05 are in bold.

3.5. Analysis of Relations between Inflammation-Driven Parameters in COPD Patients and Identification of COPD Clusters Regarding Systemic Inflammation

Based on the differences obtained in cytokines' concentrations between healthy participants and COPD patients, cytokine network analysis and evaluation of predicting potential of investigated cytokines, IL-1β, IL-6 and TNFα showed statistically the most significant results. As systemic inflammation in COPD goes beyond increased production of cytokines, we wanted to broaden our view regarding complexity and networking of inflammatory parameters in blood of patients. Therefore, based on our previous research, common inflammatory parameters CRP and Fbg as well as DAMPs eATP and eHsp70 were included together with cytokines IL-1β, IL-6 and TNFα in further analysis. Now, we wanted to assess the relations between all those parameters, so additional network analysis was performed (Figure 2). Potential relations between them were also investigated in three groups of participants (healthy non-smokers, healthy smokers and COPD patients) with reference values of the 95th percentile of each parameter in healthy non-smokers as well (see Supplementary

Table S2). Nodes were small in their size in healthy non-smokers, and only two links were present—one between CRP and IL-6 and the other between IL-1β and TNFα. Nodes with IL-1β ($p < 0.01$), TNFα ($p < 0.01$), eATP ($p < 0.001$) and eHsp70 ($p < 0.001$) were larger in healthy smokers in comparison to healthy non-smokers, and there were more links between all the parameters. Similar to cytokine network analysis, the most developed network could be seen in COPD patients where nodes of IL-1β, IL-6, TNFα, CRP, Fbg, eATP and eHsp70 were significantly larger in comparison to both healthy non-smokers ($p < 0.001$ for all except for CRP whose p value is <0.01) and healthy smokers ($p < 0.001$ for all except for CRP whose p value is <0.05, and Fbg whose p value is <0.01).

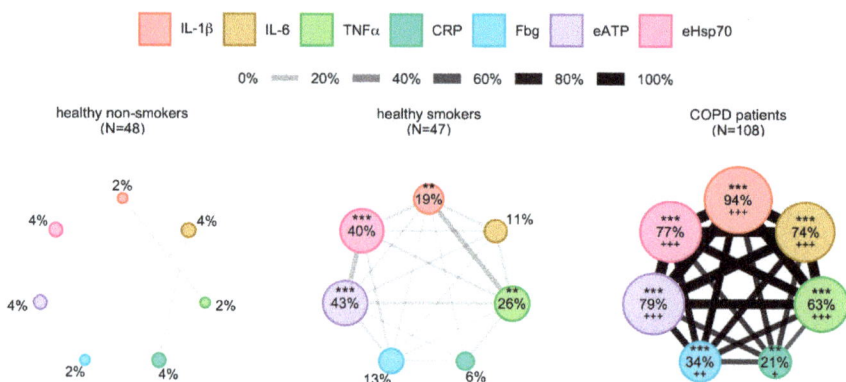

Figure 2. Network layout of cytokines combined with common inflammatory parameters and DAMPs in healthy non-smokers, healthy smokers and COPD patients. Parameters are shown as different nodes of the network whose size is in proportion with the prevalence of their abnormal values defined by 95th percentile of healthy non-smokers. Two nodes are linked when more than 1% of participants in the network share abnormal values of these two parameters, and width of a line is proportional to that proportion. DAMP—damage-associated molecular pattern; IL-1β—interleukin-1beta; IL-6—interleukin-6; TNFα—tumor necrosis factor alpha; CRP—C-reactive protein; Fbg—fibrinogen; eATP—extracellular adenosine-triphosphate; eHsp70—extracellular heat shock protein 70. ** $p < 0.01$, *** $p < 0.001$ in comparison to healthy non-smokers; +++ $p < 0.001$ in comparison to healthy smokers.

In addition, hierarchical cluster analysis was conducted with seven variables and clinical data obtained from COPD patients (Figure 3, see Supplementary Table S3). FEV_1 (% predicted) was included for the evaluation of airflow limitation-based severity. However, FEV_1 is insufficient for the disease severity assessment, and there was a need for additional assessment by DLCO (as a measure of the diffusion properties of the alveolar capillary membrane), number of exacerbations, mMRC (for dyspnoea severity), CAT and SGRQ-C (for more comprehensive assessment of symptoms and quality of life related to health status) and multicomponent index CODEx that incorporates several variables with great emphasis on comorbidities. Division of COPD patients based on FEV_1 was defined by GOLD guidelines [4], and there were four groups of COPD patients according to the severity of airflow limitation, as already described. Criteria for the diffusion limitation severity assessed by DLCO was defined by literature as well [30]. According to Fragoso et al., in our cluster analysis COPD patient that experienced two or more exacerbations or at least one exacerbation which led to hospitalization were considered to have a phenotype of exacerbator, while those that had less than two exacerbations during the previous year without hospitalization were considered to be non-exacerbators [31]. The division criteria for other parameters (mMRC, CAT, SGRQ-C, CODEx) were established by median values in COPD patients from the study.

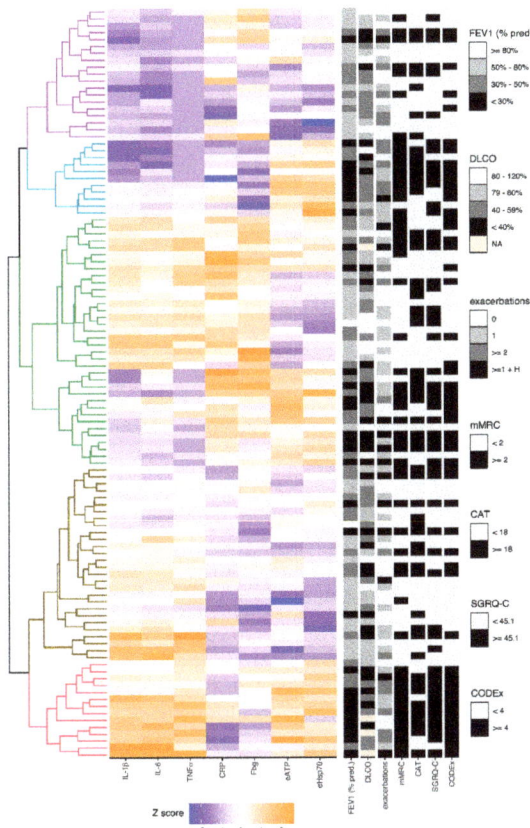

Figure 3. The heatmap of clusters of COPD patients regarding concentrations of cytokines (IL-1β, IL-6, TNFα), common inflammatory parameters (CRP, Fbg) and DAMPs (eATP, eHsp70). Hierarchical clustering analysis was used to characterize different phenotypes in COPD patients based on concentrations of cytokines (IL-1β, IL-6, TNFα), common inflammatory parameters (CRP, Fbg) and DAMPs (eATP, eHsp70). All concentrations were rank-based inverse normal transformed, and Euclidian correlation test with complete linkage was used for the clustering analysis. The heatmap shows colored squares, which present values of each parameter in each COPD patient. Five clusters of COPD patients were identified (left), and their clinical data (right) was included in the analysis, too. DAMP–damage-associated molecular pattern; IL-1β—interleukin-1beta; IL-6—interleukin-6; TNFα—tumor necrosis factor alpha; CRP—C-reactive protein; Fbg—fibrinogen; eATP—extracellular adenosine-triphosphate; eHsp70—extracellular heat shock protein 70; FEV_1 (% pred.)—forced expiratory volume in one second (% predicted); DLCO—diffusing capacity for carbon monoxide; exacerbations–number of exacerbations reported in previous year; mMRC—modified Medical Research Council; CAT–COPD Assessment Test; SGRQ-C—St George's Respiratory Questionnaire for COPD patients; CODEx—comorbidities, obstruction, dyspnoea, previous exacerbations; NA—not applicable; H–hospitalization.

Patients from cluster group 1 showed to have decreased concentrations of all three cytokines as well as mostly lower concentrations of eATP and eHsp70, while levels of CRP and Fbg seemed to be heterogeneous. Based on clinical data, those were predominantly the patients with mild clinical phenotype. COPD patients from cluster group 2 shared decreased values of all cytokines and they also mostly had lower levels of common inflammatory parameters, yet they had increased levels of DAMPs.

All the patients from cluster group 2 were in GOLD 3 or GOLD 4 stages of the disease and were above the median of mMRC score. Most of them had a phenotype of exacerbator. Predominantly, patients in cluster group 2 had higher scores of CAT, SGRQ-C and CODEx. Cluster groups 3 and 4 showed to have various changes of all parameters included in the analysis, and there was no unambiguous clinical phenotype regarding observed changes. However, cluster group 4 showed to recruit more patients with milder clinical phenotype. Patients in cluster group 5 showed mostly lower values of CRP and Fbg and increased levels of all cytokines, eATP and eHsp70. All of them were in GOLD 3 and GOLD 4 stages of the disease, had at least one exacerbation in the previous year as well as lower DLCO (a few patients could not perform this analysis due to their severe symptoms; therefore, not applicable (NA) was designated for them on the heatmap). Almost whole group had great impact of dyspnoea on everyday life assessed by mMRC and great impact of comorbidities assessed by CODEx score, while most of the patients from the group had more severe symptoms that affect their quality of life.

3.6. Model Combined of IL-1β, eATP and eHsp70 as the Best Combination for Identifying COPD Patients

Finally, evaluation of predictive performances of additional parameters was performed by univariate logistic regression analysis, and it was shown that all parameters had potential in identifying COPD patients. CRP showed to have OR of 1.24 (95% CI = 1.09–1.41, $p = 0.001$), OR of Fbg was 2.55 (95% CI = 1.65–3.95, $p < 0.001$), while eATP showed to have OR of 20.16 (95% CI = 8.40–48.38, $p < 0.001$), and eHsp70 OR of 5.20 (95% CI = 3.02–8.96, $p < 0.001$). Based on all statistically significant results from univariate logistic regression analysis (cytokines in Table 3 as well as CRP, Fbg, eATP and eHsp70), multivariate logistic regression analysis suggested a model composed of IL-1β (OR = 3.58, 95% CI = 1.71–7.47), eATP (OR = 6.08, 95% CI = 1.79–20.64) and eHsp70 (OR = 3.10, 95% CI = 1.59–6.03). This model showed the greatest predictive performance in comparison to other models and successfully classified 91% of cases, while area under the curve (AUC) was 0.966 (95% CI = 0.931–0.987, $p < 0.001$) which was the highest one when compared to other AUCs of all investigated models.

4. Discussion

Our study showed that all investigated cytokines (IL-1α, IL-1β, IL-6, IL-8 and TNFα) were increased in plasma of COPD patients, yet there was no association with airflow obstruction and symptoms severity. Inflammation was more developed in healthy smokers when compared to healthy non-smokers, and even more in COPD patients which was assessed by two network analyses–one including only cytokines, and the other conducting IL-1β, IL-6 and TNFα as well as additional inflammation-associated parameters CRP, Fbg, eATP and eHsp70. Moreover, when all parameters and clinical data were included in cluster analysis, different COPD clusters were observed. Finally, our study suggested combination of IL-1β, eATP and eHsp70 as the best model in identifying COPD patients with 91% correctly classified cases.

COPD is characterized by persistent inflammation predominantly localized to the peripheral airways and lung parenchyma, but it is also recognized that systemic inflammation might have an important role in development and progression of the disease and its comorbidities. Underlying mechanism of systemic inflammation in COPD include oxidative stress and altered circulating levels of inflammatory mediators [6,7]. It was shown that IL-1α and IL-1β were increased in lung samples and sputum of COPD patients. Additionally, it has been established that IL-1β was increased in peripheral circulation, while no study, to the best of our knowledge, investigated levels of blood IL-1α in patients with COPD [32,33]. IL-6 was increased in blood samples as well as in samples obtained from respiratory system of COPD patients when compared to controls [2,12]. In addition, IL-8 was increased in plasma [7] and sputum [8] of COPD patients as well as TNFα [5,7]. Increased cytokine levels in patients with COPD from the current study in comparison to controls might be more related to the systemic inflammation present in stable COPD than to pulmonary function impairment. Cytokines are the markers of low-grade inflammation, which was significantly developed in COPD patients. This was observed from network analysis of all cytokines, and IL-1β, IL-6 and TNFα were the best discriminators of COPD patients with cytokine levels being >95th percentile of the group of healthy non-smokers. However, one should have in mind that those cytokines are not specific to COPD and that systemic inflammation develops later in the disease course. Therefore, association of cytokines with disease severity parameters and/or outcomes would be preferable. It was shown that IL-1β from peripheral circulation positively correlated with CRP and negatively with FEV_1 [33]. Additionally, IL-1β is a dominant part of systemic pro-inflammatory response in COPD, and its high levels in sputum were associated with impaired lung function [11,34]. Negative correlation was also observed between IL-6 and FEV_1 [35]. However, IL-6 was not associated with decline in lung function in COPD patients from the ECLIPSE cohort [11]. Cytokines IL-1β, IL-6 and TNFα showed to be associated with the severity of COPD [10,16,36,37]. Our study did not show an increase in cytokine concentration regarding the severity of airflow obstruction or symptoms severity and history of exacerbations. Association of cytokines with disease severity was not successfully replicated either in some other studies, which might indicate heterogeneity within patient populations [6,17,38]. Kleniewska et al. showed that COPD patients had increased IL-1β, IL-6 and TNFα in induced sputum, but there was no difference in their concentration in serum in comparison to healthy subjects. However, CRP and Fbg showed to be increased in serum of COPD patients from the same study [39]. Cigarette smoking is one of the main environmental contributors to the development and progression of COPD. Still, our results indicate that the elevation of plasma cytokine levels was a consequence of COPD rather than smoking status. Similar observation was present in the study by Selvarajah et al. [40]. Besides cytokines, other parameters significantly contribute to the inflammatory processes as well, so they should be also explored as potential diagnostic and/or therapeutic targets. Additionally, it is considered that spirometry, symptoms assessment and data regarding exacerbations are not sufficient to reflect entirely the heterogeneity of COPD [31], and similar levels of airflow obstruction might result with different outcomes depending on the presence or absence of persistent systemic inflammation [21]. Therefore, investigation of biomarkers is important because of the possible distinction of COPD patients based on various patterns in alteration of investigated biomarkers. In our previous publications that included the same subjects as the current study, common inflammatory parameters CRP and Fbg were increased in COPD patients, and their predictive potential was observed as well [22]. Additionally, in the same patients we also assessed eATP and eHsp70 and showed that both of those DAMPs were associated with smoking status, airflow obstruction severity as well as symptoms severity and history of exacerbations [23,24]. Moreover, their great predictive values and association with multicomponent clinical parameters used for COPD assessment indicate there might be eATP- and eHsp70-driven inflammation as a part of disease progression. When all aforementioned parameters were combined with IL-1β, IL-6 and TNFα in network analysis, it was shown that not all patients with stable COPD have increased systemic inflammatory parameters, and even already well-known inflammatory parameters like CRP and Fbg were increased in only 21% and 34% of COPD patients, respectively, in comparison to the 95th percentile of healthy non-smokers. This suggest that other parameters (IL-1β, IL-6, TNFα, eATP, eHsp70) might have more important role in ongoing inflammation. In addition, increasing compactness of connected lines indicates there is a significant progression of inflammation in COPD patients. Still, systemic inflammation does not have to be persistent. It was demonstrated after three years follow-up that if duration of systemic inflammation was at least one year, it could lead to worse COPD outcomes (all-cause mortality and/or exacerbation frequency) [21]. Therefore, our suggestion for the future studies is to include a measurement of the same parameters after prolonged period with the aim to assess the persistence of systemic inflammation. Furthermore, different phenotypes of COPD might be identified with the purpose of better prognosis, diagnosis, and targeted treatment of COPD. Some of advanced statistical techniques may prove to be useful in identifying candidate phenotypes. Cluster analysis encompasses different algorithms for grouping objects without a priori hypothesis. By applying cluster data analysis, we studied concentrations of various parameters and clinical data obtained from our patients with stable COPD. Therefore, the goal was to classify overall data into relatively homogeneous cluster groups. There were previous studies with cluster analyses of various cytokines in COPD. Cluster group of COPD patients with lower cytokines values regarding statin therapy was suggested as an important one by Marević et al. [41]. Additionally, comorbidity clusters of COPD patients were associated with systemic inflammation [42], while other studies suggested several COPD subtypes after applying cluster analyses that explored clinical variables and outcomes [43–45]. Our cluster analysis joined IL-1β, IL-6 and TNFα with CRP, Fbg, eATP and eHsp70 since they were recognized as potential parameters in identifying various subgroups among COPD patients with systemic inflammation. In addition, we included clinical data as referent variables. There were several observations from cluster analysis that are worth mentioning. Cluster groups 2 and 5 showed the worst status regarding all clinical variables in the study. Cluster group 2 had increased both eATP and eHsp70, while other investigated parameters were decreased. On the other hand, cluster group 5 encompassed patients with increased cytokines as well as eATP and eHsp70, while they had mostly intermediate or decreased levels of CRP and Fbg. Patients from both cluster groups were the ones with lowest FEV_1 that was accompanied with lower health-related quality of life and possible significant impact of comorbidities assessed by CODEx. Considering that an increase in eATP and eHsp70 was accompanied by more severe clinical features, it could be suggested to include them in the assessment of COPD. Cluster groups 3 and 4 comprised most of the patients and it seems they represent the heterogeneity of COPD. All clinical variables significantly differed among these COPD patients. The heatmap shows there might be additional subgroups within groups 3 and 4 that were not separated by the cluster analysis. Finally, COPD patients from cluster group 1 had lower levels of all cytokines and mostly also of eATP and eHsp70, while CRP and Fbg differed. Predominantly, they showed to have mild to moderate clinical phenotype when the assessment of airflow limitation, exacerbations, symptoms severity and comorbidities were considered. Results from cluster analysis suggest there might be several patterns of inflammation in COPD patients, and similar was observed in the study of Rennard et al. [45]. It would be interesting to evaluate observed patterns in investigated parameters regarding commonly present comorbidities and potential effect of therapy. Cluster analysis might be a part of targeted approach towards future study designs, so the questions of interest could be directed to the specific COPD subgroups. Finally, when all statistically significant predictors from this study were included in multivariate logistic regression analysis, a combination of IL-1β, eATP and eHsp70 showed to have great performances in identifying COPD patients. The suggested model successfully classified 91% of all cases. Therefore, combined three-parameter model might have a great value in recognizing COPD patients, while patterns in concentrations of cytokines, CRP, Fbg, eATP and eHsp70 might be useful in identifying different COPD subgroups.

Several shortcomings are present in the current study. There were no patients in GOLD 1 stage or GOLD C group since COPD patients in GOLD 1 stage of the disease mostly do not contact their physician because of the very mild symptoms, while patients in GOLD C group usually do not manifest many symptoms and are not frequent exacerbators. However, larger number of participants in general should be considered in the further studies and a longitudinal study should be preferred over a cross-sectional case-control study.

5. Conclusions

Cytokines are one of the contributors in inflammatory processes present in COPD patients. However, by itself they are insufficient for the assessment of COPD, so additional biomarkers should be also evaluated. Models that include IL-1β, eATP and eHsp70 might prove to be useful in recognizing COPD patients because of its great predictive value, while combinations of IL-1β, IL-6 and TNFα with CRP, Fbg, eATP and eHsp70 might have a potential in differentiating COPD patients regarding clinical subgroups, with eATP and eHsp70 being particularly useful in identifying patients with severe COPD.

Supplementary Materials: The following are available online at http://www.mdpi.com/2075-4418/10/12/1029/s1, Table S1: Levels of cytokines in all participants regarding their smoking status, Table S2: Values of 95th percentile of the parameters determined in healthy non-smokers that are used in network analyses, Table S3: Clinical characteristics and concentrations of cytokines (IL-1β, IL-6, TNFα), common inflammatory parameters (CRP, Fbg) and DAMPs (eATP, eHsp70) in COPD patients according to the five clusters after unsupervised hierarchical clustering analysis.

Author Contributions: I.H. and L.R. wrote the main manuscript text and prepared figures and tables; L.R. and D.K. performed statistical analysis and interpreted it with I.H.; all authors contributed to the design of the work, while D.B. and M.B. performed the experiments; A.V.D. was responsible for collecting the samples, performing spirometry and DLCO analysis, and collecting data about participants; all authors reviewed the manuscript and approved the submitted version (and any substantially modified version). In addition, all authors have agreed both to be personally accountable for the author's own contributions and to ensure that questions related to the accuracy or integrity of any part of the work, even ones in which the author was not personally involved, are appropriately investigated, resolved, and the resolution documented in the literature. All authors have read and agreed to the published version of the manuscript.

Funding: This work has been fully supported by the Croatian Science Foundation under the project number IP-2014-09-1247. The work of PhD student Iva Hlapčić has been fully supported by the "Young researchers' career development project–training of doctoral students" of the Croatian Science Foundation funded by the European Union from the European Social Fund.

Conflicts of Interest: The authors declare no conflict of interest. The funders had no role in study design, data collection and analysis, decision to publish, or preparation of the manuscript.

References

1. Ramani, T.; Auletta, C.S.; Weinstock, D.; Mounho-Zamora, B.; Ryan, P.C.; Salcedo, T.W.; Bannish, G. Cytokines. *Int. J. Toxicol.* **2015**, *34*, 355–365. [CrossRef]
2. Bade, G.; Khan, M.A.; Srivastava, A.; Khare, P.; Solaiappan, K.; Guleria, R.; Palaniyar, N.; Talwar, A. Serum cytokine profiling and enrichment analysis reveal the involvement of immunological and inflammatory pathways in stable patients with chronic obstructive pulmonary disease. *Int. J. Chron. Obstruct. Pulmon. Dis.* **2014**, *9*, 759–773.
3. Boutou, A.K.; Pitsiou, G.G.; Stanopoulos, I.; Kontakiotis, T.; Kyriazis, G.; Argyropoulou, P. Levels of inflammatory mediators in chronic obstructive pulmonary disease patients with anemia of chronic disease: A case-control study. *QJM* **2012**, *105*, 657–663. [CrossRef] [PubMed]
4. Global Initiative for Chronic Obstructive Lung Disease (GOLD). *Global Strategy for the Diagnosis, Management, and Prevention of Chronic Obstructive Pulmonary Disease (2020 Report)*; Global Initiative for Chronic Obstructive Lung Disease: Fontana, WI, USA, 2019; Available online: https://goldcopd.org/gold-reports/ (accessed on 30 October 2020).
5. Bailey, K.L.; Goraya, J.; Rennard, S.L. Chronic obstructive pulmonary disease: Co-morbidities and systemic consequences. In *The Role of Systemic Inflammation in COPD*; Nici, L., ZuWallack, R., Eds.; Humana Press: Totowa, NJ, USA, 2012; pp. 15–30.
6. Karadag, F.; Karul, A.B.; Cildag, O.; Yilmaz, M.; Ozcan, H. Biomarkers of Systemic Inflammation in Stable and Exacerbation Phases of COPD. *Lung* **2008**, *186*, 403–409. [CrossRef] [PubMed]
7. Morello Gearhart, A.; Cavallazzi, R.; Peyrani, P.; Wiemken, T.L.; Furmanek, S.P.; Reyes-Vega, A.; Gauhar, U.; Rivas Perez, H.; Roman, J.; Ramirez, J.A.; et al. Lung Cytokines and Systemic Inflammation in Patients with COPD. *J. Respir. Infect.* **2017**, *1*, 4. [CrossRef]
8. Barnes, P.J. Cellular and molecular mechanisms of asthma and COPD. *Clin. Sci.* **2017**, *131*, 1541–1558. [CrossRef] [PubMed]
9. Gan, W.Q.; Man, S.F.P.; Senthilselvan, A.; Sin, D.D. Association between chronic obstructive pulmonary disease and systemic inflammation: A systematic review and a meta-analysis. *Thorax* **2004**, *59*, 574–580. [CrossRef]
10. Sapey, E.; Ahmad, A.; Bayley, D.; Newbold, P.; Snell, N.; Rugman, P.; Stockley, R.A. Imbalances Between Interleukin-1 and Tumor Necrosis Factor Agonists and Antagonists in Stable COPD. *J. Clin. Immunol.* **2009**, *29*, 508–516. [CrossRef]
11. Bradford, E.; Jacobson, S.; Varasteh, J.; Comellas, A.P.; Woodruff, P.; O'Neal, W.; DeMeo, D.L.; Li, X.; Kim, V.; Cho, M.; et al. The value of blood cytokines and chemokines in assessing COPD. *Respir. Res.* **2017**, *18*, 180. [CrossRef]

12. Barnes, P.J. The cytokine network in asthma and chronic obstructive pulmonary disease. *J. Clin. Investig.* **2008**, *118*, 3546–3556. [CrossRef]
13. Osei, E.T.; Brandsma, C.A.; Timens, W.; Heijink, I.H.; Hackett, T.L. Current perspectives on the role of interleukin-1 signalling in the pathogenesis of asthma and COPD. *Eur. Respir. J.* **2020**, *55*, 1900563. [CrossRef] [PubMed]
14. Borthwick, L.A. The IL-1 cytokine family and its role in inflammation and fibrosis in the lung. *Semin. Immunopathol.* **2016**, *38*, 517–534. [CrossRef] [PubMed]
15. Rumora, L.; Hlapčić, I.; Popović-Grle, S.; Rako, I.; Rogić, D.; Čepelak, I. Uric acid and uric acid to creatinine ratio in the assessment of chronic obstructive pulmonary disease: Potential biomarkers in multicomponent models comprising IL-1beta. *PLoS ONE* **2020**, *15*, e0234363. [CrossRef] [PubMed]
16. El-Shimy, W.S.; El-Dib, A.S.; Nagy, H.M.; Sabry, W. A study of IL-6, IL-8, and TNF-α as inflammatory markers in COPD patients. *Egypt. J. Bronchol.* **2014**, *8*, 91.
17. Wei, J.; Xiong, X.F.; Lin, Y.H.; Zheng, B.X.; Cheng, D.Y. Association between serum interleukin-6 concentrations and chronic obstructive pulmonary disease: A systematic review and meta-analysis. *PeerJ.* **2015**, *2015*, e1199. [CrossRef]
18. Aghasafari, P.; George, U.; Pidaparti, R. A review of inflammatory mechanism in airway diseases. *Inflamm. Res.* **2019**, *68*, 59–74. [CrossRef]
19. Cao, Y.; Gong, W.; Zhang, H.; Liu, B.; Li, B.; Wu, X.; Duan, X.; Dong, J. A Comparison of Serum and Sputum Inflammatory Mediator Profiles in Patients with Asthma and COPD. *J. Int. Med. Res.* **2012**, *40*, 2231–2242. [CrossRef]
20. Karadag, F.; Kirdar, S.; Karul, A.B.; Ceylan, E. The value of C-reactive protein as a marker of systemic inflammation in stable chronic obstructive pulmonary disease. *Eur. J. Intern. Med.* **2008**, *19*, 104–108. [CrossRef]
21. Agustí, A.; Edwards, L.D.; Rennard, S.I.; MacNee, W.; Tal-Singer, R.; Miller, B.E.; Vestbo, J.; Lomas, D.A.; Calverly, P.M.A.; Wouters, E.; et al. Persistent systemic inflammation is associated with poor clinical outcomes in copd: A novel phenotype. *PLoS ONE* **2012**, *7*, e37483. [CrossRef]
22. Hlapčić, I.; Somborac-Bačura, A.; Popović-Grle, S.; Vukić Dugac, A.; Rogić, D.; Rako, I.; Žanić Grubišić, T.; Rumora, L. Platelet indices in stable chronic obstructive pulmonary disease—Association with inflammatory markers, comorbidities and therapy. *Biochem. Med.* **2020**, *30*, 60–73. [CrossRef]
23. Hlapčić, I.; Hulina-Tomašković, A.; Somborac-Bačura, A.; Grdić Rajković, M.; Vukić Dugac, A.; Popović-Grle, S.; Rumora, L. Extracellular adenosine triphosphate is associated with airflow limitation severity and symptoms burden in patients with chronic obstructive pulmonary disease. *Sci. Rep.* **2019**, *9*, 15349. [CrossRef] [PubMed]
24. Hlapčić, I.; Hulina-Tomašković, A.; Grdić Rajković, M.; Popović-Grle, S.; Vukić Dugac, A.; Rumora, L. Association of Plasma Heat Shock Protein 70 with Disease Severity, Smoking and Lung Function of Patients with Chronic Obstructive Pulmonary Disease. *J. Clin. Med.* **2020**, *9*, 3097. [CrossRef] [PubMed]
25. Morales, D.R.; Flynn, R.; Zhang, J.; Trucco, E.; Quint, J.K.; Zutis, K. External validation of ADO, DOSE, COTE and CODEX at predicting death in primary care patients with COPD using standard and machine learning approaches. *Respir. Med.* **2018**, *138*, 150–155. [CrossRef] [PubMed]
26. Simundic, A.M.; Bölenius, K.; Cadamuro, J.; Church, S.; Cornes, M.P.; van Dongen-Lases, E.C.; Eker, P.; Erdeljanovic, T.; Grankvist, K.; Tiago Guimaraes, J.; et al. Joint EFLM-COLABIOCLI Recommendation for venous blood sampling. *Clin. Chem. Lab. Med.* **2018**, *56*, 2015–2038. [CrossRef] [PubMed]
27. GenABEL Project Developers. GenABEL: Genome-wide SNP association analysis. R package version 1.8-0. Available online: http://CRAN.R-project.org/package=GenABEL (accessed on 24 April 2020).
28. Charrad, M.; Ghazzali, N.; Boiteau, V.; Niknafs, A. Nbclust: An R package for determining the relevant number of clusters in a data set. *J. Stat. Softw.* **2014**, *61*, 36. [CrossRef]
29. 3.5.1. RDCT. A Language and Environment for Statistical Computing. Vol. 2, R Foundation for Statistical Computing. Available online: http://www.r-project.org (accessed on 27 April 2020).
30. Landsberg, J. Pulmonary Function Testing. In *Clinical Practice Manual for Pulmonary and Critical Care Medicine*, 1st ed.; Elsevier: Philadelphia, PA, USA, 2018; pp. 23–27.
31. Fragoso, E.; André, S.; Boleo-Tomé, J.P.; Areias, V.; Munhá, J.; Cardoso, J. Understanding COPD: A vision on phenotypes, comorbidities and treatment approach. *Rev. Port. Pneumol.* **2016**, *22*, 101–111. [CrossRef]

32. Botelho, F.M.; Bauer, C.M.T.; Finch, D.; Nikota, J.K.; Zavitz, C.C.J.; Kelly, A.; Lambert, K.N.; Piper, S.; Foster, M.L.; Goldring, J.J.P.; et al. IL-1α/IL-1R1 Expression in Chronic Obstructive Pulmonary Disease and Mechanistic Relevance to Smoke-Induced Neutrophilia in Mice. *PLoS ONE* **2011**, *6*, e28457. [CrossRef]
33. Zou, Y.; Chen, X.; Liu, J.; Zhou, D.B.; Kuang, X.; Xiao, J.; Yu, Q.; Lu, X.; Li, W.; Xie, B.; et al. Serum IL-1β and IL-17 levels in patients with COPD: Associations with clinical parameters. *Int. J. Chron. Obstruct. Pulmon. Dis.* **2017**, *12*, 1247–1254. [CrossRef]
34. Donaldson, G.C.; Seemungal, T.A.R.; Patel, I.S.; Bhowmik, A.; Wilkinson, T.M.A.; Hurst, J.R.; Maccallum, P.K.; Wedzicha, J.A. Airway and Systemic Inflammation and Decline in Lung Function in Patients with COPD. *Chesty* **2005**, *128*, 1995–2004. [CrossRef]
35. Zhang, J.; Dai, R.; Zhai, W.; Feng, N.; Lin, J. The efficacy of modified neutrophil alkaline phosphatase score, serum IL-6, IL-18 and CC16 levels on the prognosis of moderate and severe COPD patients. *Biomed. Res.* **2017**, *28*, 7651–7655.
36. Singh, S.; George, K.; Kaleem, M.; King, A.; Kumar, S.; King, S. Association between serum cytokine levels and severity of chronic obstructive pulmonary disease in Northern India. *Innov. Sp. Sci. Res. J.* **2015**, *18*, 357–361.
37. Pinto-Plata, V.; Toso, J.; Lee, K.; Park, D.; Bilello, J.; Mullerova, H.; De Souza, M.M.; Vessey, R.; Celli, B. Profiling serum biomarkers in patients with COPD: Associations with clinical parameters. *Thorax* **2007**, *62*, 595–601. [CrossRef] [PubMed]
38. Queiroz, C.F.; Lemos, A.C.M.; de Lourdes Sanatana Bastos, M.; Neves, M.C.L.C.; Camelier, A.A.; Carvalho, N.B.; de Carvalho, E.M. Inflammatory and immunological profiles in patients with COPD: Relationship with FEV_1 reversibility. *J. Bras. Pneumol.* **2016**, *42*, 241–247. [CrossRef] [PubMed]
39. Kleniewska, A.; Walusiak-Skorupa, J.; Piotrowski, W.; Nowakowska-Świrta, E.; Wiszniewska, M. Comparison of biomarkers in serum and induced sputum of patients with occupational asthma and chronic obstructive pulmonary disease. *J. Occup. Health.* **2016**, *58*, 333–339. [CrossRef]
40. Selvarajah, S.; Todd, I.; Tighe, P.J.; John, M.; Bolton, C.E.; Harrison, T.; Fairclough, L.C. Multiple Circulating Cytokines Are Coelevated in Chronic Obstructive Pulmonary Disease. *Mediators Inflamm.* **2016**, *2016*, 9. [CrossRef]
41. Marević, S.; Petrik, J.; Popović-Grle, S.; Čepelak, I.; Grgić, I.; Gorenec, L.; Stjepanović, G.; Laskaj, R.; Židovec Lepej, S. Cytokines and statin therapy in chronic obstructive pulmonary disease patients. *Scand. J. Clin. Lab. Investig.* **2018**, *78*, 533–538.
42. Vanfleteren, L.E.G.W.; Spruit, M.A.; Groenen, M.; Gaffron, S.; van Empel, V.P.M.; Bruijnzeel, P.L.B.; Rutten, E.P.A.; Op 't Roodt, J.; Wouters, E.F.M.; Franssen, F.M.E. Clusters of Comorbidities Based on Validated Objective Measurements and Systemic Inflammation in Patients with Chronic Obstructive Pulmonary Disease. *Am. J. Respir. Crit. Care. Med.* **2013**, *187*, 728–735. [CrossRef]
43. Garcia-Aymerich, J.; Gomez, F.P.; Benet, M.; Farrero, E.; Basagana, X.; Gayete, A.; Paré, C.; Freixa, X.; Ferrer, J.; Ferrer, A.; et al. Identification and prospective validation of clinically relevant chronic obstructive pulmonary disease (COPD) subtypes. *Thorax* **2011**, *66*, 430–437. [CrossRef]
44. Burgel, P.R.; Paillasseur, J.L.; Caillaud, D.; Tillie-Leblond, I.; Chanez, P.; Escamilla, R.; Court-Fortune, I.; Perez, T.; Carré, P.; Roche, N.; et al. Clinical COPD phenotypes: A novel approach using principal component and cluster analyses. *Eur. Respir. J.* **2010**, *36*, 531–539. [CrossRef]
45. Rennard, S.I.; Locantore, N.; Delafont, B.; Tal-Singer, R.; Silverman, E.K.; Vestbo, J.; Miller, B.E.; Bakke, P.; Celli, B.; Calverley, P.M.A.; et al. Identification of Five Chronic Obstructive Pulmonary Disease Subgroups with Different Prognoses in the ECLIPSE Cohort Using Cluster Analysis. *Ann. Am. Thorac. Soc.* **2015**, *12*, 303–312. [CrossRef]

Publisher's Note: MDPI stays neutral with regard to jurisdictional claims in published maps and institutional affiliations.

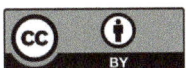

© 2020 by the authors. Licensee MDPI, Basel, Switzerland. This article is an open access article distributed under the terms and conditions of the Creative Commons Attribution (CC BY) license (http://creativecommons.org/licenses/by/4.0/).

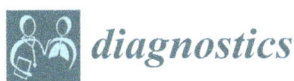

Article

Salivary Metabolic Profile of Patients with Lung Cancer, Chronic Obstructive Pulmonary Disease of Varying Severity and Their Comorbidity: A Preliminary Study

Lyudmila V. Bel'skaya [1,*], Elena A. Sarf [1], Denis V. Solomatin [2] and Victor K. Kosenok [3]

1. Biochemistry Research Laboratory, Omsk State Pedagogical University, 14, Tukhachevsky str, 644043 Omsk, Russia; nemcha@mail.ru
2. Department of Mathematics and Mathematics Teaching Methods, Omsk State Pedagogical University, 14, Tukhachevsky str, 644043 Omsk, Russia; denis_2001j@bk.ru
3. Department of Oncology, Omsk State Medical University, 12, Lenina str, 644099 Omsk, Russia; victorkosenok@gmail.com
* Correspondence: belskaya@omgpu.ru

Received: 14 November 2020; Accepted: 14 December 2020; Published: 15 December 2020

Abstract: The aim of the work was to study the features of the salivary biochemical composition in the combined pathology of lung cancer and chronic obstructive pulmonary disease (COPD) of varying severity (COPD I, COPD II). The study group included patients with lung cancer (n = 392), non-malignant lung pathologies (n = 168) and healthy volunteers (n = 500). Before treatment, the salivary biochemical composition was determined according to 34 indicators. Survival analysis performed by the Kaplan-Meier method. Biochemical parameters (catalase, imidazole compounds ICs, sialic acids, lactate dehydrogenase (LDH)) that can be used to monitor patients at risk (COPD I) for timely diagnosis of lung cancer are determined. A complex of salivary biochemical indicators with prognostic value in lung cancer was revealed. For patients with lung cancer without COPD, a group of patients with a favorable prognosis can be distinguished with a combination of ICs < 0.478 mmol/L and LDH > 1248 U/L (HR = 1.56, 95% CI 0.40–6.07, p = 0.03891). For COPD I, a level of ICs < 0.182 mmol/L are prognostically favorable (HR = 1.74, 95% CI 0.71–4.21, p = 0.07270). For COPD II, combinations of pH < 6.74 and LDH > 1006 U/L are prognostically favorable. In general, for patients with lung cancer in combination with COPD I, the prognosis is more favorable than without COPD.

Keywords: lung cancer; chronic obstructive pulmonary disease; saliva; biochemistry; diagnostics; prognosis

1. Introduction

Lung cancer is one of the predominantly diagnosed cancers (11.6% of the total number of cases); it was the leading cause of cancer death in 2018 (18.4% of the total number of cancer deaths) [1,2]. Another common lung disease is a chronic obstructive pulmonary disease (COPD) [3]. Recently, COPD has become the focus of attention due to increased morbidity, mortality and increased risk of lung cancer [4]. COPD and lung cancer have common features: high mortality and risk factors such as smoking, some genetic background, environmental exposure and major common inflammatory processes [5]. Several studies have shown that COPD is a risk factor for lung cancer, regardless of exposure to smoking, with a four to six times increased risk of lung cancer [6]. This risk increases with a progressive decline in FEV1, regardless of smoking history [7]. In addition, COPD worsens the prognosis of lung cancer due to higher morbidity and mortality [8]. There are numerous studies confirming the role of chronic inflammation in the genesis of cancer in general and lung cancer in particular [9]. It was found that various dysregenerative changes in the pulmonary epithelium against the background of chronic inflammatory lung disease have a malignant potential [10]. This explains the fact of frequent development of lung cancer against the background of COPD, in which dysplastic changes and metaplasia of the bronchial epithelium are clinical manifestations. Until now, no biomarker has been identified that would unequivocally determine the presence of lung cancer and/or COPD using both sputum and exhaled air and blood serum [11–13]. In previous studies, including ours, we have shown that the composition of saliva reflects metabolic changes occurring against the background of lung cancer [14–16]. However, a study of the effects of the combined pathology of lung cancer and COPD on the metabolic profile of saliva has not yet been conducted. The aim of the work was to study the characteristics of the biochemical composition of saliva in combined pathology, lung cancer and COPD of varying severity.

2. Materials and Methods

2.1. Study Design and Group Description

The study included 593 patients hospitalized in the thoracic department of the Clinical Oncological Dispensary in Omsk in the period 2014–2017. The inclusion criteria were: the age of the patients 30–75 years, the absence of any treatment, including surgery, chemotherapy or radiation. The collection of saliva samples was carried out strictly before the start of treatment.

A detailed description of the study group is given in Table 1. After histological verification, 168 people (28.3%) were diagnosed with non-malignant lung pathologies, including 51—hamartoma, 30—sarcoidosis, 28—tuberculoma, 39—fibrosis/pneumosclerosis, 13—inflammatory tumor, 4—pneumonia, 2—papilloma, 1—lipoma. These patients made up the comparison group. In 425 patients (71.7%), lung cancer of various histological types was confirmed, including 189—adenocarcinoma (ADC), 135—squamous cell carcinoma (SCC), 8—mixed (ADC + SCC), 68—neuroendocrine cancer (NEC) and 25—undifferentiated lung cancer. The NEC group included 16 patients with a diagnosis of typical and atypical carcinoid (low-grade G1 + G2) and 45 patients with small cell lung cancer, and 7 patients with large cell lung cancer (high-grade G3). Patient groups with mixed and undifferentiated cancers were subsequently excluded from the study. The control group consisted of 500 healthy patients, in whom no lung pathology was detected during routine clinical examination.

Table 1. The structure of the study group.

Feature	Lung Cancer, n (%)			Non-Malignant Lung Diseases, n = 168
	ADC, n = 189	SCC, n = 135	NEC, n = 68	
Age, years	61.0 (56.0; 65.0)	59.0 (55.0; 66.5)	55.0 (52.0; 60.0)	55.0 (45.5; 60.5)
Gender				
Male	129 (68.3)	128 (94.8)	50 (73.5)	98 (58.3)
Female	60 (31.7)	7 (5.2)	18 (26.5)	70 (41.7)
Stage				
St IA	16 (8.5)	3 (2.2)	5 (7.4)	-
St IB	52 (27.5)	28 (20.7)	10 (14.7)	-
St IIA+B	23 (12.2)	19 (14.1)	6 (8.8)	-
St IIIA	25 (13.2)	34 (25.2)	10 (14.7)	-
St IIIB	17 (9.0)	24 (17.8)	17 (25.0)	-
St IV	56 (29.6)	27 (20.0)	20 (29.4)	-
COPD				
No	113 (59.8)	69 (51.1)	41 (60.3)	141 (83.9)
Yes GOLD I	57 (30.2)	40 (29.6)	17 (25.0)	27 (16.1)
GOLD II	18 (9.5)	23 (17.1)	10 (14.7)	-
GOLD III	1 (0.5)	3 (2.2)	-	-

To describe the severity of COPD, a classification based on FEV1 as a percentage of predicted was used [17]. GOLD criteria were used to classify the severity of COPD (GOLD I; FEV1 > 80% of predicted, GOLD II; FEV1 = 50–79% of predicted, GOLD III; FEV1 = 30–49% of predicted, and GOLD IV; FEV1 < 30% of predicted). In this work, we examined groups of patients without COPD, with mild and moderate COPD (GOLD I, GOLD II), designated, respectively NO COPD, COPD I and COPD II.

The study was approved at a meeting of the Ethics Committee of the Omsk Regional Clinical Hospital "Clinical Oncology Center" on 21 July 2016 (Protocol No. 15). All of the volunteers provided written informed consent.

2.2. Collection, Processing, Storage and Analysis of Saliva Samples

Saliva (5 mL) was collected from all participants prior to treatment. Collection of saliva samples was carried out on an empty stomach after rinsing the mouth with water in the interval of 8–10 am by spitting into sterile polypropylene tubes; the salivation rate (mL/min) was calculated. Saliva samples were centrifuged (10,000× g for 10 min) (CLb-16, Moscow, Russia), after which biochemical analysis was immediately performed without storage and freezing using the StatFax 3300 semi-automatic biochemical analyzer [16].

2.3. Statistical Analysis

Statistical analysis was performed using Statistica 13.3 EN software (StatSoft, Tulsa, OK, USA); R version 3.6.3; RStudio Version 1.2.5033; FactoMineR version 2.3. (RStudio, version 3.2.3, Boston, MA, USA) by a nonparametric method using the Mann-Whitney U-test and the Kruskal-Wallis H-test. At the preliminary stage, the character of distribution and homogeneity of dispersions in groups was checked. According to the Shapiro-Wilk test, the content of all determined parameters does not correspond to the normal distribution ($p < 0.05$). The test for the homogeneity of variances in groups (Bartlett's test) allowed us to reject the hypothesis that variances are homogeneous across groups ($p = 0.00017$). Therefore, nonparametric statistical methods were used to process the experimental data. The description of the sample was made by calculating the median (Me) and the interquartile range as the 25th and 75th percentiles (LQ; UQ). Differences were considered statistically significant at $p < 0.05$.

The Kruskal-Wallis test is a nonparametric alternative to one-dimensional (intergroup) ANOVA. It is used to compare three or more samples. With a high significance of the Kruskal-Wallis test (H), the characteristics of different experimental groups significantly differ from each other ($p < 0.05$). Using the Kruskal-Wallis test, we compared several groups (3 groups in Tables 2 and 3; 5 groups in Table 4) and selected indicators whose change was significant at $p < 0.05$. These indicators were subsequently used for the principal component analysis (PCA). In addition, we included indicators in the PCA analysis, the values of which differ at the 0.10 significance level. In the case of $0.05 < p < 0.10$, the limit of significance is slightly exceeded, which means that there is a tendency towards the manifestation of a pattern. If a significant pattern is identified, to identify groups that are significantly different from each other, it is necessary to test all groups in pairs. The Mann-Whitney test was used only for pairwise comparison of the differences between the COPD and NO COPD groups in different histological types of lung cancer; in all other cases, the Kruskal-Wallis test was used to compare the groups.

A principal component analysis (PCA) was performed using the PCA program in R [18]. The significance of the correlation is determined by the correlation coefficient (r): strong—$r = \pm 0.700$ to ± 1.00, medium—$r = \pm 0.300$ to ± 0.699, weak—$r = 0.00$ to ± 0.299. The rate of change of individual biochemical parameters was quantified using the ratio of natural logarithms (LnRR), with LnRR (indicator) = ln (COPD / NO COPD value). Medians and interquartile range presented in figures were calculated using nontransformed data.

The survival curve was calculated by the Kaplan-Meier method and compared using the Log-rank test for univariate analysis (Statistica 10.0, StatSoft). Prognostic factors were analyzed by multivariate analysis using Cox's proportional hazard model in a backward stepwise fashion to adjust for potential confounding factors. Overall survival (OS) was computed from the date of diagnosis to the date of death or the date of the last follow-up. Survival data were obtained until December 2019.

Table 2. Biochemical markers of saliva in patients with lung cancer, depending on the presence/absence and severity of cancer, chronic obstructive pulmonary disease (COPD).

Indicators	Lung Cancer (LC)	LC + COPD I	LC + COPD II		Kruskal-Wallis Test (H, p)
Flow rate, mL/min	0.85 (0.72; 0.99)	0.81 (0.74; 0.94)	0.78 (0.64; 0.97)	↓↓	0.8541, 0.7596
Electrolytes					
pH	6.46 (6.20; 6.68)	6.57 (6.32; 6.85)	6.63 (6.28; 7.03)	↑↑	11.20, 0.0037 *
Calcium (Ca), mmol/L	1.48 (1.07; 1.92)	1.41 (1.02; 1.80)	1.19 (0.83; 1.51)	↓↓	8.900, 0.0117 *
Phosphorus (P), mmol/L	4.61 (3.37; 5.78)	4.00 (2.97; 5.32)	4.55 (3.37; 6.01)	↓↑	3.979, 0.1368
Ca/P-ratio, c.u.	0.32 (0.23; 0.47)	0.33 (0.23; 0.51)	0.28 (0.17; 0.39)	=↓	4.737, 0.0936 **
Sodium (Na), mmol/L	9.0 (5.4; 13.5)	9.6 (6.1; 13.8)	8.3 (5.9; 16.5)	↑↓	0.9659, 0.6170
Potassium (K), mmol/L	12.9 (9.4; 16.0)	13.0 (8.5; 15.9)	12.8 (9.3; 16.6)	==	0.3176, 0.8532
Na/K-ratio, c.u.	0.73 (0.45; 1.23)	0.87 (0.48; 1.31)	0.76 (0.46; 1.19)	↑↓	1.058, 0.5892
Chlorides, mmol/L	28.3 (22.3; 35.7)	27.5 (21.0; 37.2)	29.8 (21.0; 36.4)	↓↑	0.1096, 0.9467
Magnesium, mmol/L	0.311 (0.248; 0.381)	0.286 (0.220; 0.361)	0.279 (0.213; 0.346)	↓↓	5.981, 0.0503 **
Protein Metabolism					
Protein, g/L	0.64 (0.33; 1.10)	0.65 (0.36; 0.94)	0.64 (0.40; 0.96)	==	0.7507, 0.6870
Albumin, g/L	0.313 (0.154; 0.475)	0.286 (0.153; 0.462)	0.311 (0.178; 0.485)	↓↑	0.9102, 0.6344
Urea, mmol/L	8.06 (5.34; 11.60)	7.78 (6.09; 11.64)	7.34 (4.49; 11.60)	↓↓	0.4845, 0.7849
Uric acid, μmol/L	90.4 (45.0; 181.0)	76.7 (34.7; 133.7)	100.0 (24.8; 195.2)	↓↑	4.346, 0.1138
Sialic acids, mmol/L	0.189 (0.110; 0.287)	0.134 (0.079; 0.238)	0.180 (0.093; 0.314)	↓↑	6.161, 0.0459 *
Seromucoids, c.u.	0.104 (0.056; 0.159)	0.097 (0.060; 0.149)	0.081 (0.039; 0.134)	↓↓	3.464, 0.1770
α-amino acids, μmol/L	4.16 (3.87; 4.66)	4.12 (3.86; 4.53)	4.16 (3.93; 4.49)	↓↑	0.5360, 0.7649
Imidazole compounds, mmol/L	0.296 (0.197; 0.478)	0.319 (0.182; 0.455)	0.341 (0.266; 0.531)	↑↑	1.995, 0.3688
Lactate, μmol/L	2.32 (1.59; 3.50)	2.75 (1.71; 3.96)	3.12 (1.85; 4.14)	↑↑	2.702, 0.2590
Enzymes					
ALT, U/L	4.00 (2.69; 6.00)	3.77 (2.62; 4.96)	4.15 (2.69; 6.54)	↓↑	2.651, 0.2657
AST, U/L	5.58 (3.33; 8.08)	4.96 (3.25; 6.99)	4.58 (3.04; 6.75)	↓↓	3.854, 0.1456
AST/ALT, c.u.	1.29 (1.01; 1.70)	1.32 (1.03; 1.66)	1.07 (0.86; 1.55)	↑↓	5.026, 0.0810 **
ALP, U/L	76.06 (49.98; 117.34)	63.02 (47.81; 97.79)	73.88 (52.15; 130.38)	↓↑	2.284, 0.3192
LDH, U/L	1248.5 (604.3; 1907.0)	1165.0 (605.2; 1715.0)	764.4 (481.0; 1206.3)	↓↓	9.210, 0.0100 *
GGT, U/L	22.3 (18.5; 26.1)	20.6 (17.5; 25.5)	21.1 (18.5; 23.1)	↓↑	3.603, 0.1651
α-amylase, U/L	317.4 (198.6; 655.7)	287.6 (99.9; 600.9)	303.3 (139.7; 680.2)	↓↑	1.529, 0.4656
Catalase, ncat/mL	2.66 (2.04; 4.36)	2.78 (2.13; 4.13)	2.41 (1.73; 3.17)	↑↓	5.986, 0.0501 **
SOD, c.u.	60.5 (26.3; 121.1)	61.8 (34.2; 110.5)	65.8 (39.5; 92.1)	↑↑	0.1997, 0.9050
Lipoperoxidation products and endogenous intoxication rates					
Diene conjugates, c.u.	4.01 (3.83; 4.20)	3.91 (3.75; 4.13)	3.97 (3.79; 4.15)		6.136, 0.0465 *
Triene conjugates, c.u.	0.892 (0.775; 1.004)	0.879 (0.792; 0.967)	0.907 (0.793; 1.009)	↓↑	0.7660, 0.6818
Schiff bases, c.u.	0.561 (0.494; 0.675)	0.529 (0.474; 0.638)	0.556 (0.509; 0.652)	↓↑	5.054, 0.0799 **
MDA, μmol/L	7.14 (5.81; 9.32)	6.67 (5.60; 9.27)	8.46 (6.15; 10.17)	↓↑	4.258, 0.1189
MM 280/254 nm	0.897 (0.806; 1.002)	0.875 (0.794; 0.989)	0.906 (0.832; 1.055)	↓↑	1.878, 0.3914

*—differences between 3 groups are statistically significant, $p < 0.05$; **—differences between 3 groups are statistically significant, $p < 0.10$; the first arrow shows the change in the parameter when switching from the LC group to the LC + COPDI, the second—when changing from the LC + COPDI to LC + COPD II; ↑—the indicator value increases; ↓—the indicator value decreases; =—the indicator value does not change; SOD—superoxide dismutase; MDA—malondialdehyde; MM 280/254—middle molecular toxins; AST—aspartate aminotransferase; ALT—alanine aminotransferase; LDH—lactate dehydrogenase; GGT—gamma glutamyltransferase; ALP—alkaline phosphatase.

Table 3. Metabolic profile of saliva in patients with lung cancer of various histological types depending on the presence/absence of COPD.

Indicator	HT	NO COPD	COPD I	COPD II	Kruskal-Wallis Test (H, p)
pH	ADC	6.47 (6.22; 6.72)	6.57 (6.32; 6.85)	6.60 (6.29; 7.00)	2.508, 0.2853
	SCC	6.45 (6.23; 6.64)	6.61 (6.43; 6.90)	6.76 (6.13; 7.15)	9.085, 0.0106 *
	NEC	6.33 (6.03; 6.50)	6.43 (6.14; 6.60)	6.74 (6.28; 6.81)	2.706, 0.2584
Calcium, mmol/L	ADC	1.40 (1.03; 1.88)	1.60 (1.11; 1.84)	1.24 (0.77; 1.51)	2.239, 0.3264
	SCC	1.58 (1.14; 2.08)	1.27 (0.85; 1.68)	1.02 (0.83; 1.47)	10.49, 0.0053 *
	NEC	1.44 (1.28; 1.80)	1.25 (1.03; 1.57)	1.24 (0.98; 1.55)	1.948, 0.3776
Magnesium, mmol/L	ADC	0.320 (0.259; 0.406)	0.285 (0.216; 0.389)	0.245 (0.161; 0.343)	5.441, 0.0658 **
	SCC	0.302 (0.254; 0.378)	0.292 (0.228; 0.336)	0.277 (0.213; 0.349)	2.117, 0.3471
	NEC	0.299 (0.230; 0.342)	0.298 (0.219; 0.328)	0.287 (0.275; 0.398)	0.3195, 0.8524

Table 3. Cont.

Indicator	HT	NO COPD	COPD I	COPD II	Kruskal-Wallis Test (H, p)
AST/ALT, c.u.	ADC	1.38 (1.01; 1.73)	1.30 (1.08; 1.81)	1.03 (0.76; 1.28)	4.566, 0.1020
	SCC	1.17 (0.92; 1.56)	1.34 (1.01; 1.60)	1.05 (0.94; 1.58)	1.107, 0.5750
	NEC	1.31 (1.08; 1.69)	1.34 (0.99; 1.88)	1.32 (0.97; 1.54)	0.3129, 0.8552
LDH, U/L	ADC	1253.0 (655.1; 1842.0)	1185.0 (665.7; 1647.0)	572.3 (497.9; 1095.0)	5.428, 0.0663 **
	SCC	1193.0 (566.0; 1893.0)	1205.5 (492.4; 1918.5)	795.8 (437.7; 1108.0)	3.955, 0.1384
	NEC	986.8 (446.5; 1940.0)	1165.0 (1007.0; 1616.0)	1148.0 (724.3; 1430.0)	0.2333, 0.8899
Catalase, ncat/mL	ADC	2.74 (2.12; 4.42)	2.81 (2.18; 4.08)	2.29 (1.81; 3.04)	3.506, 0.1733
	SCC	2.69 (2.00; 4.29)	2.65 (2.12; 3.48)	2.68 (1.90; 3.17)	1.522, 0.4673
	NEC	2.36 (2.04; 3.38)	3.48 (2.60; 4.33)	1.72 (1.65; 3.24)	3.137, 0.2083
Sialic acids, mmol/L	ADC	0.159 (0.098; 0.275)	0.125 (0.092; 0.226)	0.168 (0.079; 0.323)	2.103, 0.3493
	SCC	0.201 (0.125; 0.281)	0.150 (0.069; 0.269)	0.183 (0.098; 0.232)	3.468, 0.1766
	NEC	0.204 (0.101; 0.336)	0.128 (0.092; 0.323)	0.293 (0.092; 0.488)	1.103, 0.5761
Diene conjugates, c.u.	ADC	4.01 (3.83; 4.18)	3.90 (3.67; 4.17)	4.00 (3.79; 4.15)	3.541, 0.1702
	SCC	4.03 (3.85; 4.21)	3.92 (3.78; 4.07)	3.96 (3.78; 4.23)	3.957, 0.1383
	NEC	4.05 (3.80; 4.15)	3.99 (3.85; 4.16)	3.88 (3.84; 3.92)	1.135, 0.5669
Schiff bases, c.u.	ADC	0.559 (0.499; 0.671)	0.529 (0.478; 0.638)	0.551 (0.495; 0.665)	2.627, 0.2688
	SCC	0.573 (0.490; 0.669)	0.538 (0.476; 0.646)	0.556 (0.507; 0.627)	1.402, 0.4960
	NEC	0.557 (0.495; 0.641)	0.487 (0.417; 0.633)	0.570 (0.532; 0.662)	1.589, 0.4517
α-amylase, U/L	ADC	316.5 (178.7; 645.0)	323.3 (184.7; 929.3)	377.1 (266.5; 680.2)	0.4174, 0.8116
	SCC	270.7 (198.6; 857.0)	232.3 (56.4; 360.3)	232.8 (90.1; 284.7)	6.986, 0.0304 *
	NEC	349.6 (223.9; 458.8)	477.1 (74.8; 965.0)	796.8 (379.5; 1278.0)	2.126, 0.3454
Lactate, nmol/mL	ADC	2.14 (1.66; 3.12)	2.75 (1.59; 4.41)	3.12 (1.31; 3.43)	1.032, 0.5971
	SCC	2.23 (1.29; 3.36)	2.74 (1.77; 3.96)	4.14 (2.79; 4.74)	2.887, 0.2361
	NEC	3.76 (2.68; 6.44)	3.01 (2.28; 7.97)	1.77 (0.76; 1.85)	5.381, 0.0479 *

HT—histology type; ADC—adenocarcinoma; SCC—squamous cell carcinoma; NEC—neuroendocrine cancer; AST—aspartate aminotransferase; ALT—alanine aminotransferase; LDH—lactate dehydrogenase; *—differences between 3 groups are statistically significant, $p < 0.05$; **—differences between 3 groups are statistically significant, $p < 0.10$.

Table 4. Biochemical markers of saliva in patients with lung cancer, noncancerous pathologies of the lung and control group.

Indicator	Control Group		Lung Cancer	Comparison Group	Kruskal-Wallis Test (H, p)
Electrolytes					
pH	6.50 (6.30; 6.72)	1 2	6.46 (6.20; 6.68) 6.59 (6.32; 6.89)	6.49 (6.24; 6.80) 6.34 (6.08; 6.82)	14.11, 0.0070 *
Calcium, mmol/L	1.33 (1.05; 1.66)	1 2	1.48 (1.07; 1.92) 1.30 (0.97; 1.76)	1.36 (1.02; 1.69) 1.44 (1.16; 2.35)	13.75, 0.0081 *
Phosphorus, mmol/L	4.53 (3.58; 5.85)	1 2	4.61 (3.37; 5.78) 4.13 (3.25; 5.53)	4.74 (3.47; 5.64) 4.80 (3.17; 6.54)	5.955, 0.2026
Ca/P-ratio, c.u.	0.29 (0.22; 0.39)	1 2	0.32 (0.23; 0.47) 0.31 (0.21; 0.47)	0.29 (0.20; 0.40) 0.34 (0.17; 0.53)	11.34, 0.0230 *
Sodium, mmol/L	8.4 (5.5; 12.4)	1 2	9.0 (5.4; 13.5) 9.3 (6.1; 15.0)	7.8 (5.9; 10.7) 9.5 (4.8; 15.3)	5.546, 0.2357
Potassium, mmol/L	11.8 (9.3; 14.7)	1 2	12.9 (9.4; 16.0) 12.8 (8.9; 15.9)	12.4 (9.4; 14.8) 9.7 (7.2; 13.9)	6.576, 0.1601
Na/K-ratio, c.u.	0.72 (0.49; 1.15)	1 2	0.73 (0.45; 1.23) 0.83 (0.48; 1.30)	0.74 (0.47; 1.08) 0.90 (0.55; 1.49)	3.033, 0.5524
Chlorides, mmol/L	26.1 (21.2; 32.2)	1 2	28.3 (22.3; 35.7) 28.2 (21.0; 36.8)	25.4 (20.7; 33.5) 23.3 (19.2; 34.3)	9.383, 0.0522
Mg, mmol/L	0.300 (0.246; 0.350)	1 2	0.311 (0.248; 0.381) 0.286 (0.220; 0.349)	0.295 (0.241; 0.366) 0.313 (0.221; 0.400)	6.389, 0.1719

Table 4. Cont.

Indicator	Control Group		Lung Cancer	Comparison Group	Kruskal-Wallis Test (H, p)
Protein metabolism					
Protein, g/L	0.80 (0.50; 1.23)	1	0.64 (0.33; 1.10)	0.69 (0.49; 1.11)	20.78, 0.0004 *
		2	0.65 (0.36; 0.95)	0.69 (0.54; 1.02)	
Albumin, g/L	0.258 (0.171; 0.435)	1	0.313 (0.154; 0.475)	0.337 (0.178; 0.543)	7.562, 0.1090
		2	0.295 (0.162; 0.474)	0.304 (0.178; 0.498)	
Urea, mmol/L	7.84 (5.40; 11.03)	1	8.06 (5.34; 11.60)	7.78 (5.27; 10.78)	4.087, 0.3944
		2	7.57 (5.81; 11.60)	6.12 (3.84; 9.06)	
Uric acid, µmol/L	86.5 (28.2; 154.8)	1	90.4 (45.0; 181.0)	84.9 (30.4; 163.4)	6.472, 0.1666
		2	80.4 (34.7; 146.8)	85.0 (22.3; 176.6)	
Sialic acids, mmol/L	0.195 (0.134; 0.299)	1	0.189 (0.110; 0.287)	0.165 (0.104; 0.238)	35.35, 0.0000 *
		2	0.146 (0.085; 0.262)	0.134 (0.079; 0.201)	
Seromucoids, c.u.	0.090 (0.060; 0.130)	1	0.104 (0.056; 0.159)	0.105 (0.066; 0.149)	6.607, 0.1582
		2	0.092 (0.055; 0.141)	0.095 (0.046; 0.146)	
α-amino acids, µmol/L	4.12 (3.83; 4.50)	1	4.16 (3.87; 4.66)	4.25 (4.00; 4.60)	13.05, 0.0110 *
		2	4.13 (3.87; 4.51)	4.02 (3.77; 4.50)	
Imidazole compounds, mmol/L	0.281 (0.175; 0.379)	1	0.296 (0.197; 0.478)	0.326 (0.212; 0.448)	30.09, 0.0000 *
		2	0.326 (0.212; 0.478)	0.448 (0.197; 0.660)	
Lactate, µmol/L	2.36 (1.61; 3.48)	1	2.32 (1.59; 3.50)	2.65 (1.65; 3.24)	3.357, 0.5000
		2	2.81 (1.77; 4.10)	1.54 (0.36; 4.21)	
Enzymes					
ALT, U/L	3.62 (2.54; 4.92)	1	4.00 (2.69; 6.00)	3.96 (2.85; 6.31)	13.56, 0.0088 *
		2	3.88 (2.62; 5.38)	3.58 (2.54; 5.23)	
AST, U/L	5.50 (3.67; 7.33)	1	5.58 (3.33; 8.08)	6.00 (4.17; 8.67)	12.22, 0.0158 *
		2	4.92 (3.17; 6.99)	4.29 (3.08; 6.75)	
AST/ALT, c.u.	1.42 (1.13; 1.92)	1	1.29 (1.01; 1.70)	1.42 (1.08; 1.83)	23.45, 0.0001 *
		2	1.25 (0.97; 1.64)	1.25 (1.00; 1.76)	
ALP, U/L	58.7 (41.3; 82.6)	1	76.1 (50.0; 117.3)	71.7 (52.2; 115.2)	38.57, 0.0000 *
		2	69.5 (47.8; 108.7)	69.5 (50.0; 117.3)	
LDH, U/L	1127.5 (652.1; 1838.0)	1	1248.5 (604.3; 1907.0)	1291.0 (762.0; 1902.0)	10.17, 0.0377 *
		2	1060.0 (545.5; 1616.0)	883.2 (527.7; 1443.0)	
GGT, U/L	20.3 (17.5; 24.0)	1	22.3 (18.5; 26.1)	21.6 (18.1; 25.4)	15.29, 0.0041 *
		2	20.8 (18.0; 25.1)	20.1 (16.2; 25.0)	
α-amylase, U/L	201.6 (100.5; 404.4)	1	317.4 (198.6; 655.7)	316.0 (178.6; 468.4)	23.54, 0.0001 *
		2	287.6 (122.2; 618.1)	168.1 (27.9; 804.2)	
Catalase, ncat/mL	4.32 (3.20; 5.57)	1	2.66 (2.04; 4.36)	3.28 (2.34; 5.06)	160.5, 0.0000 *
		2	2.70 (1.97; 3.62)	2.57 (1.76; 3.52)	
SOD, c.u.	57.9 (34.2; 103.9)	1	60.5 (26.3; 121.1)	63.2 (42.1; 131.6)	2.971, 0.5627
		2	63.2 (39.5; 110.5)	63.2 (52.6; 84.2)	
Lipoperoxidation products and endogenous intoxication rates					
Diene conjugates, c.u.	3.92 (3.78; 4.06)	1	4.01 (3.83; 4.20)	3.97 (3.76; 4.13)	21.50, 0.0003 *
		2	3.92 (3.77; 4.14)	4.04 (3.77; 4.25)	
Triene conjugates, c.u.	0.870 (0.793; 0.944)	1	0.892 (0.775; 1.004)	0.901 (0.824; 1.010)	7.994, 0.0918
		2	0.890 (0.792; 0.981)	0.861 (0.792; 0.958)	
Schiff bases, c.u.	0.528 (0.492; 0.565)	1	0.561 (0.494; 0.675)	0.555 (0.492; 0.686)	38.33, 0.0000 *
		2	0.541 (0.480; 0.640)	0.563 (0.470; 0.661)	
MDA, µmol/L	6.84 (5.81; 8.38)	1	7.14 (5.81; 9.32)	7.39 (5.94; 9.44)	8.374, 0.0788
		2	7.35 (5.64; 9.91)	6.03 (5.13; 9.10)	
MM 280/254 nm	0.847 (0.749; 0.948)	1	0.897 (0.806; 1.002)	0.892 (0.812; 0.970)	28.88, 0.0000 *
		2	0.894 (0.802; 1.020)	0.893 (0.776; 1.075)	

1—Groups without COPD, 2—groups with COPD; *—differences between the 5 groups are statistically significant ($p < 0.05$); SOD—superoxide dismutase; MDA—malondialdehyde; MM 280/254—middle molecular toxins; AST—aspartate aminotransferase; ALT—alanine aminotransferase; LDH—lactate dehydrogenase; GGT—gamma glutamyltransferase; ALP—alkaline phosphatase.

3. Results

3.1. Metabolic Features of Saliva in Lung Cancer Depending on the Presence/Absence of COPD

At the first stage, the biochemical composition of the saliva of patients with lung cancer was studied to identify metabolic changes (Table 2). It was found that the differences between the three groups are significant in the following indicators: pH, calcium concentration, the level of diene conjugates, sialic acids, and lactate dehydrogenase (LDH) activity (Table 2).

High values of the Kruskal-Wallis criterion were also noted for the Ca/P-ratio, magnesium concentration, catalase activity, alanine aminotransferase (ALT)/AST (aspartate aminotransferase)-ratio, and the level of Schiff bases ($p < 0.10$). All these indicators were used further for analysis by the PCA method (Figure 1). The first two dimensions of the analysis represent 34.25% of the total inertia of the dataset; this means that 34.25% of the total cloud variability is explained by the plane (Figure 1B). Estimating the correct number of axes for interpretation suggests limiting the analysis to describing the first five axes (principal components) (Figure 1B,D,F).

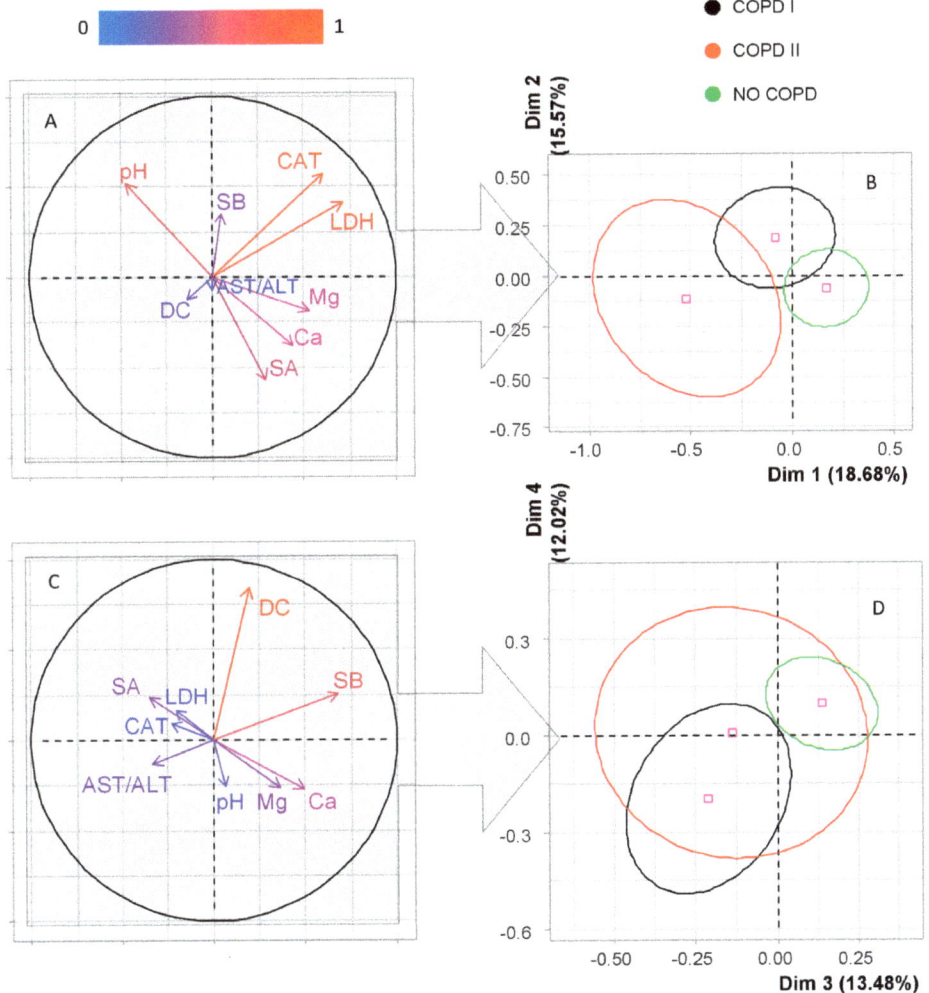

Figure 1. *Cont.*

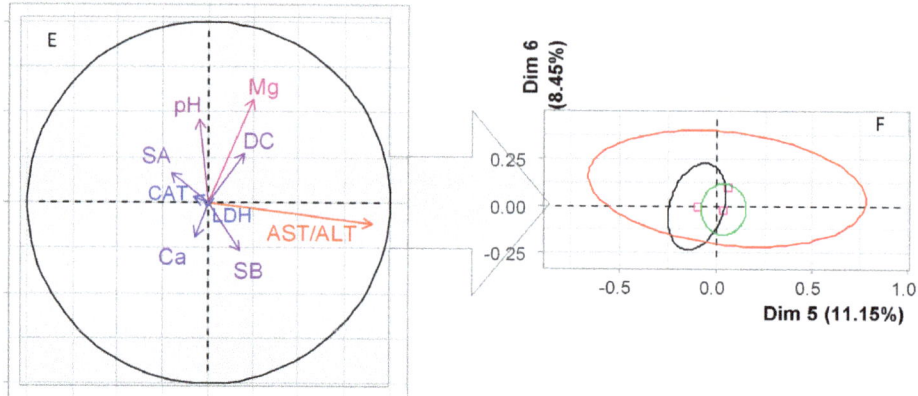

Figure 1. Principal component analysis (PCA)—Factor plane (**B,D,F**) and the corresponding correlation circle (**A,C,E**) in the first five dimensions for three groups (lung cancer without COPD, lung cancer with COPD I, lung cancer with COPD II). The color of the arrows on the correlation circle changes from blue (weak correlation) to red (strong correlation), as shown on the color bar. The orientation of the arrows characterizes positive and negative correlations (for the first principal component, we analyze the location of the arrows relative to the vertical axis, for the second principal component—relative to the horizontal axis). LDH—lactate dehydrogenase; CAT—catalase; SB—Schiff bases; DC—diene conjugates; SA—sialic acids; Ca—calcium; Mg—magnesium; AST/ALT—aspartate aminotransferase to alanine aminotransferase ratio.

For the first principal component (PC1), high correlation coefficients ($p = 0.001$) were obtained only for LDH ($r = 0.71$), average strength for catalase ($r = 0.61$), magnesium ($r = 0.53$), calcium ($r = 0.44$) and pH ($r = -0.47$). For PC2, high correlation coefficients were not revealed, correlations of average strength were confirmed for catalase ($r = 0.57$), pH ($r = 0.52$), LDH ($r = 0.41$), Schiff bases ($r = 0.35$), calcium ($r = -0.38$) and sialic acids ($r = -0.57$). For PC3, correlations of average strength were established with Schiff bases ($r = 0.68$), calcium ($r = 0.50$), magnesium ($r = 0.37$), sialic acids ($r = -0.35$) and the AST/ALT-ratio ($r = -0.33$). For PC4 and PC5, only one strong correlation was revealed: with diene conjugates ($r = 0.84$) and the AST/ALT-ratio ($r = 0.90$), respectively (Figure 1). Thus, the given factor planes make it possible to divide the studied groups among themselves, but it should be borne in mind that the ellipses in the diagrams cover only 60% of the values that make the greatest contribution (Figure 1B,D,F). Thus, the most significant indicators affecting the composition of saliva in COPD are the activity of enzymes (LDH, catalase) (Figure 1B), then the level of lipid peroxidation products (diene conjugates, Schiff bases) (Figure 1D) and the value of AST/ALT-ratio are significant (Figure 1F).

3.2. Influence of Histological Type of Lung Cancer on Metabolic Indicators of Saliva in Patients with COPD

Since the group of patients with lung cancer is heterogeneous in its composition, at the next stage, each of the groups under consideration was divided into subgroups in accordance with the histological type of lung cancer (Table 3).

It was found that some of the indicators change unidirectionally for different histological types of lung cancer (Table 3). Regardless of the histological type of lung cancer, the pH increases in the presence of COPD. The maximum increase in pH was observed in COPD II. For adenocarcinoma, there is the smallest increase in pH (+2.0%), the largest for neuroendocrine lung cancer (+6.5%). For squamous cell lung cancer, the pH increases by 4.8%; it is for this group that the difference between the subgroups is statistically significant ($p = 0.0106$). The concentration of calcium and magnesium decreases in the presence of COPD. The decrease in calcium concentration is more pronounced for squamous cell carcinoma (-35.4%, $p = 0.0053$), while magnesium for adenocarcinoma (-23.4%, $p = 0.0658$).

For diene conjugates and Schiff bases, a pronounced minimum is observed in COPD I, and then a sharp increase in their content. For LDH, on the contrary, there is a different nature of the change in activity depending on the histological type of lung cancer. Thus, for adenocarcinoma, LDH activity decreases (−5.4% for groups NO COPD vs. COPD I; −51.7% for COPD I vs. COPD II). For squamous cell and neuroendocrine cancers, LDH activity first increases (+1.0 and +18.1%, respectively) and then decreases (−34.0 and −1.5%, respectively). Lactate levels increase for adenocarcinoma and squamous cell carcinoma (+45.8 and +85.7%, respectively) but decrease for neuroendocrine lung cancer (−52.9%). The α-amylase activity increases for adenocarcinoma and neuroendocrine cancer (+19.1 and +127.9%, respectively) but decreases for squamous cell lung cancer (−14.0%).

For a visual representation of how the indicators change while taking into account the histological type of lung cancer and the severity of COPD, diagrams of the intensity of changes are plotted in comparison with the corresponding groups without COPD (Figure 2). To plot the diagram, only those biochemical indicators of saliva were selected, the change in which is statistically significant according to the Kruskal-Wallis test (Table 3). As can be seen from Figure 2, for all indicators except LDH and α-amylase, a wide scatter of data is observed. Changes in these indicators against the background of COPD of varying severity most reliably show the differences between histological types of lung cancer.

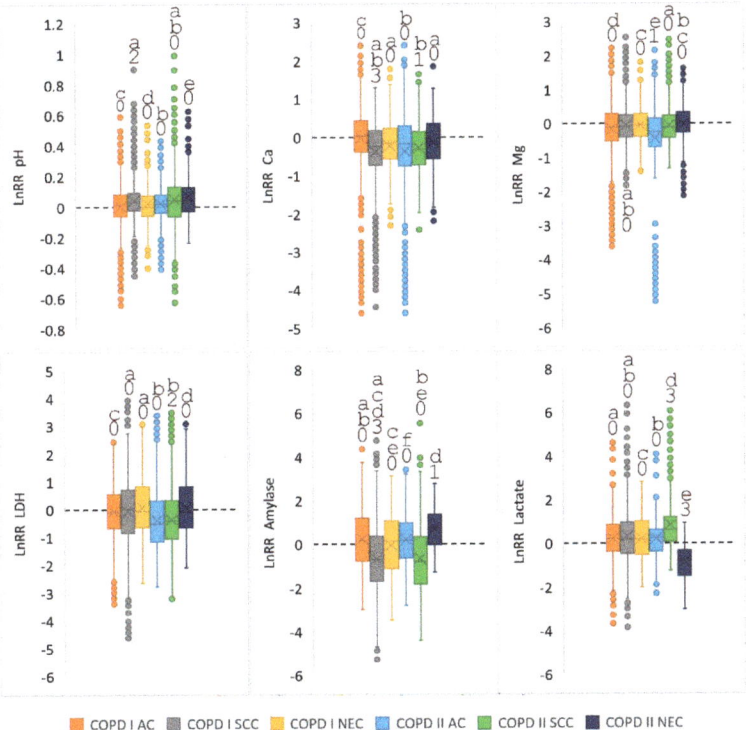

Figure 2. The intensity of the difference (LnRR = Ln (COPD/NO COPD)) in saliva biochemical parameters for different histological types of lung cancer, depending on the presence/absence of COPD. The rectangles show the mean (line) and median (cross); individual points show values outside the interquartile range. The same letters (a, b, c, d, e, f) denote groups, the differences between which were not revealed ($\alpha = 0.05$). The dotted line represents the zero level (LnRR = 0). Significance of difference from 0 was checked using the t-test of one sample and indicated by numbers ("0": not significant; "1": $p < 0.05$; "2": $p < 0.01$; "3": $p < 0.001$). AC—adenocarcinoma; SCC—squamous cell carcinoma; NEC—neuroendocrine lung cancer.

3.3. Biochemical Markers of Saliva in Patients with Lung Cancer, Noncancerous Pathologies of the Lung and Control Group Depending on the Presence/Absence of COPD

The differences between the groups with and without COPD are significant even within the group of patients with lung cancer; nevertheless, at the next stage of the study, the results obtained were compared with the control group and the comparison group. Table 4 shows the values of the indicators for each of the five groups and the corresponding value of the Kruskal-Wallis test. It was shown that the number of indicators by which the studied groups differ is significantly greater than for differences within the lung cancer group (Table 2).

The indicators, which turned out to be statistically significant according to the Kruskal-Wallis test (Table 4), were used for the analysis by the PCA method (Figure 3). It is shown that the first two dimensions of the analysis express 25.23% of the total inertia of the data set; therefore, for correct interpretation of the data, it is necessary to limit the analysis to the description of the first four axes (Figure 3).

For PC1, strong correlations were found only with protein content ($r = 0.71$), correlations of average strength with the activity of the enzymes LDH ($r = 0.64$), catalase ($r = 0.58$), GGT ($r = 0.52$) and ALP ($r = 0.42$), as well as with the content of α-amino acids ($r = 0.49$) and sialic acids ($r = 0.31$). For the other axes, high correlation coefficients were not found. For PC2, correlations of average strength were found for pH ($r = 0.52$), LDH enzymes ($r = 0.36$) and catalase ($r = 0.44$), diene conjugates ($r = 0.33$), and Schiff bases ($r = 0.43$), negative correlations were noted for protein metabolites: imidazole compounds ($r = -0.41$) and sialic acids ($r = -0.45$). For PC3, correlations of medium strength with imidazole compounds ($r = 0.51$) remain, correlations with diene conjugates ($r = 0.56$) and Schiff bases ($r = 0.46$) become more significant, and a correlation with the level of middle molecular toxins MM 280/254 ($r = 0.37$) is added. For PC4, the indicators of mineral metabolism are significant: pH ($r = 0.34$), calcium ($r = 0.41$), Ca/P-ratio ($r = 0.56$), as well as the level of α-amino acids ($r = 0.32$), diene conjugates ($r = -0.35$) and AST/ALT-ratio ($r = -0.33$).

As seen in Figure 3, the horizontal axis divides the study groups into a control group and a comparison group without COPD (above the axis), and patients with lung cancer, regardless of the presence/absence of COPD (below the axis) and a comparison group with COPD (below the axis). At the same time, the differences between the control group, the comparison group without COPD, and patients with lung cancer without COPD are less pronounced. In the diagram, these groups are located to the right of the vertical axis, while both groups of patients with COPD (lung cancer and the comparison group) are located to the left of the vertical axis (Figure 3B). The division into the listed groups provides differences in the content of protein metabolites (protein, α-amino acids, sialic acids and imidazole compounds) and enzymes (LDH, catalase, GGT, ALP and AST/ALT-ratio) in saliva. According to the severity of intoxication (indicators of lipid peroxidation and the level of medium molecular weight toxins), a control group can be distinguished both relative to the vertical and relative to the horizontal axes (Figure 3D).

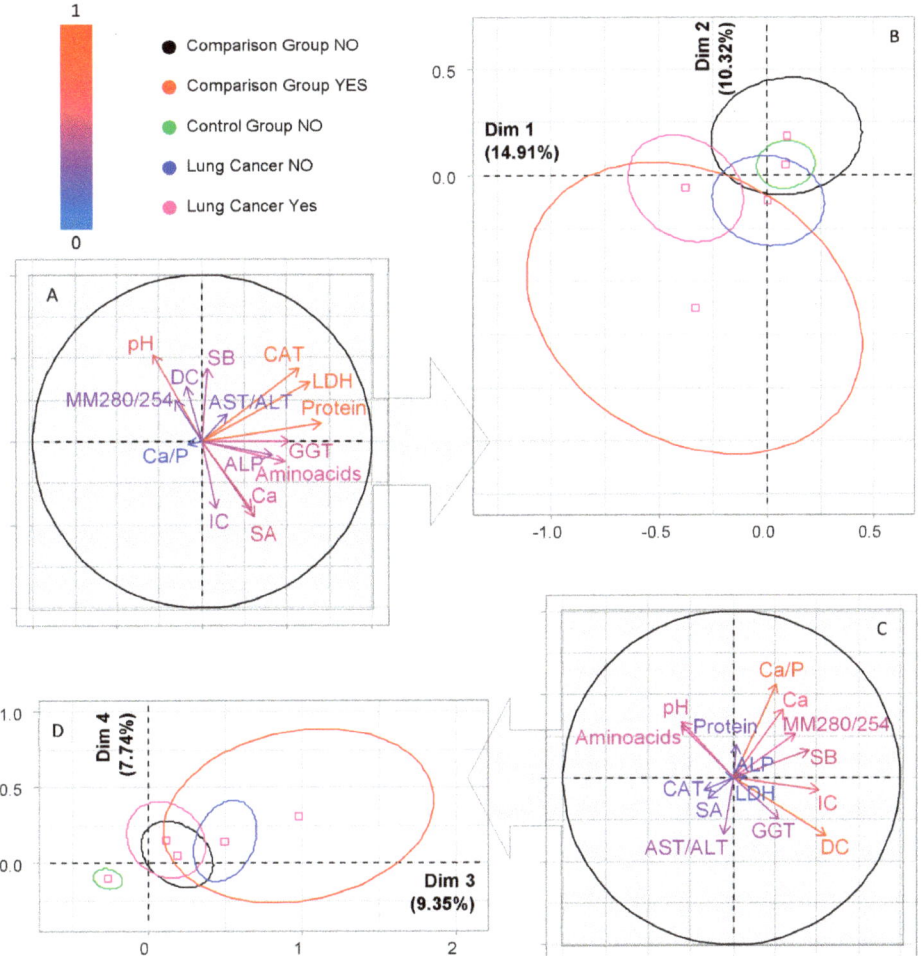

Figure 3. PCA—Factor plane (**B,D**) and the corresponding correlation circle (**A,C**) in the first four dimensions for five groups (control, lung cancer without COPD, lung cancer with COPD, comparison group without COPD, comparison group with COPD). The color of the arrows on the correlation circle changes from blue (weak correlation) to red (strong correlation), as shown on the color bar. The orientation of the arrows characterizes positive and negative correlations (for the first principal component, we analyze the location of the arrows relative to the vertical axis, for the second principal component-relative to the horizontal axis). LDH—lactate dehydrogenase; CAT—catalase; SB—Schiff bases; DC—diene conjugates; SA—sialic acids; Ca—calcium; Mg—magnesium; Ca/P—calcium to phosphorus ratio; IC—imidazole compounds; GGT—gamma glutamyltransferase; MM 280/254—middle molecular toxins; AST/ALT—aspartate aminotransferase to alanine aminotransferase ratio; ALP—alkaline phosphatase.

3.4. Predictive Value of Saliva Biochemical Parameters Taking into Account the Presence/Absence of COPD

At the first stage of the study, we compared the overall survival rates (OS) of patients with lung cancer, as well as patients with concomitant pathology: lung cancer and COPD I and II (Figure 4A,B).

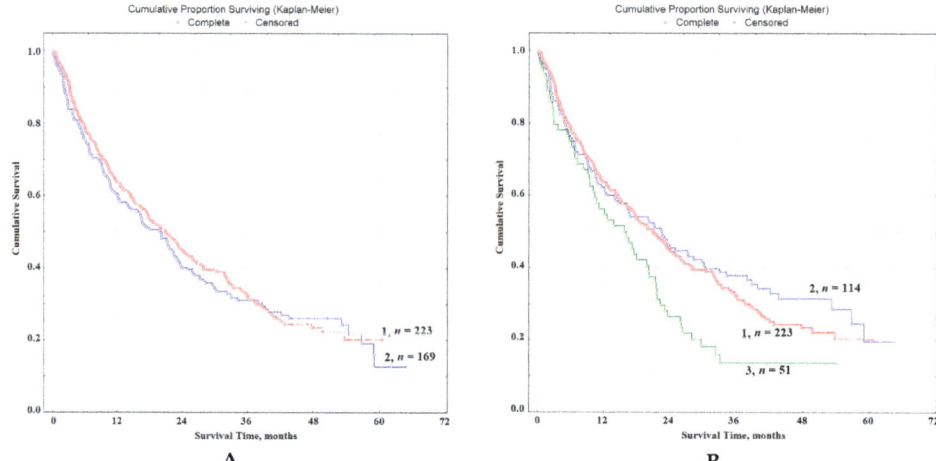

Figure 4. Overall survival of patients with lung cancer: (**A**) without COPD (curve 1) and in the presence of COPD (curve 2); (**B**) without COPD (curve 1), lung cancer with COPD I (curve 2) and lung cancer with COPD II (curve 3). n is the number of patients in each group.

It was shown that, without taking into account the severity of COPD, the differences between OS indicators are insignificant HR = 1.17, 95% CI 0.79–1.74, p = 0.34185 (Figure 4A); in the case of combined pathology, the indicators of 1-year-old (63.9 vs. 60.8%), 3-year (32.3 vs. 31.1%) and 5-year survival rates (20.2 vs. 12.6%) decrease slightly. The median OS was 18.1 and 17.4 months, respectively. Taking into account the severity of COPD, it was found that the differences between patients with only lung cancer and those with COPD I are not significantly expressed HR = 0.86, 95% CI 0.56–1.32, while the differences between the groups of patients with lung cancer and COPD II statistically significant HR = 2.52, 95% CI 1.22–5.13, p = 0.05250 (Figure 4B). Differences between groups with COPD I and COPD II are also significant; HR = 2.94, 95% CI 1.37–6.20, p = 0.03878 (Figure 4B). It was found that the 1-year survival rates for patients with lung cancer, as well as patients with a combination of lung cancer with COPD I and COPD II, were 63.9, 62.3 and 56.3%, while the 3-year survival rates were 32.3, 38 and 13.7% and 5-year-old were 20.2, 19.7 and 13.7%, respectively (Figure 4B). The median of OS for the group of patients with COPD I increased slightly and amounted to 20.5 months, while against the background of COPD II, it decreased to 16.2 months.

For groups of lung cancer patients without COPD and with COPD (COPD I, II), the prognostic value of saliva biochemical indicators was determined by the method of multivariate regression. For the group of patients with lung cancer without COPD, such indicators were the level of imidazole compounds (ICs) and the activity of salivary LDH (Figure 5A).

It has been shown that the level of ICs less than 0.478 mmol/L and the LDH activity more than 1248 U/L are prognostically favorable signs. The selected values correspond to the median for LDH and the upper value of the interquartile range for ICs (Table 2). When combining indicators ICs < 0.478 and LDH >1248, a group of patients with a favorable prognosis can be distinguished (HR = 1.56, 95% CI 0.40–6.07, p = 0.03891), for which the median of OS is 11.8 months higher than for the group with a poor prognosis (Figure 5A). The differences between the other groups are not statistically significant.

For the group of patients with COPD of varying severity, the indices were divided: for COPD I, only the ICs level is significant, while for COPD II, the LDH activity and pH are significant (Figure 5B,C). For COPD I, the prognostically favorable ICs level is less than 0.182 mmol/L (HR = 1.74, 95% CI 0.71–4.21 and HR = 1.87, 95% CI 0.65–5.28, p = 0.07270, Figure 5B), while the median of OS with a favorable prognosis reaches 34.5 months. For COPD II, pH values less than 6.74 and LDH activity less than 1006 U/L are predictively favorable. In this case, we identified a group of patients with a poor prognosis HR = 2.17, 95% CI 0.43–10.79, $p = 0.08977$ (pH > 6.74 and LDH > 1006 U/L), for which the median of OS was 7.3 months; this is 2.2 times lower than the average for the group of patients with COPD II (Figure 5C). Some groups contain a small number of patients; therefore, the differences are not statistically significant and can be considered as preliminary data requiring verification on more representative samples of patients.

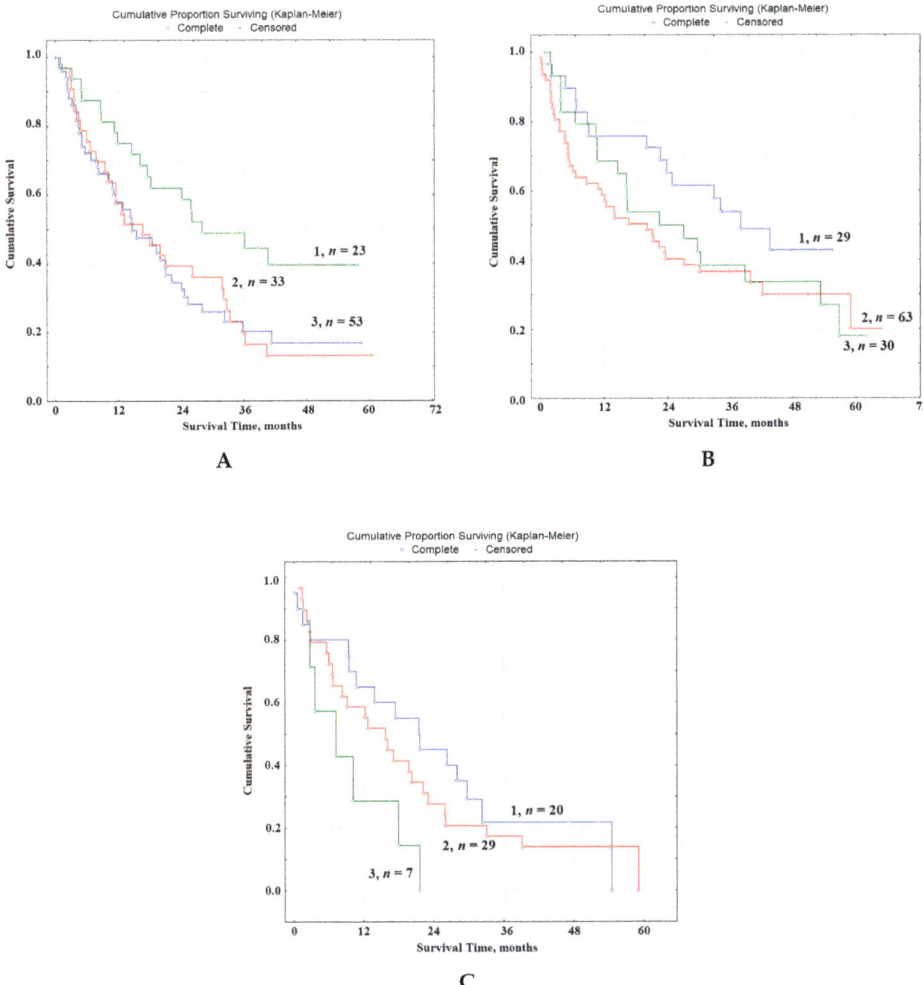

Figure 5. Multivariate regression analysis of overall survival: (**A**) ICs < 0.478 mmol/L and LDH > 1248 U/L (curve 1, favorable prognosis, median 26.3 months), ICs > 0.478 mmol/L and LDH < 1248 U/L (curve 2, poor prognosis, median 16.9 months), other combinations (curve 3, median 14.5 months); (**B**) ICs < 0.182 mmol/L (curve 1, median 34.5 months), 0.182 < ICs < 0.455 mmol/L (curve 2, median 14.3 months), ICs > 0.455 mmol/L (curve 3, median 16.7 months); (**C**) pH < 6.74 and LDH < 1006 U/L (curve 1, favorable prognosis, median 21.9 months), pH > 6.74 and LDH > 1006 U/L (curve 3, poor prognosis, median 7.3 months), other combinations (curve 2, median 16.0 months). n is the number of patients in each group.

4. Discussion

It has long been assumed that there is a link between persistent chronic inflammation and lung cancer. Complex inflammatory processes involving many types of immune cells can cause tissue damage, leading to the development of COPD and lung cancer [19]. Over the past decade, there has been an increase in interest in the identification of biomarkers, in particular in COPD [20]. Some studies have observed a reduction in the risk of lung cancer in patients using inhaled corticosteroids [21]. Consequently, the likelihood of lung cancer due to COPD is increased, especially in cases where chronic inflammation is present along with the action of carcinogenic compounds of tobacco.

We have shown that in the group of patients with lung cancer, 43.1% have COPD of varying severity as a concomitant pathology, while in the comparison group, this percentage is significantly lower than 16.1%. In accordance with the histological type of lung cancer, COPD was detected in 40.2% of patients with adenocarcinoma, 48.9% with SCC, and 39.7% with neuroendocrine lung cancer. It is known that inflammatory processes in squamous cell lung cancer are more pronounced, which may explain the higher proportion of patients with concomitant COPD. Our data, however, somewhat contradict the literature, according to which 98% of lung cancer cases in patients with COPD are non-small cell lung cancer [22]. In our case, the share of patients with COPD accounts for 84% of non-small cell lung cancer, but this may be due to the characteristics of the sample.

The saliva composition of patients with lung cancer and COPD of varying severity has its own characteristics. Thus, the most pronounced differences between the groups in terms of electrolyte balance (pH, calcium and magnesium) and enzyme activity (catalase, LDH). The same parameters remain important when considering the histological type of lung cancer. It is known that hypercalcemia is relatively common in patients with lung cancer [23,24]; however, we have shown that, against the background of combined pathology of lung cancer and COPD, the level of calcium in saliva decreases. Some studies have shown that oxidative stress, defined as an imbalance between antioxidant defenses and the production of reactive oxygen species, is exacerbated in lung cancer in combination with COPD and can cause cellular dysfunction, DNA damage, and protein and lipid peroxidation [25–28]. This fact is confirmed by the high correlation coefficients for diene conjugates and Schiff bases (Figure 1C), as well as by a decrease in the activity of the main antioxidant enzyme in saliva, catalase [29]. Sialic acids play an important role in the differentiation of the studied groups; against the background of COPD, their content significantly decreases, which is consistent with our earlier data [30]. The literature describes the use of 13 glycans for differentiating lung cancer, COPD and their comorbidity from control and lung cancer from COPD [31]. In the cited work, it was shown that changes in the subclasses of N-glycans, in particular sialylation, can carry interesting diagnostic information.

It should be noted that when taking into account the histological type of tumor, two additional parameters appear, the activity of α-amylase and the level of lactate in saliva. Earlier, we showed that the activity of salivary α-amylase significantly increases against the background of lung adenocarcinoma, which coincides with the literature data, and the level of salivary amylase is increasing [32]. For neuroendocrine lung cancer, we have shown an increase in salivary amylase activity for the first time. In this case, the revealed patterns persist against the background of COPD. Hyperlactatemia can be considered as part of the stress response, which includes an increase in metabolic rate, activation of the sympathetic nervous system, accelerated glycolysis, and modified bioenergy reserves [33]. An increase in lactate levels may also be due to a corresponding decrease in LDH activity in the presence of COPD.

Despite the differences within the lung cancer group, when trying to compare the metabolic saliva profile of this group with the control group and the comparison group, it was likely that the division of groups with COPD of different severity would not occur. Nevertheless, it has been shown that, first, groups of patients without COPD are distinguished (control group and comparison group), and indicators of protein metabolism (protein, α-amino acids, sialic acids and imidazole compounds), as well as metabolic enzymes. All this indicates significant metabolic changes that are observed in lung cancer, including in combination with COPD. Against the background of COPD, there is a more pronounced change in the content of individual components in saliva (Table 2). Thus, it has been shown that it is possible to monitor metabolic changes in lung cancer by saliva, while the presence of COPD as a concomitant disease does not radically change the metabolic profile but increases the range of changes in the corresponding biochemical parameters.

We have found that some of the studied biochemical parameters may have a prognostic value in lung cancer. Therefore, for the group of patients without COPD, these indicators include imidazole compounds and LDH, with COPD I—only imidazole compounds, with COPD II—pH and LDH. In the first two cases, groups with a favorable prognosis were identified, for which the median overall survival was significantly higher (26.3 vs. 18.1 months and 34.5 vs. 20.5 months, respectively). In the case of COPD II, we managed to identify a group with a poor prognosis: the median was 7.3 vs. 16.2 months. Such prognostic results using saliva were obtained for the first time. Earlier, a comparison was made of the mortality rate in the groups of patients with COPD and patients with combined pathology of COPD and NSCLC [34,35]. NSCLC has been shown to have a higher mortality rate in patients with mild to moderate COPD (HR = 2.62, 95% CI 1.47–4.68), while in patients with severe/very severe COPD, mortality rates in lung cancer increased insignificantly (HR = 1.22, 95% CI 0.71–2.08) [36]. In general, according to the literature, COPD is associated with a poor prognosis; for example, 3-year mortality among patients with COPD in the GOLD 4 group was 25.8% compared to 4% in the group of patients with COPD in the GOLD 1 group [37].

In our study, only four cases of severe COPD were identified, so they were not taken into account in statistical processing. We obtained data according to which the survival rates of patients with mild COPD were not only not worse but also even better than those of the group with lung cancer without COPD. One of the probable reasons is the uneven distribution of different histological types of lung cancer in groups. Thus, the group without COPD includes 50.7% adenocarcinomas, 30.9% squamous cell and 18.4% neuroendocrine cancers, while the corresponding values for COPD I group are 50.0, 35.1 and 14.9%, for COPD II group—35.3, 45.1 and 19.6%. The median survival for adenocarcinoma calculated for the study group is 23.2 months, for squamous cell carcinoma 15.2 months, for neuroendocrine carcinoma—11.1 months. Thus, HR = 1.81 (95% CI 1.10–2.95) was for SSC and HR = 2.69 (95% CI 1.23–5.77) for neuroendocrine cancer ($p < 0.00001$). Therefore, it can be assumed that the prevalence of patients with adenocarcinoma in the COPD I group improves the survival rates for this group, while in the COPD II group, the proportion of patients with squamous cell and neuroendocrine cancers with a less favorable prognosis significantly increases. It is known that associations between COPD and worse survival outcomes were stronger in squamous cell carcinoma [38]. The group of patients with COPD II accounts for the maximum proportion of cancer with central growth (42.6%), while for the COPD I group and without COPD, the corresponding values were 33.8 and 27.3%. The share of peripheral cancer was 51.5, 62.5 and 69.2% for the groups with COPD II, COPD I and without COPD. It is also one of the factors in the less favorable prognosis for lung cancer combined with COPD II. By the nature of the treatment carried out, the study groups are comparable. Complete radical treatment was performed in 22.1, 28.1, and 26.9%, combined—in 19.1, 28.8 and 28.0%, palliative—in 39.7, 32.3 and 34.8% of patients with COPD II, COPD I and without COPD. For the group of patients with COPD II, the proportion of patients who are not indicated for special treatment methods (19.1%) is higher; for the groups with COPD I and without COPD, the corresponding values were 10.8 and 10.2%. These data show that the group with lung cancer in combination with COPD I includes a larger number of patients who are indicated for radical and combined treatment, and therefore higher survival rates are quite justified. Nevertheless, we have shown that when comparing the metabolic parameters of saliva for the group of patients with lung cancer and COPD I, the values are closer to the control than those for the group of patients with lung cancer without COPD. This may be due to the formation of compensatory mechanisms in the early stages of COPD, which requires more detailed research in the course of further work.

The limitations of the study are associated with the absence of patients with severe COPD (GOLD III and GOLD IV) and with the absence of patients with COPD without other pulmonary pathologies (control group). The small sample size of patients with lung cancer and COPD II limits the possibility of dividing this group into subgroups and reduces the statistical significance of the results.

5. Conclusions

Thus, saliva adequately reflects metabolic characteristics in lung cancer, as well as lung cancer in combination with COPD of varying severity. It has been shown that the presence of COPD as a concomitant pathology does not fundamentally change the metabolic profile of saliva but increases the range of changes in the corresponding biochemical parameters. A complex of biochemical parameters of saliva, which have prognostic value in lung cancer, was revealed. It should be noted that in the presence of COPD, the list of parameters differs from that without COPD, which must be taken into account when planning treatment tactics and assessing the prognosis of lung cancer. In general, for patients with lung cancer in combination with mild COPD, the prognosis is more favorable than without COPD, which is due to compensatory mechanisms. The revealed biochemical parameters (catalase, imidazole compounds, sialic acids, LDH) can be used to monitor patients from risk groups, for example, groups of patients with initial stages of COPD, in particular for the timely diagnosis of lung cancer.

Author Contributions: Conceptualization, L.V.B. and V.K.K.; methodology, L.V.B.; validation, L.V.B., E.A.S. and D.V.S.; formal analysis, D.V.S.; investigation, L.V.B. and E.A.S.; resources, V.K.K.; data curation, D.V.S.; writing—original draft preparation, L.V.B. and D.V.S.; writing—review and editing, V.K.K.; visualization, D.V.S.; supervision, L.V.B.; project administration, V.K.K. All authors have read and agreed to the published version of the manuscript.

Funding: This research received no external funding.

Conflicts of Interest: The authors declare no conflict of interest.

References

1. Bray, F.; Ferlay, J.; Soerjomataram, I.; Siegel, R.L.; Torre, L.A.; Jemal, A. Global cancer statistics 2018: GLOBOCAN estimates of incidence and mortality worldwide for 36 cancers in 185 countries. *CA Cancer J. Clin.* **2018**, *68*, 394–424. [CrossRef] [PubMed]
2. Siegel, R.L.; Miller, K.D.; Jemal, A. Cancer statistics. *CA Cancer J. Clin.* **2019**, *69*, 7–34. [CrossRef] [PubMed]
3. Durham, A.L.; Adcock, I.M. The relationship between COPD and lung cancer. *Lung Cancer* **2015**, *90*, 121–127. [CrossRef] [PubMed]
4. López-Campos, J.L.; Tan, W.; Soriano, J.B. Global burden of COPD. *Respirology* **2016**, *21*, 14–23. [CrossRef] [PubMed]
5. Wang, Z. Association between chronic obstructive pulmonary disease and lung cancer: The missing link. *Chin. Med. J.* **2013**, *126*, 154–165. [PubMed]
6. Young, R.P.; Hopkins, R.J.; Christmas, T.; Black, P.N.; Metcalf, P.; Gamble, G.D. COPD prevalence is increased in lung cancer, independent of age, sex and smoking history. *Eur. Respir. J.* **2009**, *34*, 380–386. [CrossRef] [PubMed]
7. Mouronte-Roibás, C.; Leiro-Fernández, V.; Fernández-Villar, A.; Botana-Rial, M.; Ramos-Hernández, C.; Ruano-Ravina, A. COPD, emphysema and the onset of lung cancer. A systematic review. *Cancer Lett.* **2016**, *382*, 240–244. [CrossRef]
8. Spyratos, D.; Papadaki, E.; Lampaki, S.; Kontakiotis, T. Chronic obstructive pulmonary disease in patients with lung cancer: Prevalence, impact and management challenges. *Lung Cancer* **2017**, *8*, 101–107. [CrossRef]
9. Shvartsburd, P.M. Chronic inflammation increases the risk of developing epithelial neoplasms, inducing precancerous microenvironment: Analysis of the mechanisms of dysregulation. *Vopr. Onkol.* **2006**, *52*, 137.
10. Hodge, S.J.; Hodge, G.L.; Reynolds, P.N.; Scicchitano, R.; Holmes, M. Increased production of TGF-β and apoptosis of T lymphocytes isolated from peripheral blood in COPD. *Lung Cell Mol. Physiol.* **2003**, *285*, 492–499. [CrossRef]
11. Chen, X.; Dong, T.; Wei, X.; Yang, Z.; Pires, N.M.M.; Ren, J.; Jiang, Z. Electrochemical methods for detection of biomarkers of Chronic Obstructive Pulmonary Disease in serum and saliva. *Biosens. Bioelectron.* **2019**, *142*, 111453. [CrossRef] [PubMed]

12. Agusti, A.; Gea, J.; Faner, R. Biomarkers, the control panel and personalized COPD medicine. *Respirology* **2016**, *21*, 24–33. [CrossRef] [PubMed]
13. Eickmeier, O.; Huebner, M.; Herrmann, E.; Zissler, U.; Rosewich, M.; Baer, P.C.; Buhl, R.; Schmitt-Grohé, S.; Zielen, S.; Schubert, R. Sputum biomarker profiles in cystic fibrosis (CF) and chronic obstructive pulmonary disease (COPD) and association between pulmonary function. *Cytokine* **2010**, *50*, 152–157. [CrossRef]
14. Wang, C.; Qian, L.; Ji, L.; Liu, S.; Wahid, A.; Jiang, X.; Sohail, A.; Ji, Y.; Zhang, Y.; Wang, P.; et al. Affinity chromatography assisted comprehensive phosphoproteomics analysis of human saliva for lung cancer. *Anal. Chim. Acta* **2020**, *1111*, 103–113. [CrossRef] [PubMed]
15. Sun, Y.; Huo, C.; Qiao, Z.; Shang, Z.; Uzzaman, A.; Liu, S.; Jiang, X.; Fan, L.Y.; Ji, L.; Guan, X.; et al. Comparative proteomic analysis of exosomes and microvesicles in human saliva for lung cancer. *J. Proteome Res.* **2018**, *17*, 1101–1107. [CrossRef]
16. Bel'skaya, L.V.; Sarf, E.A.; Kosenok, V.K.; Gundyrev, I.A. Biochemical Markers of Saliva in Lung Cancer: Diagnostic and Prognostic Perspectives. *Diagnostics* **2020**, *10*, 186. [CrossRef]
17. Vestbo, J.; Hurd, S.S.; Agusti, A.G.; Jones, P.W.; Vogelmeier, C.; Anzueto, A.; Barnes, P.J.; Fabbri, L.M.; Martinez, F.J.; Nishimura, M.; et al. Global strategy for the diagnosis, management, and prevention of chronic obstructive pulmonary disease: GOLD executive summary. *Am. J. Respir. Crit. Care Med.* **2013**, *187*, 347–365. [CrossRef]
18. Lê, S.; Josse, J.; Husson, F. FactoMineR: An R Package for Multivariate Analysis. *J. Stat. Softw.* **2008**, *25*, 1–18. [CrossRef]
19. Negrini, S.; Gorgoulis, V.G.; Halazonetis, T.D. Genomic instability—An evolving hallmark of cancer. *Nat. Rev. Mol. Cell Biol.* **2010**, *11*, 220–228. [CrossRef]
20. Agusti, A.; Sin, D.D. Biomarkers in COPD. *Clin. Chest Med.* **2014**, *35*, 131–141. [CrossRef]
21. Parimon, T.; Chien, J.W.; Bryson, C.L.; McDonell, M.B.; Udris, E.M.; Au, D.H. Inhaled corticosteroids and risk of lung cancer among patients with chronic obstructive pulmonary disease. *Am. J. Respir. Crit. Care Med.* **2007**, *175*, 712–719. [CrossRef] [PubMed]
22. Hohberger, L.A.; Schroeder, D.R.; Bartholmai, B.J.; Yang, P.; Wendt, C.H.; Bitterman, P.B. Correlation of regional emphysema and lung cancer: A lung tissue research consortium-based study. *J. Thorac. Oncol.* **2014**, *9*, 639–645. [CrossRef] [PubMed]
23. Hiraki, A.; Ueoka, H.; Takata, I.; Gemba, K.; Bessho, A.; Segawa, Y.; Kiura, K.; Eguchi, K.; Yoneda, T.; Tanimoto, M.; et al. Hypercalcemia—Leukocytosis syndrome associated with lung cancer. *Lung Cancer* **2004**, *43*, 301–307. [CrossRef] [PubMed]
24. Hiraki, A.; Ueoka, H.; Bessho, A.; Segawa, Y.; Takigawa, N.; Kiura, K. Parathyroid hormone-related protein measured at first visit is an indicator for bone metastases and survival in lung cancer patients with hypercalcemia. *Cancer* **2002**, *95*, 1706–1712. [CrossRef] [PubMed]
25. Reuter, S.; Gupta, S.C.; Chaturvedi, M.M.; Aggarwal, B.B. Oxidative stress, inflammation, and cancer: How are they linked? *Free Radical Biol. Med.* **2010**, *49*, 1603–1616. [CrossRef]
26. Gęgotek, A.; Nikliński, J.; Žarković, N.; Žarković, K.; Waeg, G.; Łuczaj, W.; Charkiewicz, R.; Skrzydlewska, E. Lipid mediators involved in the oxidative stress and antioxidant defense of human lung cancer cells. *Redox Biol.* **2016**, *9*, 210–219. [CrossRef]
27. Barreiro, E.; Fermoselle, C.; Mateu-Jimenez, M.; Sánchez-Font, A.; Pijuan, L.; Gea, J.; Curull, V. Oxidative stress and inflammation in the normal airways and blood of patients with lung cancer and CORD. *Free Radical Biol. Med.* **2013**, *65*, 859–871. [CrossRef]
28. Yigla, M.; Berkovich, Y.; Nagler, R.M. Oxidative stress indices in COPD—Broncho-alveolar lavage and salivary analysis. *Arch. Oral Biol.* **2007**, *52*, 36–43. [CrossRef]
29. Pastor, M.D.; Nogal, A.; Molina-Pinelo, S.; Meléndez, R.; Salinas, A.; González De la Peña, M.; Martín-Juan, J.; Corral, J.; García-Carbonero, R.; Carnero, A.; et al. Identification of proteomic signatures associated with lung cancer and COPD. *J. Proteom.* **2013**, *89*, 227–237. [CrossRef]
30. Bel'skaya, L.V.; Kosenok, V.K. The level of sialic acids and imidazole compounds in the saliva of patients with lung cancer of different histological types. *Sib. J. Oncol.* **2018**, *17*, 84–91. [CrossRef]
31. Mészáros, B.; Járvás, G.; Farkas, A.; Szigeti, M.; Kovács, Z.; Kun, R.; Szabó, M.; Csánky, E.; Guttman, A. Comparative analysis of the human serum N-glycome in lung cancer, COPD and their comorbidity using capillary electrophoresis. *J. Chromatogr. B* **2020**, *1137*, 121913. [CrossRef] [PubMed]

32. Bel'skaya, L.V.; Kosenok, V.K. The activity of metabolic enzymes in the saliva of lung cancer patients. *Natl. J. Physiol. Pharm. Pharmacol.* **2017**, *7*, 646–653. [CrossRef]
33. Adamo, L.; Nassif, M.E.; Novak, E.; LaRue, S.J.; Mann, D.L. Prevalence of lactic acidaemia in patients with advanced heart failure and depressed cardiac output. *Eur. J. Heart Fail.* **2017**, *19*, 1027–1033. [CrossRef]
34. Wheatley-Price, P.; Blackhall, F.; Lee, S.M.; Ma, C.; Ashcroft, L.; Jitlal, M.; Qian, W.; Hackshaw, A.; Rudd, R.; Booton, R.; et al. The influence of sex and histology on outcomes in non-small-cell lung cancer: A pooled analysis of five randomized trials. *Ann. Oncol.* **2010**, *21*, 2023–2028. [CrossRef] [PubMed]
35. Sereno, M.; Esteban, I.R.; Zambrana, F.; Merino, M.; Gómez-Raposo, C.; López-Gómez, M.; Sáenz, F.C. Squamous-cell carcinoma of the lungs: Is it really so different? *Crit. Rev. Oncol./Hematol.* **2012**, *84*, 327–339. [CrossRef] [PubMed]
36. Jeppesen, S.S.; Hansen, N.G.; Schytte, T.; Nielsenc, M.; Hansen, O. Comparison of survival of chronic obstructive pulmonary disease patients with or without a localized non-small cell lung cancer. *Lung Cancer* **2016**, *100*, 90–95. [CrossRef]
37. Lange, P.; Marott, J.L.; Vestbo, J.; Olsen, K.R.; Ingebrigtsen, T.S.; Dahl, M.; Nordestgaard, B.G. Prediction of the clinical course of chronic obstructive pulmonary disease, using the new GOLD classification: A study of the general population. *Am. J. Respir. Crit. Care Med.* **2012**, *186*, 975–981. [CrossRef]
38. Zhai, R.; Yu, X.; Shafer, A.; Wain, J.C.; Christiani, D.C. The impact of coexisting COPD on survival of patients with early-stage non-small cell lung cancer undergoing surgical resection. *Chest* **2014**, *14*, 346–353. [CrossRef]

Publisher's Note: MDPI stays neutral with regard to jurisdictional claims in published maps and institutional affiliations.

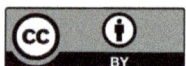

© 2020 by the authors. Licensee MDPI, Basel, Switzerland. This article is an open access article distributed under the terms and conditions of the Creative Commons Attribution (CC BY) license (http://creativecommons.org/licenses/by/4.0/).

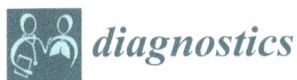

Article

Participation of *HHIP* Gene Variants in COPD Susceptibility, Lung Function, and Serum and Sputum Protein Levels in Women Exposed to Biomass-Burning Smoke

Alejandro Ortega-Martínez [1,2], Gloria Pérez-Rubio [1], Alejandra Ramírez-Venegas [3], María Elena Ramírez-Díaz [4], Filiberto Cruz-Vicente [5], María de Lourdes Martínez-Gómez [6], Espiridión Ramos-Martínez [7], Edgar Abarca-Rojano [2,*] and Ramcés Falfán-Valencia [1,*]

[1] HLA Laboratory, Instituto Nacional de Enfermedades Respiratorias Ismael Cosío Villegas, Mexico City 14080, Mexico; alex_om_scv@outlook.com (A.O.-M.); glofos@yahoo.com.mx (G.P.-R.)
[2] Sección de Estudios de Posgrado e Investigación. Escuela Superior de Medicina, Instituto Politécnico Nacional, Plan de San Luis y Díaz Mirón s/n, Casco de Santo Tomas, Mexico City 11340, Mexico
[3] Tobacco Smoking and COPD Research Department, Instituto Nacional de Enfermedades Respiratorias Ismael Cosío Villegas, Mexico City 14080, Mexico; aleravas@hotmail.com
[4] Coordinación de Vigilancia Epidemiológica, Jurisdicción 06 Sierra, Tlacolula de Matamoros Oaxaca, Servicios de Salud de Oaxaca, Oaxaca 70400, Mexico; drmariel2504@hotmail.com
[5] Internal Medicine Department. Hospital Civil Aurelio Valdivieso, Servicios de Salud de Oaxaca, Oaxaca 68050, Mexico; filitv6cv@hotmail.com
[6] Hospital Regional de Alta Especialidad de Oaxaca, Oaxaca 71256, Mexico; ane-margo68@hotmail.com
[7] Experimental Medicine Research Unit, Facultad de Medicina, Universidad Nacional Autónoma de México, Mexico City 06720, Mexico; espiri77mx@yahoo.com
* Correspondence: rojanoe@yahoo.com (E.A.-R.); rfalfanv@iner.gob.mx (R.F.-V.); Tel.: +52-55-5729-6000 (ext. 62718) (E.A.-R.); +52-55-5487-1700 (ext. 5152) (R.F.-V.)

Received: 6 August 2020; Accepted: 16 September 2020; Published: 23 September 2020

Abstract: Background: A variety of organic materials (biomass) are burned for cooking and heating purposes in poorly ventilated houses; smoke from biomass combustion is considered an environmental risk factor for chronic obstructive pulmonary disease COPD. In this study, we attempted to determine the participation of single-nucleotide variants in the *HHIP* (hedgehog-interacting protein) gene in lung function, HHIP serum levels, and HHIP sputum supernatant levels in Mexican women with and without COPD who were exposed to biomass-burning smoke. Methods: In a case-control study (COPD-BS, n = 186, BBES, n = 557) in Mexican women, three SNPs (rs13147758, rs1828591, and rs13118928) in the *HHIP* gene were analyzed by qPCR; serum and supernatant sputum protein levels were determined through ELISA. Results: The rs13118928 GG genotype is associated with decreased risk (p = 0.021, OR = 0.51, CI95% = 0.27–0.97) and the recessive genetic model (p = 0.0023); the rs1828591-rs13118928 GG haplotype is also associated with decreased risk (p = 0.04, OR = 0.65, CI95% 0.43–0.98). By the dominant model (rs13118928), the subjects with one or two copies of the minor allele (G) exhibited higher protein levels. Additionally, two correlations with the AG genotype were identified: BBES with FEV_1 (p = 0.03, r^2 = 0.53) and COPD-BS with FEV_1/FVC (p = 0.012, r^2 = 0.54). Conclusions: Single-nucleotide variants in the *HHIP* gene are associated with decreased COPD risk, higher HHIP serum levels, and better lung function in Mexican women exposed to biomass burning.

Keywords: COPD; biomass-burning; *HHIP*; sputum supernatant; lung function; indoor pollution

1. Introduction

Chronic obstructive pulmonary disease (COPD) is a common and tractable pathology characterized by persistent respiratory symptoms and limited airflow; these symptoms are commonly caused by significant exposure to noxious particles or gases [1]. Smoking tobacco is the principal risk factor associated with the development of COPD [2]. However, a range of organic materials (such as coal, animal dung, agricultural waste, and wood) are utilized for cooking and heating purposes in poorly ventilated houses [3], leading to chronic exposure to smoke from biomass burning. A study conducted in suburban areas near Mexico City observed that nearly 47% of women employ any biomass source for cooking and detected a COPD prevalence of 3% [4]; previously, the PLATINO study reported a COPD prevalence of 7.8% in Mexico City [5].

COPD is classified as a multifactorial disease, which means that in addition to the environmental factors strongly associated with the physiopathology of the disease, genetic factors, mostly single nucleotide polymorphisms (SNPs), have also been determined to contribute to the susceptibility and clinical variables of COPD [6]. In 2009, through genome-wide association studies (GWAS), several SNPs in the *HHIP* (hedgehog-interacting protein) gene were identified [7]; however, in this initial study, the results did not reach strict levels of significance. Finally, Wilk et al., in a GWAS, found polymorphisms in *HHIP* associated with a decrease in forced expiratory volume in the first second (FEV_1) in the general population of the Framingham Heart Study cohort [8].

The hedgehog pathway is the signaling route in which the HHIP protein participates, and this pathway is highly conserved from an evolutionary perspective. The hedgehog signaling cascade plays an essential role in embryonic processes in vertebrates, including tooth and lung development and hair follicle anatomical structures [9]. The gene encoding the *HHIP* protein has the same name, HHIP [10], comprises 13 exons, covers approximately 91 kb, encodes a 700 amino acid protein, and is located in the 4q31.21–q31.3.9 gene region [11].

In this study, we attempted to determine the participation of single-nucleotide variants in the *HHIP* gene in lung function, HHIP serum levels, and HHIP sputum supernatant levels in Mexican women with and without COPD who were exposed to biomass-burning smoke.

2. Materials and Methods

2.1. Case and Control Groups

Seven hundred and forty-three Mexican women were included in a case-control study. These subjects attended the COPD clinic, which is part of the Department of Smoking and COPD Research of the Instituto Nacional de Enfermedades Respiratorias Ismael Cosio Villegas (INER), Mexico.

Applying diagnostic criteria according to the Global Initiative for Chronic Obstructive Lung Disease (GOLD) recommendations [12] and considering the symptoms and the deterioration of the patient's health status, a team of pulmonary specialists completed the clinical evaluation. The diagnosis was confirmed using lung function tests (by post-bronchodilator spirometry), considering a ratio of forced expiratory volume in the first second/forced vital capacity (FEV_1/FVC) < 70% to be proof of COPD according to the reference values for Mexicans reported by Perez-Padilla et al. [13].

Women who employed firewood as an organic fuel source (biomass) for indoor cooking, were older than 40 years, were directly exposed to biomass-burning smoke, had an accumulated biomass-burning smoke exposure index (BBEI, calculated as the average number of hours spent cooking daily per the total number of years exposed) higher than 100 h/year for biomass smoke, exhibited FEV_1/FVC < 70%, were never smokers and were never exposed to second-hand tobacco smoke or other fumes or gases associated with COPD development were classified into the COPD-BS ($n = 186$) group.

All included patients were clinically stable, were not utilizing supplementary oxygen at the enrollment time, did not have a history of previous exacerbations, and had not been administered antibiotics or systemic corticosteroid treatments for at least three months. Consecutive COPD patients were enrolled from the COPD support clinic from 2015 to 2019. Additionally, GOLD stages I and II were grouped as G1, while stages III and IV were grouped as G2.

The control group consisted of participants who had been exposed to biomass-burning smoke (BBES, n = 557) and did not have COPD, including those with normal spirometry parameters ($FEV_1/FVC \geq 70\%$) and without a history of active or passive smoking or non-COPD respiratory or chronic inflammatory diseases.

All participants were part of the national program to achieve equality between women and men through the Early Diagnosis/Breath Without Smoke campaigns for women living in rural areas, primarily in the northern highlands of the state of Oaxaca and suburban areas of the Tlalpan mayoralty of Mexico City.

All participants fulfilled a family questionnaire regarding inherited pathologies, by which participants who reported suffering some pulmonary or chronic inflammatory disease were excluded, as well as those with ancestry different from Mexican (that is, with no Mexican-by-birth parents and grandparents). Participants had no biological relations among themselves or with the subjects in the corresponding comparison group, and they had no history of family pulmonary diseases.

2.2. Ethics Approval and Informed Consent

This study was reviewed and accepted by the Institutional Committees for Investigation, Ethics in Research, and Biosecurity of the Instituto Nacional de Enfermedades Respiratorias Ismael Cosío Villegas (INER) (approbation number: B11–19). All participants were informed of the protocol's aims after being given a detailed description of the study and being invited to participate as volunteers. All of the participants signed an informed consent paper and were supplied with a privacy statement describing the legal protection of personal data; both documents were approved (14 May 2019) by the Institutional Research and Ethics in Research Committees. All analyses were conducted following the relevant guidelines and regulations. The STREGA (STrengthening the REporting of Genetic Association) [14] recommendations were taken into consideration in the design of this genetic association study.

2.3. Blood Sample Processing and DNA Extraction

The sample processing began with a whole-blood 15 mL blood sample obtained by venipuncture and collected in two EDTA tubes (S-Monovette 4.9 mL K3E, Sarstedt, Nümbrecht, Germany) and another tube for obtaining serum (S-Monovette 4.9 mL Z-Gel, Sarstedt, Nümbrecht, Germany), and subsequent centrifugation was employed for 5 min at 4500 rpm to separate the peripheral blood mononuclear cells (PBMCs) and serum. Samples were stored in cryopreservation tubes at −80 °C until use.

2.4. Sputum Induction and Sample Preparation

Based on genotype analysis, we selected a subsample of participants for more in-depth characterization. To obtain sputum, we followed a previously published protocol [15]; briefly, participants were treated with a nebulizer with a sterile 7% saline solution. Treatment lasted for 5 min followed by a rest period of 5 min. Treatment and rest cycles were repeated three times.

The sample was mechanically disaggregated using 1X PBS buffer (Invitrogen; Carlsbad, CA, USA) in equal volumes to eliminate excess mucus followed by centrifugation at 4500 rpm for 10 min, and the saliva was extracted. Then, 10 mL of sterile 0.9% saline solution was added, and the sample was centrifuged again at 4500 rpm for 10 min, and the supernatant was separated into 1.8 mL aliquots. These aliquots were concentrated using a SpeedVac Concentrator (Thermo Fisher Scientific, Asheville, NC, USA) at 14,000 rpm for 12 h, resuspended in 1 mL of 1X PBS and stored at −80 °C until use.

2.5. SNP Selection

SNPs were selected based on a bibliographic search in the National Center for Biotechnology Information (NCBI) database, identifying polymorphisms previously associated with COPD in different GWAS analyses and having been positively replicated in at least two other populations. Additionally, we considered a minor allele frequency (MAF) higher than 5% in the Mexican population in Los Angeles according to the 1000 Genomes Project [16]. Supplementary Table S4 shows all selected SNPs.

2.6. SNP Genotyping

The allele discrimination of SNP variants was performed using commercial TaqMan probes (Applied Biosystems, Foster City, CA, USA) at a 20X concentration. We selected three SNPs: rs13118928 (commercial probe id: C__11375931_20), rs1828591 (C__11482211_10), and rs13147758 (C___2965080_10). These SNPs are located in intronic (noncoding) regions. Supplementary Table S4 summarizes the principal characteristics of the assessed SNPs.

Genotyping was evaluated by applying real-time PCR (qPCR) in a StepOne Real-Time PCR System (Applied Biosystems/Thermo Fisher Scientific Inc., Singapore), and genotype assignment was performed by sequence detection software (SDS) version 2.3 (Applied Biosystems, Foster City, CA, USA).

2.7. Serum and Sputum HHIP Protein Level Measurement

The determination of protein levels in serum (n = 80) and sputum supernatant samples (n = 40) was performed by a commercial ELISA kit (cat. E-EL-H0888. Elabscience, Houston, TX, USA) according to the manufacturer's specifications. The micro ELISA plate was precoated with a human HHIP-specific antibody (detection range: 0.31 – 20 ng/mL, sensitivity: 0.19 ng/mL), and the assays were performed in duplicate on the same plate.

2.8. Statistical Assessment

The demographics, clinical characteristics, pulmonary function data, protein levels, and correlations were described using SPSS v.24.0 (IBM, New York, USA). The median, minimum, and maximum values for each continuous quantitative variable were determined.

Hardy-Weinberg equilibrium (HWE) was calculated before performing genotype analysis using PLINK software v1.9 [17], and De Finetti diagrams were constructed with Finetti software v.3.0.8 [18]. The analysis of the genetic association between groups was evaluated by comparing allele and genotype frequencies through Pearson's chi-square test and Fisher's exact test using Epi Info v. 7.1.4.0 [19], Epidat statistical software version 3.1 [20], and the haplotype analysis was performed with Haploview v4.2 [21] and R version 3.6.2 (12 December 2019).

The results were considered to be significant when the p-value was <0.05; similarly, the odds ratio (OR) with 95% confidence intervals (CI) was estimated to determine the strength of the association. To adjust for potential confounding variables, a logistic regression analysis was performed using Plink v. 1.09. [17] (1 degree of freedom), including age, body mass index, and biomass-burning smoke exposure index as covariables.

Analysis of the HHIP protein levels in serum and sputum supernatant was performed with R version 3.6.2 (12 December 2019), applying the Kolmogorov–Smirnov test, the Mann–Whitney U test for two group comparisons, the Kruskal–Wallis test for three or more comparisons, and Pearson's r^2 value for correlations among protein levels and lung function.

2.9. Drugs' Metabolism in Silico Analysis for COPD and Its Interaction with HHIP

To evaluate the probable effects of pharmacological treatment on HHIP protein levels, a in silico analysis was carried out; First-line drugs were documented from clinical records, identifying the targets, carriers, enzymes, and transporters participating in the drugs' metabolism for the COPD treatment, using the DRUGBANK v.5.1.7 database [22], released 2 July 2020. The identified proteins were used for the interaction analysis, and HHIP was added in the STRING software v11.0 [23].

3. Results

3.1. Demographic and Clinical Characteristics

The clinical and demographic characteristics of the patients are outlined in Table 1. The median age in the group of women with COPD was 73 years, while biomass-burning smoke-exposed subjects (BBES) were younger by approximately ten years. The COPD group presented a lower body mass index (26.4) than the control group (27.8); this difference was determined to be significant.

Regarding the biomass-smoke exposure index (BSEI), the COPD group was exposed approximately 100 h more than the control group. As expected, the pulmonary function tests in the COPD group were lower than those in the control group. Regarding the distribution by degrees of GOLD severity, >80% of the participants were GOLD I and II.

Table 1. Demographic, clinical, exposure and lung function of participants exposed to biomass-burning smoke.

Variables	COPD-BS (n = 186)	BBES (n = 557)	p
Age (Years)	73 (47–93)	62 (45–98)	<0.001
BMI	26.47 (17.81–45.04)	27.83 (15.67–56.25)	0.020
Years of exposure to smoke biomass-burning	50 (10–80)	43 (10–87)	0.005
Hours/day exposure	8 (2–24)	7 (2–24)	0.003
BBEI	320 (108–1116)	240 (105–1050)	<0.001
Lung function post-bronchodilator			
FEV$_1$ (%)	64 (18–119)	98 (55–187)	<0.001
FVC (%)	83 (35–146)	94 (53–193)	<0.001
FEV$_1$/FVC (%)	58 (21.53–69.7)	83 (70–138)	<0.001
GOLD			
GOLD I (%)	46 (24.7)	NA	-
GOLD II (%)	103 (55.4)	NA	-
GOLD III (%)	27 (14.5)	NA	-
GOLD IV (%)	10 (5.4)	NA	-

COPD-BS: chronic obstructive pulmonary disease (COPD) related to biomass-burning exposure; BBES: biomass-burning smoke-exposed subjects. $p < 0.05$ statistical significance; BMI: body mass index; BBEI: biomass-burning smoke exposure index; FEV$_1$: forced expiratory volume in the first second; FVC: forced vital capacity; NA: not applicable. The median and minimum and maximum values are shown.

3.2. Hardy-Weinberg Equilibrium and Genotype Frequencies and Genetic Susceptibility

The three SNPs that were evaluated comply with the HWE: rs13118928 ($p = 0.23$), rs1828591 ($p = 0.16$), and rs13147758 ($p = 0.40$).

The DNA samples of 743 women with and without COPD who were exposed to biomass-burning smoke were genotyped, and three SNPs (rs13147759, rs1828591, and rs13118928) were evaluated. The relationship between cases and controls is 1 case for 2.99 controls; therefore, the statistical power of our study is 90% using the following parameters: an OR = 2, a ratio of controls to case 3:1, a MAF = 15%, and a confidence interval of 95%.

Table 2 shows the results of the genotype frequencies; in the three polymorphisms, the AA genotype was determined to be the most common genotype, and the GG genotype was the least frequently observed genotype. Interestingly, the heterozygous genotypes in both groups occurred in more than 40% of our study population.

The GG homozygous genotype of rs13118928 shows a decreased risk of developing the disease ($p = 0.038$), and the statistical test used was the χ^2 test. The analyses with the rs13147758 and rs1828591 polymorphisms did not demonstrate significant differences.

Furthermore, all significant results were adjusted for possible confounding variables (age, BMI, and BSEI) through a logistic regression model, where the rs13118928 GG genotype maintained its association with decreased risk (adjusted $p = 0.021$, OR = 0.51, 95% CI 0.27–0.97).

Table 2. Genotype frequencies among study groups.

Genotype	COPD-BS		BBES		p	OR	CI 95%	* p
	n = 186	%	n = 557	%				
rs13147758								
AA	87	46.78	243	43.63	0.49	0.13	0.89–1.28	
AG	80	43.01	243	43.63	0.93	0.97	0.69–1.36	
GG	19	10.21	71	12.74	0.43	0.80	0.49–1.29	0.42
rs1828591								
AA	90	48.38	257	46.16	0.61	1.09	0.78–1.52	
AG	77	41.41	232	41.64	1	0.98	0.70–1.38	
GG	19	10.21	68	12.20	0.51	0.81	0.47–1.40	0.13
rs13118928								
AA	88	47.32	258	46.32	0.86	1.04	0.74–1.45	
AG	86	46.23	233	41.83	0.30	1.19	0.85–1.66	
GG	12	6.45	66	11.85	0.038	0.51	0.27–0.97	0.021

COPD-BS: COPD related to biomass-burning exposure; BBES: exposed to biomass-burning smoke. $p < 0.05$ statistical significance; * p-value adjusted by age, BMI, and BBEI. Associations are shown in the full genotype model.

3.3. Genetic Models

The three polymorphisms were analyzed by the codominant and recessive genetic association models; as observed in Table 3, rs13118928, which showed a decreased risk of disease susceptibility in the genotype frequencies, maintained this result with the GG genotype in the recessive model ($p = 0.038$, adjusted $p = 0.0023$ OR = 0.51, 95% CI = 0.27–0.97). The OR and the confidence interval were maintained in both analyses, and the p-value was strengthened after the logistic regression analysis, demonstrating that minor allele homozygous carriers have a decreased COPD risk.

Table 3. Analysis by genetic models of rs13118928 in exposed to biomass-burning smoke with and without COPD.

Model/Genotype	COPD-BS		BBES		p	OR	CI 95%	* p
	n = 186	%	n = 557	%				
Codominant								
AA	88	47.32	258	46.32		1 (ref.)		
AG	86	46.23	233	41.83	0.25	1.08	0.76–1.52	0.36
GG	12	6.45	66	11.85		0.53	0.27–1.03	
Recessive								
GG	12	6.45	66	11.85	0.038	0.51	0.27–0.97	0.0023
AA + AG	174	93.55	491	88.15		1.94	1.02–3.69	

COPD-BS: COPD related to biomass-burning exposure; BBES: biomass-burning smoke-exposed subjects. $p < 0.05$ statistical significance; * p-value adjusted by age, BMI, and BBEI.

3.4. Haplotypes

Supplementary Figure S1 presents the haplotypes identified in the rs13147758 and rs1828591 polymorphisms. Four haplotypes were formed, with two showing significant trends: AA ($p = 0.07$, OR = 1.25, 95% CI = 0.98–1.60) and AG ($p = 0.06$, OR = 0.53, 95% CI = 0.27–1.02). Figure 1 shows the haplotypes formed by rs1828591 and rs13118928 ($r^2 = 0.54$); the haplotype formed by both minor alleles (G) presented a decreased risk of disease ($p = 0.04$, OR = 0.65, CI95% = 0.43–0.98). In the analysis examining the three SNPs, no haplotypes were determined to be associated.

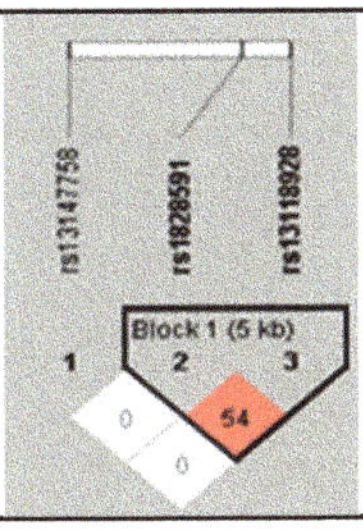

Haplotypes	COPD-BS	BBES	p	OR	CI 95%
AA	178	517	0.63	1.05	0.83–1.34
AG	84	232	0.46	1.10	0.83–1.47
GA	79	229	0.76	1.03	0.83–1.27
GG	**31**	**136**	**0.04**	**0.65**	**0.43–0.98**

Figure 1. Haplotypes of rs1828591 and rs13118928 in the *HHIP* gene. COPD-BS: COPD related to biomass-burning exposure; BBES: Biomass-burning smoke-exposed subjects: $p < 0.05$ demonstrates significance; OR: odds ratio; CI 95%: 95% confidence interval; showing r^2 values among SNPs.

3.5. Severity in COPD and Genetic Analysis

All COPD patients were clustered according to the degree of disease severity following the GOLD guidelines. Patients in GOLD grades I and II were grouped as G1 ($n = 149$), and those in the disease stages GOLD III and IV were grouped as G2 ($n = 37$). No significant differences were found in any of the 3 SNPs after comparing the genotype frequencies between these two groups. These results are shown in Supplementary Table S1.

3.6. HHIP Serum Levels

The serum HHIP protein levels were determined through ELISA assays in 80 randomly selected women exposed to burning biomass smoke (COPD-BS = 40 and BBES = 40) (Supplementary Table S2); these subgroups were derived from the main groups. COPD patients had a median age of 71.5 years, while in women without the disease, the mean age was 64 years ($p = 0.003$); for this reason, age, and BMI, were employed as a covariables to adjust.

3.6.1. HHIP Serum Level Comparison

This analysis was performed by comparing HHIP serum protein levels between both groups, regardless of polymorphism; however, this comparison was not significant ($p = 0.62$) (Figure 2).

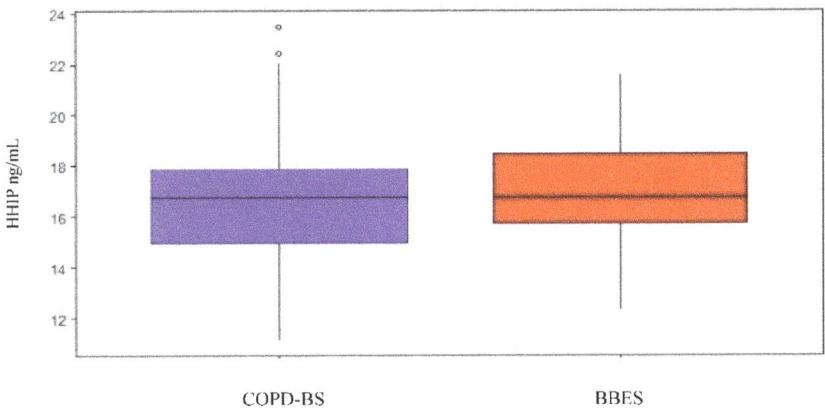

Figure 2. Comparison of protein HHIP in serum levels among COPD-BS vs. BBES.

The comparison between cases and controls depending on the polymorphism showed significant differences with the SNPs rs13147758 (AA; $p = 0.021$) and rs1828591 (AA; $p = 0.023$); however, after the logistic regression analysis, these associations were not significant. A similar result was observed in the intra-case analysis, as rs13147758 showed a difference between cases and controls with the AA genotype ($p = 0.021$), and after adjustment for covariates, it changed to $p = 0.28$. The effect same occurred with rs1828591 ($p = 0.046$, after adjustment, $p = 0.053$). In this analysis, rs13118928 did not present any significant difference before adjustment for covariates.

3.6.2. Analysis of Serum Protein Levels by Applying Genetic Models

The analysis of genetic association models was performed using the dominant and recessive models, comparing protein levels in both groups.

Among individuals exposed to biomass-burning smoke without the disease (BBES), the dominant model (AA vs. AG + GG) of rs13118928 showed that individuals who carry one or two copies of the minor allele (G) have higher protein levels compared with individuals who are homozygous for the common allele (A) ($p = 0.005$, and after adjustment, $p = 0.04$). However, in the COPD-BS group, significant differences were not observed (Figure 3).

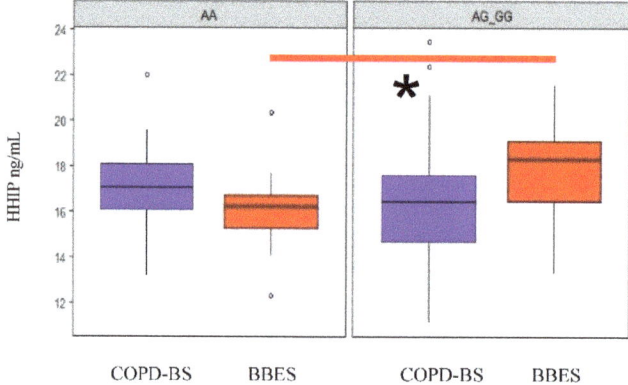

Figure 3. Levels of HHIP protein in serum by the dominant model of rs13118928. * The statistical difference between BBES with AA vs. AG+GG ($p < 0.05$).

3.6.3. Correlations of Serum Protein Levels in COPD-BS and BBES with Lung Function

The rs1828591 showed a positive correlation among heterozygosity (AG) and the FEV_1/FVC ratio in the COPD-BS group ($p = 0.01$, r2 = 0.56), and after logistic regression analysis, this value remained significant ($p = 0.02$, $r^2 = 0.52$) (Figure 4A).

Two positive correlations were observed in rs13118928: the first in the BBES group with the AG genotype and FEV_1 ($p = 0.04$, $r^2 = 0.50$; after the analysis by covariates, $p = 0.03$, $r^2 = 0.53$). In addition, in the COPD-BS group, the heterozygous (AG) genotype showed a positive correlation with FEV_1/FVC ($p = 0.006$, $r^2 = 0.56$ and adjusted values $p = 0.012$ and $r^2 = 0.54$) (Figure 4B,C).

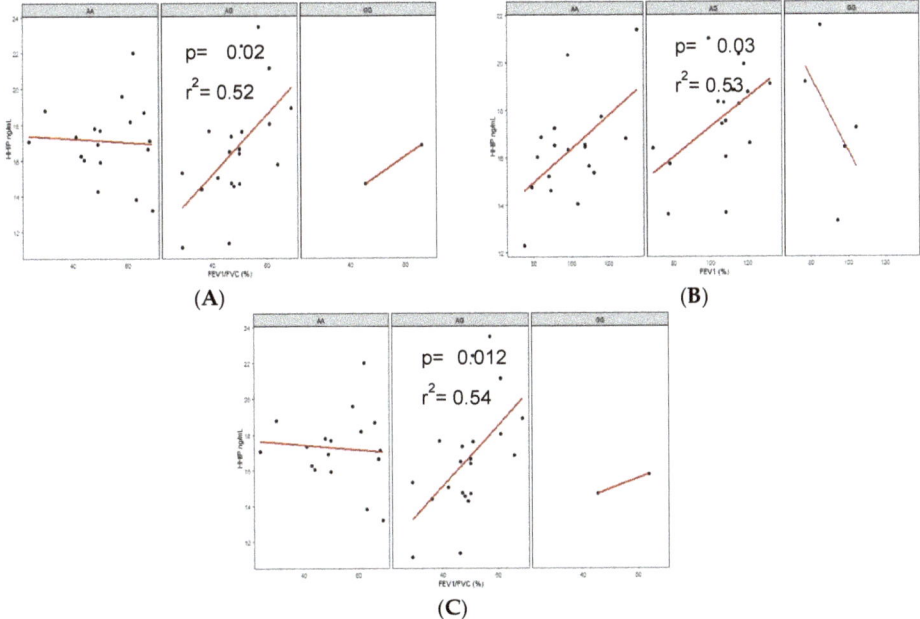

Figure 4. Correlations of protein levels and lung function. (**A**) correlation of FEV_1/FVC and protein levels in heterozygous (AG) BBES group of the rs1828591; (**B**) correlation of FEV_1 and protein levels in heterozygous (AG) BBES group; and (**C**) correlation of FEV_1/FVC and protein levels in heterozygous (AG) COPD-BS group, both in the rs13118928.

3.7. HHIP Levels in Supernatant Sputum of Smoke Biomass Burning

Analysis of HHIP protein levels in sputum supernatant (SS) from subjects exposed to smoke by biomass burning was performed in a subgroup of 40 randomly selected participants (20 COPD-BS and 20 BBES).

The age of the COPD-BS group (median = 72) was higher than that of the BBES group (median = 61.5) ~10 years, which was determined to be significant. For BBEI, the COPD group was more heavily exposed with a median = 470 h/year, and the BBES group had a median of 360 h/year; however, this difference was not significant. On the other hand, pulmonary function test results are lower in the COPD-BS group than in the BBES group, and this difference is expected in our study, since lung function tests are the diagnostic criteria (Supplementary Table S3).

Protein Level Comparison in Sputum Supernatant

In general, when comparing the protein levels between both groups, regardless of the polymorphism, the BBES group had higher protein levels than did the COPD-BS group ($p = 0.09$); however, this difference was not significant (Figure 5).

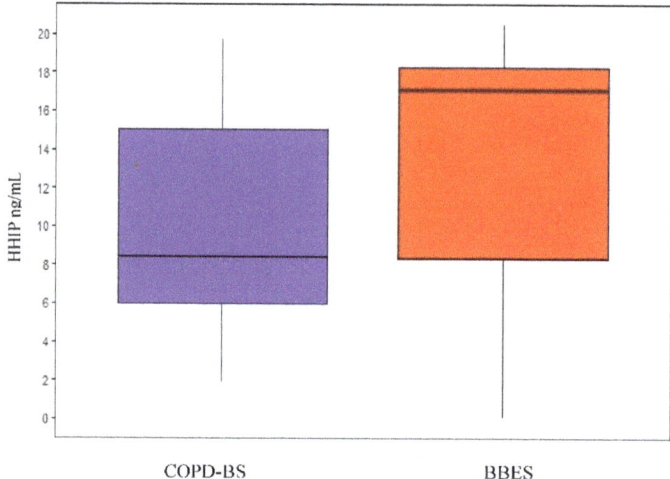

Figure 5. Comparison of HHIP protein in supernatant sputum levels among COPD-BS 4. 3.

In the analysis, according to genotypes among case-controls, no differences were found in the general association, genetic models, or correlations.

3.8. HHIP Levels and Metabolism of Drugs for COPD

Nine drugs were identified as the first-line treatment (tiotropium bromide, umeclidinium, vilanterol, fluticasone furoate, salbutamol, ipratropium bromide, budesonide, fluticasone, and/or salmeterol). Based on the above, the in silico analysis showed a strong interaction between the different drugs and the enzymes, carriers, targets, and transporters that participate in their metabolism. However, as shown in supplementary Figure S2, no interaction among the drugs used in treating COPD, and the HHIP protein was identified.

4. Discussions

COPD is caused by exposure to noxious particles or gases, such as cigarette smoke or smoke caused by the combustion of solid fuels, known as biomass, which may include coal or crop residue, grass, dry branches, animal dung, charcoal, and wood [24,25].

In the current study, three polymorphisms (rs13118928, rs1828591, and rs13147758) in the *HHIP* gene were analyzed in Mexican women exposed to biomass-burning smoke; this kind of environmental risk factor is relatively common in low- and middle-income countries, such as Mexico, in addition to women being more likely than men to be affected by this exposure [26,27]. Additionally, some authors have suggested that biomass-burning smoke has a different pathophysiological mechanism from that caused by cigarette smoke [28].

The clinical and demographic characteristics of our study group are similar to those of previous reports; Moran-Mendoza et al., in 2008, described a group of women affected by exposure to smoke from biomass burning, aged approximately 67 years, mostly residing in rural or suburban areas, who had 5 h/day of direct exposure to smoke for up to 45 years [29]. Additionally, the BSEI may reach 275 h/year [25]. In our current study, the COPD group exceeded 300 h per year for harmful particles.

Previously, two GWAS seeking to identify genetic susceptibility to COPD in the Caucasian population found two SNPs in the *HHIP* gene (rs1828591 and rs13118928) with consistent replications in three cohorts; however, the combined p-values did not reach levels of significance at the GWAS level (1.74×10^{-7} and 1.67×10^{-7}) [7]. In addition, in the Boston Early-Onset COPD (BEOCOPD) family cohort, rs1828591 and rs13118928 were associated with FEV_1 ($p = 0.0025$ and $p = 0.0014$, respectively), but neither SNP was significantly associated with COPD. Additionally, these same polymorphisms were associated with FEV_1 in the British Birth Cohort ($p = 0.039$ and $p = 0.038$, respectively) [7]. In another GWAS, rs13147758 had a genome-wide p-value associated with FEV_1/FVC and FEV_1, as well as airflow obstruction, in smokers [8].

Some studies in Asian populations have evaluated these particular polymorphisms in the HHIP gene but focused on their relationship with tobacco smoking; in the KOLD cohort, 15 SNPs were analyzed, and none was associated with COPD; however, four were significantly associated with FEV_1 value [30]. Similarly, in a Chinese Han population, none of the SNPs in HHIP had an association with COPD, but the rs12509311, rs13118928, and 1,828,591 were associated with the FEV_1/FVC ratio in COPD smokers [31]. In contrast, three SNPs (rs13147758, rs1828591, and rs13118928) were associated with a decreased COPD risk (OR = 0.57, 0.54 and 0.56, respectively) with the GG genotype in a comparative study between Chinese Han and Mongolian populations [32]. We selected these SNPs because a critical role in the disease has been observed in other populations; however, in biomass-burning smoke-exposed individuals, their participation has not been evaluated to date. In our current study in biomass-burning smoke-exposed women, we found that the rs13118928 GG genotype was associated with a decreased risk (OR = 0.51) of the disease; interestingly, these populations have a higher Amerindian component [33]. Regarding the analysis by genetic association models (recessive model), it was shown that carrying two copies of the minor allele (GG) also provides a decreased risk of disease. In a recent study in Mexican-mestizo smokers, we found an association with COPD susceptibility with rs13147758 [34] but not rs13118928. [33,34].

Interestingly, the GG haplotype (rs13118928–rs1828591) shows that both SNPs' minor alleles confer a decreased risk of COPD. Previously, we reported that rs13147758 (not associated in the current exposure comparison) and the haplotype formed with rs1828591 are associated with smokers' COPD susceptibility. In the current study, we did not observe any genetic association with susceptibility at the allele or haplotype level. This lack of association is probably due to the minimal differences in the genotype frequencies among cases and controls (approximately 3% between groups), which is in contrast to the tobacco-smoking study, where the difference in genotype frequencies reached 10%. [33,34].

The *HHIP* gene encodes a protein with the same symbol; this protein is a regulatory component of the Hedgehog pathway for embryonal development in vertebrates. HHIP is a transmembrane protein that attenuates the signals of this pathway and, from an evolutionary perspective, it is highly conserved. HHIP plays an essential role in embryogenesis processes, such as lung development and the development of other organs [11]. In a haploinsufficient murine model exposed to cigarette smoke, the importance of the HHIP protein in lung development was demonstrated; homozygous (Hhip-/-) mice died in the short term after birth due to defects in lung morphogenesis. In contrast, heterozygous mice (Hhip+/−) were viable with normal lung development but with an approximately 33% decrease in protein expression and an increase in functional and histological emphysema [35].

The diagnosis of COPD is performed through the spirometry test, and no other procedures are indicated (such as bronchoalveolar lavage or lung tissue biopsy) [1]. We believe that the biological sample closest to the pulmonary microenvironment is sputum; therefore, in this study, we decided to determine protein levels in sputum supernatant and serum. In addition, these measurements have not been previously reported for this pathology.

Interestingly, most of the results associated with the disease were obtained in serum protein levels; however, comparing cases and controls, regardless of polymorphisms, no significant differences were found.

In the case-control comparison, depending on the genotype/polymorphism, with rs13118928 being associated at the genetic level, no differences at the serum protein level were observed. Interestingly, among non-COPD exposed subjects, according to the dominant model (AA vs. AG + GG), the HHIP serum levels are increased among subjects carrying one or two copies for the minor allele (G). Notably, the GG genotype was associated with decreased risk. In this work, we observe that all subjects with one or two copies of the minor allele have higher levels of the protein, which acquires relevance at the biological level, since previous investigations in murine models observed that the protein may play a protective role against harmful stimuli, such as exposure to cigarette smoke [36]. However, this protective role has not been previously described in people exposed to smoke from biomass burning.

In the lung function correlations with serum protein, the HHIP levels correlated positively with the FEV_1 and FEV_1/FVC parameters. Additionally, the rs13118928 AG genotype showed that both in controls with FEV_1 and in cases with FEV_1/FVC, lung function was better at higher serum protein levels, suggesting that the protein is stimulated by the oxidative stress caused by noxious particles or gases, such as those contained in the smoke from biomass combustion, similar to that described in murine models of tobacco smoke exposure [36]. Our findings with the AG genotype but not with the GG genotype could be due to the reduced number of subjects carrying the GG genotype.

On the other hand, supernatant sputum protein levels did not exhibit significant differences, either in the first case-control comparison or in subsequent analyses, where comparisons depend on genotypes/SNPs. Notably, the HHIP protein levels in the sputum supernatant were consistently lower than those in serum samples.

According to the databases and software consulted [22,23], no direct or indirect interactions of the different pharmacological drugs with the HHIP protein were identified; this allows us to presume so far HHIP levels are not they are altered by the pharmacological treatment used.

Our study has a number of limitations, among which we consider the small number of sputum supernatant samples obtained for protein level determination; although the statistical power for serum and supernatant protein levels is 68% and 60%, respectively, in a study such as the one that we conducted and in a poorly explored population, this approach presents good statistical power between protein levels and lung function.

Finally, our study analyzed three polymorphisms that had been previously associated with COPD in other populations. However, to the best of our knowledge, no previous association studies have investigated populations exposed to smoke due to biomass burning. Additionally, our study is the first to describe the protein levels in serum and sputum in subjects exposed to smoke by biomass burning with and without COPD. Our results may pave the way for further studies investigating COPD pathophysiology, where the HHIP participates at the gene-variation and protein levels.

5. Conclusions

The rs13118928 GG genotype and the rs13118928–rs1828591 (GG) haplotype are associated with decreased COPD risk in Mexican women exposed to smoke from biomass burning.

In addition, the HHIP serum protein levels in subjects harboring the rs13118928 AG genotype exposed to smoke by biomass burning, both with and without COPD, are associated with better lung function.

Supplementary Materials: The following are available online at http://www.mdpi.com/2075-4418/10/10/734/s1, Figure S1: Haplotypes of the rs13147758 and rs18285918 in the HHIP gene, Figure S2: In silico analysis from the metabolism of drugs in the treatment of COPD, and the interaction of HHIP with pharmacological treatment, Table S1: Genotype frequencies comparison among COPD patients, according to G2 vs. G1 groups, Table S2: Characteristics of selected women for serum protein levels analysis, Table S3: Demographical, clinical, exposition and lung function of exposed to biomass-burning smoke of the subgroup for protein levels in supernatant sputum; Table S4: General characteristics of SNPs included in the analysis.

Author Contributions: Conceptualization, A.O.-M., E.A.-R. and R.F.-V.; data curation, A.O.-M.; formal analysis, A.O.-M.; funding acquisition, A.R.-V. and R.F.-V.; investigation, A.O.-M., M.E.R.-D., F.C.-V., M.d.L.M.-G., E.R.-M. and E.A.-R.; methodology, A.O.-M., M.E.R.-D., F.C.-V., M.d.L.M.-G., E.R.-M. and E.A.-R.; project administration, G.P.-R., A.R.-V. and R.F.-V.; resources, G.P.-R., A.R.-V. and R.F.-V.; software, A.O.-M.; supervision, G.P.-R., A.R.-V. and R.F.-V.; validation, R.F.-V.; visualization, M.E.R.-D., F.C.-V., M.d.L.M.-G., E.R.-M., E.A.-R. and R.F.-V.; writing—original draft, A.O.-M. and R.F.-V.; writing—review and editing, A.O.-M., G.P.-R., A.R.-V., E.R.-M. and R.F.-V. All authors have read and agreed to the published version of the manuscript.

Funding: This work was supported by the budget allocated to research (RFV-HLA Laboratory) from the Instituto Nacional de Enfermedades Respiratorias Ismael Cosío Villegas (INER). This paper constitutes a partial fulfillment of the Graduate Program in Maestría en Ciencias de la Salud of the Instituto Politécnico Nacional (IPN) for

A.O.-M. A. Ortega-Martínez acknowledges the scholarship (920256) and financial support provided by the National Council of Science and Technology (CONACyT). The authors acknowledge the support received from physicians and technicians from the COPD clinic at INER for confirmation of diagnosis, acquisition of data on lung function, and clinical care of the study participants.

Conflicts of Interest: The authors declare no conflict of interest. The funders had no role in the design of the study; in the collection, analyses, or interpretation of data; in the writing of the manuscript, or in the decision to publish the results.

Data Availability Statement: The datasets generated and analyzed for this study can be found in ClinVar SCV001423136, SCV001423137, and SCV001423138.

References

1. Global Initiative for Chronic Obstructive Lung Disease. *Global Strategy for the Diagnosis, Management, and Prevention of Chronic Obstructive Pulmonary Disease (2018 Report)*; Global Initiative for Chronic Obstructive Lung Disease, 2018. Available online: http://www.goldcopd.org (accessed on 1 January 2019).
2. Montes de Oca, M.; Zabert, G.; Moreno, D.; Laucho-Contreras, M.E.; Lopez Varela, M.V.; Surmont, F. Smoke, biomass exposure, and COPD risk in the primary care setting: The PUMA study. *Respir. Care* **2018**, *62*, 1058–1066. [CrossRef] [PubMed]
3. Mannino, D.M.; Buist, A.S. Global burden of COPD: Risk factors, prevalence, and future trends. *Lancet* **2007**, *370*, 765–773. [CrossRef]
4. Ramírez-Venegas, A.; Velázquez-Uncal, M.; Pérez-Hernández, R.; Guzmán-Bouilloud, N.E.; Falfán-Valencia, R.; Mayar-Maya, M.E.; Aranda-Chávez, A.; Sansores, R.H. Prevalence of COPD and respiratory symptoms associated with biomass smoke exposure in a suburban area. *Int. J. COPD* **2018**, *13*, 1727–1734. [CrossRef] [PubMed]
5. Perez-Padilla, R.; Fernandez, R.; Lopez Varela, M.V.; Montes de Oca, M.; Muiño, A.; Tálamo, C.; Brito Jardim, J.R.; Valdivia, G.; Baptista Menezes, A.M. Airflow Obstruction in Never Smokers in Five Latin American Cities: The PLATINO Study. *Arch. Med. Res.* **2012**, *43*, 159–165. [CrossRef] [PubMed]
6. Perez-Rubio, G.; Cordoba-Lanus, E.; Cupertino, P.; Cartujano-Barrera, F.; Campos, M.A.; Falfan-Valencia, R. Role of genetic susceptibility in nicotine addiction and chronic obstructive pulmonary disease. *Rev. Investig. Clin.* **2019**, *71*, 36–54. [CrossRef]
7. Pillai, S.G.; Ge, D.; Zhu, G.; Kong, X.; Shianna, K.V. A Genome-Wide Association Study in Chronic Obstructive Pulmonary Disease (COPD): Identification of Two Major Susceptibility Loci. *PLoS Genet* **2009**, *5*, 1000421. [CrossRef]
8. Wilk, J.B.; Chen, T.H.; Gottlieb, D.J.; Walter, R.E.; Nagle, M.W.; Brandler, B.J.; Myers, R.H.; Borecki, I.B.; Silverman, E.K.; Weiss, S.T.; et al. A genome-wide association study of pulmonary function measures in the framingham heart study. *PLoS Genet.* **2009**, *5*, 1000421. [CrossRef]
9. Murone, M.; Rosenthal, A.; De Sauvage, F.J. Hedgehog signal transduction: From flies to vertebrates. *Exp. Cell Res.* **1999**, *253*, 25–33. [CrossRef]
10. HGNC SUB1P1 Gene Symbol Report. HUGO Gene Nomenclature Committee. Available online: https://www.genenames.org/data/gene-symbol-report/#!/hgnc_id/HGNC:14866 (accessed on 1 March 2020).
11. Bak, M.; Hansen, C.; Friis Henriksen, K.; Tommerup, N. The human hedgehog-interacting protein gene: Structure and chromosome mapping to 4q31.21–>q31.3. *Cytogenet. Cell Genet.* **2001**, *92*, 300–303. [CrossRef]
12. Global Initiative for Chronic Obstructive Lung Disease (GOLD) Global Strategy for The Diagnosis, Management, and Prevention of Chronic Obstructive Pulmonary Disease (Updated 2013). 2013. Available online: https://goldcopd.org/ (accessed on 1 January 2020).
13. Pérez-Padilla, R.; Valdivia, G.; Muiño, A.; López, M.V.; Márquez, M.N.; Montes de Oca, M.; Tálamo, C.; Lisboa, C.; Pertuzé, J.; Jardim, J.R.B.; et al. Spirometric Reference Values in 5 Large Latin American Cities for Subjects Aged 40 Years or Over. *Arch. Bronconeumol. (Engl. Ed.)* **2006**, *42*, 317–325. [CrossRef]

14. Little, J.; Higgins, J.P.T.; Ioannidis, J.P.A.; Moher, D.; Gagnon, F.; von Elm, E.; Khoury, M.J.; Cohen, B.; Davey-Smith, G.; Grimshaw, J.; et al. STrengthening the REporting of Genetic Association studies (STREGA)–an extension of the STROBE statement. *Eur. J. Clin. Investig.* **2009**, *39*, 247–266. [CrossRef] [PubMed]

15. Ambrocio-Ortiz, E.; Pérez-Rubio, G.; Ramírez-Venegas, A.; Hernández-Zenteno, R.; Del Angel-Pablo, A.D.; Pérez-Rodríguez, M.E.; Salazar, A.M.; Abarca-Rojano, E.; Falfán-Valencia, R. Effect of SNPs in HSP Family Genes, Variation in the mRNA and Intracellular Hsp Levels in COPD Secondary to Tobacco Smoking and Biomass-Burning Smoke. *Front. Genet.* **2020**, *10*, 11. [CrossRef] [PubMed]

16. Zerbino, D.R.; Achuthan, P.; Akanni, W.; Amode, M.R.; Barrell, D.; Bhai, J.; Billis, K.; Cummins, C.; Gall, A.; Girón, C.G.; et al. Ensembl 2018. *Nucleic Acids Res.* **2017**, *46*, D754–D761. [CrossRef] [PubMed]

17. Purcell, S.; Neale, B.; Todd-Brown, K.; Thomas, L.; Ferreira, M.A.R.; Bender, D.; Maller, J.; Sklar, P.; de Bakker, P.I.W.; Daly, M.J.; et al. PLINK: A Tool Set for Whole-Genome Association and Population-Based Linkage Analyses. *Am. J. Hum. Genet.* **2007**, *81*, 559–575. [CrossRef]

18. Henschke, H. De Finetti Diagram. Available online: https://web.archive.org/web/20110719103301/https://finetti.meb.uni-bonn.de/downloads/finetti_3.0.5_windows.zip (accessed on 2 June 2020).

19. CDC Epi Info Epi Info™ 7. Available online: https://www.cdc.gov/epiinfo/esp/es_pc.html (accessed on 18 April 2020).

20. de Galicia, X. Organización Panamericana de la Salud EPIDAT, Versión 3.1. 2006. Available online: https://extranet.sergas.es/EPIWB/EPIWB/SolicitudeEpidat.aspx?IdPaxina=62715&idv=1&lng=es (accessed on 25 April 2020).

21. Barrett, J.C.; Fry, B.; Maller, J.; Daly, M.J. Haploview: Analysis and visualization of LD and haplotype maps. *Bioinformatics* **2005**, *21*, 263–265. [CrossRef]

22. Wishart, D.S.; Feunang, Y.D.; Guo, A.C.; Lo, E.J.; Marcu, A.; Grant, J.R.; Sajed, T.; Johnson, D.; Li, C.; Sayeeda, Z.; et al. DrugBank 5.0: A major update to the DrugBank database for 2018. *Nucleic Acids Res.* **2018**, *46*, D1074–D1082. [CrossRef]

23. Szklarczyk, D.; Gable, A.L.; Lyon, D.; Junge, A.; Wyder, S.; Huerta-Cepas, J.; Simonovic, M.; Doncheva, N.T.; Morris, J.H.; Bork, P.; et al. STRING v11: Protein-protein association networks with increased coverage, supporting functional discovery in genome-wide experimental datasets. *Nucleic Acids Res.* **2019**, *47*, D607–D613. [CrossRef]

24. Torres-Duque, C.A.; García-Rodriguez, M.C.; González-García, M. Enfermedad pulmonar obstructiva crónica por humo de leña: ¿un fenotipo diferente o una entidad distinta? *Arch. Bronconeumol.* **2016**, *52*, 425–431. [CrossRef]

25. Pérez-Padilla, R.; Ramirez-Venegas, A.; Sansores-Martinez, R. Clinical Characteristics of Patients With Biomass Smoke-Associated COPD and Chronic Bronchitis, 2004–2014. *Chronic Obstr. Pulm. Dis. J. COPD Found.* **2014**, *1*, 23–32. [CrossRef]

26. Regalado, J.; Pérez-Padilla, R.; Sansores, R.; Ramirez, J.I.P.; Brauer, M.; Paré, P.; Vedal, S. The effect of biomass burning on respiratory symptoms and lung function in rural Mexican women. *Am. J. Respir. Crit. Care Med.* **2006**, *174*, 901–905. [CrossRef]

27. Ramírez-Venegas, A.; Sansores, R.H.; Pérez-Padilla, R.; Regalado, J.; Velázquez, A.; Sánchez, C.; Eugenia Mayar, M.; Mayar, M.E. Survival of patients with chronic obstructive pulmonary disease due to biomass smoke and tobacco. *Am. J. Respir. Crit. Care Med.* **2006**, *173*, 393–397. [CrossRef]

28. Silva, R.; Oyarzún, M.; Olloquequi, J. Mecanismos patogénicos en la enfermedad pulmonar obstructiva crónica causada por exposición a humo de biomasa. *Arch. Bronconeumol.* **2015**, *51*, 285–292. [CrossRef]

29. Moran-Mendoza, O.; Pérez-Padilla, J.R.; Salazar-Flores, M.; Vazquez-Alfaro, F.; Moran-Mendoza, O. Wood smoke-associated lung disease: A clinical, functional, radiological and pathological description. *Int. J. Tuberc. Lung Dis.* **2008**, *12*, 1092–1098.

30. Kim, W.J.; Oh, Y.M.; Lee, J.H.; Park, C.S.; Park, S.W.; Park, J.S.; Lee, S. Do Genetic variants in HHIP are associated with FEV1 in subjects with chronic obstructive pulmonary disease. *Respirology* **2013**, *18*, 1202–1209. [CrossRef]

31. Zhang, Z.; Wang, J.; Zheng, Z.; Chen, X.; Zeng, X.; Zhang, Y.; Li, D.; Shu, J.; Yang, K.; Lai, N.; et al. Genetic Variants in the Hedgehog Interacting Protein Gene Are Associated with the FEV1/FVC Ratio in Southern Han Chinese Subjects with Chronic Obstructive Pulmonary Disease. *Biomed Res. Int.* **2017**, *2017*, 1–10. [CrossRef]

32. Xu, G.; Gao, X.; Zhang, S.; Wang, Y.; Ding, M.; Liu, W.; Shen, J.; Sun, D. Comparison of the role of HHIP SNPs in susceptibility to chronic obstructive pulmonary disease between Chinese Han and Mongolian populations. *Gene* **2017**, *637*, 50–56. [CrossRef]
33. Pérez-Rubio, G.; Ambrocio-Ortiz, E.; López-Flores, L.A.; Juárez-Martín, A.I.; Jiménez-Valverde, L.O.; Zoreque-Cabrera, S.; Galicia-Negrete, G.; Ramírez-Díaz, M.E.; Cruz-Vicente, F.; de Castillejos-López, M.J.; et al. Heterozygous genotype rs17580 AT (PiS) in SERPINA1 is associated with COPD secondary to biomass-burning and tobacco smoking: A case-control and populational study. *Int. J. COPD* **2020**, *15*, 1181–1190. [CrossRef]
34. Ortega-Martínez, A.; Pérez-Rubio, G.; Ambrocio-Ortiz, E.; Nava-Quiroz, K.; Hernández-Zenteno, R.; Abarca-Rojano, E.; Rodríguez-Llamazares, S.; Hernández-Pérez, A.; García-Gómez, L.; Ramírez-Venegas, A.; et al. The SNP rs13147758 in the HHIP gene is associated with COPD susceptibility, serum and sputum protein levels in smokers. *Front. Genet.* **2020**, *11*, 882.
35. Wan, E.S.; Li, Y.; Lao, T.; Qiu, W.; Jiang, Z.; Mancini, J.D.; Owen, C.A.; Clish, C.; Demeo, D.L.; Silverman, E.K.; et al. Metabolomic profiling in a Hedgehog Interacting Protein (Hhip) murine model of chronic obstructive pulmonary disease. *Sci. Rep.* **2017**, *7*, 2504. [CrossRef]
36. Lao, T.; Jiang, Z.; Yun, J.; Qiu, W.; Guo, F.; Huang, C.; Mancini, J.D.; Gupta, K.; Laucho-Contreras, M.E.; Naing, Z.Z.C.; et al. Hhip haploinsufficiency sensitizes mice to age-related emphysema. *Proc. Natl. Acad. Sci. USA* **2016**, *113*, E4681–E4687. [CrossRef]

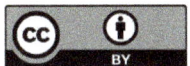

© 2020 by the authors. Licensee MDPI, Basel, Switzerland. This article is an open access article distributed under the terms and conditions of the Creative Commons Attribution (CC BY) license (http://creativecommons.org/licenses/by/4.0/).

MDPI
St. Alban-Anlage 66
4052 Basel
Switzerland
www.mdpi.com

Diagnostics Editorial Office
E-mail: diagnostics@mdpi.com
www.mdpi.com/journal/diagnostics

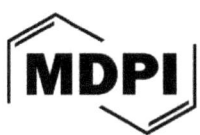

Disclaimer/Publisher's Note: The statements, opinions and data contained in all publications are solely those of the individual author(s) and contributor(s) and not of MDPI and/or the editor(s). MDPI and/or the editor(s) disclaim responsibility for any injury to people or property resulting from any ideas, methods, instructions or products referred to in the content.

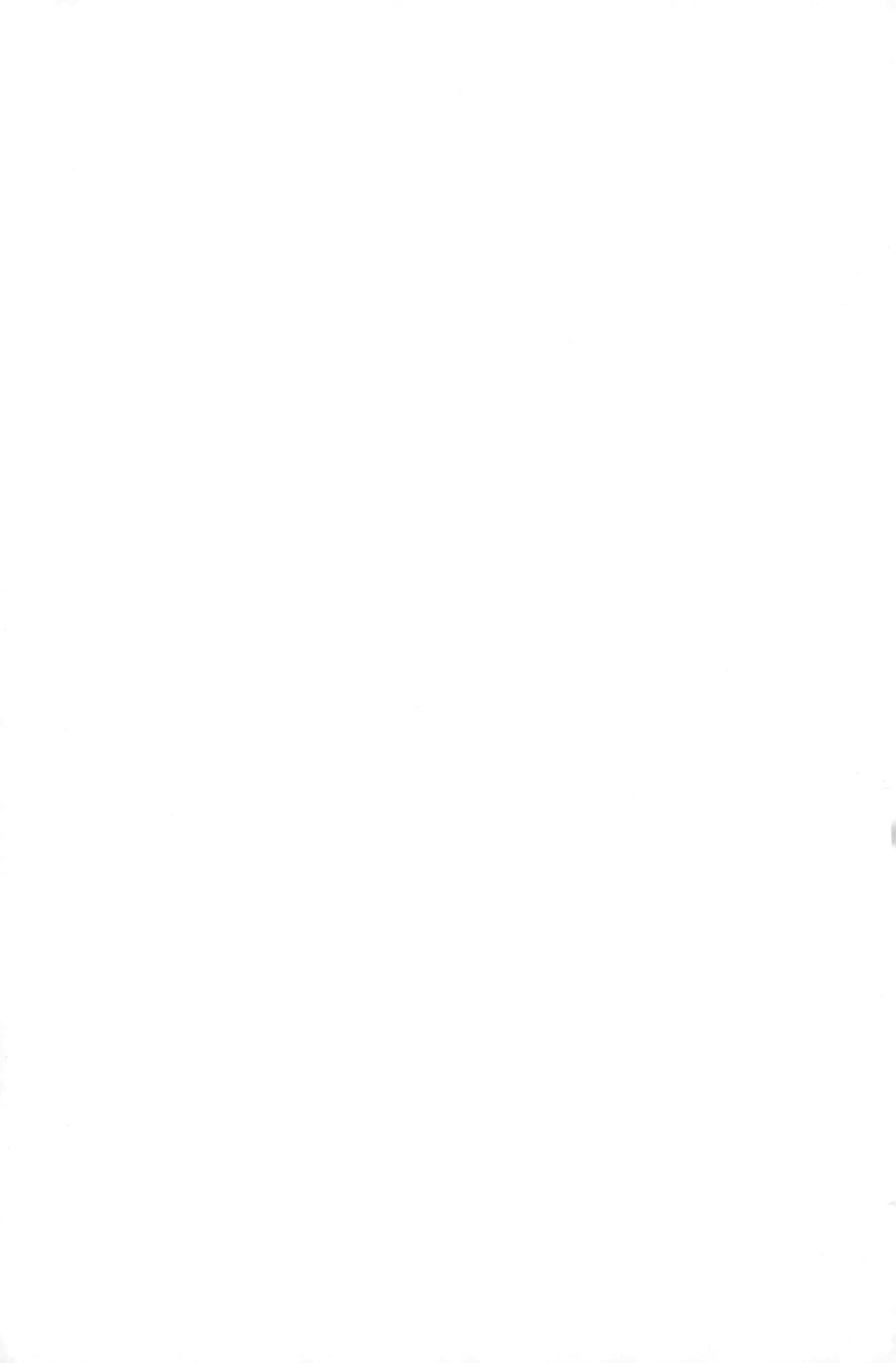

www.ingramcontent.com/pod-product-compliance
Lightning Source LLC
LaVergne TN
LVHW070142100526
838202LV00015B/1877